HEALTHFUL LIVING:
A TEXTBOOK OF PERSONAL AND COMMUNITY HEALTH

NINTH EDITION

HEALTHFUL LIVING

A TEXTBOOK OF PERSONAL AND COMMUNITY HEALTH

HAROLD S. DIEHL, M.A., M.D., Sc.D.
Emeritus Professor of Public Health and
Dean of the Medical Sciences
University of Minnesota
Consultant to the American Cancer Society, Inc.
Diplomat, American Board of Preventive Medicine
Fellow and former member Governing Council
American Public Health Association
Past President, American College Health Association

WILLARD DALRYMPLE, A.B., M.D.
Director of University Health Service
Princeton University
President, American College Health Association
Assistant Clinical Professor of Medicine
Rutgers Medical School

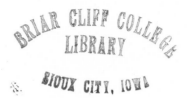
McGRAW-HILL BOOK COMPANY
New York   St. Louis   San Francisco   Düsseldorf   Johannesburg
Kuala Lumpur   London   Mexico   Montreal   New Delhi
Panama   Rio de Janeiro   Singapore   Sydney   Toronto

LIBRARY OF CONGRESS CATALOGING IN PUBLICATION DATA
Diehl, Harold Sheely, 1891–
Healthful living.

Includes bibliographies.
1. Hygiene. I. Dalrymple, Willard, joint
author. II. Title.
RA776.D52 1973   613   72-10455
ISBN 0-07-016835-0

HEALTHFUL LIVING: A TEXTBOOK OF PERSONAL AND COMMUNITY HEALTH

1 2 3 4 5 6 7 8 9 0 M U R M 7 9 8 7 6 5 4 3

This book was set in Melior by Black Dot, Inc.
The editors were Robert C. Morgan and Susan Gamer;
the designer was Nicholas Krenitsky;
and the production supervisor was Thomas J. Lo Pinto.
The drawings were done by Danmark & Michaels, Inc.
The printer was The Murray Printing Company;
the binder, Rand McNally & Company.

CONTENTS

Preface   vii

1   Better Health and a Long Life   1
2   Health Problems in the College Years   11
3   Human Ecology   21
4   Modern Medical Services   43
5   Heart Disease, Stroke, and Cancer   59
6   Accidents, Arthritis, and Rehabilitation   79
7   Tobacco   91
8   Alcohol and Other Mind-altering Drugs   109
9   Mental Health   125
10   Mental Disturbances   139
11   Food for the World's Health and Yours   155
12   Obesity and Digestive Disorders and Diseases   171
13   Some Health Factors in Daily Life   187
14   Eyes, Ears, Nose, and Throat   201
15   Teeth, Skin, and Hair   219

16   Communicable Diseases   239
17   Immunizations of Value   259
18   Respiratory Diseases   273
19   Hormones   289
20   Sex and Sexuality   299
21   Social and Emotional Aspects of Sex   313
22   Reproduction: Having a Family and Being a Parent   327
23   Aging and Dying   345
24   Community and Occupational Health   363
25   The Schools and Health   379
26   Government and Health   387
27   Voluntary Health Organizations   403
28   Critical Health Problems of the Future   415

Appendix: Nutritive Values of Foods   423
Index   447

PREFACE

This ninth edition of *Healthful Living* includes many more changes from the previous edition than is customary in revisions. Considerable new information has been incorporated concerning population and pollution of the environment. The hazards of population growth and ways to control it are discussed; as are the pollution of streams, lakes, rivers, oceans, and the atmosphere and the impact on the environment of industry, pesticides, detergents, human wastes, and noise.

The changing attitudes toward human sexuality are considered, as are methods of contraception, the increase in voluntary sterilization, and the rapid changes in laws regulating abortion.

The chapters on tobacco, alcohol, marijuana and other mind-altering drugs have been revised and expanded.

A new section on death and dying has been introduced. The chapters on the major causes of chronic illness—heart disease, cancer, stroke, chronic bronchitis, emphysema, arthritis, and mental illnesses—have been extensively revised to include new scientific information and control measures.

A new chapter—Health in the College Years—has been added.

The index and glossary have been combined, to simplify their use. Reading suggestions have been updated and reduced in number.

The discussion and self-examination questions for each chapter have been revised. The purpose of these questions is to check comprehension of the facts presented in the chapter and also of the reasoning and the purpose behind all major parts of the chapter. This purpose has been accomplished with fewer questions than appeared in the eighth edition.

My coauthor of this book, Dr. Dalrymple, in 1972 became President of the American College Health Association, a position I held in the early years of the Association. Dr. Dalrymple and I are both indebted to Nancy Marcus, who has been especially helpful in the preparation of the manuscript and in the production of the book.

Harold S. Diehl

HEALTHFUL LIVING:
A TEXTBOOK OF PERSONAL AND COMMUNITY HEALTH

1

BETTER HEALTH AND A LONG LIFE

Students today are asking serious questions about the meaning and the values of life. They are striving for personal identity and for freedom from pressures to conform to patterns of living which to them seem superficial and empty. They are seeking purposes in life other than security and material success.

To achieve satisfactions in this turbulent world requires clarity of objectives, steadfastness of purpose, and health both of body and of mind. Francis Bacon, who knew ill health, wrote, "A healthy body is the soul's guest chamber; a sick body, its prison." Health is not an end in itself, but rather a means to accomplishment and to the enjoyment of life.

It is essential that people be accurately informed about matters of health. And information about health is not dull. These complex and mysterious bodies of ours are fascinating, as are the things that can go wrong with them and what we can do to keep them functioning smoothly, efficiently, and happily. This does not imply that people need become health prigs or health cranks who make life miserable for themselves and are a nuisance to friends and associates. Intelligent people follow a different course. They acquaint themselves with the facts, face their problems realistically, and proceed to get the most out of life.

LENGTH OF LIFE

Probably the most important achievement of man is the progress he has made in the prevention of disease and the prolongation of life. From superstition, ignorance, and early death man has advanced in a few centuries to understanding and solution of many of his health problems.

Figure 1.1 Trend in life expectancy of white men and women at birth. Source: Data for 1790–1930, Massachusetts State Department of Health; data for 1930–1970, U.S. Public Health Service.

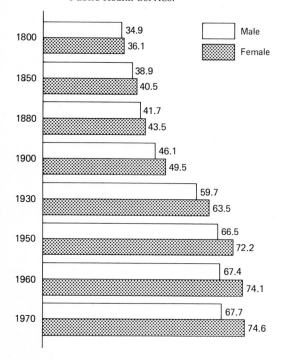

development of modern medical services. This improvement means that today at birth a child has a better chance of surviving to the age of 60 than a child had of surviving to the age of 10 a century ago.

Notable also is the progressive increase in the life expectancy of women as compared with men. As a result, the ratio of men to women in the population declined from 106 men for every 100 women in 1910 to 95 men for every 100 women in 1970 (Figure 1.2). The principal explanations for the increases in deaths among males in recent years vary with age. Among younger men, there were sharp increases in violent deaths, particularly automobile accidents, suicide, other accidents, and murder. Among older men, deaths from lung cancer have increased greatly as have deaths from coronary heart disease, other circulatory diseases, cirrhosis of the liver, and other diseases.

MORTALITY, MORBIDITY, AND FATALITY RATES

In order to compare the *mortality* (number of deaths) or the *morbidity* (amount of sickness) in different groups of the population, the frequency of occurrence is expressed as a ratio or rate, i.e., the number of deaths or the amount of sickness that occurs per unit of the population, usually per 1,000 or per 100,000. Since various factors—such as age, sex, race, occupation, and place of residence—influence mortality and morbidity, comparisons are more meaningful if rates are specific for such

In the sixteenth century in western Europe, life expectancy at birth is said to have been 19 years; in the seventeenth century, 25 years; in the eighteenth century, 32 years. In the nineteenth century in this country it was approximately 40 years; at the beginning of the present century it had increased to 47 years; and by the end of the first quarter of the twentieth century it was approximately 57 years for men and approximately 60 years for women. By 1970 life expectancy at birth in the United States had increased to 67.7 years for white men and 74.6 years for white women. (See Figure 1.1.)

Studies of the factors responsible for the reduction in death rates over the past several centuries suggest that about one-third is attributable to improvements in nutrition, agriculture, and engineering; about one-third to public health measures, particularly to the provision of safe drinking water and safe foods and to the control of communicable diseases; and about one-third to the

Figure 1.2 Ratio of men to women in the United States, 1860 to 1970. Source: National Center for Health Statistics.

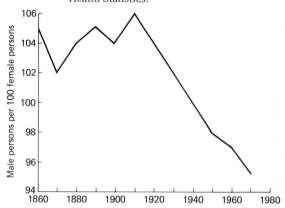

Figure 1.3 Cancer death rates, United States, by age, sex, and color. Source: U.S. Public Health Service.

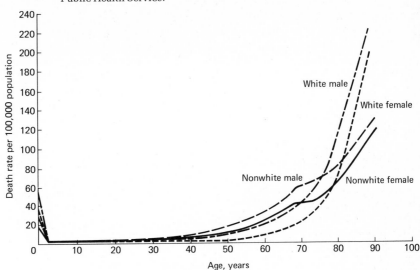

factors. For example, in 1970 the total death rate per 100,000 population was 153.5, but the rate for cancer was 162 per 100,000: with the rate for men 167 and the rate for women 136. However, if we make the rates specific for age and sex, we find that up to the age of 50, the rates for males and females are essentially equal; but after 50, the rate for males increases more rapidly than that for females. (See Figure 1.3.)

Death rates are also related to occupation and social class. For example, among men 25 to 64 years of age, professional workers have the lowest mortality rate of any occupational group. Second come technical, administrative, and managerial workers; third, agricultural workers; fourth, proprietors, clerical, sales, and skilled workers; and fifth, semiskilled workers, with rates of 4, 5, 14, and 19 percent, respectively, higher than that of professional men. Highest of all are unskilled laborers, among whom death rates are 96 percent higher than among professional men.

In a similar manner morbidity rates may be computed either for total populations or for specific groups or subgroups within the population.

Another rate frequently used is the *fatality rate*. This means the average number of deaths that occur among patients with a given disease. The number of patients usually taken as a basis is 100. The rates, therefore, are expressed as percentages. For example, with the development of antibiotic drugs, the fatality rate for pneumococcic pneumonia decreased from about 30 percent to about 5 percent; while the fatality rate for rabies has remained at almost 100 percent since the disease was first known.

Fatality rates, like mortality and morbidity rates, may be made specific for age, sex, residence, occupation, type of treatment, and other factors.

LIFE EXPECTANCY

The term *life expectancy* means the number of additional years that persons of a given age may expect, on the average, to live beyond that age. Thus a person 80 or 90 years of age still has some life expectancy, small though it may be. An increase in life expectancy, or in the average length of life, occurs when there is a decrease in the diseases or conditions which destroy life. Increases in the average length of life, however, are not necessarily proportionate to decreases in death rates, for a reduction in the death rate of children has a much greater effect on the average length of life than a similar reduction in the death rate of older people.

CHANGES OF LIFE EXPECTANCY WITH AGE

Between 1900 and 1965, when life expectancy at birth in our country increased from 47.3 to 70.2 years, the death rate for people of all ages decreased 45 percent. During this same period, however, the death rate among children under 1 year of age dropped 83 percent. Among adults the reductions became smaller with advancing age until this reduction was only 38 percent in the age group 75 to 84.

Because of the smaller reductions in death rates of older persons, their life expectancy shows but little increase. In other words, the life expectancy of a man or woman of 60 living today is very little longer than the life expectancy of a man or woman of 60 living 30 years ago.

The average life expectancy of children at 1 year of age is greater than that of newborn babies. This is true because more children die in the first year of life than in any other single year of childhood. At the age of 20 life expectancy is 50.2 years for men and 56.6 years for women, and at the age of 65 the average remaining life expectancy is 13.0 years for men and 16.3 years for women.

OTHER FACTORS IN LIFE EXPECTANCY

Improved living conditions and better health care contribute greatly to an increased life expectancy. Family life apparently contributes to good health: in 1960 the death rate, adjusted for age, of unmarried men was 74 percent higher than that of married men of the same age; and that of unmarried women was 51 percent higher than that of married women of the same age.

Since the expectation of life rises when death rates fall, and falls when death rates rise, life expectancy in states which are considered health resorts and thus have a high invalid population is adversely affected. Climate is another factor in the differences in life expectancy among the states, but industrialization appears to be much more important. Life expectancy is significantly higher in the highly agricultural states than in the industrial states.

INTERNATIONAL DIFFERENCES IN LONGEVITY

Great differences exist in longevity in the various countries of the world. In general, where social and economic conditions are good and health standards are high, longevity is high; while in countries where social and economic conditions are poor and health standards are low, longevity is little better today than it was in ancient times.

For example, in 1965, when life expectancy at birth in the United States was 70 years, it was 73 in Norway and Sweden; 72 in Israel, the Netherlands, Italy, Czechoslovakia, and Portugal; 71 in France, Belgium, Denmark, and New Zealand; 70 in England, Scotland, Ireland, West Germany, Switzerland, Japan, and Australia; 68 in the Soviet Union; 63 in Taiwan; 60 in Argentina and Peru; 53 in Brazil; 52 in Chile; 51 in Mexico; 50 in Southern Rhodesia; 37 in the Congo; and 32 in India.[1]

The relatively favorable position of the United States in respect to longevity, or life expectancy at birth, is due to the saving of lives in infancy and childhood, for death rates in this country between the ages of 40 and 65 are higher than those in much of western Europe and English-speaking countries elsewhere. The high death rate in the middle years of life in the United States is particularly disturbing since these are usually the years of greatest responsibility and achievement.

IS LONG LIFE DESIRABLE?

The great increase in the average length of life from less than 20 years in the sixteenth century in Europe to approximately 70 years in the United States today has made an enormous difference in the welfare of the race and the possibilities of human progress. With an average life span of 20 or 30 years, many of the potential leaders in every field died in childhood and the average person had relatively few years of maturity in which to contribute to his family and to the progress of the race. Under such circumstances an occasional genius stood out, but the lives of most persons were cut short before they could make their contributions to society.

To be sure, scientists, artists, and authors frequently do their most brilliant work in their early years; but Thorndike reports that the period

---

[1]Data from *United Nations Demographic Yearbook*, 1965.

of greatest achievement for authors, artists, scientists, and scholars averages just under 50. Sorenson agrees that most scholars and scientists do their best intellectual work at about 50 years of age but says that there is considerable variability within 10-year periods before and after 50. During the late forties a slight downward trend usually begins in the curve of individual accomplishment, but the average drop is so slight that at the age of 60 the curve has dropped little from its highest peak of 10 years before. There are, however, many notable exceptions: Darwin was 50 when he published his greatest work, *On the Origin of Species;* William James, foremost of American psychologists, had published not a single book and few articles by the age of 40; Benjamin Franklin helped to frame the Consitution at 81; Goethe completed *Faust* at 82; Edison was busy in his laboratory at 83; Toscanini was conducting at 87; and Titian painted his greatest masterpieces between 80 and his death at 99.

BIOLOGICAL LIMITS TO THE SPAN OF LIFE

In spite of the increases in the average length of life, the potential span of life—the length of life attained by the oldest persons—has changed little or not at all since antiquity.

The number of persons who have reached the venerable age of 100 years is small, about 13,000 in 1970, but is increasing annually. There are authoritative records of persons who have attained the age of 120 years, and one person may have lived to be 140. Whether such unusual cases represent the upper biological limit for the race or are merely "freaks" of nature we do not know.

Several recent studies of insects and animals suggest that a hormonelike substance, which usually decreases with age, may prevent certain of the physiological changes that result in aging. Other studies indicate that animals live longer on diets which supply basic nutritional needs but are restricted in amount to less than the animals would normally eat; these studies indicate also that regular physical and mental activities delay the aging process.

Studies of tissue cells suggest that under ideal conditions individual cells from the animal body may continue to live indefinitely. For example, although the normal life span of a chicken is 3 to 7 years, Dr. Alexis Carrel was able to keep the heart of an embryo chick alive in his laboratory for over 20 years. To do this he supplied the food which it needed, removed waste products, and regulated environmental conditions of temperature and moisture.

Unfortunately, the communities of cells which constitute the human body are not provided with such ideal conditions of existence. They are exposed to the weakening influence of imperfect diets, the wear and tear of activity, the toxins of infections, the burden of overeating, and the effects of alcohol and tobacco. No matter how great the biological possibilities of life may be, the practical upper limit for the average person probably is not much beyond the age now attained by a reasonable percentage of the population.

Today the life expectancy at birth of approximately 70 years has reached the biblical "three-score and ten" but is 20 years short of the age attained by approximately 20 percent of our population. How much further improvement is possible there is no way of knowing; but it is conservative to estimate that if people make reasonable use of currently available scientific knowledge, not only will some years be added to the average length of life, but even greater gains can be made in health and happiness.

Preventive medicine and health promotion make use of this scientific knowledge which can add years to life and life to years. Good diet, regular exercise throughout life, good safety habits, an adequate amount of sleep, and other good general health habits are measures for which the scientific basis will be given in later chapters. The prevention of specific diseases is the goal of much of the important medical research going on today.

PREVENTABLE CAUSES OF DEATH

In 1970 some of the leading causes of death were diseases of the heart, cancer, stroke, influenza and pneumonia, diseases of early infancy, diabetes, and arteriosclerosis. At the beginning of the century the list of executioners was quite different, with tuberculosis in the lead, and pneumonia, diarrhea and enteritis, and diseases of the heart following in that order (see Table 1.1).

Table 1.1   Changes in the leading causes of death in the United States since 1900

Causes of death in 1900	Death rate per 100,000 population, all ages	Causes of death in 1970	Death rate per 100,000 population, all ages
1 Tuberculosis	194.4	1 Diseases of the heart	360.3
2 Pneumonia	175.4	2 Cancer	162.0
3 Diarrhea and enteritis	139.9	3 Stroke (apoplexy)	101.7
4 Diseases of the heart	137.4	4 Accidents	34.2
5 Nephritis*	88.7	5 Influenza and pneumonia	30.5
6 Diseases of infancy	72.3	6 Diseases of infancy	20.9
7 Apoplexy (stroke)	72.0	7 Diabetes mellitus	18.5
8 Accidents	66.6	8 Arteriosclerosis†	15.9
9 Cancer	64.0	9 Cirrhosis of liver	15.8
10 Bronchitis	45.3	10 Emphysema	11.1
11 Meningitis	40.6	11 Suicide	11.1
12 Diphtheria	40.3	12 Congenital malformations	8.1
13 Typhoid fever	31.3	13 Homicide	7.6
14 Influenza	26.7	14 Hypertension without mention of heart	6.0
15 Paralysis	26.2	15 Nephritis*	3.9

*Nephritis, also called *Bright's disease,* is the medical term for inflammation of the kidney.
†Medical term for hardening of the arteries.
SOURCE: U.S. Public Health Service.

The shifts in the relative importance of these diseases have resulted, first, from the reduction of the communicable diseases of infancy and childhood and, second, from the increasing proportion of older people in the population, with men and women who have escaped the hazards of infancy and childhood entering upon a period of life in which they are subject to new hazards.

INDIVIDUAL CAUSES OF DEATH

Of the fifteen leading causes of death today only influenza and pneumonia are communicable (see Chapter 16). Accidents are principally a man-made hazard, and by man they can be reduced (see Chapter 6). Most of the others—heart disease, cancer, arteriosclerosis, and stroke—are chronic degenerative diseases and present a radically different public health problem.

The fundamental cause of cancer is still largely a mystery which research is seeking to unravel. It is estimated, however, that more than 100,000 lives might be saved annually in this country if presently available medical knowledge about the prevention, diagnosis, and treatment of cancer was effectively utilized.

Heart diseases, apoplexy, arteriosclerosis, and nephritis represent to a large degree the breakdown of one vital system of the body, the circulatory or "cardiovascular" system. A susceptible system may be inherited and then may suffer from improper diet, from the toxins of tobacco, alcohol, and infectious diseases, and from the stresses of high-pressure modern living. Thus it is small wonder that diseases of the cardiovascular system have come to occupy a leading position in present-day mortality.

DEATHS OF INFANTS AND CHILDREN

What about the possibilities of preventing deaths of children and young people? Saving young lives means much more than does the postponement for a short while of the deaths of the aged.

Deaths from diseases of early infancy and from congenital malformations have decreased but, with proper prenatal and obstetrical care, can be reduced still more (see Chapter 22). A century ago parents knew that serious epidemic diseases might occur at any time, and they fervently hoped that their children would survive the hazards of infancy and childhood. Today the situation is vastly different, but there are still many unnecessary deaths and disabilities from these causes among children. At no other period of life does the relative impor-

Table 1.2 Leading causes of death in the United States: under 45 years of age,* 1965 and 1950, per 100,000 estimated population in each age group

Cause of death	Number of deaths, 1965	Death rate 1965	Death rate 1950
Under 1†:			
Certain diseases of early infancy	55,375	1,926	1,926
Congenital malformations	13,433	349	435
Influenza and pneumonia	8,036	208	269
Accidents	3,316	86	115
Gastritis, enteritis, colitis‡	1,709	44	123
Hernia and intestinal obstruction	852	22	30
Meningitis	844	22	36
1–14:			
Accidents	12,661	23	28
Cancer	3,996	7	8
Congenital malformations	2,805	5	6
Influenza and pneumonia	2,712	5	9
Meningitis	588	1	1
Gastritis, enteritis, colitis‡	483	1	2
Diseases of heart	449	1	1
Homicide	438	1	1
15–24:			
Accidents	18,688	62	61
Homicide	2,504	8	6
Cancer	2,485	8	9
Suicide	1,876	6	4
Diseases of heart	895	3	6
Congenital malformations	737	2	2
Influenza and pneumonia	652	2	3
25–34:			
Accidents	10,913	49	52
Cancer	4,200	19	20
Diseases of heart	3,094	14	20
Suicide	2,722	12	8
Homicide	2,635	12	10
Stroke	1,065	5	4
Influenza and pneumonia	803	4	5
35–44:			
Diseases of heart	17,692	73	86
Cancer	14,780	61	62
Accidents	11,315	47	50
Suicide	4,064	17	13
Stroke	3,745	15	18
Cirrhosis of liver	3,649	15	10
Homicide	2,402	10	9

*For rates of higher age groups, see Table 23.2, page 351.
†Note that the deaths for this age group are for a single year, the next group for a 14-year period, and subsequent groups for 10-year periods.
‡Formerly called *diarrhea and enteritis*.
SOURCE: U.S. Public Health Service.

tance of the various diseases change so rapidly as in childhood. From 1 to 14 years of age, accidents, cancer, congenital malformations, influenza, and pneumonia head the list of causes of death. From 15 to 24 years, the order has changed to accidents, homicide, cancer, suicide, and diseases of the heart. (See Table 1.2.)

These major health problems of childhood and youth are for the most part acute conditions. The number of accidents should be minimized. Pneumonia and meningitis usually can be cured if treated promptly and properly. Cancer and diseases of the heart present more difficult problems, but much can be done even now to prevent their development and to diagnose and treat them successfully.

ILLNESS AND DISABILITY

The goal of health work is not only to reduce death rates but also to improve the quality of human life. All too frequently both the usefulness and the joy of living are seriously impaired years before life is ended.

The National Health Survey conducted by the U.S. Public Health Service shows that in 1964 the population of the United States, excluding people in nursing homes and other institutions, experienced more than 3 billion days of restricted activity because of illness—an average of 16 days for every man, woman, and child. This includes more than a billion days of confinement to bed, 385 million days lost from work, and more than 200 million days lost from school. The survey shows also that the average person made 4.5 visits to a physician and 1.6 visits to a dentist during the year and that 128 persons in every 1,000 were admitted to a hospital.

HEALTH AND THE NATIONAL WELFARE

Health is such a personal matter that in normal times few people think of it as having national importance. Yet in times of national emergencies, everyone realizes that good health is essential for the national welfare and even for national survival. Illness destroys the effectiveness of the armed forces, hampers industrial production, undermines morale, and places an enormous burden of medical care upon a weakened populace.

The U.S. Public Health Service estimates that approximately 350 million man-days are lost annually because of illness and accidents among industrial workers in this country. This corresponds to the total working time of more than a million workers for a whole year. Other surveys of illness among industrial workers show that the average loss of time on account of illness is 8 days per year for men and 12 days per year for women.

THE HEALTH OF THE ARMED FORCES
During World War II and the wars in Korea and Vietnam, United States troops have lived and fought in areas of the world exceedingly hazardous to health. They were able to do this because insecticide sprays, new antimalarial drugs, and modern sanitary engineering methods prevented malaria, which previously had infected most human beings in the area; because vaccines and DDT protected them against typhus fever, which always before had accompanied the devastation of war; because modern methods of food processing, food sanitation, and transportation ensured adequate and safe nutrition from the arctic to the tropics; because new vaccines and new drugs, such as the sulfonamides and the antibiotics, helped to prevent and combat infections and infectious diseases; and because blood plasma and whole blood were flown to battlefields in the most remote corners of the globe.

The result of these improved health programs was less illness among our military forces than ever before. In medical care, too, the record was unbelievably good, for only 4.5 percent of wounded men who received medical care died during World War II, compared with 8 percent during World War I. The figure was further reduced to 2.3 percent during the war in Korea and to less than 1 percent in Vietnam, although the weapons of warfare were the most destructive and deadly ever known.

These excellent results were due not only to new scientific discoveries but even more to the excellent quality of the professional medical service which was available to the wounded. This service extended from the beachheads and battlefields through emergency dressing stations and field hospitals to the large general hospitals which offered long-term definitive treatment.

POSSIBILITIES, OPPORTUNITIES, AND OBLIGATIONS

The analysis of the health status of the United States population presented in this chapter shows that there are possibilities, opportunities, and obligations for improvement. The realization of these opportunities will depend primarily on interest, understanding, and action of individuals and groups to prevent disease and disabilities and to improve health. This book will present the essential health information on which such interest, understanding, and action must depend.

In planning a campaign or program for better health, a health officer surveys the situation of the community and concentrates first on problems of major importance. The measures of importance which he uses are death rates and sickness and disability rates of various diseases and conditions. Accidents, heart diseases, and cancer are leading causes of death in most age groups; yet mental illnesses, colds, emphysema and other respiratory diseases, and conditions affecting the muscular, nervous, and skeletal system (such as arthritis) are even more important as causes of disability and time lost from school and work than many of the more deadly diseases.

Both the incidence of disease and the suffering it brings to its victims and their families increase with poverty. Many of the improvements in health and in longevity in the past have been due to the rise in standards of living. Much more must be done in this respect.

Health in old age is determined largely by heredity and by what has happened before. Inherent traits cannot be modified, nor can damage already done be repaired.

The moving Finger writes; and having writ,
Moves on: nor all your Piety nor Wit
  Shall lure it back to cancel half a Line
Nor all your Tears wash out a Word of it.[2]

Realizing this makes it obvious that the health practices and habits developed in youth—in regard to eating, drinking, smoking, exercising, adjusting to life—are of vastly greater importance for the future than they are for the present. When one is endowed with the exuberant health and vitality of youth, 20, 30, 40, or 50 years ahead seems so remote that it takes unusual perspective and strength of character to forego immediate pleasures or satisfactions in the interest of health later on. However, as the years slip by, diseases and disabilities which are the result of unsound health practices take their inevitable toll.

[2]From Edward Fitzgerald (translator), *The Rubáiyát of Omar Khayyám.*

QUESTIONS FOR DISCUSSION AND SELF-EXAMINATION

1 Imagine that you and your husband or wife have two children, 6 months and 2 years old. Compare their chances for survival to the age of 75 today with their chances of survival to the age of 75 if they had been born about 1900.

2 What is the relationship of morbidity to mortality, and of each to longevity?

3 Compare longevity at age 50 today: first, with longevity at age 1 week today, and second, with longevity at age 50 in 1900. Account for the differences.

4   Does improved medical care account for most of the improved health enjoyed by Americans today (as compared with previous generations)? Defend your answer.

5   What five problems of society at large will affect your health to the greatest extent? Would the effect be different if you were (a) a Chicano living in San Antonio, (b) a rancher in Wyoming, or (c) a black in Harlem, New York?

6   Discuss the relations among health, personal income, and medical services. How may each affect the others?

7   How does the United States compare with other countries in health, longevity, and infant mortality? What accounts for the differences?

8   What do you consider the most important responsibility of the United States with respect to health and disease in the next 10 years? Where do you think this responsibility lies, most appropriately? Defend your answer.

9   Compare the ten leading causes of death today with the ten leading causes in 1900. Account for the changes.

10   Discuss limits to the possible extension of human life.

REFERENCES AND READING SUGGESTIONS

BOOKS

Dublin, Louis I.: *Fact Book on Man from Birth to Death,* 2d ed., The Macmillan Company, New York, 1965.

A gold mine of information on every aspect of health, presented in the form of questions and answers by a world-recognized authority.

Dubos, Rene J.: *Mirage of Health: Utopias, Progress, and Biological Change,* Harper & Row, Publishers, Incorporated, New York, 1959. (Also in paperback, Doubleday & Company, Inc., Garden City, N.Y., 1961.)

A delightful and thought-provoking series of discussions of man's successful struggle against disease, other destructive forces of nature, and the problems associated with the aging and loss of vigor of a society.

PAMPHLETS AND PERIODICALS

Graber, Joe Bales: "Preventing Dependence: Protective Health Services," *American Journal of Public Health,* vol. 59, p. 1413, August 1969.

Perceptions and goals with respect to health and illness change over time. What might be done in terms of present problems and our knowledge of how to prevent illness and consequent dependency is considered in this article.

Indicators, U.S. Department of Health, Education, and Welfare, monthly.

Feature articles on key problems and issues in health, education, and welfare; with current statistics, presented in charts, tables, brief text, and source notes.

Johnson, Harry J.: *Your Health Is Your Business,* Public Affairs Pamphlet, New York.

The president of the Life Extension Institute discusses why keeping healthy is good business.

Linder, F. E.: "Health of the American People," *Scientific American,* June 1966, p. 21.

Some of the important findings of the National Health Survey conducted over the previous 10 years by the U.S. Public Health Service.

Trends, U.S. Department of Health, Education, and Welfare.

An annual supplement to *Indicators,* with feature articles on major national trends and expenditures, plus statistical perspectives on long-term developments and projections in health, education, welfare, and related fields.

2

HEALTH PROBLEMS IN THE COLLEGE YEARS

During the college years, muscular, mental, and sexual powers are generally high. The susceptibility of the immature individual to serious infections has passed, and the increasing incidence of degenerative and malignant diseases that comes with age has not begun. The college-age person can often withstand greater physical, psychological, or environmental stress than younger or older people. His physiology and metabolism are strong, and his psychological traits are usually flexible, so that he can change them if he gives the matter determined effort. Indeed, it may be this *relative* immunity to weakness and disease that creates feelings of omnipotence and omniscience in some people. These feelings contribute to two of the three leading causes of death in this age group: automobile accidents and drug abuse or overdose (the number one killer in New York City). Suicide is also a leading cause of death in the college years.

EXERCISE AND HEALTH

Exercise tests show that one can attain good physical training or "shape" most readily when one is still in the teens. The Harvard or Brouha step test, which demonstrates the ability of the heart to recover from the stress of exercise, is a good measure of physical fitness. In this test, a person steps up and down on a 20-inch step at a given pace for 5 minutes (or less if he cannot go the full time); his pulse is then taken for 30-second intervals at certain points in the next 5 minutes. If he is in "good shape" his heart rate and pulse slow rapidly; if he is in "poor shape" his heart rate and pulse return to normal very slowly. Regular, vigorous exercise will bring a poorly trained person into a state of good training. Through the late teens and usually into the early twenties, one can attain a state of good training in a short period—several weeks—but gradually the length of time taken to attain good training becomes longer and the efficiency of heart and muscle function which one can attain is less.

The goal of exercise for most of us is not great competitive performances, but the regular and frequent stimulation of the heart, blood vessels, endocrine glands, and other body systems, which promotes general health and makes most people feel more healthy and vigorous. Exercise also allows partial release of anxieties and tensions, particularly those resulting from unexpressed anger, hostility, or annoyance. Furthermore, people in good physical training seem to recover from infections more rapidly than those in poor shape, particularly prolonged infections such as infectious mononucleosis.

YOUTH VERSUS AGE

Psychological tests show that the ability to learn new intellectual material rapidly is at its maximum in the teens and twenties. However, some older people may have more motivation than some younger ones and so may outperform them in practical situations.

Kinsey's researches showed that men reach the peak of their sexual activity at 19; this is confirmed by the studies of Masters and Johnson. Men's ability to have *frequent* intercourse begins to decrease after the age of 30. Many women do not reach the peak of their sexual activity until the late twenties; however, cultural factors influence women more than men in their sexual activity.

These capacities are felt as both psychological and physical strengths by most people, and the relative absence of natural disease in youth has the same effect. Diseases of the heart and blood vessels, the most serious degenerative diseases in the United States, are infrequent in young people. The various forms of cancer are far more common after the age of 40 than before. Degenerative arthritis, which stiffens and slows so many older people, rarely makes its appearance before the age of 40.

PSYCHOLOGICAL PROBLEMS IN YOUTH

With natural vigor at its peak and fatal disease rare, why are there health problems in the college years? A prime reason is the psychological difficulties of youth.

Adolescence is often portrayed as a stormy period of life, beset with conflicts, with rapid changes of motivation and drive, and with difficulties in handling new sexual urges. Though this is a familiar portrait, it is one which does not apply to everyone, for many reach adulthood without crises. Nevertheless, even people who pass through adolescence without much surface turmoil can look back when the period is finished and see that they have made great strides. They have matured rapidly not only in knowledge and performance, but in subtle ways of dealing with other people, in understanding themselves, and in capacities for love and work. Adolescence is not a set period, starting on a certain birthday and terminating so many years and months afterward. Some people may have more or less completed adolescence by the time they go to college; still others may be in some ways still adolescents when they are graduated from college.

People in this age group, including college students, have four important ways in which to grow and change. They may be more or less successful in any of these ways.

First, they develop a clearer picture of themselves. What kind of people are they? What are their chief characteristics and chief goals in college and in life? To be motivated, they must become consistent in these goals and not be influenced by campus fads, by transient pressures from friends and acquaintances, and by the temptations which stem from minor successes and failures. This kind of growth has been called *stabilizing ego identity*.

Second, as people mature, they develop a greater ability to form appropriate relationships with many kinds of people, both young and old. They can understand better what other people are actually feeling, and they no longer see others in a stereotyped way.

Next, maturing human beings deepen their interests. This involves an increased absorption in subjects and objects of interest, and increased ability and desire to do a thing for its own sake without regard for outside support or praise.

Finally, people develop their value systems, or sense of what is important and worthwhile in life. They develop priorities in responsibilities and relationships. Values are increasingly related to social purposes and community life; they are related one to another, and are fitted into a person's past and possible future experience.

To some extent, people continue to develop in these ways throughout life, revising value systems, developing character and personality, and becoming more confident in personal identity. But the tasks are most important and most intense during the years in which many young people are in college. Performing these tasks is easy. Even if a college student is not conscious of these processes, he probably cannot proceed with them smoothly and uneventfully under all circumstances. Some students have major difficulties, perhaps accompanied by disruption in other areas of life. Others, who accomplish much during their college years, give no outward signs of turmoil over the inward growth they have worked hard to gain.

That these are formative years means that character and personality disorders are less likely to be fixed and inflexible than they are later. They are more susceptible to treatment and to change, in a person who desires treatment and change. The nature of personality disorders, psychologically caused symptoms, and psychological and psychiatric treatment receives more extensive investigation in Chapter 10.

Because the personality is changing so rapidly in these years, one is susceptible to stresses from the environment. Academic failure, rejection by a boy friend or a girl friend, quarrels with parents, or the threat of undesired military service find the personality less able to cope with these difficult events at this age than a few years later. Temporary disabilities, breakdowns, acting out (accidents, drug abuse, etc.), and even suicide may result.

Aside from such serious problems, ordinary pressures of the environment may lead to a genuine need for counseling. A study of members of student councils (governments) at three Eastern liberal arts colleges, who were considered to have a relatively high degree of mental health, showed that one in four sought psychiatric counseling at some time to cope with the stresses of everyday living.

The most serious psychological illnesses of college students, schizophrenia and depression, are described in Chapter 10. Schizophrenia causes most of the sudden psychiatric hospitalizations which college students require, although its onset is usually slow. Most depressions are also of slow onset. People who commit suicide have usually talked about the possibility with friends or relatives in the past. Depression can be very serious in the college years, and suicide is a leading cause of death among college students, with about $1\frac{1}{2}$ successful suicides annually for each 10,000 students in the United States. Depression and suicide are discussed in Chapter 10.

Recognizing the frequency of psychological and emotional problems among students, most colleges and universities today provide a psychiatric service or a counseling service or both. When such services are readily available, from 10 to 40 percent of students receive help from them during the college years. Many intelligent, sensitive students recognize their own problems and seek help promptly. Students who voluntarily seek help are likely to be helped and so overcome their difficulties. Talking to an appropriate professional person helps them to make fundamental advances in understanding the emotional causes of their problems, and they may eliminate the problems by direct confrontation. In some cases, tranquilizers or antidepressant medicines are useful during a particularly difficult period of life.

Although many students are aware of their problems, others see their struggles only dimly. The best examples of this are situations in which self-destructive behavior is the result of psychological conflict. Not infrequently this involves careless or dangerous automobile driving.

TRAFFIC RISKS

Psychiatrists report that cars may have particular psychological implications. Many people are selfish and intolerant of one another in the use of their cars. Many forget that the strength and vitality of youth does not make them immune to accident and to death. A few regard cars as extensions of themselves, particularly of their own aggressive tendencies, and display these aggressive or competitive urges on the highway; when they do so with the unconscious delusion that they are invulnerable, severe injury to themselves or others may result.

The anonymity of the highway encourages freer expression of emotion than face-to-face contact. A man or a woman who would be too polite to rebuke a salesman or to cut into a check-out line in a supermarket might not hesitate to cut into a traffic line or to push ahead if someone tried to pass him. A man who dodges down the street in his car, cutting dangerously from lane to lane, may well be thoughtful when he deals personally with people he knows. Since he does not know who the other drivers are and since personal contact with them is impossible, he permits himself to express feelings that otherwise would be well hidden.

The greatest risk to the lives of college students comes from traffic accidents. Men die at four times the rate that women die in this age group. In 1970, 23,200 drivers under the age of 25 were involved in fatal accidents; they accounted for more than a third of all the fatal accidents in the United States. The proportion of young people dying in automobile accidents has gradually increased since 1942.

Like other accidents, many traffic accidents are preventable. The causes of traffic accidents fall into two categories: first, those directly under the control of the driver, such as not using seat belts, using alcohol, failing to practice safe driving skills, and driving at an inappropriate speed; and second, those completely or relatively out of his control, such as badly designed automobiles, poor roads, and bad weather conditions.

Alcohol and excessive speed are two major factors in accidents, each being involved in from one-fourth to one-half of fatal accidents, often simultaneously. Routine police accident reports often do not show the use of alcohol accurately. As many as half of the fatal automobile accidents which have been studied specifically and thoroughly with reference to alcohol consumption appeared to be due to alcohol, at least in part. Even small amounts of alcohol may impair coordination; moderate amounts impair judgment as well as coordination and reflex, despite the bravado of the driver who boasts of his ability to "hold it."

A 1968 study prepared for the United States Congress showed the contribution of heavy drinkers to traffic accidents. Each year, according to this report, 25,000 Americans were dying on the highways and at least 800,000 crashes were occurring because of the use of alcohol by drivers and pedestrians. More than half of the people involved had drunk alcohol heavily, chronically, or both. In one-car accidents (not involving a second vehicle) occurring between 9 P.M. and midnight, the chances were eight to one that the driver had been drinking heavily.

Strict laws aimed at controlling drinking before driving have succeeded in lowering accident rates and fatalities. Sweden has had stringent laws and a lower accident rate for years. In 1967 Great Britain made it mandatory for any driver suspected of driving under the influence of alcohol to have a measurement of the alcohol on his breath; within a month the enforcement of this law, the accident rate dropped by 10 percent.

By 1970, forty-six states had passed implied-consent laws which permit police authorities to test drivers for the amount of alcohol in their blood or in the air they exhale, on suspicion of driving under the influence of alcohol. *Implied consent* means that when the driver applies for a license to drive or when he uses public roads, he implies that he is willing to accept the test if requested. The breathing test, often called *Breatholator*, is the most commonly used; it is based on the fact that air expired from the lungs will contain alcohol in proportion to the amount of alcohol in the blood; usually the results are given in terms of the percentage of alcohol in the blood. This calculation of blood alcohol on the basis of breath checked is reliable except when the subject has had alcohol in his mouth in the few minutes prior to the test. Criteria vary from state to state, but usually drivers with 0.15 percent of alcohol in the blood are assumed to be driving under the influence of alcohol (such levels can be produced readily by four or five drinks). Only if the blood level is below 0.05 percent is the driver presumed to be sober; more than one drink would be likely to raise the blood alcohol above this level. Between these levels, sobriety or intoxication is judged by the driver's actions and self-control. In some states additional categories are defined.

Smoking, too, is related to driving accidents. In one study, smokers were involved in four times as many accidents as nonsmokers. The reasons are probably multiple.

Speed is another, more obvious cause of accidents. According to some studies, it contributes to about two out of five fatal accidents and to an even higher proportion of accidents fatal to young drivers. Many of these deaths are single-vehicle accidents, in which the car overturns or collides with a tree or abutment rather than another car. The National Safety Council's figures for 1970 showed that about a third of fatal accidents involved cars which were being driven too fast, at least too fast for the local conditions. Speed is much more often a factor in deaths in the country than in the city.

An alarming phenomenon is the growing prevalence of high speeds on rural roads. In the 12 years from 1956 to 1968 the percentage of vehicles traveling over 60 miles per hour on main rural roads more than tripled, rising from 13 percent to 45 percent. The chances of being killed rise with increased speed, too: one is twice as likely to be killed in an accident going 55 miles per hour as in an accident going only 45 miles per hour.

Despite the dangers of speed, "Drive at a reasonable rate" is probably better advice than "Drive slowly." Driving much more slowly than the rest of the traffic going your way can lead to accidents, though not as many as driving faster. Furthermore, on the Pennsylvania Turnpike during World War II, when the speed limit was lowered from 60 miles per hour to 35 miles per hour to save gasoline, the accident rate went up.

Alcohol, smoking, and speed are factors under the control of individual drivers which contribute heavily to accidents and deaths. Other such factors also contribute to safety. Safety devices such as seat belts and adjustable headrests already save many lives and prevent many injuries; they could save many more lives if used regularly. In 1966, a

University of Michigan study reconstructed 139 accidents which had resulted in 177 deaths in the Ann Arbor area in the previous 4 years. The conclusions were:

1 Forty percent of those killed could have lived had they merely worn lap belts.
2 Another 13 percent would have lived had they worn both lap belts and shoulder straps.
3 Because of high speed at the time of collision, 37 percent would have died even with belts.
4 Only three people who were wearing belts died.

Although other studies show similar facts, unfortunately only about 40 percent of passenger-car occupants were using seat belts in 1970. This means that about 2,800 to 3,000 lives were saved each year by seat belts, but that 8,000 to 10,000 lives would have been saved if everyone had used seat belts at all times.

Is wearing seat belts dangerous? Not nearly as dangerous as not wearing them. Only rarely will a person be trapped dangerously in a car because he is unconscious and unable to release his seat belt. It is much more likely that a nonbelted person will be thrown from the car and have permanent brain damage from a blow to the head or be killed instantly by the blow. There are, however, dangerous ways to wear a seat belt. If it is loose or worn around the mid-abdomen instead of snugly across the pelvis at the hips, it may damage the contents of the abdomen or even the chest in case of accident. A lap belt gives good protection, but it gives maximum protection only when used with a shoulder strap. A shoulder strap should not be used alone.

In the early 1970s, attention was being given to the development and use of inflatable bags which would cushion drivers and front-seat passengers in case of any impact to the car.

Driving skills are conscious and learnable. By 1970, over 2 million high school students were enrolled in driver-education programs, and the number was increasing every year. According to several studies, graduates of driver-training schools or courses have better safety records than drivers who have not had formal training. Insurance companies recognize this and often charge

Table 2.1 Highways and death rates per 100 million miles

Highway	Rate
United States highways, general average	5.7
Toll roads, general average	2.5
Pennsylvania Turnpike	2.4
Garden State Parkway (New Jersey)	1.4
Maine Turnpike	0.8
Hutchinson River Parkway (New York)	0.8
Miami Airport Expressway	0.6

lower premiums to such drivers. In a study in South Africa, a training program for truck drivers cut accidents by a third.

Defensive driving is a technique and philosophy taught in many of the most successful driving programs. A defensive driver anticipates situations of increased hazard and expects other drivers to drive carelessly. He slows appropriately on curves and at difficult intersections. When anxious or preoccupied, he drives more cautiously than usual, if he must drive at all. On long trips, he knows his route numbers beforehand in order to avoid indecision (especially at the poorly marked intersections which too often mar many highways today). He does not tailgate. If someone tailgates him, he drops farther behind the car next ahead in order to provide the extra space needed for sudden stops for both vehicles. Such principles are taught in a defensive-driving course organized by the National Safety Council. In 1969 the United States Navy joined various industrial and business companies in using this course for its personnel.

SAFE ROADS AND SAFE CARS

Good roads save lives. The Interstate System of national highways saved approximately 3,300 lives in 1970. The death rate per 100 million miles traveled on the Interstate System was only 2.8, but it was 4.9 for all roads. Had the Interstate System not been available, 3,300 more Americans would have died in 1970. (See Table 2.1.)

Carefully designed cars save lives. During the late 1960s a national highway safety agency came into being and established standards for safety for both new and used cars. Improved windshield glass was required in 1966, for example: glass much less likely to cut when broken than previous glass. Headrests to prevent the whiplash injuries which occur in rear-end collisions, latches to prevent doors from flying open on impact, and minimum standards for windshield wiping and defrosting all were required in 1969. Standards for tires were introduced. All these engineering advances cost money but saved lives. Obviously, however, it is the responsibility of the car owner to maintain his car in safe condition, with emphasis on effective braking and on tires with adequate treads and optimum inflation. For proper control of a car in turning corners and changing speed, tire pressure should be maintained at the upper limit recommended by the manufacturer.

Not surprisingly, different makes of cars have different safety records. These safety records, however, depend not only on the safety features and engineering of the car, but on its size, its weight, and the personality and habits of the average driver of that make. In a New York State study, heavy, expensive, American-made cars had a low incidence of accidents with serious injury and fatalities, but small, foreign-made cars had a high incidence of such accidents.

In 1970, 2,330 motorcycle riders died in accidents, at a rate over four times as high as the rate at which drivers of automobiles died, per mile traveled. Driving a motorcycle safely requires more skill than driving a car safely. Unfortunately, many automobile drivers fail to observe motorcyclists on the road and do not respect their rights. Not only should motorcyclists wear safety helmets, leather garments to prevent skin damage if they are thrown off the cycle, and protective footgear; but they should learn the various techniques for handling slippery surfaces, turns, and passing.

INFECTIONS COMMON TO COLLEGE STUDENTS

While traffic accidents are the most frequent cause of death in college students, infections cause the majority of illnesses. Respiratory infections, particularly the common cold and influenza, cause more visits to college health centers and infirmaries than any other problem; infections of the intestinal tract come second. Infectious mononucleosis often causes the most apprehension among college students.

Other infections which may be important to

college students are discussed in other chapters: veneral disease in Chapter 20, respiratory diseases (including tuberculosis) in Chapter 18, hepatitis in Chapter 12, some other communicable diseases in Chapter 16, and certain diseases which can be prevented by immunizations in Chapter 17.

RESPIRATORY INFECTIONS

Caused by at least six different major groups of viruses, the common cold produces more illness and disability in college students and the American population at large than any other illness in our society. Fortunately, it rarely causes serious complications or severe illness, except when the victim is already feeble because of underlying chronic disease or old age.

There is much folklore about colds. One myth is that they result from getting wet or chilled. Thomas Jefferson exploded this one almost two centuries ago when he wrote, "A person not sick will not be injured by getting wet. It is but taking a cold bath, which never gives a cold to anyone." Modern scientists have done experiments which corroborate Jefferson's statement; volunteer subjects chilled but not exposed to cold germs will not develop colds, and subjects chilled and deliberately exposed to cold germs will *not* develop colds more readily than those not chilled but still deliberately exposed to cold germs.

In the college community, there are several times during the year when colds are rampant. First, when students gather in the fall, they bring cold viruses (to which they themselves may be immune) from their home communities to the college communities. The viruses immediately begin to spread from student to student and an epidemic of colds starts. This may coincide with an early touch of cool weather, which will lead some to blame the colds on chilling. Second, during the winter, students spend more time indoors in closed spaces and pass cold germs from one to another more readily than when they are outdoors. This is the season of cold and stormy weather, and so once again epidemics of colds are blamed on being chilled.

The causes, natural course, and treatment of colds are discussed at length in Chapter 18. The important practical points for college students and their communities are that since colds are infectious, it is unfair to others to circulate socially when you have a cold; that no treatment specifi-

cally "cures" a cold; that antibiotics are slightly dangerous rather than helpful; and that the bacterial complications, particularly sinusitis, ear infections, and lower-respiratory diseases such as bronchitis and pneumonia, are what you should guard against when you have a cold.

INFLUENZA AND GRIPPE

Because it may occur in epidemics during examination periods and incapacitate students at critical times, influenza is a feared disease on campuses. The term *flu* is often used, mistakenly, to refer to *any* acute infection. True influenza is a 3- or 4-day feverish illness, usually with a slight cough, which often leaves its victims tired and debilitated. It is caused by any of a small group of influenza viruses. The viruses are closely related but have the property of changing their characteristics every few years (as indicated by the fact that a new influenza virus stimulates slightly different antibodies, or immune proteins, in the human body). This capability for change accounts for the worldwide epidemics of influenza which occur from time to time. The most serious such epidemic occurred in 1918–1919. (On this and subsequent major epidemics, see pages 279–281.)

In addition to these major epidemics most communities, including colleges and universities, suffer outbreaks of influenza or grippe every second year. In these outbreaks, the disease is usually milder and affects smaller numbers of people, but the nature of the disease is similar to that in most widespread epidemics.

Vaccines are available against influenza, though unfortunately they are only 50 to 70 percent effective. They confer immunity on that percentage of people who receive them at least a few weeks before an epidemic. Once an epidemic has started in a community, it is useless to get an influenza shot. Because influenza is incapacitating for a few days, many students choose to receive the vaccine in years when the Public Health Service predicts influenza in their area. A relatively new drug, amantadine, will prevent influenza from developing when given *after* exposure to the disease but *before* symptoms develop. Unfortunately it has deleterious side effects, and it is therefore usually used only for feeble people to whom influenza might be very dangerous or for those whose exposure has been intense and certain, as within a family.

Feverish illnesses similar to influenza occur sporadically, especially during the winter and early spring months in temperate climates. Often called *grippe,* some of these are nonepidemic cases of influenza, while many result from other viruses, such as the adenoviruses. Since the laboratory demonstration of viruses is much more difficult and much slower than the isolation of bacteria, specific identification of the type of virus responsible for a particular illness cannot be made by the clinical laboratories of college health services or of general hospitals.

With any of the infections which cause fever and respiratory symptoms, the most important treatment is bed rest, fluids, aspirin to reduce fever, and warmth until the fever has gone. A doctor can determine whether bacterial infection is present. If the disease is caused by a virus, the use of antibiotics will merely lead to the development of antibiotic-resistant strains of bacteria which may invade the lungs and cause dangerous complications. (See Chapter 18 for a more detailed discussion of influenza and grippe.)

GASTROENTERITIS

Familiar in any college community is the acute illness consisting of violent vomiting and retching, followed by loose bowel movements. The vomiting is usually over in a few hours, and the diarrhea in a day or two. Often, it is wrongly attributed to food poisoning; but if others have eaten the same meals and have not developed intestinal symptoms at the same time, the illness cannot be due to food eaten. Food poisoning and its attributes are described in Chapter 12.

This acute vomiting-and-diarrhea illness is referred to by doctors as *gastroenteritis,* meaning "inflammation of the stomach and intestines." The disease appears to be caused by viruses, although it is not known how many different kinds of viruses can cause it. Many lay people refer to it as *flu* or *intestinal flu,* but it has no relationship to influenza. The proper treatment consists of resting the body and intestinal tract by staying in bed and taking a liquid diet; certain new drugs related to tranquilizers can calm the vomiting if it persists, and drugs such as paregoric can stop the diarrhea.

INFECTIOUS MONONUCLEOSIS

Mononucleosis, a common disease among all young people, is surrounded by folklore on the college campus. Causing, not caused by, fatigue; called *infectious,* but of uncertain transmission; and usually lasting but a week or 10 days, it is feared beyond reason by many college students.

Possibly caused by a virus (the Ebstein-Barr virus) identified in 1967, it produces variable combinations of sore throat, fever, fatigue, jaundice, swelling of lymph nodes, enlargement of the spleen, and characteristic changes in the blood. A typical case might run as follows: A college undergraduate, after 3 or 4 days of fatigue and lack of energy, develops a moderate sore throat and a fever of 101°. The physician whom he consults finds several small whitish patches in his throat, notes that the lymph nodes in the neck are enlarged, and finds that the spleen, which is usually hidden underneath the left side of the rib cage, can now be felt easily. The student enters the college infirmary, where he is moderately uncomfortable for 3 or 4 days. He then improves gradually and is able to return to classes at the end of a week, although he has diminishing amounts of fatigue for the next month and needs somewhat more sleep than usual. Laboratory tests, which confirmed the diagnosis after 3 days in the infirmary, remain positive for a lengthier period than his symptoms of illness.

Stories about people who have had infectious mononucleosis for 3 months or even a year abound in college circles. Such cases are very rare. Only a tenth to a quarter of patients with mononucleosis even feel any excess fatigue 6 weeks after the beginning of their disease; only a tiny fraction still have any symptoms after 3 months. As many as a quarter of patients never have to be confined to bed at all.

How mononucleosis spreads is unknown. It has been called "the kissing disease"; a very careful study of a large number of patients by Dr. A. S. Evans, then at the University of Wisconsin, showed that about twice as many paitents with mononucleosis had engaged in deep or "French" kissing within a few weeks of the onset of their symptoms as had patients with other types of feverish illness. It seems likely that kissing is one way in which mononucleosis can be spread; but the disease is usually contracted from a "carrier" rather than from an active case. Students who are married and come down with infectious mononucleosis rarely, if ever, give it to their spouses.

There is substantial evidence that many people have infectious mononucleosis but continue to feel very well. In a survey of the entire freshman class at Princeton University approximately 2 percent had evidence of recent infectious mononucleosis in their blood, but less than half of these knew that they had had it. Furthermore, a few patients come to the doctor because of swelling of the lymph nodes and turn out to have infectious mononucleosis; but they do not *feel* ill in any way.

No antibiotics or other drugs "cure" mononucleosis, in the sense that penicillin cures a streptococcal sore throat. Even rest is of limited use; in a study of 186 college students, those who exercised as they felt able recovered slightly faster than those who were kept on strict bed rest until their tests were almost normal. In some cases, cortisone derivatives are useful in suppressing symptoms. Serious complications and recurrences are rare.

SETTING GOOD HEALTH PATTERNS IN COLLEGE

It is not hard to stay healthy in college. Avoiding a few obvious hazards, coping with psychological change, and acting sensibly during temporary illness will preserve health and life.

It is much harder to establish patterns of good health behavior for later life while you are in college. Poor nutrition, lack of sleep, lack of exercise, and poor mental health patterns can often be withstood for short periods, even for a few years at the college age level, but they establish the likelihood of serious illness, disability, premature death, or some combination of these later on. Some of these factors are discussed earlier in this chapter, and others elsewhere (nutrition in Chapters 11 and 12; tobacco and health in Chapter 7; alcohol and other mind-altering drugs in Chapter 8; some health factors in daily life in Chapter 13). The temptation

for college students is to follow immediate impulses and desires rather than to adhere to healthy long-term patterns. By their mid-twenties, the great majority of human beings have started to decline in physical and even in mental powers; only persistent effort and attention to health promotion will maintain these powers and minimize the decline. To neglect the promotion of health until discomfort and other symptoms appear may be to delay until irreversible change, however minor, has occurred.

To be sure, failure to follow careful health habits seems common. Though there are numbers of pleasures and satisfactions in life which do not damage health, sometimes it is necessary to give up or postpone other gratifications in order to have reasonable health habits.

HEALTH IN COLLEGES

College life presents special problems and opportunities in regard to health. In college, many students are on their own and must manage their own health matters for the first time in their lives. They have been dependent on parents for guidance, even in minor illness, but unless they live at home they must now be independent. They must overcome or compensate for any health or other deficits which existed before their college careers.

They must learn what to do in the event of acute illness, where to seek competent medical care, and how to make reasonable decisions about diet, activity, rest, and other principles of healthful living. They must find sound sources of medical information and must learn how to use them to solve their physical and emotional problems and to promote health.

To help meet these needs, colleges and universities have established health services to provide infirmary care; preventive inoculations; medical consultations and services for all sorts of physical and emotional problems; assistance in the correction of physical defects and handicaps; and a healthful and safe environment in classrooms, dormitories, athletic facilities, and other areas. The good health service aims not only at the best of medical care but also at the best of community health maintenance, at the best of preventive medicine, and at helping students to recognize good medicine. Each encounter between student and health service should be an educational as well as a diagnostic and therapeutic experience.

About half the colleges also provide courses in personal and community health. The goals of such courses are apparent from the content of this book. The course should derive impetus not only from the student's need for adequate health knowledge but also from the fact that today's college generation will be giving both professional and lay leadership to tomorrow's society in health as well as other matters.

By utilizing college health services and the educational opportunities related to health, students not only learn to deal effectively with their immediate health problems but also build a foundation for meeting the future health responsibilities of their families and of the communities in which as college men and women they should exert constructive leadership.

QUESTIONS FOR DISCUSSION AND SELF-EXAMINATION

1 In what ways is health at its best during the college years?
2 What is the relationship between adolescence and the college years? Defend your answer.
3 How does "stablizing ego identity" correspond to the entire process of maturation?
4 What is the relationship of value systems to psychological health and to maturity?
5 How are emotional stresses and supports in early childhood related to emotional stresses and supports during the college years? Be specific.
6 Describe three ways in which psychological problems are commonly manifested in the college years.
7 How do psychological factors, alcohol, and driving techniques act and interact to cause or promote traffic accidents?
8 Discuss the relationship of speed to traffic accidents.
9 What virus infections are common among college students? What measures of protection against them are effective or partly effective and what are known to be ineffective?
10 What effect do health and health habits in college years have on health in middle age and afterward?

REFERENCES AND READING SUGGESTIONS

BOOKS

Blaine, Graham G., and MacArthur, Charles C. (eds.): *Emotional Problems of the Student*, 2d ed., Appleton-Century-Crafts, Inc., New York, 1971. A practical, down-to-earth discussion of common problems and how to handle them.

Brody, Eugene B.: *Minority Group Adolescents in the United States*, The Williams & Wilkins Company, Baltimore, 1968. Emphasizes psychological aspects of adolescence, particularly the identity crises which are particularly difficult for minority-group adolescents.

PAMPHLETS AND PERIODICALS

Bliven, Bruce: "The Most Creative Years of Our Lives," *The New York Times Magazine*, May 6, 1962, p. 24.

A report of a number of studies and surveys which show that talented men are likely to produce their most significant achievements earlier in their careers than is commonly realized.

3

HUMAN ECOLOGY

Until recent years the word *ecology* was relatively unknown. Rachel Carson's book *Silent Spring* in 1962 and innumerable articles and books since that time have changed this. Today practically everyone is concerned about the effects of man and the environment on each other—plants, trees, birds, fish, animals, and especially men himself. That is human ecology. It includes the harmful effects of our increasingly polluted environment not only upon health but also upon the quality of life. Experience has shown that human beings can exist under unbelievably bad conditions; but is this living?

The environment with which we are primarily concerned in this chapter includes the air we breathe and by which we are surrounded, the water we drink, the foods we eat, the human and industrial wastes which must be disposed of, the noises to which we are exposed, and the tensions and pressures under which we live. These factors act upon and interact with each other as well as man.

But the common factor basic in the pollution of the environment is man himself.

It is people who build, buy, drive, and ride in automobiles, trucks, airplanes, and other fuel-using vehicles. It is people and the industries that supply their needs and wants that use larger and larger amounts of water and increasingly pollute the air and the water. It is people who develop and use the pesticides, herbicides (weed killers), detergents, and fertilizers that have been shown to be harmful to many forms of life. It is people who make and operate the machines that create noise intolerable to urban areas. It is people who use the electricity produced by power plants that pollute the atmosphere by burning coal and oil and by using atomic energy. And it is people who produce the waste products and the litter that are creating hazards to health and detracting from the quality of our environment.

Therefore, we consider first the problem of population and its effects upon ecology.

OVERPOPULATION

One of the greatest menaces to health and welfare is overpopulation. If food supplies and other resources are insufficient to provide the minimum basic needs of the population, hunger and disease are inevitable. In certain areas of the world, overpopulation has long been recognized as a serious problem, but only in recent years has its ominous portent for the entire world been generally understood.

The population of the world at the beginning of the Christian era is estimated to have been about 250 million. It took about 1,800 years for the population to reach a billion. It took less than 100 years to add the next billion and only about one-third as long to add the third billion. And it is estimated that if current rates continue, the population of the world will be 4 billion in 1980 and 7 billion by the year 2000. In other words, in 35 to 40 years, the world's population will be double what it is today. (See Figure 3.1.)

Currently, the population of the world is increasing about 70 million a year—8,000 every hour. Yet more than half the world's population is chronically hungry, and approximately two-thirds of the people of the world today do not have enough food to provide the energy necessary to do a day's work. Hungry, sick people cannot build an

independent, growing economy or stable government.

Furthermore, the most rapid population increases are in underdeveloped and overpopulated countries which already have very low standards of living. Even in wealthier countries, such as the United States, birth rates are highest in the poorer and less-educated segments of the population. In 1970 more than half of all children born in New York City were born into indigent families.

The situation in the United States (Figure 3.2) has been summarized by stating that the burden of unwanted children among impoverished and uneducated mothers in the United States is much like that experienced by mothers in underdeveloped countries. This situation all too frequently leads to what is known as the "cycle of dependency." The cycle is sad, but not surprising. Poor people tend to have more children than they want or can afford, and the larger the number of children in a family, the less chance the children have to receive the education and training they need to break the cycle. More than 40 percent of parents whose children receive funds from the Aid for Dependent Children program themselves had parents who received relief checks. Thus succeeding generations tend to appear on public relief rolls.

The increasing population is due in part to increases in the birth rate; but in the underdeveloped countries a more important factor is the reduction in death rates, especially in the death rates of infants and children from communicable diseases. (See Table 3.1.) The result is that *in many areas living standards are getting worse* instead of better, in spite the local successes in technology and the material assistance that the United States has been giving to these countries since the end of World War II.

Where no private or government provision for old age is available, elderly couples need children, particularly sons, to help support them. In India it is calculated that, because of the high death rates in infancy and childhood, families need an average of 6.3 children to be reasonably certain that one son will be alive when the father grows old. In such situations new programs of social security, and perhaps economic inducements to limit families

Figure 3.1 Population of the United States, 1790 to 1970. Source: Bureau of the Census, 1960 PC(1)-1A, page 4, Table 2, and 1970 projection by the Statistical Bureau of the Metropolitan Life Insurance Company.

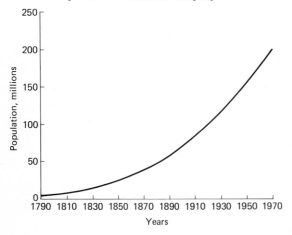

Figure 3.2 Population increase in the United States, 1915 to 1970. Source: U.S. Census.

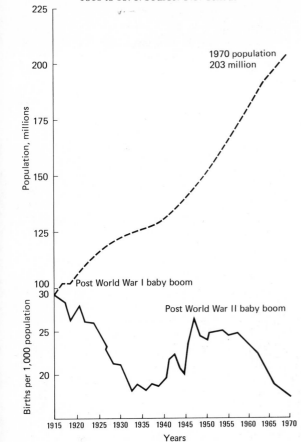

The population of underdeveloped countries is mounting at an annual rate of 2.4 percent. This means that there are 70 million more impoverished people in the world each year. The control of population increase, therefore, has become a health problem of paramount importance for the entire world. Even in the United States with its immense resources and productivity, the annual population increase of 3 million persons—the equivalent of a city the size of Chicago—is a matter for concern. To provide housing for a population increase of this size would require the equivalent of a new city of 250,000 every month.

In the United States the birth rate and the number of births have been declining steadily in recent years. Yet, because the birth rate is still almost double the death rate, the population continues to increase. For example, in 1970 in the United States 18 babies were born and only 10 persons died per 1,000 population. Continued for 10 years this would result in a population increase of 25 million persons. In addition, the population is increased by immigration, about 400,000 a year. The decrease in the birth rate, however, is encouraging: from 23.7 births per 1,000 population in 1960 to 18.2 in 1970. And this decrease occurred in spite of an increase in the number of marriages. The obvious conclusion to be drawn is that many married couples have decided to have fewer children.

The Population Reference Bureau states that 7 million American girls have it within their power to set a new marriage and fertility vogue that could significantly alter the nation's future. These young women are now in the peak marriage years, 18 to 21. The attitudes toward population control and family planning in this group could greatly in-

must go hand in hand with programs to produce the medical means of preventing conception.

Latin America, where most people have always lived under unbelievably poor conditions, is experiencing an annual population increase of nearly 3 percent and now has an annual per-capita income substantially lower than before World War II. This situation leads to increasing poverty and ill-health. (See Figure 3.3.)

The situation is serious because "poor health means lower productivity; lower productivity means lower standards of living; lower standards of living means less food, less education, and poorer living conditions; these in turn mean poor health. Thus the cycle of misery is completed."[1]

[1]Francis T. P. Plimpton, *Population, The U.N. and the U.S.*, Planned Parenthood Federation of America, New York.

Table 3.1 Annual world population increase by area, 1960 to 1970

Areas	Current annual increase, percent
Latin America	2.8
Asia, excluding Japan	2.5
Africa	2.4
United States and Canada	1.7
U.S.S.R.	1.5
Japan	1.0
Europe	0.9

SOURCE: United Nations.

Figure 3.3 Population growth in Latin America. Source: After *Population Bulletin,* vol. 23, no. 3.

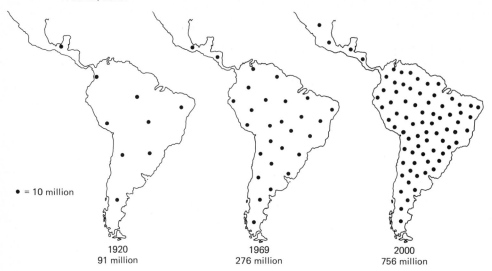

• = 10 million

| 1920 | 1969 | 2000 |
| 91 million | 276 million | 756 million |

fluence the future for this country. There were 6 million more potential mothers of childbearing age (15 to 44) in 1970 than in 1960. Concerning these facts, the president of the Population Reference Bureau stated that the United States birth rate is definitely a controlled birth rate. What has motivated this decline is mainly a matter of conjecture. It is unquestionably related to a recognition on the part of the young people who have embarked on matrimony that rearing children and educating them, especially through college, is an expensive undertaking.

With the large increase in potential mothers, the number of children desired becomes of crucial importance. If women choose the two- to four-child family, the fashion in the 1950s, then the nation will have a baby boom of unprecedented magnitude. Such a fertility rate during the 1970s could result in a total United States population of nearly 400 million by the year 2000—twice the present population of the country.

The possibility of a population of such magnitude has for years alarmed students of demography, but today people everywhere are coming to realize what this would mean to society, not only in terms of the provision of food and housing but also in terms of education; transportation; air and water pollution; sewage, garbage, and waste disposal; noise; and overcrowding, with accompanying

physical and mental stresses, strains, and illnesses. Overpopulation would result in a deterioration in the quality of life for everybody. The deprived, uneducated, and unskilled would suffer first and most severely, but no group of society would be unaffected. Therefore it is everybody's responsibility and in everybody's interest to help bring the population increase under control.

ZERO POPULATION GROWTH

In a zero increase in population, the number of births would not exceed the number of deaths. That would occur if the birth rate were two children per couple and every child grew to maturity and became a parent of two. Since some children do not grow to adulthood and some adults do not have children, an average of two children per family would result eventually in a slight decrease in population. However, because there is a larger number of young persons of childbearing age today than there was a generation or two ago—there were nearly 2.2 million marriages in 1970, a figure exceeded only in 1946—an average of two children or less per family will result in an increasing population in the United States until about the year 2000. Furthermore, this analysis does not take into account migration of people from other countries to the United States.

PREVENTING BIRTHS

Charles F. Westoff of Princeton University's Office of Population Research has reported that in the mid-1960s about 750,000 children born in the United States each year were conceived contrary to the wishes of both parents and another 250,000 were unwanted by at least one parent. Measures are available to prevent this.

The methods of preventing births are: abstinence from sexual activity, utilization of effective contraception methods, abortion, and sterilization.

CONTRACEPTION

The most acceptable and the most effective measure to prevent unwanted pregnancies is contraception. Contraceptive measures currently available are effective but not ideal. (See page 332.) They require intelligence, strong motivation, and dedication. Research into better methods of contraception is essential. Some projects currently being investigated include a pill to take after intercourse, an injection that will prevent conception for a far longer time than "the pill," and better pills to replace the ones currently in use. Such measures are needed for both the literate and the illiterate millions in the world.

ABORTION

Abortion, used since earliest times to prevent the birth of unwanted children, is also an effective method of population control.

In Japan after World War II, the increase in birth rates caused a great increase in population. Recognizing this trend as a serious threat to Japan's survival as a nation, the Japanese, through education, legislation, contraception, and legalized abortion successfully reduced the rate of population growth and brought it into line with the capacity of the economy. This has contributed greatly to the rising industrial and commercial development and the mounting standard of living which have made Japan the most prosperous nation in the East.

An abortion performed by a qualified physician or osteopath under proper conditions carries very little risk to life or to health (though still a greater risk than the pill). On the other hand, the vast majority of illegal abortions are performed by medically unqualified persons under poor conditions and involve hazards to future fertility, to health, and even to life. It is estimated that each year in this country there are 1 million illegal abortions, and that 1,000 women die and 350,000 are admitted to hospitals because of complications from such abortions. That so many women are willing to take such a well-recognized risk to health and to life indicates how desperately they need to avoid bearing unwanted children.

Over the period of 15 years before legalization of abortion in New York State, more than 90 percent of the therapeutic abortions performed in hospitals in New York City were on white women in private rooms. The upper- and middle-income-class women who had these abortions are also the ones who could afford to go to other countries, such as Japan, Sweden, Poland, Hungary, and England, where abortions by licensed physicians in good hospitals are legal. The result is that the abortion laws in this country which permit abortions only to save the life of the mother discriminate against the poor, the socially disadvantaged, and the socially oppressed—the group least able to afford more children.

In 1970 the New York State Legislature replaced its century-old law, which permitted abortions only to save the life of the mother, with the most liberal abortion law in the United States. This law legalized abortions during the first 24 weeks of pregnancy on the grounds that women have a right to bear children only when they are willing to do so. The new law makes the question whether an abortion should be performed a matter of decision between the woman and her physician. Abortions may be performed only by licensed physicians or osteopaths under conditions and in facilities approved by the department of public health.

During the first year of this law almost 165,000 legal abortions were performed in New York City and about 40,000 in the rest of the state. About half the patients in New York City and a quarter in the rest of the state were nonresidents. About half were from the so-called underprivileged social and economic portion of the population. Most of the latter group were residents of New York City.

During the seventh and eighth months of the law 77 percent of the operations were performed during the first 3 months of pregnancy as compared to 69 percent during the first and second months of the law. These figures indicate a trend toward termination of pregnancy during the early months when the risk and the attendant disability are minimal. Clearly, early abortions are safer than late ones. Complications occured in only 6.3 per 100 abortions performed during the first 3 months of pregnancy, but in 30.6 per 100 for later abortions.

Hospital records indicate that the mortality rate in New York City for abortions during the first year was 8 per 100,000 legal abortions. This is less than half the fatality rate of women who give birth to live babies in the United States. It also is much lower than the 17 deaths per 100,000 abortions in Britain and 40 per 100,000 in Scandanavia, during the first years of their permissive abortion laws. Hospital records indicate also that the number of patients admitted to municipal hospitals for the treatment of complications of illegal abortions during this period was only about half the number admitted during a corresponding period a year before. The primary purposes of liberalized abortion laws are to permit women to make their own decisions concerning childbearing, and to prevent tragic physical and mental suffering and economic and social disaster for countless women, families, and unwanted children.

Opponents of these laws frequently speak of them as "abortion on demand." This is misleading. No woman can obtain an abortion by demanding it. She can request a physician or a clinic to perform an abortion; and if her reasons justify an abortion, it will be performed. However, physicians or clinics or hospital groups are not required to perform abortions if for medical or other reasons they are unwilling to do so. And no ethical physician will perform an abortion or other surgical procedure unless he considers it in the best interest of his patient.

The states of Colorado, Maryland, California, Hawaii, and Washington (by referendum) also have liberalized their abortion laws, and many other states are considering similar action. (See also page 397.) In the first 12 months after liberalization of the Maryland abortion law, the John Hopkins University Hospital in Baltimore performed more than 1,100 abortions. Although court decisions and legislative acts permitting abortion are not made for the purpose of controlling population, they are nevertheless effective in so doing.

STERILIZATION
Another effective method of population control is the sterilization of persons, men or women, who do not want additional children. (See Chapter 22.)

The operations to accomplish this are very simple, for both men and women. For men it is frequently performed in a clinic or doctor's office. For women the facilities of a hospital are necessary, but only a few days of hospital care are required. This is a safe, medically accepted method of terminating fertility. Sterilization does not interfere with sexual potency or activity in either men or women. In fact, with the possibility of pregnancy removed, sexual response is frequently increased.

Because of their safety, effectiveness, acceptability, and low cost—nothing beyond the initial operation—sterilization programs are being vigorously promoted in many countries. Voluntary sterilization is legal in all states, although Utah limits its use to "medical necessity." Authorities estimate that several million Americans have been voluntarily sterilized. The Department of Defense has approved voluntary sterilization in military hospitals, and all but one of the states operating Medicaid programs pay for voluntary sterilization under this program.

BIRTH CONTROL AS NATIONAL POLICY
In China birth control is state policy, with contraceptive pills and intrauterine devices provided by the state. Government programs of family planning have been adopted by several overpopulated countries of Asia: Japan, India, Pakistan, Singapore, Korea, and the Philippines. Population control in these countries is a question not of religion or politics but simply of human welfare.

Similar efforts in Latin America and in other parts of the world are encouraging, but they are mere beginnings. (See Figure 3.3.) To meet this ominous threat to the future of the world, individual governments and the United Nations must establish and implement policies designed to limit population growth the world over in order that human beings everywhere may develop their highest capacities and may enjoy individual freedom, health, privacy, security, and the beauty and wonder of the world.[2]

Unfortunately, at the present time no methods of birth control exist which are simple enough, cheap enough, and effective enough to meet the desperate need in the less-developed countries. The development of such methods should be given top research priority.

[2] After A Statement of Conviction about Overpopulation, signed by distinguished citizens of seventeen countries, including thirty-four Nobel Laureates.

URBANIZATION

The tremendous and continuing migration from rural communities to cities the world over is giving rise to increasingly serious health and social problems. A report by the recently organized metropolitan group of the World Health Organization lists Paris as the most overcrowded city, with Tokyo, New York, London, and Berlin following in that order. This group predicts that, with the continued mechanization of agriculture, by the end of this century only 10 percent of the world's people will be working on farms. In the United States in 1900, the total population was 90 million, most of them in rural areas; in 1950, 97 million lived in urban areas, and in 1970, the figure was more than 125 million. (Figure 3-4.)

The health implications of living in overcrowded communities are many. Inadequate and polluted water supplies, unhygienic and inadequate housing, polluted air, and nerve-wracking noise are some of the conditions that contribute to a general degradation of man's physical and social environment.

Dr. Desmond Morris, curator of mammals for the Zoological Society of London, says:

Under normal conditions, in their normal habitats, wild animals do not mutilate themselves, mastur-bate, attack their offspring, develop stomach ulcers, suffer from obesity, form homosexual pair bonds, or commit murder. But in zoos, as in urbanized human society, all these things occur. . . . The modern human animal is no longer living under conditions natural for his species. Trapped by his own brainy brilliance he has set himself up in a huge, restless menagerie where he is in constant danger of cracking.[3]

What effect crowded living conditions may have on increases in acts of violence, in mental illness, and in certain diseases is not known; but the effects of abnormal living situations on human beings need to be given serious consideration in connection with increasing urbanization.

HOUSING

Poor health and poor housing (Figure 3.5) cannot fail to be associated in the mind of any physician, nurse, or social worker who has been called upon to see patients in the slums or blighted areas of our cities. Associated with poor housing are other factors and conditions prejudicial to health:

[3]Desmond Morris, *The Human Zoo*, McGraw-Hill Book Company, New York, 1971.

Figure 3.4   Increasing urbanization in the United States.

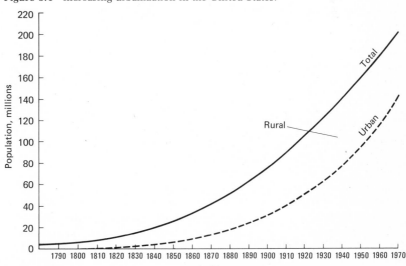

poverty, overcrowding, and ignorance about nutrition, hygiene, sanitation, and other basic principles of personal health. The communicable diseases of childhood, as well as tuberculosis and pneumonia, are more prevalent in crowded than in uncrowded houses. Accident rates are consistently higher in old, dilapidated houses than in newer, well-maintained ones.

NOISE

Contributing to nervous disorders, insomnia, nervous tension, ill temper, and accidents, noise has become a serious problem in most urban communities. Automobiles, trucks, buses, motorcycles, airplanes, and certain industries are producing noise of increasing intensity and universality. Functions of the body affected by noise are those of the nervous system, particularly disturbing sleep and producing tension and fatigue, and of the cardiovascular system, with constriction of the blood vessels and increases in pulse rate and blood pressure. Much more research is needed concerning these and other effects of noise upon the functioning of the body.

Impairment of hearing is the most obvious physiological damage caused by noise. Many studies have shown that prolonged exposure to intense noise produces permanent hearing loss. A

Figure 3.5   Poor housing in a rural area of the South. (U.S. Department of Agriculture.)

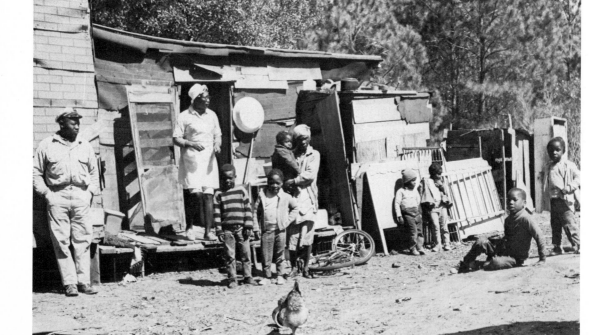

government report estimates that the number of United States workers experiencing conditions unsafe to hearing is in excess of 6 million and may be as high as 16 million. The report also says that the overall loudness of environmental noise is doubling every 10 years and that man can no longer escape from it, even in the privacy of his vacation retreats. Generally speaking, the government report said, traffic noise from automobiles, buses, motor-cycles, and trucks, particularly trailer trucks, on freeways and expressways and in downtown areas, and air traffic in the vicinity of airports disturb more people than other sources of outdoor noise. Noise levels in dwellings, particulary in kitchen areas, are beginning to approach those of factories, the report said. And modern building design and construction materials were criticized for not protecting against inside and outside noise.

WATER SUPPLIES

For centuries epidemics of waterborne diseases—cholera, typhoid fever, and dysentery—were common occurrences. Then came the discovery and identification of the bacterial causes of these diseases and the engineering developments to remove them from water supplies.

The World Health Organization estimates that 200 million urban dwellers in the world lack adequate safe drinking water and that 300 million will soon be in this predicament unless greater preventive efforts are made. With increased urbanization and industrialization, demands upon water supplies will substantially increase. Add to this the needs of a 50 percent increase in population, and the result may well be a chronic water shortage that it will be difficult to remedy at any price. There will also be the continuing problem of providing water supplies that are safe for drinking purposes.

For public health purposes water supplies may be divided into two general groups: surface and underground. Surface water supplies are obtained from lakes and streams and are not considered safe for drinking unless purified. Underground water supplies are obtained from wells and springs. Such supplies are practically always safe, provided they are properly located, properly constructed, and properly operated.

The water supplies of large communities are usually obtained from lakes and streams. Unless such surface water supplies are grossly polluted, they may be rendered safe for drinking purposes by adequate treatment. (See Figure 3.6.) However, the massive contamination of rivers and lakes that in the past have been considered sources of limitless supplies of water for human use and recreation is raising a new and serious problem. For example, the water of the Hudson River as it flows past New York is contaminated by more than half a billion gallons of raw sewage daily from cities and towns along the course of the river. And into Lake Erie the states of Pennsylvania, New York, Ohio, Indiana, and Michigan are reported to dump each day 1.5 billion gallons of sewage and 9.6 billion gallons of industrial wastes. Most other major lakes and rivers are in similar situations; edible fish are rapidly disappearing from their waters, and shellfish, such as oysters, clams, and shrimp, taken from them or from the bays or oceans into which they empty, are likely to be contaminated.

At least twice as much industrial waste (in volume) as sewage is dumped into the nation's waters. Some of these wastes are chemicals known to be toxic either directly or through the fish taken from contaminated waters. Furthermore, some of the chemicals exert delayed toxic effects.

When contaminated waters are supplied for human use, special treatment is required. Research concerning toxic materials that cannot be removed by present treatment methods must be continued.

In the usual method of purification of surface water supplies, water is taken from the source of supply, and a small amount of aluminum sulfate (commonly called *alum*) is added. This, when thoroughly mixed with the water, reacts with some of its chemical constituents, producing a slightly gelatinous precipitate known as *floc*. The precipitate envelops the suspended material and carries it to the bottom of the sedimentation basin. From this basin the water passes on to filters, which usually consist of approximately 3 feet of sand, gravel, and crushed rock, with the fine sand

Figure 3.6 Typical water-purification system.

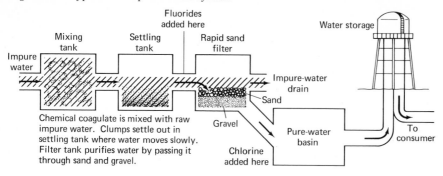

Fluorides added here

Water storage

Mixing tank

Settling tank

Rapid sand filter

Impure water

Impure-water drain

Sand

Chemical coagulate is mixed with raw impure water. Clumps settle out in settling tank where water moves slowly. Filter tank purifies water by passing it through sand and gravel.

Gravel

Chlorine added here

Pure-water basin

To consumer

on the surface and the gravel and crushed rock at the bottom. The treatment up to this point removes the suspended material and a large part of the color from the water and materially reduces its bacterial content. As the water leaves the filter, chlorine, usually in the form of gas, is added to destroy any bacteria that may have passed through the filter. If the source of the water supply is badly contaminated, chlorine is used before as well as after filtration. Water filtration does not remove some toxic chemicals, such as mercury and DDT that may have contaminated the water supply.

Treatment of community water supplies has practically eliminated waterborne diseases in the Western world. However, occasional serious waterborne outbreaks of typhoid fever, dysentery, salmonella infection, and infectious hepatitis in recent years are evidence that the safety of water supplies needs constant attention.

In fact, in 1969 the Bureau of Water Hygiene of the U.S. Public Health Service surveyed approximately 1,000 community water supply systems and reported that many systems are delivering water of marginal quality and that some are delivering water of poor quality in one or more areas of their distribution system. Furthermore, many systems, particularly the smaller ones, do not have adequate surveillance to assure their efficient operation. Many of these systems were constructed 50 or more years ago and are operating beyond the capacities for which they were planned.

The increase in pollution of the sources of many public water supplies and the greater need for water by our increasing population and by an expanding industry are creating potentially dangerous situations that demand more public concern than they are receiving.

Even underground water supplies, from dug, bored, driven, or drilled wells and from springs, may be contaminated. If wells are located in limestone subsoil, they may be polluted by seepage from cesspools or privies located nearby or even at a considerable distance. In most soil, however, it is possible with care to construct wells that will not be polluted. For safety, all water supplies should be inspected periodically by appropriate authorities.

Water from unknown or questionable sources, such as the camper or traveler must use, can be rendered safe for drinking purposes by boiling it for a few minutes or by treatment with water-disinfecting tablets which are available at many drugstores. The boiling of water, however, drives off dissolved air and gases, with the result that the water has a flat taste. Shaking the water in a bottle or stirring it with an egg beater will correct this. Boiled water should be kept in covered pails or well-stopped bottles. If ice is used to cool the water, it should be placed around the container, not in it, unless the source of the ice is known to be free of contamination.

Travelers to tropical countries should not depend on chlorine for the disinfection of drinking water, since small amounts of chlorine will not destroy the cysts of amebic dysentery, but should either boil their drinking water or treat it. For the purification of small quantities of drinking water the army is now using iodine tablets, each of which gives 8 parts per million of iodine when added to a canteen or bottle containing approximately a quart of water.

FOOD HAZARDS

The foods which constitute the chief potential hazards to health, and the infections and food poisonings which may result from them, are discussed in Chapter 12. Against most of these hazards the individual must provide his own protection rather than relying on society. There is, of course, federal control of food products sold in interstate commerce or for export. The prompt removal of cyclamates from the market and from food products, when it was shown that these chemicals could cause cancer in certain laboratory animals, is an example of protective measures applied by the federal government.

Mercury is another highly toxic chemical which in recent years has been shown to be so widely disseminated in the environment as to be a hazard to animals, including many birds and fish. Late in 1970 an order from the U.S. Food and Drug Administration withdrew more than a million cans of tuna from the American market because of a dangerous level of mercury in certain shipments. In 1971 when a large percentage of swordfish were found to contain high mercury levels, the Food and Drug Administration advised people not to eat swordfish. Mercury gets into water primarily from insecticides and from industries which use mercury in certain manufacturing processes, particularly of chemicals, plastics, and paper. Intensive studies of this potentially serious hazard are now in progress.[4]

[4]See Peter Montague and Katherine Montague, "Mercury: How Much Are We Eating?" *Saturday Review*, Feb. 6, 1971, p. 50.

Some protection of food supplies is provided by the inspection of meats by the Bureau of Animal Industry of the U.S. Department of Agriculture. Such inspection, however, applies only to meat which is butchered and sold by companies that do an interstate business. Some states and a few cities have their own meat inspection laws; but these are not general, nor are they usually effective.

The licensing of restaurants and hotels by state or local departments of health gives considerable health protection to the public if adequate standards of sanitation are required and efficient inspection and law enforcement are provided. The same holds true for manufacturing plants and stores, wholesale and retail, which process or sell foods.

MILK

Milk and milk products constitute a special situation because they are commodities which are so susceptible to contamination and adulteration that the only way to obtain protection against fraud and against the diseases which may be transmitted through milk is by community action. The first step in achieving such protection is education, followed by the passage of a satisfactory milk ordinance. The next step is to make sure that this ordinance is enforced. That milk should be clean and safe from disease is the aim of programs for milk sanitation. Pasteurization—heating milk to destroy disease-producing bacteria—does not impair its nutritional value.

DISPOSAL OF WASTES

The disposal of human waste material is an age-old problem. It was of concern in ancient days and is still important. Human excreta are not necessarily dangerous. However, since disease-producing organisms in some excretory products are a menace to health, all excreta must be disposed of properly.

A distinction should be made between the terms *sewage* and *sewerage*. *Sewage* is made up of liquid wastes from buildings to which ground and surface water entering the sewers is added. It is a more or less homogeneous suspension of material

with both mineral and organic matter in solution. The liquid waste from business buildings, industrial concerns, and residences is known as *domestic sewage*. It consists of wash water, water from kitchens, and human waste materials and is about 99.9 percent water. The term *sewerage* refers to the system provided for the collection of sewage.

Sewerage systems collect domestic and industrial wastes and carry them to a sewage-treatment plant or directly to a point of discharge. Usually the discharge is into a river or large lake, but rarely is there sufficient dilution to permit this without serious objection. In most situations, therefore, sewage treatment is necessary. Such treatment may be no more than a settling process which removes the solids from the sewage and permits the liquid part to drain off into a lake or river. On the other hand, the sewage treatment may be so complete that the end product is neither objectionable nor dangerous to health. Complete sewage treatment involves first a settling process, then oxidation, filtration, and finally chlorination of the liquid effluent.

Unfortunately many sewage-treatment plants, although well designed and constructed, are no longer adequate to meet the needs of the increasing population. To remedy this will require large expenditures of funds—federal, state, and local— and these will have to be provided in the immediate future to prevent potentially catastrophic pollution of water supplies.

The current widespread use of detergents is giving rise to a new problem. Detergents contain a chemical, phosphoric oxide, that is not removed by sewage treatment but which provides food for and stimulates growth of a weed of the plankton family. In rivers and lakes that are contaminated with sewage the growth of this weed smothers other forms of life and creates odoriferous, unsightly, and otherwise objectionable conditions. So extensive and alarming has this problem become in many areas that legislation has been proposed in a number of states to ban the use of all phosphate detergents. The U.S. Public Health Service, however, is questioning the prohibition of phosphate detergents because of the possibility that the proposed substitutes may be more dangerous to human health.

In the absence of sewerage systems, other methods of disposal, such as those listed below, can be utilized.

CHEMICAL TOILETS

In the absence of running water, chemical toilets may be used inside the house. They consist of a jar or an iron tank. The excreta are received into a strong solution of caustic soda which liquefies and disinfects the material. Tanks which permit several months' storage may be emptied by drainage or some other way, as into a scavenger wagon. These toilets, which are nearly free from odor, are sold by many manufacturers. In homes they can be used as a temporary expedient until a water-carriage system can be installed.

PRIVIES

A sanitary privy requires a pit of proper depth and capacity; a tight building so constructed as to protect the excreta from flies, chickens, domestic animals, rats, etc.; a floor above the ground level; a tight door that closes automatically; seat covers that close when not in use; and durable screens over all openings for ventilation. The provision of such elementary conditions of sanitation and decency would seem simple enough, but the primitive conditions of waste disposal which still exist in certain areas throughout this country are almost unbelievable.

CESSPOOLS

Cesspools are deep holes in the ground to receive drainage or sewage from sinks, toilets, etc. Although cesspools have been widely used in rural areas, they are not recommended by health authorities. If located in limestone they are sources of danger because sewage may travel through crevices in the limestone for a considerable distance. Also, cesspools may clog up and overflow, and may contaminate water supplies.

SEPTIC TANKS

Where sewers are not available, septic tanks are quite often used for sewage disposal from residences or other buildings where running water is available. The purpose of a septic tank is to receive household wastes. The solid particles settle to the bottom of the tank and form a semiliquid called *sludge*. Some particles form "floating scum" on the surface of the liquid. The solids thus retained are digested by the action of bacteria so that the volume of the solids is reduced. Some of the solids are converted by the digestion process to liquids and gases that pass off with the tank overflow, which is called the *effluent*. That solids are retained in the septic tank makes it necessary for the tank to have a removable cover to afford access for cleaning. A distribution box receives the effluent; and from it the liquid material enters the subsurface disposal field, which is also known as the *absorption field*. Sometimes one hears such statements as "The liquid as it flows from a septic tank is pure." That is not true. Bacteria in the soil are important in removing impurities from the effluent.

The maintenance of a septic tank is important. It should be inspected at least once a year. Where a household garbage grinder is used, the cleaning must be more frequent unless the tank is large enough for the extra material. The removed solids should be buried or disposed of in ways approved by the local health department.[5]

Connection to an adequate public sewerage system is the most satisfactory way of disposing of sewage. But sometimes it is necessary to construct individual sewage-disposal systems. Before a person has such a sewage-disposal system constructed, he should seek advice from the local health authorities in the area, because state and local health departments may have developed requirements which must be met. Septic tanks and subsurface tile filter systems are often advised as means of treating and disposing of sewage in rural situations. Proper location, design, and maintenance of such facilities are essential considerations for the protection of private water supplies and the elimination of nuisance conditions.[6]

GARBAGE
The disposal of animal and vegetable wastes, commonly called *garbage*, is accepted as one of the responsibilities of a community. The odors from fermenting garbage is objectionable, and garbage may serve as a breeding place for flies and a feeding place for rats and other vermin.

Garbage disposal is usually accomplished by collecting the garbage and then disposing of it by incineration, by hog feeding, by utilizing the material for a "sanitary land fill," or by dumping at

[5]See *Septic Tank Care*, U.S. Public Health Service Publication 73.
[6]See *Manual of Septic-tank Practice*, U.S. Public Health Service Publication 526.

sea. Other methods include using a reduction process, from which revenue may be obtained by the sale of grease and tankage.

Individual citizens may use garbage grinders which discharge into a sewer. This is a convenient and practical way of disposing of garbage. However, communities must provide sufficient sewage-treatment plants if garbage grinding is widespread.

Outbreaks of a serious disease of hogs have focused attention on the dangers of feeding uncooked garbage to hogs. This has led to requirements in all fifty states that garbage be cooked before being fed to hogs. A by-product of this should be the reduction or elimination of human trichinosis.

SOIL AND DISEASE
Soil may be related to poor health because it lacks some essential elements, such as iodine or fluorides, or because it contains disease-producing bacteria or parasites. Decomposition of animal and vegetable matter in fertile soil is the result of bacterial action, but these organisms are harmless to man. The ones which produce disease reach the soil with the intestinal discharges of man or animals.

Most of these organisms produce bacterial diseases of the intestinal tract, such as typhoid fever or dysentery, or intestinal parasitic infections. Except for hookworm, the larvae of which most commonly enter the body through the skin, man can become infected from the soil with these diseases only through contamination of his food or drink. If human excreta are used for fertilizer, as is the custom in the Orient and certain sections of the tropics, contamination of vegetables is likely. The germs of tetanus and gas gangrene are found in soil which contains animal excreta. They produce disease only when they enter the body through wounds. Otherwise, the danger of contracting disease from the soil is slight.

AIR POLLUTION

The envelope of air surrounding the earth, upon which all life depends, is only a few miles thick. Furthermore, this thin covering of air is apparently unique in the solar system. Without it our earth

would be like the barren mountains of the moon or the polar regions of Mars.

Oxygen, the essential ingredient of air, is not replaceable from any source other than the earth itself. Photosynthesis in the leaves of plants takes from the air the carbon dioxide that is formed in animal bodies and from other sources and converts it into oxygen for animal use. If the oxygen supply is exhausted or so heavily polluted as to be damaging to health, a deterioriation in the quality of life and eventually an end to life will result.

At the present time, however, under all but extreme circumstances, the greatest atmospheric hazard to health comes not from variations in oxygen, heat, or humidity but from air pollution. Under such varied terms as *fog, smog, smaze, haze,* and *fallout,* gross pollution of the outside air by smoke, dust, and gases exists in almost all urban and suburban communities. In many cities, including New York and Chicago, 50 to 100 tons of dirt fall on each square mile in most months. Even that dramatic figure does not tell the whole story, for there are many harmful chemicals which never reach the ground to be measured by weight.

There are at least two major types of urban air pollution. In one, best exemplified in London, heavy smoke plus cold, damp weather with frequent natural fog combine to produce a smog which has water droplets, dirt, and sulfur dioxide as its main ingredients. In the other, best known for its occurrence in Los Angeles, sunlight acts on automotive exhaust products to produce a photochemical fog. In many cities, including New York, these two types are usually combined when smog occurs.

In a few dramatic instances the damage to human beings from air pollution has been overwhelming: 63 dead in the Meuse Valley of France in 1930; 2,000 ill and 12 dead in Donora, Pennsylvania, in 1948; the heaviest toll, 4,000 dead, in London due to a series of fogs in December 1952. According to studies made in London and in New York in 1953, such deaths occur mostly in the very young and the old, and in those with some preceding disease of heart or lungs.

Attacks of smog occur readily when a peculiar atmospheric condition known as *inversion* is present. Cool air with much moisture is "trapped" under a layer of warm air; the cool air retains the industrial, automobile, and other wastes spewed into the atmosphere. Inversion is a frequent phenomenon when surrounding hills hamper the movement of air, as in Los Angeles.

The air we breathe has been polluted increasingly by smoke, soot, chemicals, and the fumes from the combustion of gasoline and fuel oil. There is evidence that these air pollutants contain substances known to be carcinogenic, i.e., cancer-producing. Air pollution therefore has been suspected as a cause of lung cancer and also as a cause of chronic bronchitis and emphysema, the chronic lung disease in which dilated and destroyed air sacs in the lungs make the victim shorter and shorter of breath. (See page 284.)

An investigation of the effects of air pollution upon health in Buffalo, New York, involved 77,800 men, 50 to 70 years of age, about half of whom lived in areas of the city with a high degree of air pollution, while the others lived in areas of low pollution. The results showed that the overall death rate was nearly one-third higher in areas of heavy pollution and that deaths from bronchitis and emphysema were three times as high. There was no difference in deaths from lung cancer, and the conclusion was that, if air pollution is related to lung cancer, its effect is so small that it is obscured by cigarette smoking. (See Figure 3.7.)

In addition to containing substances that irritate and destroy tissues of the respiratory tract, both cigarette smoking and direct inhalation of automobile exhaust fumes cause an accumulation of carbon monoxide in the blood. (See page 93.) A survey in July 1966 of air pollution in Newark, New Jersey, showed that the carbon monoxide in the atmosphere ranged from 3.8 parts per million to 23.4 parts per million, a level sufficient to inactivate 2 percent of a person's hemoglobin as carboxyhemoglobin (see page 372), thereby significantly reducing the capacity of the blood to transport oxygen.

Nitrogen dioxide, NO_2, was identified some years ago as the toxic agent in "silo-fillers disease." (See page 373.) More recently it has been shown to be a major component of smog. The source of this is the colorless nitrous oxide which reacts with oxygen in the air to form yellow-brown nitrogen dioxide, a gas which in appropriate concentration reduces visibility, is toxic to plants and animals, and reacts with hydrocarbons in photochemical smog to form ozone. The inhalation of high concentration of NO_2 has been shown to produce serious lung damage. The damage caused by the inhalation of low concentrations of photochemical smog over long periods of time has not been clearly demonstrated, but alert physicians in areas of air pollution are convinced that chronic exposure to smog is deleterious to pulmonary functions and that efforts to reduce air pollution are in the interest of health.[7]

A study in New York City reported in 1970 by Cornell Medical College and the City Health Department showed that air pollution and high temperature are associated with increased death rates, particularly in persons over 65.

Smoke and soot, called *particulate matter*, from power plants, incinerators, and industries are visible types of air pollution and are therefore the ones people are most concerned about. Their effects upon health, however, are not nearly so great as those of the invisible gases. Visible particulate matter can be rendered invisible by passing the smoke through a hot flame or by diluting the smoke with a large amount of air. Unfortunately, the flame aggravates the air-pollution problem by oxidizing nitrogen, thus adding nitrogen oxide to the air.

Although human illness is the most serious consequence of air pollution, the dollar costs of pollution are also substantial. It has been estimated that if the total cost of air pollution were divided equally, each citizen of the United States would have a loss of between $10 and $30 each year. Obviously, however, the damage to house paint, house funishings, exposed metals, and even stone and brickwork is greater in some areas than in others. The motto of the Department of Air Pollution Control of the City of New York reads, "Clean air costs money, dirty air costs more."

It is estimated that 60 percent of the air pollution in this country, and 80 percent in urban areas, is caused by motor cars; it is also estimated that the 90 million private automobiles exhaust 90 million tons of waste products into the atmosphere each year—three times as much as any other source.

The rapid increase in the number of both automobiles and industrial plants contaminating the atmosphere is so great that some experts feel that the control measures now available will be insufficient to bring real reduction in the amount of this contamination. Fundamental changes in our modes of transportation and manufacture will be

[7]"Nitrogen Dioxide: The New Yellow Peril," Editorial, *Journal of the American Medical Association*, vol. 212, no. 8, p. 1368, May 25, 1970.

Figure 3.7 Air pollution and lung cancer; death rates in urban and rural areas: nonsmokers and cigarette smokers. Source: Hammond and Horn, *Journal of the American Medical Association*, vol. 166, pp. 1159, 1295, 1958.

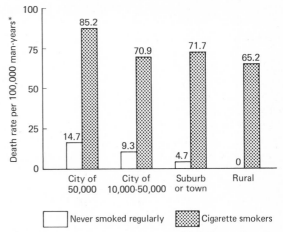

*Man years = number of men observed, multiplied by number of years over which the observations were made

needed: a more efficient internal-combustion engine (perhaps a turbine engine), substitution of electric motors in automobiles, much greater construction and use of public transportation (subways and electric trains in particular), and the use of sources of heat and energy other than coal and oil.

With the increasing population and the expansion of industry, the control of air pollution, particularly in urban areas, demands strong community action. The President's Science Advisory Committee stated: "There should be no right to pollute the public air. . . . The pressure to pollute has been an economic one; the pressure to abate in the future must be an economic one." In Palm Beach Shores, Florida, polluters are charged $20 a ton for the "junk they dump into the sky." The Science Advisory Committee recommended similar legislation on a national basis.

Federal, state, and city governments are finally taking cognizance of this problem and are initiating programs to control it. The Clean Air Amendments Act of 1970, passed overwhelmingly by both houses of Congress, greatly strengthens federal controls over air pollution and, if implemented properly, has the potential of reversing the steady deterioration of air quality. Among other provisions, the act orders automobile manufacturers to produce nearly pollutionfree cars by 1976, authorizes national air-quality standards, and sets up a $1.1 billion government research program.

Also in 1970 President Nixon's reorganization of the executive branch of the government established the Environmental Protection Agency as the major federal agency responsible for administration and enforcement of environmental legislation.

PESTICIDES—BIOLOGICAL BUILDUP

The chemical DDT (dichloro-diphenyl-trichloroethane) was developed by a Swiss chemist, Dr. Paul Mueller, during World War II. It proved dramatically effective in controlling epidemics of typhus fever, transmitted by the body louse, and of malaria, transmitted by the anopheles mosquito. In 1948 Dr. Mueller was awarded a Nobel Prize in chemistry for his work.

DDT is much more effective and much less toxic than earlier insecticides that contained arsenic or nicotine. Unfortunately, over a period of years its residues have proved to be toxic not only to insects but to other forms of animal, bird, and fish life. Much of this effect is indirect and difficult to detect. For example, if trees are sprayed with DDT to destroy insects, residues remain on the leaves which fall to the ground and are eaten by earthworms. Birds may eat the worms and build up poisonous amounts of the chemical in their bodies. Or the residues on the leaves may be washed by rains into streams and other bodies of water where they are eaten by fish. Man may ingest the toxic residues with various foods. DDT and related pesticides, some of them more toxic than DDT, are so widespread in the environment that it is impossible to avoid them. Even some mothers' milk has been found to contain several times the amount of DDT that is considered safe in cows' milk by the Food and Drug Administration.

Some countries, including Russia, have banned this insecticide. The U.S. Department of Agriculture proposed limitations on its use, but court actions have prevented their enforcement. The use of DDT is decreasing, but an order by the U.S. Public Health Service to phase out DDT is being challenged. Meanwhile related toxic chemicals, such as dieldrin and endrin, are being produced in increasing amounts.

DDT is exceedingly valuable in the control of certain widespread and serious diseases in many areas of the world, notably typhus fever and malaria. (See pages 254 and 256.) Its most important use in the control of these diseases, however, is for the spraying of clothing (Figure 3.8) and of the interior of buildings to destroy body lice and mosquitoes. Such use, says the 1971 report of the World Health Organization, presents no

significant risk to man or to wild life and withdrawal of DDT from malaria programs would be unjustifiable in the light of present knowledge. At the same time it is recognized that the outdoor use of DDT in public health programs should be avoided as far as possible. Pesticides are important in agriculture also. Current United Nations Food and Agriculture Organization (FAO) programs for increased food production in many parts of the world are dependent to a large extent on the use of pesticides. Collaboration between FAO and WHO is helping to ensure that this will result in no hazard to man or his domestic animals, and the association between the two organizations should be further enhanced as the "green revolution" develops. . . .

A scientific paper published in 1968 reported that DDT slows down the life processes of microscopic marine plants—the most numerous food and oxygen producers on our planet. "To scientists," reports Dr. Paul Ehrlich, the eminent Stanford University biologist, "the announcement smacked of doomsday."

Amounts of DDT in seawater are even greater today than they were in 1968, and DDT can be found in the bodies of virtually every marine animal, even penguins in Antarctica and starfish on the ocean floor, hundreds of miles from the nearest inhabited land. The brown pelican, which is the state bird of Louisiana, and the Bermuda petrel appear headed for extinction because their eggshells are weakened by the DDT that females absorb from the sea. Ospreys have been drastically reduced in

Figure 3.8 DDT dusting teams in a campaign against typhus. (United Nations.)

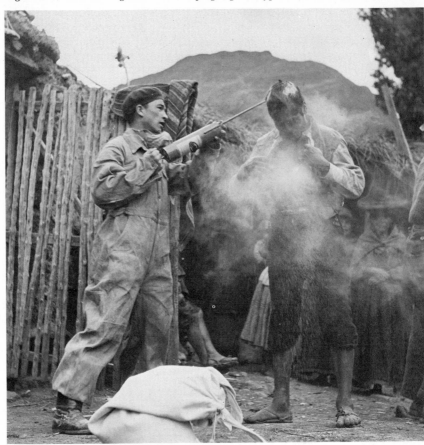

number. Much more research, regulation, and enforcement concerning these ubiquitous toxic chemicals are essential to protect us from serious, long-time ill effects.

The widely used weed killers (herbicides) have been considered harmless to man if used as directed. However, the herbicide 2,4,5T, which has been used as a defoliant in Vietnam, has been found to cause birth defects in animals, and may be a hazard to pregnant women.

LEAD POISONING

Although lead poisoning had been virtually eliminated as an occupational hazard, it is occurring with increasing and alarming frequency among children. A recent report estimates that 112,000 children each year in this country suffer from lead poisoning. Of reported cases 20 to 30 percent die and an even larger number suffer serious and permanent brain damage: mental retardation, cerebral palsy, recurrent seizures, etc. Most victims are children under 6, and 85 percent of the cases are children between 1 and 3 years of age.

Paints containing lead are no longer on the market in the United States; however, older buildings frequently have lead paint exposed. The poisoning occurs when children eat chips of such paint from walls and woodwork in old, dilapidated housing. "High-risk" areas are almost synonymous with the slums, but the risk is by no means limited to such areas. (See also page 371.)

A more generalized source of exposure to lead that is beginning to cause concern is the lead in the atmosphere of cities due to the use of gasolines containing lead. This is one of the types of contamination of the environment that is under scientific scrutiny.

RADIATION HAZARDS

Health hazards can arise from the careless or unintelligent handling of radioactive materials, through external irradiation or ingestion and inhalation of radioactive isotopes. Control measures of the Atomic Energy Commission and local radiological health programs have provided this industry with an enviable safety record.

The nuclear age was ushered in with the discovery and isolation of radium from pitchblende in 1898 by Marie Sklodowska Curie and Pierre Curie. The first sustained chain reaction at the University of Chicago in 1941 was the signal for the beginning of a new industry which may well modify our way of life. However, this development has created potential health problems by introducing a somewhat new facet to the environment: the hazards of exposure to ionizing radiation.

Today nuclear reactors propel submarines, as well as surface craft, and provide economically competitive electric power. Radioactive isotopes are being used extensively in medical diagnosis and therapy. They serve as an invaluable research tool in a broad variety of projects.

The centering of attention on radiation hazards, associated with the "atomic age," has led to studies also of the use of x-rays for diagnosis and treatment. These studies show that certain leukemias, cancers of the thyroid and the central nervous system, and other diseases and abnormalities are related to the use of x-rays. The risk is particularly great for an unborn child exposed to radiation. A Harvard School of Public Health study of 450,000 infants showed an incidence of cancer of up to 30 percent following prenatal irradiation. Some Japanese children exposed before birth to atomic bomb radiation were born with abnormally small heads and mental defects. Elsewhere prenatal exposure to x-rays has been blamed for similar anomalies.

Today x-ray procedures that have produced clearly documented harmful effects are either no longer used or are used only when the risk of not using them is greater than the risk of giving them. Current medical opinion is that unnecessary exposure to x-rays should be avoided, that such practices as the use of fluoroscopes by shoe salesmen should be eliminated, and that x-rays and other types of radiation should be utilized only by physicians trained and experienced in their use. However, under the proper conditions, there is no reason to forego the use of x-rays when indicated for medical diagnosis or treatment.

The effects of exposure of an entire population to radioactive pollution of the environment is a different problem. This major health hazard is the one that is least easy to document: that is, the long-term degeneration of human genes. In "Report to the Public" the National Academy of Sciences makes these points:

> Of all the biological systems, the inheritance mechanism is by far the most sensitive to radiation.

> Any radiation that reaches the reproductive cells causes mutations that are passed on to succeeding generations.

> Human gene mutations that produce observable effect are believed to be generally harmful.

> Even the smallest amount of radiation increases the number of mutations in a large group.

> The harm is cumulative and depends on the total gonad dose received by people from their own conceptions to the conceptions of their last children—that is, the dose to the testes and the ovaries.

The possibility of exposure to tiny doses of environmental radiation, as well as the possibility of catastrophic accidents, is responsible for the increasing fear concerning the construction of atomic powered electric plants around the country. Currently there are only twenty-three nuclear power plants in operation, and these produce only about 2 percent of the nation's electricity supply. However, many more plants are under construction or are being planned, many of them near large metropolitan centers. The chairman of the Atomic Energy Commission insists that nuclear reactors can provide mankind with a source of power in "a clean environment where resources are efficiently used and reused and pollution is never a problem." Other scientists raise the question whether the values of nuclear power are worth the hazards involved in its use.

Dangerous amounts of radioactive particles may be scattered over the earth by the explosion of atomic or hydrogen (thermonuclear) bombs. The international nuclear test-ban treaty has greatly reduced radiation fallout from the atmosphere. Furthermore, these hazards are monitored and evaluated by well-trained scientists who from time to time supply the public with information and advice. As yet, the amount of radiation exposure from fallout does not equal ordinary "background" radiation from the ground, cosmic rays, stone or brick buildings, people, etc.

The destructive power of atomic and thermonuclear bombs and the harmful effects of the radiation which they generate upon all living things are well known. However, x-rays and radioactive chemicals are essential for medical diagnosis and treatment, and nuclear reactors are being built as sources of power for many uses. This is desirable progress. But the possible harmful effects of radiation from these sources presents a continuing health problem of tremendous importance.

ENVIRONMENT AND HEALTH

The environment has always been an important factor in the survival of life. As Charles Darwin noted, the animals and plants that are best able to adapt to their environment are the ones that survive.

For man the need for sanitation began when he left his nomadic ways and took to settling down in one spot to live and reproduce. As urbanization developed, it became imperative to provide for adequate and safe water supplies, for the disposal of human wastes, and for the safeguarding of food supplies. These are still acute needs in underdeveloped countries.

The enormity of the pollution problem is indicated by the following data:

More than 142 million tons of toxic matter released into the air each year from automobiles, factories, power plants, municipal dumps, and backyard incinerators

More than 3.5 billion tons of solid wastes discarded in automobile graveyards; mountains of trash created by no-return bottles, cans, and other packaging that is not or cannot be recycled; and rat breeding in uncollected garbage in low-income urban areas

Pesticide residues on food crops; traces of veterinary drugs in meat, milk, and eggs; and more than 500 new chemicals introduced into industry each year

In view of this, the next generation may well be confronted with a situation that is essentially hopeless: the air too foul to breathe in safety, the water too polluted to sustain life, and most natural beauty lost forever.

Such appraisals of our environment and the speed with which it is deteriorating are causing alarm and demands for action by government, by industry, and by the public. Some types of environmental pollution are a greater hazard to health than others and so should be given top priority in the application of control measures.

WHAT CAN BE DONE
ABOUT POLLUTION

Few of the major health or social problems with which we are faced can be so greatly influenced by the actions of individuals and of citizen groups as protection of the environment. Pollution begins with people and people can stop pollution. To do so, however, will require a much more widespread awareness of and concern about the situation and much more deterimination to do something about it than exists at the present time.

In the past decade many citizen groups concerned with the environment have been formed. Some are national, some local. A number of good laws have been enacted. Unfortunately, some of these have not been enforced or funded adequately to make them effective. The accomplishments, however, and these have not been inconsiderable, have been the result of individual citizens and citizen groups making their wishes known to their representatives in government—national, state, and local.

Special-interest groups, with powerful lobbies, have frequently opposed the enactment of legislation or the support of laws which they consider to be contrary to their special interests. Yet it has been demonstrated that the public interest can prevail if citizens demand it.[8]

Another way to improve the environment is by personal practices and actions. The control of

population growth depends upon the practices of people in the peak childbearing years.

Less use of paper products will result in less cutting of timber and less waste to be disposed of. Less use of electricity will mean less air pollution: electricity does not pollute, but the production of power to provide electricity from the burning of coal or oil does. Less waste of water will conserve water for essential needs. Less use of automobiles, particularly in urban areas where driving is slow, will reduce the major cause of air pollution. Individuals can aid in the enforcement of laws and regulations by reporting observed pollution from power plants or incinerators to the proper authorities. The development of neighborhood groups to keep sidewalks clean in front of homes or places of business will make our towns and cities less littered.

It may seem that what one person can do is insignificant, but multiplied by hundreds or thousands or millions it becomes significant. Also, simple practices such as those mentioned help make the safeguarding of the environment a way of life which will eventually influence others to join in making this world a better place in which to live.

[8]"What You Can Do about Pollution of the Environment," Common Cause Report, April 1971, 2100 M Street, N.W., Washington 20037.

QUESTIONS FOR DISCUSSION AND SELF-EXAMINATION

1   What is the effect of variations in birth rate and death rate on size of population?

2   Discuss the absolute and relative importance of contraception, abortion, and sterilization to (a) limitation of family size and (b) limitation of total population in a country.

3   In what ways have rapid or merely excessive increases in population impaired individual and community health?

4   What is the role of urban areas in population increases and the problems created by them?

5   What are the two major sources of water supply? What are their advantages and disadvantages? Discuss ways of preventing contamination of each.

6   Why is milk the most readily contaminated food product, and what is the importance of this fact?

7   What is the difference between sewage and sewerage, and what is the significance of each to human health and civilization?

8   What types of air pollution subject human beings to which health hazards?

9   How do pesticides compare with other pollutants of the environment in their risks and dangers?

10   In what ways and in what forms has radiation come to be a hazard to human health?

REFERENCES AND READING SUGGESTIONS

BOOKS

Camus, Albert: *The Plague* (translated from the French by Stuart Gilbert), Alfred A. Knopf, Inc., New York, 1952.

Camus, winner of the 1957 Nobel Prize for literature, tells a story which involves an outbreak of the plague and holds the attention of the reader to the last page.

Commoner, Barry: *The Closing Circle: Nature, Man and Technology*, Alfred A. Knopf, Inc., New York, 1971.

A summary of the essential aspects of pollution of the air, earth, and water, with consideration of the relative importance of population growth and technological growth. The conclusion is that even if we are able to achieve zero population growth, the environment will soon become unbearable if industrial growth continues at the present rate.

Ehrlich, Paul R., and Ehrlich, Anne H.: *Population, Resources and Environment—Issues in Human Ecology.* W. H. Freeman and Company, San Francisco, 1970.

A comprehensive source book of important information relative to the problems that mankind faces for continued survival on this planet; special consideration is given to the increasing population, food supplies, pollution and poisoning of the environment, and the possibilities of controlling these hazards. It is a fascinating but frightening story.

Graham, Frank: *Since Silent Spring*, Houghton Mifflin Company, Boston, 1969.

An appraisal, 7 years later, of Rachel Carson's sensational and frightening book *Silent Spring* and a story of the advances in scientific knowledge stimulated largely by that book concerning the serious hazards to life and to health resulting from the increasing pollution and poisoning of the environment.

Hauser, Philip M. (ed.): *The Population Dilemma*, The American Assembly, Columbia University Press, New York, 1970.

Papers by eight distinguished students of population concerning the present situation and prospects for the future.

Loder, Lawrence: *Breeding Ourselves to Death*, Ballantine Books, Inc., New York, 1971 (1972).

An interesting story of the pioneering efforts being made by small groups of men and women throughout the world to control the population increase that is a threat to the reality of life everywhere.

Snow, John: *On the Mode of Communication of Cholera*, 2d ed., John Churchill, London, 1855. (Reprinted together with a biographical memoir by The Commonwealth Fund, New York, 1936.)

Of much historical interest, this book includes interesting maps in connection with the discussion of the Broad Street pump incident; in which an epidemic of cholera was stopped by removing the handle of a pump drawing water from a contaminated well that was used as the main source of water by a large population.

PAMPHLETS AND PERIODICALS

Annual Report, Population Reference Bureau, Washington.

This includes an excellent list of reports and studies of the population problem.

Craig, Paul P.: "Lead, the Inexcusable Pollutant," *Saturday Review*, Oct. 2, 1971, p. 68.

An interesting history of lead poisoning and an appraisal of its current importance and prevention.

Curtis, Richard, and Fisher, David: "The Seven Wonders of the Polluted World," *The New York Times*, sec. 10, p. 1, Sept. 26, 1971.

"Environment and the Quality of Life," *Saturday Review*, July 3, 1971, pp. 37–48.

A series of articles concerning the disposal of solid wastes, garbage, cans, batteries, paper, etc. This is the third most costly public expenditure in the United States, exceeded only by schools and roads, with a description of some new methods of waste disposal that are proving effective in Sweden and in a few experimental situations in this country.

"Population and Family Planning in the People's Republic of China," The Victor-Bastrom Fund and The Population Crisis Committee, 1730 K St., N.W., Washington.

A splendid series of brief reports on birth-control policies and practices in China—a country with about 20 percent of the world's total population.

Population—The U.S. Problem; The World Problem," *The New York Times*, sec. 12, Apr. 30, 1972.

This special supplement is a comprehensive yet concise consideration of the current status of this problem.

Rosenfeld, Albert: "The Global Dimensions of Health," *Family Health*, April 1971, p. 15.

Looking at the damage that has already been done to the environment, man is discovering that he and his environment are one and that the future is in his hands.

4

MODERN MEDICAL SERVICES

Michael Creighton describes the case of John O'Connor in his book *Five Patients*. O'Connor had a vague pain in his abdomen, vomited once, and had some diarrhea. In the afternoon, he felt warm, had shaking chills, and then collapsed as he tried to telephone to his doctor. His wife brought him to the emergency room of the hospital, where he was found to have a fever of 108°F, to be completely delirious, and to be very seriously ill.

Thirty-one days later John O'Connor was discharged from the hospital, well. It was not known precisely what had caused his illness. He had been seen by a large number of physicians and had had a large number of x-rays and laboratory examinations. His hospital bill, printed out by a computer, was 17 feet long, and the total on it was $6,172.55, almost as much as his annual wages. Fortunately, his hospital insurance was better than most patients' and he had to pay only $357 from his own pocket.

Was John O'Connor poorly treated? Were the doctors negligent in not making a definite diagnosis? Was his hospital bill excessive? The answer to each of these questions is a resounding "no." He had the very best of care and attention. He was lucky to live through his first few days, and did so only because of the skill devoted to his care and because of modern procedures and medications available to his physicians. In many cases, specific diagnoses are not possible. The costs of O'Connor's care, like the costs of medical care in general, were frighteningly high, but necessary to modern, complete medical care in a crisis situation.

In the last century more progress has been made in medical science, including the diagnosis, treatment, and prevention of disease, than in all the preceding thousands of years of recorded history. Yet the practice of medicine is not today and never can be an exact science, in the sense that chemistry or physics is, for medical practice is in part an art and in part a science. The best practitioners of medicine, therefore, are physicians who are thoroughly informed concerning the scientific aspects of medicine but who apply their knowledge with wisdom, sympathy, and understanding of the emotional factors involved.

To provide the quality of health services which modern medical science has made possible, society needs an adequate number of physicians, properly located, with the necessary facilities and associated staffs of health professionals such as the following:

1   Medical specialists of many sorts, such as surgeons, psychiatrists, and ophthalmologists, each of whom has special knowledge of a particular field, or special ability for specific procedures, or both.

2   Dentists, who give therapeutic and preventive attention to the teeth and the mouth.

3   Nurses, who take care of the sick and provide expert assistance in the doctor's consulting room, hospital ward, or operating room.

4   Laboratory technologists, who analyze specimens of blood, urine, and other products or parts of the body, usually under the supervision of a physician called a *pathologist*.

5   X-ray technicians, who take x-ray films and otherwise assist the x-ray specialists known as *radiologists* or *roentgenologists*.

6   Physician's assistants and associates: men and women especially trained to do many aspects of diagnosis and treatment under physicians' supervision. This is a relatively new group, many of whom are former military service corpsmen.

7   Physical therapists, who utilize whirlpools, baths, diathermy, ultrasound sources of heat, exercise, and other methods to aid damaged musculoskeletal systems.

8   Occupational therapists, who teach skills to people with damaged bodies or damaged minds, helping them to overcome their handicaps and recover the ability to live effectively.

9   Social workers, who assist people in dealing with the many material problems of life and often with the psychological aspects of these problems.

10   Clinical psychologists, who test and treat the psychological and intellectual functions of the mind.

11   Pharmacists in hospitals and private pharmacies, who fill prescriptions accurately and with scientific skill.

12   Dietitians, who ensure that the doctor's dietary prescriptions are filled.

13   Public health engineers, who are concerned with environmental hygiene.

14   Epidemiologists, who investigate the spread of disease.

15   Health educators.

16   Other technically and nontechnically trained men and women; administrators, secretaries, and many others.

The efforts of physicians and other health professionals are supplemented by the many institutions dealing with health and disease. Among these are (1) hospitals, private or public, which utilize the many types of personnel listed above; (2) clinics, laboratories, and other special organizations, which are available particularly in large cities; (3) local service organizations, such as the visiting-nurse associations which provide home nursing care; (4) health departments, local, state, and national; (5) foundations, the volunteer health organizations, and governmental agencies which support health education, medical care, and research.

The term *modern medical services* means even more than the increasing specialization and technical competence of modern medicine. It means that both the health of the individual and the health of the community depend on a wide range of people and institutions that bring the benefits of medical science to the individual and his community.

SCIENTIFIC MEDICINE

Scientific medicine is built upon careful observation and research. The admonition of the ancient Greek physician Hippocrates to his pupils "to observe and record for mankind" has been followed through the ages. From observations at the bedside and in the laboratory have come new knowledge, new theories, and new practices—each carefully tested before acceptance.

Many ideas held first by lay people have been investigated and have passed the tests of scientific scrutiny. A general practitioner in Gloucestershire, Edward Jenner, after more than 20 years of study, proved by scientific methods the truth of an idea held by some of the country people of his region that those who had had cowpox would not develop smallpox. This was the beginning of vaccination, which has saved and is still saving millions of human lives through the prevention of smallpox. More recently, medical scientists discovered that the extract of a root traditionally used in India for the treatment of high blood pressure is indeed effective; today in one form or another rauwolfia and its derivatives are widely used in the United States and elsewhere.

Progress in scientific medicine is proceeding at an accelerating rate. New discoveries, observations, conclusions, and techniques are constantly being made available to physicians to enable them to deal with mankind's diseases more effectively.

These advances belie the occasional accusations that the medical profession is unsympathetic to new forms of diagnosis and treatment. New forms of treatment are constantly finding acceptance, as witnessed by insulin treatment for diabetes, the use of liver and then of vitamin B_{12} in pernicious anemia, the sulfonamides and many antibiotics which now control most bacterial infections, the anticoagulants to prevent or treat clotting in blood vessels, and, of course, magnificent surgical advances such as open-heart surgery.

On the other hand, the public would be in a sorry plight if physicians adopted every proposal made in the name of health. The worth and safety of a proposal must be scientifically tested before it is used. Carefully controlled studies have to be made before new methods of treatment can be accepted.[1] Although, to borrow Alexander Pope's familiar words, physicians are reluctant to be "the first by whom the new are tried," they are by no means "the last to lay the old aside." Physicians are anxious to use any form of treatment that will benefit their patients. All that they ask is evidence that the treatment is safe and has real merit.

[1]See the description of scientifically controlled studies of the prevention and treatment of colds, pages 277–279.

MEDICAL EDUCATION

In the early days of this country, as well as in Europe at that time, medical education was conducted under a preceptorial or apprentice system. That is, a physician interested in training young men for the practice of medicine would accept a few trainees; lend them his books; and teach them about the structure and function of the body, its diseases, and the treatment of disease. The trainee would frequently live with his preceptor and serve as his coachman and general assistant. Under this system some wise and dedicated physicians were educated.

Today, however, the training of physicians is much more highly organized. Almost all American medical schools are associated with large universities. In contrast, all the schools for training practitioners of the healing cults are without university affiliation. States require that, to be eligible for licensure to practice medicine, physicians must be graduates of medical schools which meet the standards established by the Association of American Medical Colleges and the Council on Medical Education of the American Medical Association.

In 1970, there were 8,367 physicians graduated from the medical schools in the United States. This was about 3,000 more than had been graduated 15 years earlier. This increase in doctors has been insufficient to keep up with the increase in population and the increased utilization of medical services. More physicians are constantly needed, both in family practice and in the several specialties in which the application of advanced techniques requires more manpower. In addition to the physicians needed for patient care, more physicians are constantly needed in research, in teaching, in public health work, etc. (Figure 4.1.)

The deficiencies in medical care are most serious in rural areas and in the central cores of cities. It is in these areas that people are most likely to have difficulty in finding personal physicians. To eliminate the estimated present shortage of physicians and to keep pace with the growing population, most medical schools are increasing the size of their classes, new medical schools are being developed, and still more are in the planning stage. The time needed for graduating students from medical schools and for training physicians

in hospitals is being shortened in many institutions. A critical major problem, however, is in the shortage of funds for medical school construction and expansion, for faculty salaries, for scholarships and loan funds for medical students, and for the training of specialists, teachers, and research scientists. Increases in federal appropriations for these purposes, as well as for the training of nurses, dentists, pharmacists, and other members of the health team, are essential if the health needs of the nation are to be met.

THE MEDICAL COURSE

For admission to medical school the usual requirement is 3 or 4 years of college education. The purpose of this requirement is to provide medical students with a sound foundation in the biological and physical sciences on which medicine is based, to give them a knowledge of the social sciences concerned with human relationships, and to acquaint them with other fields of knowledge contributing to a liberal education.

The medical school course itself traditionally has taken 4 years, but some schools have shortened this to 3 years. The graduate then takes 1 or more years of hospital training, in which he cares for patients under the supervision of experienced practitioners and teachers. On completion of this hospital training, the physician may enter medical practice or may continue graduate training in one of the specialties, including family medicine.

To shorten this long period of education and training, several medical schools have instituted programs in which selected students earn the M.D. degree in 6 years of study after high school.[2]

Two or three times as many students have applied to United States medical schools in each recent year as the schools have been able to accept. Still, there remains great need for able and dedicated young men and women to enter medicine.

Shortages also exist in most of the other health professions listed above, and properly qualified applicants have little or no difficulty in obtaining entrance to training programs. Most notably there is a great need for more young people to enter the nursing profession.

Figure 4.1 Physicians in the United States, by types of practice. SOURCE: *Health Manpower SOURCE Book,* U.S. Public Health Publication, 1962.

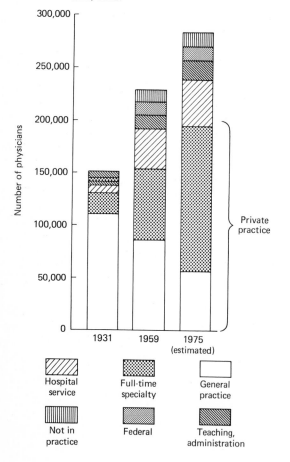

[2]For details see Admission Requirements of Medical Colleges, Association of American Medical Colleges, Evanston, Ill.

It is not enough for a physician to have a good medical education and hospital training before starting practice. In these days of rapid advances in medical knowledge, he needs continuing education to prevent obsolescence of his professional information. An alert physician learns from every patient. He learns also by consultations with other physicians and by conducting or observing operations and postmortem examinations.

Some persons are reluctant to request or even to permit postmortem medical examinations on their relatives. This shows a lack of understanding of the purpose and value of such examinations. Physicians are able to practice better medicine because of what they learn from postmortem examinations. Occasionally a medical discovery,

such as insulin, of value to millions of persons grows out of observations made in connection with such examinations. Through a postmortem examination the death of one person contributes to the life and health of others.

There are few individuals whom people must depend upon and trust so fully as the doctor. A survey by Louis Harris, sponsored by *Newsweek*, asked college seniors to rate professional and other occupational groups in the order of those in whom they had "a great deal of confidence." They ranked physicians first, followed by scientists, bankers, U.S. Supreme Court justices, educators, and corporation heads. Such esteem should be merited and perpetuated. The selection of students for medical school is a tremendous responsibility.

THE PHYSICIAN

CHOOSING A PHYSICIAN

The casual way in which many people select a physician to act as personal or family health adviser suggests that they have little appreciation of the importance of this choice.

For minor or imaginary illnesses any sort of medical service may seem satisfactory, but when major illnesses occur everybody wants the best. This is natural, but it could lead to neglect of the early stages of disease. The diagnosis of cancer, tuberculosis, and other diseases is easy after they become advanced, but by that time even the best of care is usually unavailing. Of far greater value is the recognition of these conditions when they are just beginning. At this stage diagnosis is difficult, but most can be done for the patient.

Since physicians differ in competence, in many communities a choice may be difficult. Popularity is a poor guide. Several sources of information are helpful in making a wise selection.

1 State medical licensing boards provide the public with considerable protection against incompetent and dishonest physicians. Before a physician is licensed to practice medicine, he must present evidence of graduation from an approved medical school, of good moral character, and in most states, of hospital experience. Then he must pass examinations in the various

branches of fundamental science and medical practice. Another safeguard is set up by the county medical society, which has its own qualifications for admission and occasionally refuses membership to a physician even though he is licensed to practice.

2 Leading hospitals choose their staff physicians carefully; their superintendents can furnish lists of staff members.

3 Secretaries of county medical societies, listed in the telephone book of the community, can furnish details of hospital training, medical school attended, special appointments, and length of time in practice of various physicians in the area.

4 Friends may be able to indicate what physician they would call if their own doctor were not available (this diminishes the prejudices of personal attachment in their advice).

5 Specialists may be willing to indicate what personal physician they endorse or choose themselves.

6 Inquiry may reveal which physicians often takes care of other physicians and their families. Doctors rarely care for their own families, since personal concern may interfere with sound medical judgment.

7 The dean of a nearby medical school or the

director of a nearby college health service will often recommend able physicians.

8 A physician in another community, such as the community one has lived in previously, may often be able to recommend a physician.

THE FAMILY PHYSICIAN

The old-time general practitioner, who diagnosed all the family ills, brought the children into the world, pulled grandfather and babies through pneumonia and father through typhoid fever, removed tonsils and appendixes, and served as veterinarian, clergyman, and mailman, belongs to a past generation. Medical science has advanced too rapidly and too far for one man to be proficient in all fields. This has led inevitably to specialization in medical practice.

This does not mean that the family physician is an institution of the past. On the contrary, in this age of specialization the need for a family health adviser is greater than ever before. The modern family physician, however, no longer attempts to do everything himself. He knows his patients, provides most of the medical care they need, and advises the services of specialists when necessary.

Many family physicians are specialists in internal medicine, commonly called *internists;* i.e., they are physicians who have had 3 to 5 years of graduate study and hospital training in diagnosis and in treatment by measures other than surgery or radiation. Other family physicians are general practitioners or have had special hospital training for family practice, now recognized as a specialty in its own right. It is estimated that a family physician can provide at least 80 percent of the medical services which a family requires.

Everyone should have a personal or family physician who can render medical care, can act as a counselor, can conduct physical examinations, and will provide or arrange for emergency services when needed. Many medical centers now offer special programs of study and training for students who wish to become family physicians.

SPECIALISTS

Specialization has been developed in medicine in response to needs. The more a physician concentrates his attention on one particular system of the body or one diagnostic or therapeutic procedure,

the more proficient he will become in that field. There is frequent need for specialists in the broad areas of internal medicine, surgery, obstetrics and gynecology, pediatrics, and diseases of the eye, ear, nose, and throat. The services of other specialists are less frequently needed, but the skill of the highly specialized bronchoscopist or the brain surgeon occasionally means the difference between life and death.

But when should one go to a specialist, and how is one to know which specialist can best render the service needed? On these points the family physician can give valuable advice. Many conditions for which patients go directly to specialists could be treated just as satisfactorily—and in some cases more satisfactorily—by the family physician. It is important for the patient that the specialist whom he selects be thoroughly competent in his special field. State licensing boards do not set up specific requirements for practice of the specialties of medicine, but physicians in the various specialties do so themselves. In general, 3 to 5 years of special graduate study and hospital training in an approved institution are required in order to qualify for the rigorous examinations by the *specialty boards.* The physician who meets all the requirements and passes the examinations is granted a certificate by the board before which he has qualified, such as the American Board of Ophthalmology. There are similar boards of surgery, of obstetrics and gynecology, of internal medicine, of urology, and of roentgenology. One can be certain that a physician who possesses the certificate of one of these boards is thoroughly qualified for the practice of his particular specialty.

GROUP CLINICS

Increasingly, physicians in various parts of the country have grouped themselves together into clinics in order to practice medicine on a cooperative basis. These clinics usually include physicians in general medicine as well as specialists needed by the community. By frequent consultations and the pooling of laboratory and x-ray facilities the group should be able to provide better service than the patient would ordinarily receive if these same physicians were practicing independently. The numbers of physicians on the staffs of group clinics vary from a few to several hundred. In addition some clinics have considerable numbers of young physicians on a fellowship or residency basis in training for careers in the various specialties of medical practice.

Charges for services rendered to patients are usually in accord with a fixed schedule, with adjustments according to the patient's ability to pay. Some patients pay little or nothing. Today many patients' bills are covered at least in part by insurance: Medicare, Blue Cross, Blue Shield, commercial insurance companies, workmen's compensation insurance, company or union plans, etc.

Compensation to physicians in such clinics may be on a salary basis or on an agreed-upon percentage of the net earnings of the clinic. In either case the incomes of the individual doctors on the staff are not directly related to the fees paid by the patients for whom they care.

Some fear that in the clinic type of organization, personal interest in the patient may be submerged to the efficient functioning of the organization as a whole. This may occur, but it can be avoided if the clinic makes adequate plans to provide personalized service for each patient.

WHAT TO EXPECT
FROM A PHYSICIAN

Having selected a physician, what should one expect from him? In the first place, he should render careful, conscientious, interested service during illness, utilizing such facilities and obtaining such consultations as are necessary to arrive at a diagnosis and to provide adequate treatment. In so doing he can be expected "to cure sometimes, to relieve often, to comfort always," and thus to contribute to the extension of a meaningful and rewarding life.

Some diseases can be accurately diagnosed on first examination, but others require careful study and observation before the nature of the illness can be determined. In addition, the doctor should give advice on minor problems of health and illness. He should advise and administer vaccinations of established value, and he should perform periodic health examinations.

It is important that the patient have what Hippocrates called "contentment with the physician"—in other words, confidence in his physician. If he does not find this in one physician or a particular clinic group of physicians, he should seek another. Having found a good physician in whom he has confidence, he would be wise to remain under his care.

When you have established confidence in your physician, follow his advice concerning diagnosis and treatment. He will rarely perform miracles, but he will steer you on the best course to health. In difficult situations, he will often call for consultations; you are always entitled to ask for a consultation yourself if you feel the need of one. If you lose confidence in your physician, you should discuss with him the reason for your doubt; if you cannot regain confidence, you should change physicians after notifying him of your intention.

Many of the difficulties in obtaining the services of a physician, particularly to make house calls and for care at night, can be avoided by selecting and becoming acquainted with a physician and his policies on house calls before illness strikes. You will then have a personal physician who will feel responsible for you and your family.

People sometimes boast that they have not consulted a physician in years. This is unfortunate, for the most valuable service that physicians can render lies in the field of prevention. The physician of today has infinitely more to offer as a health adviser than did the doctor of the past. Given an opportunity in this capacity, he will render invaluable service.

OSTEOPATHY

Osteopathy was originally a system of treatment based upon the theory that diseases can be remedied by manipulation of the bones, muscles, nerves, blood vessels, etc. Its founder was Andrew Still, its birthplace Baldwin, Kansas. The first school was started by its founder at Kirksville, Missouri, in 1891. This school is still in existence, although most of the others that were subsequently established have disappeared. There are at present seven schools of osteopathy in the United States, all approved by the Bureau of Education of the American Osteopathic Association.

Over the years osteopathy has progressively raised its standards of education and expanded its methods of treatment until today the graduates of its schools receive an education patterned upon that provided by schools of medicine. In view of this many states now license osteopaths to practice general medicine and surgery, and the military services commission osteopaths as officers in the medical corps. In civilian life osteopaths are helping to provide needed medical services in many areas where there are shortages of doctors.

PERIODIC HEALTH EXAMINATIONS

Increasingly people go to their doctors when they do not feel ill but merely wish to prevent illness. This is individual preventive medicine at its best. The American Medical Association recommends a lifelong schedule of regular health checkups, more frequent at the extremes of life than during the middle. This schedule appears in Table 4.1.

Between examinations the patient must take responsibility by seeking the physician's help for any significant symptoms, and by following the physician's advice. Together, physician and patient should take measures to prevent disease. The periodic health survey is the backbone of these preventive efforts. It involves not only a complete examination to discover any existing disease, but also a review of the patient's habits and life.

On the basis of a thorough health examination the doctor can advise corrective measures and discuss ways in which the patient can best promote his own health and prevent future disease. At the same time, the doctor can teach the patient which symptoms are significant. For both preventive and therapeutic medicine, the doctor-patient relationship is important.

A continuing record of health examinations provides information that is valuable both to the patient and to the physician when appraising the inevitable changes that occur in health and physical condition over the years.

Far too many people regard health as "being doctored." They therefore hope that with unlimited access to physicians and hospitals, they will be healthy. Surely "doctoring" is a necessary element in health, but it is not sufficient. The provision of health service to all citizens will result in some improvement in health; that improvement, however, may be disappointingly small. There are large contributors to sickness and death about which physicians and hospitals can do little. Accidents are the greatest cause of both morbidity and mortality for Americans between the ages of 1 and 37 years. Other important causes for all age groups are obesity, smoking, abuse of alcohol and other drugs, environmental pollution, and life-styles that lead to psychosomatic disease. With the exception of environmental pollution, there is little society could do to control these causes without imposing intolerable restrictions on personal liberty. Control can come only from the individual. Only his decisions and his actions can eliminate these causes of disability and death. His physician can advise, but only he can act.

We should accept the concept that health deserves the highest priority but realize that society can guarantee only access to health service. Personal health must remain a personal responsibility.

FINANCING MEDICAL CARE

The rapid rise in the costs of medical care is causing serious family and national problems. Total national expenditures for health services increased almost sixfold from 1950 to 1970, from approximately $13 billion in 1950 to almost $80 billion in 1970. The reasons for the increase include population growth, the decrease in the purchasing value of the dollar, the greater use and expense of hospitalization, the complexity and costs of new scientific procedures for diagnosis and treatment, and most important, more adequate salaries, wages, and fees for all types of medical personnel. In the past the greater part of expenditures for personal health services went to physicians. Today physicians' fees are about one-fifth of the total, and of this less than half represents direct payment to physicians, the rest being provided by insurance, by various types of prepayment and group arrangements, or by government.

Table 4.1 Recommended frequency of health examinations*

Age	Frequency
First 6 months of life	Biweekly
Second 6 months	Monthly
1– 2 years	Every 3 months
2– 5 years	Every 6 months
5–15 years	Every 2–3 years
15–35 years	Every 2 years
35–60 years	Every year
60 on	Every 6 months

*American Medical Association.

Every owner of an automobile assumes a heavy risk for possible damage to the person or property of others, a risk which may exceed almost any possible expense for medical care. Responsible automobile owners, for the protection of themselves and of those whose property or persons might be injured by the cars they own, take out liability insurance.

This same principle applies to the financial risks incident to illness. For people with adequate incomes the problem of providing for the cost of medical care can be solved by budgeting. Disability insurance can be carried as protection against the major hazards of prolonged illness and unemployment; regular medical and dental service can be provided without hardship either on a similar insurance basis or by budgeting or regularly saving for this purpose. Figure 4.2 shows how the consumer's dollar is divided to pay for living expenses; only 7 cents out of every dollar is used for health care.

Medicare provides insurance coverage for hospitalization and certain other medical services for persons over 65 or otherwise eligible for social security benefits which are financed by payroll deductions matched by contributions from employers during the years of active employment. Commercial insurance companies, as well as the Blue Cross and Blue Shield organizations, offer various types of policies for persons of all ages.

The system of private medical practice which has always existed in this country is founded upon the free choice of physician by the patient and the payment of professional services on an individual-fee basis. The amount of the fee usually depends on the type of service rendered, the eminence of the physician, and the ability of the patient to pay. (In Figure 4.3, the patient's dollar is dissected to show where each part goes in paying for medical services.)

This system of medical practice has included the best medical care found anywhere in the world. Yet it does not adequately meet the needs of all groups. During the past decade the problem of providing medical care for low-income groups has been receiving increasing attention. European countries have developed various types of plans to meet this problem. Some such plans are on a compulsory insurance basis; others are supported out of tax funds and administered by the government.

In the rural provinces of western Canada,

Figure 4.2 Where the consumer dollar goes. Source: U.S. Department of Commerce, Office of Business Economics, 1966.

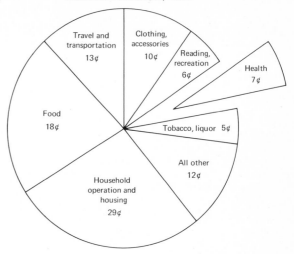

where it would be impossible for physicians to earn a living in private practice, various communities have arranged to pay physicians out of public funds. In the United States also, various modifications of the system of private practice have grown up to meet special situations. Medical schools and the larger hospitals have long maintained free clinics for those unable to pay. In many localities relief funds can be used to provide necessary medical services, and the federal government now offers matching funds (Medicaid) to states to pay for medical care for persons financially unable to provide it for themselves. Certain industries have established their own medical departments to safeguard the health of and provide medical care for their employees. Most colleges and universities have developed excellent health services for their students. States operate public hospitals for patients with tuberculosis, mental illnesses, and contagious diseases; and health departments aid physicians in the provision of better care for mothers and infants and in the diagnosis and treatment of such diseases as tuberculosis, diphtheria, syphilis, gonorrhea, and tetanus.

PREPAYMENT GROUP HEALTH PROGRAMS

Over the past 30 or 40 years a considerable number of group programs have been organized throughout the country to provide health services on a prepayment basis. Some programs provide complete

Figure 4.3 Distribution of personal expenditures for medical care in the United States in 1970. Source: *Source Book of Health Insurance Data,* Health Insurance Institute, New York, 1971.

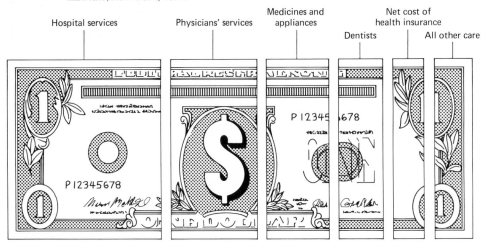

medical care in their own clinics and hospitals. Others provide more limited services, sometimes on a contractual basis with community hospitals.

The largest prepayment medical care plan in the United States is operated by the Kaiser Medical Care Foundation. Its nonprofit programs now operate in northern California; southern California; Portland, Oregon; Hawaii; Cleveland, Ohio; and Denver, Colorado. These programs provide comprehensive, prepaid medical care for more than 2 million members on a direct service basis through nineteen hospitals, two extended-care facilities, and fifty-two clinics.

This program was started when the Kaiser Corporation and several other construction companies jointly contracted to build the Hoover Dam near Las Vegas, Nevada, then a town of less than 5,000 population. To house the construction workers and their families, a town for some 15,000 people was built at the dam site. To provide medical care for this community the construction companies built a hospital and employed a staff.

Later, in a similar situation, when the Grand Coulee Dam on the Columbia River in Washington was under construction, a per-capita prepayment plan was proposed. The union approved the plan with full coverage for families. After some trial-and-error adjustments, both employers and employees were pleased with its services. Shortly thereafter, just prior to the beginning of World

War II, the Kaiser Company developed ship-building yards in the San Francisco Bay area and in the Portland, Oregon–Vancouver, Washington area, each of which employed over 100,000 workmen. For these workmen and their families, homes, hospitals, and clinics were built, and medical services were provided on the basis that had proved satisfactory at Grand Coulee. Since these locations are relatively near San Francisco and Portland, where medical services are available, enrollment in the plan was made optional. However, during the war the program served some 90,000 workers and their families in each area. After the end of the war membership in this medical-care plan was opened to the public.

Under this program medical service is provided by an autonomous group of physicians in each region. Hospital service is provided by the Kaiser Foundation hospitals and through arrangements with a number of independent hospitals. The professional and organizational independence of the physicians is preserved by a contractual relationship in each region between the health plan and the medical group. Compensation to the medical group is negotiated annually on a per-capita basis, so much per member per month. How the doctors share that compensation is their responsibility, just as the provision of professional care is their responsibility.

Wherever this program is operating, membership is voluntary for Kaiser industry employees and for members of other groups that contract with the Kaiser Foundation Health Plan to provide medical care for their members.

Other prepayment plans, such as the Health Insurance Plan of Greater New York, with some 600,000 members, are organized and operated on different bases. This is true also of several community service plans being developed by medical schools and their teaching hospitals.

In Boston, Harvard Medical School for several years has conducted a complete prepayment medical service program for persons in the area who joined the plan. During this initial period financing has been provided in part by membership fees and in part by grants from foundations and government. However, the program has been so well accepted and is having such an increase in annual memberships that it was expected to be able to continue without subsidy by 1972. These and other programs represent significant experimental efforts to provide high-quality medical care on a voluntary prepayment basis.

While these and other plans are being studied, Congress is debating the best way to make medical services, preventive as well as curative, available to all who need them. Whatever plan or plans are adopted, it is essential that provision be made to safeguard the quality of the service rendered. To fail to do so would lead to catastrophe both for the public and for the medical profession.

HEALING CULTS

Healing cults consist of groups of practitioners or followers of an unscientific theory of the causation and the treatment of disease. Such cults flourish when a considerable portion of the population lacks an understanding of the fundamental principles of health and disease. This does not necessarily imply an ignorant population, for many people who are intelligent and well-informed on other subjects regard health as they regard life hereafter, a matter for conviction and belief rather than for study and investigation.

The reasons the cults are able to hold patients and build reputations are several. One is that they promise a cure if the patient takes an adequate number of treatments. The number considered adequate is variable, but the duration is always sufficiently prolonged to give plenty of time for recovery. Most of man's illnesses are acute and self-limited, with recovery occurring in the natural course of events. For such natural recoveries the cults take full credit.

Another reason for their success is that many persons who go from one doctor to another have nothing organically wrong. Their complaints are real, but they are occasioned by emotional disturbances and made worse by concentration on them. Improvement in such cases frequently follows elaborate, mystical, and suggestive treatments which take the patient's mind off himself and his troubles. But this is only temporary, and then the pathetic victim drifts on, groping blindly for some other miraculous cure.

Other patients who, for a time, sing the praises of the cults are those with chronic illnesses which go through alternating periods of improvement and relapse. The physician, understanding the condition, may advise the patient that there is nothing that can be done for him. But the cultist, because of his lack of knowledge, is optimistic; and when improvement occurs both he and the patient are jubilant. Relapse often follows later; and if this occurs after treatments have been discontinued, arrangements for further treatments are made.

Still other cures obtained by irregular methods of treatment are cures of diseases which never existed. It is not difficult to cure "pneumonia" which is nothing more than grippe, or "cancer" which is only indigestion. Most such incorrect diagnoses are made by cultists who examine the patient, possibly even by x-ray, and then announce that some serious condition exists. In so doing the cultist may be entirely sincere. He was told certain things during his training, and having inadequate scientific or educational background for critical thinking or sound judgment, he accepts them unquestioningly and in all sincerity applies them in his practice.

CHIROPRACTIC

Chiropractic, a widespread cult in the United States, was founded at Davenport, Iowa, by D. D. Palmer, who prior to his "discovery of the principles of chiropractic" had been a magnetic healer. It was defined by his son B. J. Palmer, its "developer," as "a philosophy, science and art of things natural, and as a system of adjusting subluxated vertebra of the spinal column by hand for the elimination of disease, and the restoration of health."

This cult had a rapid growth, with schools established in most cities in this country. The courses varied from evening classes over a few months to full-time "study" for 2 years. The course at the Palmer School covered "eighteen consecutive calendar months, comprising three collegiate years of six months each, all of which are continuous, there being no vacation periods."[3]

The theory upon which chiropractic is based, namely, that disease results "from either an excess or deficiency of mental impulse flow, caused by pressure upon nerves which interfers with normal transmission," has no basis in scientific fact. This alleged flow of vital energy is nonexistent, and medical examinations, x-ray studies, and autopsy findings fail to reveal the "subluxations" which chiropractic treatments are alleged to correct.

Yet this cult has many followers, and chiropractors are licensed to practice chiropractic (but not medicine) in most states. However, the efforts of this cult to be recognized by the federal government with authorization of payment for chiropractic services from Medicare funds resulted in several independent investigations of chiropractic. The findings of these investigations led to the following public statements.

The Secretary of Health, Education, and Welfare reported to Congress that

. . . chiropractic theory and practice are not based upon the body of basic knowledge related to health, disease and health care that has been widely accepted by the scientific community. Moreover, irrespective of its theory, the scope and quality of chiropractic education do not prepare the practitioner to make an adequate diagnosis and provide appropriate treatment.

The representative of the AFL-CIO stated before the U.S. Senate Finance Committee that

. . . care of patients should be entrusted to those who have a sound scientific knowledge of disease

and whose experience and competence render them capable of diagnosing and treating patients by utilizing all the resources of modern medicine. Since neither chiropractic theory nor the quality of chiropractic education equip chiropractors to do this, the AFL-CIO opposes the coverage of chiropractors in the Medicare program.

The National Council of Senior Citizens in its official publication states,

Chiropractic treatment, designed to eliminate causes that do not exist while denying the existence of the real causes, is at best worthless—and at worst mortally dangerous.

Many other organizations have come to similar conclusions. For references see References and Reading Suggestions at the end of this chapter.

QUACKERY IN MEDICINE

The medical quack may be a physician, he may be a practitioner of one of the cults, or he may lay no claim to any sort of medical education whatsoever. His only purpose is to exploit human misery for personal gain. His technique may be to promote a dietary fad, sell reducing salts, give electrical treatments, or twist feet; or he may proclaim himself a "specialist" in cancer or some other condition. Ignorance and gullibility make many persons easy victims.

Diseases providing the greatest opportunities for the quack are chronic, painful afflictions which resist medical treatment. Prominent among these are arthritis and cancer. Pain, crippling, resistance to treatment, and discouragement lead many persons with such diseases to become victims of promised "cures."

It is estimated that people spend over $250 million a year on worthless arthritis remedies; and cancer quackery takes some $50 million a year from desperate cancer patients and their frantic families. The waste of this money is scandalous; but much more tragic is the time lost while the disease progresses, in the case of arthritis until it is more crippling and more difficult to treat effectively and in the case of cancer until it has passed the "point of no return." Nutritional quackery, already of gigantic size, is continuing to grow,

---

[3]Quotations from the announcement of the Palmer School of Chiropractic, Chiropractic Fountain Head, Davenport, Iowa.

costing an estimated 10 million Americans a half-billion dollars each year.

The quack usually claims to employ a secret form of treatment with which he obtains miraculous cures. This in itself should be a warning that his motive is selfish personal profit. Otherwise he would not keep his treatment secret but would publish his discovery, as is the custom of physicians and scientists, so that it might be utilized to relieve the suffering of mankind everywhere. But this he dares not do, for he knows that his methods will not stand the light of day and that they are of value only to him—and then only so long as they are kept secret.

Protection against quackery The people themselves are responsible for quackery because they are looking for magic, for an easy way out of sickness. Only when every patient learns to look behind glittering promises and false facades will there be an end to this crime that takes people's money and lives.

MEDICATIONS

Drugs or druglike concoctions have been used from primitive times to the present day. Some of these medicines, such as the juice of the opium poppy for the relief of pain and the bark of the cinchona tree for the treatment of malaria, were utilized for centuries before their effective medicinal ingredients were recognized.

Derivatives of opium and quinine from cinchona bark have continued to be useful to the present time. In fact, in Vietnam in the mid-1960s, a strain of malaria appeared which was resistant to all antimalarial drugs except quinine. Other old drugs have disappeared as more effective modern agents have become available.

In previous generations, an air of mystery surrounded prescriptions, fostered by the long-accepted practices of writing prescriptions in Latin and including on the container's label only the patient's name and the dosage of the medicine. However, the rising level of education among the American people, their great interest in matters of sickness and health, and the change from the "doctor-priest" to the "doctor-scientist" are contributing to the patient's expectation that his illness will be explained to him and that he will be told about the proposed treatment and what to expect from it.

A small but significant part of this trend is the growing practice of indicating the name of the drug on the label of the box or bottle of medicine that the patient takes home from the pharmacy. This information on the label is helpful when the patient has symptoms which may be due to reaction to a drug or which may result from too high a dosage. It is invaluable also when the patient changes doctors, moves to another locality, or contacts the doctor when his records are not at hand. The name of the drug and its strength on the label may save precious minutes and spell the difference between life and death in cases of attempted suicide, accidental overdosage, or accidental poisoning of children. Furthermore, naming the drug, or at least indicating its purpose on the label, helps to prevent mixups between two or more drugs that are being taken concurrently, or between drugs that are being taken by different members of the family.

The drugs available to physicians today constitute a tremendous armamentarium, and some of them are truly "wonder drugs." Many of them, however, can cause serious toxic reactions in some people or under certain conditions. Also, many of them are similar to one another, if not identical, even though they may have very different names. For example, aspirin is still aspirin, whatever names it is sold under and whatever prices are charged for it.

Drugs for the home medicine cabinet are best selected and used according to the advice of one's physician. A warning should be given concerning the all too frequent practice of deciding to use for oneself or family members a medicine prescribed for someone else either recently or months before. Many times such medicines have been used with serious results. A doctor's prescription is meant only for the person for whom he has designated it, and the dosage is calculated for that particular person. The prescription is not intended for another person, even though his illness, to the untrained observer, may appear to be "just the same." It should also be remembered that drugs may deteriorate. It is essential, therefore, that they be used only in accord with instructions and destroyed when the illness is over.

Drugs which may be toxic to some persons in the usual dosage or which may be habit-forming can be sold only on a doctor's prescription. Others may be purchased without restriction.

The manufacture of prescription drugs is a highly scientific and efficient industry; the physician and his patient are assured of the quality and potency of these drugs. The federal Food and Drug Administration (see page 392), with the cooperation of the pharmaceutical industry, supervises the manufacture of prescription drugs.

SELF-MEDICATION

People have always had a blind faith in medicines, and until recently the more complicated a medicine was and the worse it tasted, the better it was supposed to be. Today we no longer wear asafetida bags around our necks to prevent diphtheria, nor do we carry horse chestnuts to ward off rheumatism, but we waste millions of dollars on medicines and "health products" that are just as worthless as these primitive cure-alls. Actually, it is said that the amount of money spent in this country for self-medication is several times as much as that which is spent for drugs prescribed by physicians.

The preparations used for self-medication vary enormously in content, purpose, and importance. Some are standard drugs of known composition, such as aspirin, the use of which in general is safe. Claims that aspirin will prevent or cure colds are unfounded; but it relieves pain and headache, lowers fever, and is somewhat sedative. On the other hand, aspirin causes gastric bleeding or severe allergic reactions in some people. Also, aspirin is sometimes taken in toxic amounts by children who think it is candy. It is estimated that aspirin causes about 1,000 deaths a year in this country.

Preparations of unknown composition with copyrighted names belong to a different category. Some of these products are harmless but entirely worthless—just plain fakes. Some consist of standard drugs packaged to sell at fancy prices. Others, mostly prohibited in this country, contain drugs that are actually dangerous, such as aminopyrine and the potentially toxic and habit-forming acetanilid found in certain headache and cold remedies. Still others, particularly tonics to revitalize the aged, owe their popularity to the alcohol which they contain.

It is important to realize also that, except for the sulfonamides and the antibiotics in certain bacterial infections, iron for iron-deficiency anemia, and various drugs to treat tropical parasitic infections, few of the drugs we use are specific *cures* for disease. They are of value because they control undesirable reactions, support some body function, or alleviate suffering; and the physician who prescribes them does so for specific reasons in an individual case. One patient with abdominal cramps may be relieved by a cathartic, while another may suffer a ruptured appendix from the same treatment.

On television, radio, and billboards, in public conveyances, and in newspapers and magazines, advertising of preparations for self-medication induces people to waste hundreds of millions of dollars each year—much of it by people who can ill afford to lose it. Some of these preparations may do actual harm, either by making the condition worse or by suppressing symptoms and delaying treatment of serious disease. Few if any of them are ever recommended by physicians. People therefore would be wise to get the advice of their physicians before spending their money and risking their health on preparations skillfully promoted not for the improvement of health but for the enrichment of those who produce and sell the products.

Furthermore, a person should not depend on the assistance of a druggist in making his own diagnosis and planning his own treatment. A person who doctors himself when he is ill or uses a pharmacist as his consultant is indulging in self-medication which is both unscientific and unsound. It may well be said of him, "He who hath himself for a doctor, hath a fool for a patient."

QUESTIONS FOR DISCUSSION AND SELF-EXAMINATION

1 How have the relationships of physicians to others who help sick people changed in recent years?

2 What education and training do modern physicians have?

3 Compare the role of family physicians with the role of specialists. How are the two related? What differences of training and experience do they have?

4 What other health personnel can be helpful to individuals and to society, and in what ways? What personnel may be harmful and in what way?

5 Describe some of the ways in which new methods of treatment have been developed.

6 How may a person new to a community get reliable advice on the choice of a personal physician? What safeguards can he have that the physician he chooses will be a competent professional?

7 How does group practice affect the relationship between patient and physician?

8 What principles should a patient keep in mind in order to utilize his physician's services optimally?

9 What changes have been made in recent years in paying for medical care?

10 Discuss the ideal relationships among symptoms, physician, pharmacist, and medications.

REFERENCES AND READING SUGGESTIONS

BOOKS

Health Careers Guidebook, Superintendent of Documents, Washington.

This guidebook by the Manpower Administration of the U.S. Department of Labor, an updated version of the National Health Council publication, provides information on some 200 health career opportunities.

Holbrook, Stewart: *The Golden Age of Quackery*, The Macmillan Company, New York, 1959. (Also in paperback, Collier Books, a division of Crowell-Collier Publishing Co., New York, 1962.)

A fascinating story of the most famous medical quacks in the United States and how they have operated.

Smith, R. I.; *At Your Own Risk: The Case against Chiropractic*, Trident Press, a division of Simon & Schuster, Inc., New York, 1969.

A probing study of chiropractors and their methods of treatment. The author spent years investigating both as a patient and as a visitor in many of the nation's chiropractic schools and clinics. He explains why in the public interest he recommends that chiropractic be the subject of immediate legislative reviews.

Sommers, Anne R.: *Health Care in Transition: Directions for the Future*, Hospital Research and Educational Trust, 1971.

Will be used as the most important source book for discussions about health care for years. Well written, crammed with facts and figures in understandable form.

Van Anken, William B. D.: *How To Get the Best from Your Physician*, Charles C Thomas, Publisher, Springfield, Ill., 1967.

This small book considers the choice of a good physician and the development of a patient-doctor relationship that will result in the best possible medical care.

University Health Services, World Health Organization Technical Report Series No. 320, Columbia University Press, New York.

A broadly based consideration of the objectives, programs, services, organization, and financing of college and university health services.

PAMPHLETS AND PERIODICALS

Block, Irvin: *How to Get Good Medical Care*, Public Affairs Pamphlet, New York.

Emergency Health Care, U.S. Office of Civil Defense and Public Health Service, Washington.

A splendid and concise summary of what an individual can do to maintain health and alleviate suffering when professional care and normal services are not available.

Schwartz, Harry: "Health Care in America: A

Heretical Diagnosis," *Saturday Review*, Aug. 14, 1971.

A thoughtful analysis of some of the major things that are wrong or said to be wrong with medical care in this country.

What They Say about Chiropractic, American Medical Association, 535 No. Dearborn St., Chicago, Ill.

A compilation of statements about the value of chiropractic by the U.S. Department of Health, Education, and Welfare, the American Public Health Association, the AFL-CIO, the Consumer Federation of America, the National Council of Senior Citizens, and numerous other health and consumer organizations.

5

HEART DISEASE, STROKE, AND CANCER

In *The New York Times* a few years ago, an obituary appeared whose beginning read something like this: "Donald Dame, 38-year-old tenor with the Metropolitan Opera Company, collapsed and died yesterday in Minneapolis; he had been on tour. . . ."

Previously, Mr. Dame had had several attacks of squeezing pain in the chest when exercising or under emotional stress, but they had lasted only a short time. Then, there was the final attack—the same pain, which lasted only a few moments before he collapsed and was dead. If an electrocardiogram had been taken at the time, it would have showed that the heart muscle had gone into a type of random electrical activity called *ventricular fibrillation*, in which the heart is unable to pump blood out and death occurs quickly.

Had Donald Dame gone home after the earlier attacks and rested under a physician's care, he might not have had a fatal attack. Furthermore, today, if an expert first-aid man or physician had been present, the technique called *closed-chest heart message* could have been used to keep his circulation going, and Mr. Dame might have survived.

Heart disease, stroke, and cancer are responsible for about 70 percent of all deaths in this country. Diseases of the heart and circulatory system—a broad category that includes strokes—claim about a million lives each year. Cancer takes about 300,000 more. In addition, the amount of disability and suffering, both physical and mental, caused by these diseases is staggering.

HEART DISEASES

Deaths from diseases of the heart and blood vessels —cardiovascular diseases—have increased progressively each year and for a considerable number of years have ranked as the leading cause of death in this country. (See Table 1.1.) The increase in the death rates from these diseases has been due primarily to the larger proportion of older people in the population.

Since 1940 death rates from heart disease have decreased for young persons but increased for people over the age of 45. An exception is women 45 to 64 years of age, who now have 40 percent fewer deaths from heart disease than in 1940.

The major types of cardiovascular disease in order of their importance as causes of death are coronary heart disease (56 percent) and stroke (20 percent). This is a remarkable change from 50 years ago when infections—rheumatic fever, infections of the heart valves, and syphilis—were responsible for about half the deaths from heart disease. Antibiotic drugs, particularly penicillin, are primarily responsible for this change.

CORONARY HEART DISEASE

The type of heart disease that causes most deaths in this country is coronary heart disease, also called *coronary thrombosis* or *myocardial infarc-*

tion. Coronary heart disease occurs when a coronary artery or one of its branches becomes plugged or obstructed. The heart muscle receives its oxygen and nourishment not from the blood that passes through the heart cavity, but from the blood that is carried by the coronary arteries. (See Figure 5.1.)

The basic reason for obstruction of the coronary arteries is arteriosclerosis (hardening of the arteries), a chronic degenerative process that frequently develops in the walls of arteries. The most common type of arteriosclerosis is atherosclerosis—a condition in which the inner lining of the artery is made thick and irregular by deposits of fatty materials. (See Figure 5.1.) This may begin in youth and usually progresses with age. It may occur in arteries in all parts of the body but its results are particularly serious when it affects the arteries that supply the heart and the brain.

Arteriosclerosis begins when small globules or plaques of fatty substances, such as cholesterol, form in the walls of the arteries. Later, calcium may be deposited in these plaques. As the inner walls of these arteries become thicker and the openings (the lumens) in them become smaller, there is a gradual reduction in the amount of blood that can pass through them. The heart, brain, kidneys, lower extremities, and other organs or groups of

Figure 5.1 The coronary arteries supply blood to the heart muscle. Clots in narrowed, irregular portions of the coronary arteries are likely to result in heart attacks.

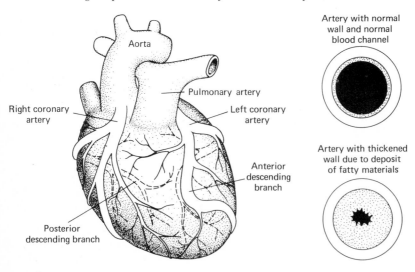

cells supplied by such arteries then suffer from a diminished blood supply. When the brain does not receive its necessary blood supply, strokes or mental disorders, including senility, may result. Arteriosclerotic arteries in the kidneys may interfere with the removal of waste products from the blood and cause a serious chronic disease of the kidneys, called *chronic nephritis* or *Bright's disease*. When the heart is involved, coronary artery disease results.

Along with the problem of diminished blood supply, another serious consequence of arteriosclerosis is clotting within a blood vessel, a condition called *thrombosis*. Blood which flows through normal blood vessels has little tendency to form a clot. However, as blood flows through arteriosclerotic vessels with roughened linings, clots are likely to form. When clots, or *thrombi*, occur in blood vessels of the brain, the condition called *cerebral thrombosis* results. When thrombi occur in the blood vessels which supply the heart muscle, *coronary thrombosis* results. When a portion of the heart muscle loses its supply of blood due to a thrombus, it dies. If one of the larger branches of a coronary artery is plugged, the heart may stop contracting or beating effectively, thereby causing sudden death.

Between 60 and 70 percent of persons who have coronary thrombosis survive the first attack. The affected muscle, called a *myocardial infarct,* dies and is replaced by scar tissue. However, enough functioning heart muscle remains to meet the body's needs. Subsequent attacks usually occur, but they may be delayed many years, so that during the period between attacks, the patient is usually able to live a relatively normal life.

The obstruction, partial or complete, of the coronary arteries is frequently accompanied by severe attacks of pain called *angina pectoris*. This pain usually originates in the region of the heart and radiates to the left shoulder and down the left arm.

Coronary thrombosis is the most common cause of death from heart disease. The younger victims are frequently those who were once strong and active, but who, for various reasons, allowed themselves to slip into a kind of muscular retirement. Sedentary living seems to predispose to coronary heart disease.

Sometimes a piece of a clot in a blood vessel may break loose and be carried along in the bloodstream. This is called an *embolus*. When it reaches a vessel too small for it to pass through, it plugs the vessel, cutting off the blood supply to whatever tissues lie beyond it, resulting in the death of such tissues. Emboli may destroy large or small areas of tissue in kidneys, spleen, lungs, liver, and the brain. Although most emboli are detached portions of thrombi, any foreign substance, such as fat or air, which is carried along in the bloodstream until it blocks a passageway, can produce embolism.

High-risk factors No single factor has been identified as the cause of atherosclerosis or of coronary heart disease and the strokes that result from it. However, various studies indicate that a number of factors are associated with an increased risk of these diseases. (See Figure 5.2.) These include advanced age, being male, heredity (having a family history of heart disease), cigarette smoking, hypertension (high blood pressure), abnormally large amounts of cholesterol in the blood, obesity, excess fat in the diet, emotional stress, and lack of exercise. Diabetes mellitus, gout, and hypothyroidism also increase the risk of coronary heart disease.

Age Death rates from cardiovascular diseases increase progressively with age. However, 45 percent of American soldiers in their early twenties who were killed in action in Vietnam showed evidence of beginning coronary artery disease, and 5 percent showed evidence of severe disease even though they had been unaware of the problem. Other studies of the coronary arteries of children in their early teens and even younger revealed surprising evidence of beginning atherosclerosis. Hence, for most Americans, especially males, the question seems to be not "Who has atherosclerosis?" but rather "How much atherosclerosis, in what arteries, and how rapidly will it progress?" We cannot control age, but we can control some of the important factors that contribute to the progress of atherosclerosis into serious, disabling, and frequently fatal diseases.

Sex Coronary heart disease is much more common in men than in women. The lower rate among women probably is due to some protection by hormones secreted by the ovaries.

Heredity Still another risk factor which we cannot change is heredity. How heredity influences coronary heart disease is not known. However, if close relatives have had high blood pressure or coronary heart disease, one should be especially careful in the ways indicated later in this chapter.

Cigarette smoking Coronary heart disease occurs three times more frequently in men and two times more frequently in women who smoke cigarettes than in nonsmokers of the same age. The risk of contracting this disease increases with the amount of smoking and degree of inhalation and decreases with the cessation of smoking. The avoidance of cigarette smoking greatly reduces the risk of coronary heart disease.

Fatal first heart attacks are more likely to occur in young cigarette smokers than in older smokers. In fact, although the risk of coronary heart disease for men of all ages is three times as great for two-

pack-a-day smokers as for nonsmokers, this risk is 5.6 times as great for men *under 40* who smoke two packs a day.

Hypertension *Blood pressure* is the pressure of the blood within the larger arteries of the body. It is usually measured in the arm. When the heart contracts and pumps blood into the arteries the blood pressure rises. Between beats the blood is prevented from flowing back into the heart by valves at the junction of the heart with the large arteries: the aorta on the left side and the pulmonary artery on the right.

The pressure at the time of the heartbeat is called the *systolic pressure*. This pressure causes the elastic walls of the arteries to stretch. Between beats the contraction of the arterial walls keeps the blood under constant, though diminishing, pressure, thereby producing a smooth, uninterrupted flow of blood through the small arterioles and capillaries in the organs and tissues of the body where the exchange of oxygen, food, and waste matter between the blood and the body cells takes place.

Figure 5.2 The combination of (a) high blood pressure, (b) high blood cholesterol, and (c) consumption of a pack or more of cigarettes a day increases the risk of dying from coronary heart disease between sixfold and sevenfold for persons 45 to 54 years of age. Source: (a) and (b) *Cardiovascular Diseases in the United States—Facts and Figures*, American Heart Association and U.S. Public Health Service, 1965; (c) E.C. Hammond, *Smoking in Relation to the Death Rates of One Million Men and Women*, National Cancer Institute monograph no. 19, pp. 146–147, 1966.

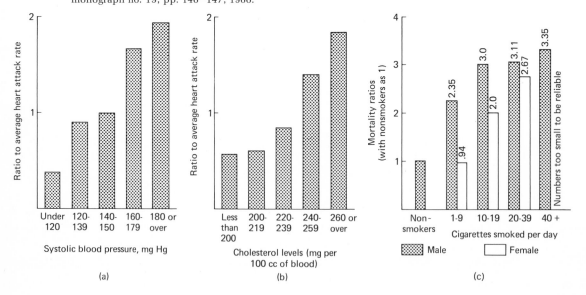

The lowest pressure between heartbeats is called the *diastolic pressure.*

Blood pressure normally increases with physical activity, with excitement, and with emotional tension. In some people the blood pressure rises and persists at abnormally high levels, frequently without known cause. This condition is called *hypertension.* When hypertension occurs the heart must work harder to keep the blood circulating in adequate amounts against the increased pressure. This extra work causes the heart to enlarge and may eventually lead to heart failure. Coronary thromboses leading to myocardial infarctions are much more likely to occur in people with elevated blood pressure. Another possible result of high blood pressure is rupture of one of the tiny blood vessels in the brain, with hemorrhage into the brain tissue, which causes a stroke. Continued high blood pressure may also interfere with the proper functioning of the kidneys or other organs.

Heredity, overweight, and emotional tension are factors in the development of hypertension. Hypertension is more common in black people than in whites; it develops earlier in life, is frequently more severe and has a higher fatality rate at a younger age—more commonly from strokes than from coronary heart disease. Arteriosclerosis is not caused by high blood pressure, but the two diseases frequently occur in the same person. When this happens the hypertension tends to accelerate the progress of the arteriosclerosis, including coronary artery disease.

Physicians have long recognized the relation of salt intake to hypertension and have restricted salt in the diet of patients with high blood pressure. The possibility that salt intake may be a factor in the development of high blood pressure is suggested by a recent study of a large population group which showed that 7 percent of persons who ate moderate amounts of salt had hypertension as comparted to less than 1 percent of persons who used little salt. It has been noted also that Eskimos, Chinese, and the Masai of Africa, who eat little salt, have almost no hypertension, while Indians, Negroes, and Japanese, who eat salt fish and salt pork, have a high incidence of this disease. It has been suggested also that the relatively high salt content of cows' milk and most baby foods may contribute to hypertension in this country, both by direct action and by conditioning babies to eat unnecessarily large amounts of salt as they grow into childhood and adulthood. Measures to control hypertension, including the use of some relatively new drugs, reduce the risk of heart disease and of stroke. Hypertension is discussed further in Chapter 23.

Cholesterol Cholesterol is a crystalline fatlike substance which occurs in many animal tissues and which our bodies need. Some cholesterol is taken into the body as food, but most of it is manufactured by the body from saturated fats, the type of fat that occurs primarily in animal tissues and their by-products such as milk, butter, and cheese. Fats from vegetable sources and from fish and poultry are "unsaturated" and do not stimulate the body to produce cholsterol.

Most persons, particularly if they are physically active, are able to use the cholesterol and saturated fats ingested. In some persons, however, the amount of cholesterol in the blood may become excessive and be deposited in the arterial walls, thereby contributing to the risk of atherosclerosis and coronary heart disease. The amount of cholesterol in one's blood, therefore, should be determined at least once in 5 years. In a large, careful study, men with blood cholesterol levels of 240 and over—that is, 240 milligrams of cholesterol in 100 cubic centimeters of blood—had three times the risk of heart attacks as men with cholesterol levels of under 200. If the level is excessive, it should be reduced by substituting unsaturated fats for saturated fats in the diet, i.e., by eating only lean meat, fewer eggs and dairy products, and more fish, chicken, calves' liver, Canadian bacon, Italian and Chinese foods, and fresh fruits and vegetables. (See Appendix.)

Obesity Middle-aged men who are 30 percent or more over normal weight have twice the risk of coronary heart disease that middle-aged men of normal weight have. Obesity also means greater likelihood of hypertension, increased amounts of cholesterol in the blood, stroke, diabetes, and kidney disease. This is another risk factor that can be controlled.

Diet Diets high in fats, particularly saturated fats, contribute to obesity and frequently produce increased amounts of cholesterol in the blood. Also, physicians are becoming persuaded that the rich diet of affluent Americans—steaks, chops, butter, and eggs—is a major factor in the high rate of coronary artery disease in this country.

Exercise In this country the risk of coronary thrombosis is reported to be one-third higher among people with physically inactive occupations than among the general population; higher among men in sedentary occupations than among farmers; higher among postal clerks than among postmen; higher among railroad clerks than among railroad maintenance men. Thus, regular, moderate physical activity appears to lessen the hazards of atherosclerosis. This holds true for people who have had a coronary thrombosis and infarction as well as for those who have never had any heart trouble. Having taken regular exercise before a coronary heart attack improves the chances of recovery.

Chronic emotional stress Studies of human beings and research on animals indicate that emotional stress may increase the amount of cholesterol in the blood. This correlates with the observation that coronary attacks and hypertension are more common among people whose occupations involve excessive amounts of emotional strain and nervous tension.

Treatment It is clear that although many factors and complex interactions are involved in the development of arteriosclerosis, atherosclerosis, and other related diseases, much can be done to reduce these risk factors and at the same time to increase health, vigor, and well-being.

Surgery for coronary heart disease is discussed later in this chapter. New drugs that reduce elevated blood pressure are not only saving lives but also making it possible for many people who suffer from hypertension to lead normal lives. Research on methods of dissolving clots holds promise of even greater lifesaving procedures for the future.

Prevention In summary, to reduce the risk of coronary heart disease: (1) Do not smoke cigarettes. (2) Keep cholesterol blood levels low, preferably below 200. (3) Maintain ideal weight. (4) Keep blood pressure down. (5) Exercise regularly and reasonably. (6) Avoid chronic emotional stress.

RHEUMATIC HEART DISEASE

Rheumatic fever is a general inflammatory disease of the entire body caused by a preceding streptococcal infection of the pharynx. Although the effects on the rest of the body subside, damage to the heart valves may be permanent and the patient may die from heart failure.

The disease is most common in cold, damp climates, such as the Rocky Mountain region and Alaska. Nationwide, 1 to 5 percent of all children develop rheumatic fever and 25 to 50 percent of these develop rheumatic heart disease. However, in the past 15 to 20 years the incidence of this disease (about 100,000 cases) and the deaths from it (about 16,000) have fallen sharply. Much of this decline is due to the prompt treatment of streptococcal infections with penicillin (or with other drugs when the patient is allergic to penicillin) and to penicillin prophylaxis against recurrences of rheumatic fever. Prompt eradication of the streptococci means that rheumatic fever cannot occur. When a patient has rheumatic fever, he should take penicillin under his doctor's supervision for at least 5 years; if his heart has been damaged, in most instances he should take it for the rest of his life. This penicillin prophylaxis is highly effective in preventing recurrence of rheumatic fever.

In the acute phase of rheumatic fever, the heart may share in the general inflammation which involves joints and other tissues through the body. This in itself may render the heart so inefficient that the patient dies, fortunately a rare occurrence nowadays. More common is the permanent scarring of heart valves which follows this inflammation and which renders the valves ineffective so that blood runs back through the valve, or is impeded in its flow through the valve, or both. With proper care, the patient can still survive this damage for many years, and modern heart surgery has made it possible to restore many valves to partial or full effectiveness, or to substitute artificial valves.

Heart murmurs The rapid flow of blood under pressure through damaged heart valves usually produces characteristic sounds called *murmurs*. The timing and quality of the murmur can tell the examining physician a great deal about the nature of the valve damage. However, most murmurs occur in normal hearts. These murmurs have no significance for health and are caused by the rapid flow of blood through the chambers and valves of the heart.

CONGENITAL HEART DISEASE

Each year more than 40,000 children—1 in 120 births—are born in this country with defects in the structure of their hearts or of the large blood vessels connected to their hearts. A minority of these defects cause a mixing of arterial and venous blood, with a resultant bluish color of the skin; hence the name "blue babies." Until a few years ago, practically all these children died in infancy or early childhood.

The first successful operation for the correction of a cogenital heart defect was performed in 1938. Since that date, dramatic advances in heart surgery have opened new horizons for these patients. Today a considerable proportion of these children not only survive but live normal and happy lives.

The rate of growth of a child whose congenital heart defect has been corrected by surgery is astounding. Such a child may have fallen 4 years behind his contemporaries in bodily development, but within 6 months after surgery, in a burst of growth, he can make up the 4-year lag.

SURGERY FOR CORONARY HEART DISEASE

HEART TRANSPLANTS

Dramatic advances in surgical techniques and in supportive measures during and following operations have occasionally made possible successful transplants of the hearts of persons who have died from causes that did not damage the heart into persons whose hearts were unable to sustain life. Many of these patients have survived for days, weeks, or months, but few have been restored to normal living. (See Figure 5.3.)

Most of the difficulties encountered have been due not to the surgery but to the rejection by the patient of the transplanted heart and to a lesser extent to other complications. One patient who received a transplant of a heart and both lungs lived 10 days but then succumbed. Dramatic as these transplants are, other types of surgery are more important.

PACEMAKERS

Some patients with coronary heart disease develop irregular and either abnormally rapid or abnormally slow heart rates. These reduce the efficiency of the heart and may result in heart failure. The cause of this is improper functioning or transmission of the electrical stimuli that control the heartbeat. To correct this, electrical transistors—called *pacemakers*—have been developed. These are implanted under the skin and in certain patients improve heart function and save lives.

Figure 5.3 The rise and fall of heart transplantation. Source: *Medical World News*, August 13, 1971.

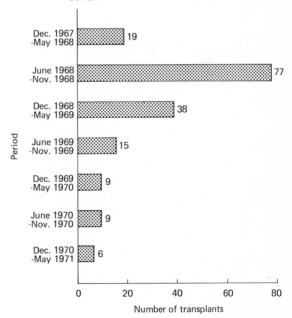

ARTERIAL TRANSPLANTS

In some patients who have had a coronary thrombosis the remaining heart muscle does not receive
a sufficient supply of blood to function normally.
This is sometimes corrected by connecting a small
artery from the inside of the chest wall to the heart
muscle. The additional blood which the heart receives from this artery improves heart function.

VENOUS TRANSPLANTS

Another surgical procedure for providing blood to
the heart muscle is the transplantation of a piece of
blood vessel, usually from the saphenous vein in
the leg, to carry the blood past an occluded or partially occluded area of the coronary artery. This
bypassing of the thrombus provides blood through
the normal portions of the coronary artery to the
heart muscle beyond the occlusion. Many encouraging results are being reported from this type of
operation; some patients previously incapacitated

are able to carry on their usual activities. Experimental studies are in progress relative to the possible use of plastic tubes instead of pieces of a vein
in this operation.

ARTIFICIAL HEARTS

In 1971 an auxiliary pump was first implanted in
the aorta of a man with heart failure. Some observers feel that these auxiliary pumps have more
potential for helping patients with heart disease
than heart transplants.

It now seems that auxiliary pumps or mechanical hearts could not be a major factor in dealing
with the vast problem of heart disease, although
technology is advancing rapidly. The prevention
of heart disease is vastly more important.

HEART MASSAGE

By direct massage of the heart, surgeons have been
able to save the lives of certain patients whose

Figure 5.4   Closed-chest heart massage. (a) The subject should be on a
firm surface. (b) Pressure is applied to the lower sternum.
(c) The heel of one hand is the point of transmission of
force.

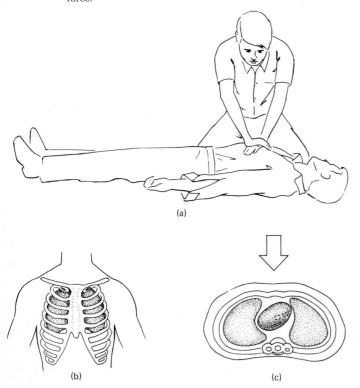

(a)

(b)   (c)

hearts have stopped beating during surgical operations. Recently it has been demonstrated that indirect massage of the heart by pressure upon the sternum will maintain the circulation of the blood and revive a considerable proportion of patients whose hearts have suddenly stopped beating. The cause of such sudden heart stoppage may be any of a variety of conditions or circumstances, such as heart attacks, electrical shock, asphyxiation, submersion in water, or failure of the heart during anesthesia or surgery.

In a collected series of 1,270 such patients a survival rate of 25 percent has been reported. However, resuscitation must be instituted within 5 or 6 minutes because lack of oxygen for even a few minutes will do irreparable damage to the brain. To carry out resuscitation, the patient should be laid on the floor or other solid support, face up and head tilted back. (See Figure 5.4.) Sufficient pressure is then applied to the patient's sternum (breastbone) to depress it 1 or 1¼ inches. This is most effectively done by placing the heel of one hand on the sternum, placing the other hand on top of the first one, and using the weight of the body to get the necessary pressure. After the pressure has been applied, it should be released immediately, and the procedure repeated 60 to 80 times a minute, approximately the heart rate.

Certain hospitals have organized cardiovascular resuscitation units with teams of trained personnel and the necessary facilities and equipment constantly available. The success of these programs has led to the recommendation that all hospitals establish resuscitation committees composed of an anesthesiologist, a surgeon, an internist, a nurse, and an administrative recorder. These groups would have the responsibility for organizing training programs, setting up standards and policies, obtaining resuscitation equipment and seeing that it is at hand when needed, evaluating the results of attempted resuscitation, and devising ways to improve techniques.

STROKES

Strokes, also called "apoplexy," produce sudden damage to the brain, often with paralysis and total or partial loss of consciousness and sensation. The cause may be the breaking of a blood vessel of the brain or an obstruction in an artery in the brain. If a blood vessel breaks, the resulting hemorrhage causes pressure on the cells of the brain, with impairment of blood flow and brain damage. Obstruction, which may be due to a thrombus or to an embolus, impedes or prevents the flow of blood to the portions of the brain served by the artery in which the obstruction occurs. In either case, if the brain cells do not receive sufficient oxygen, permanent damage will result.

Strokes cause the death of more than 200,000 Americans a year. (See Figure 5.5.) Of these, 80 percent are people 65 years old and older. Thus, strokes more than coronary heart disease or cancer affect primarily the aged. In younger persons strokes are less likely to be fatal but they may cause years of disability. It is estimated that almost 2 million people now alive in the United States have suffered major strokes and that many more have had little strokes, some diagnosed but many unrecognized.

The major causes of strokes are atherosclerosis and hypertension. Preventive measures are similar to those outlined for coronary heart disease and high blood pressure. Many strokes can be prevented. Regular health examinations can discover the presence of elevated blood pressure before it becomes dangerous; treatment of the blood-pressure elevation often prevents a stroke. Three out of four patients who develop strokes because of atherosclerosis have symptoms that forewarn of an attack. Warning symptoms include slurring of

Figure 5.5 Death rates for stroke in the United States from 1930 to 1970, by sex.

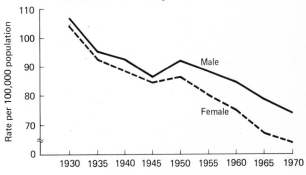

speech, weakness of limbs, staggering, and loss of consciousness. In many persons, narrowing of the blood vessels which supply the brain can be detected, and in some patients adequate circulation can be restored by surgical procedures or medical treatment.

Although severe disability may occur following a stroke, in some victims the disability recedes and in many others rehabilitation treatments make possible a useful life. (See pages 87–88.) Some fight their way back through will power and determination. Goya, at 46, had a stroke, becoming deaf and losing the use of his hands. He fought back and gradually learned to make his hands work, going on to paint some of his greatest works of art later in

his life. Louis Pasteur also suffered a stroke at the age of 46. His left leg was permanently paralyzed and the use of his left hand and arm was greatly impaired. Yet, he returned to his laboratory and carried on the research which provided the clues to the control of communicable diseases, thereby engraving his name everlastingly on the rolls of the great men of science.

Many are helped by rehabilitation programs, which, if started early and carried through, can make the difference between total dependency and self-sufficiency. The problem of stroke is truly staggering, but the possibilities of prevention, treatment, and rehabilitation are brighter today than ever before.

CANCER

Cancer is a word that strikes fear into the hearts of most persons. This is not surprising, for cancer takes more than 300,000 lives a year—almost 900 a day—in this country alone. Cancer is the second largest cause of death in the United States. (See Tables 1.1 and 1.2.) The chance that a person now under the age of 20 will develop cancer some time during his or her life is about one in four for males and slightly higher for females. Thus at present rates more than 50 million persons in this country will eventually get cancer and 30 million will die from it. (See Figure 5.6.) On the other hand, approximately 2 million who have had cancer are living and well; and it is estimated that, if measures currently available for prevention, early diagnosis, and treatment were effectively utilized, more than 150,000 cancer deaths could be prevented annually.

Twenty-five years ago, one out of seven persons who developed cancer was saved; today one out of three is saved; and one out of two could be saved by early diagnosis and prompt treatment. In addition, at least 50,000 lives a year might be saved by prevention of the cancers due to cigarette smoking.

Some of the increase in the cancer death rate is due to the larger proportion of older persons in the population. However, if we adjust for this factor, we find that there was a steady rise in the cancer death rate until 1950 but that since 1950 it has tended to level off.

Figure 5.6 (a) Most frequent sites of fatal cancers, by sex, in the United States in 1968. (b) Total cancer death rates, by age and sex, in the United States in 1965. Source: American Cancer Society and U.S. Public Health Service.

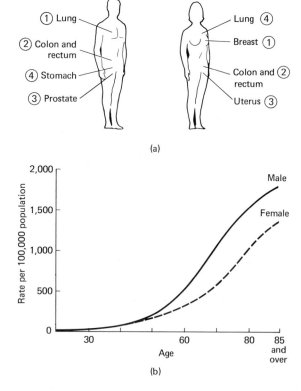

Although cancer is primarily a disease of older people (see Figure 5.6), it causes more deaths than any other disease among persons between 1 and 35 years of age (see Table 1.2) and is the leading cause of death of women between 30 and 54 years of age. Approximately half the cancer deaths in children are due to leukemia, a type of cancer involving the white blood cells.

In recent years, cancer death rates among women have decreased in almost every age group, but this reduction has been more than offset by the increase in cancer deaths among men—primarily from cancer of the lung.

THE NATURE OF CANCER

Cancer is a condition in which certain cells of the body begin to reproduce wildly and without limit. It is a disease, or rather a group of diseases, found in all ages and all races of man and was known to the early Egyptians many centuries ago. The Romans were well acquainted with the appearance of cancer; they observed how it extended into surrounding tissues. The word *cancer* in Latin means "crab," and from its appearance the condition derived its name. The columns of invading cancer cells in surrounding tissues resembled the appendages of a crab; the center of growth corresponded to the body of the crab.

The words *cancer* and *tumor* are not synonymous. A tumor, or neoplasm ("new growth"), is an overgrowth of tissue which serves no useful purpose. Tumors may be benign or malignant. Benign tumors never spread to distant parts of the body, and unless they cause pressure on vital organs, they are not generally dangerous to life. Malignant tumors, or cancers, infiltrate and destroy adjacent tissues, and spread to distant organs through blood vessels and lymph channels. This process of colonization is known as *metastasis* (derived from a Greek word which means "standing after" or "placing in another way"). Cancers may spread to nearby tissues directly as well as by metastasis.

THE EPIDEMIOLOGY OF CANCER

Studies of the occurrence of cancer are exceedingly important and are contributing to a better understanding of factors involved in cancer and to the development of preventive measures. Among the aspects being examined are the high rates of stomach cancer in Scandinavia, Iceland, and Japan; the high rates of liver cancer in South and West Africa; the high rates of cancer of the nasopharynx (the upper throat) in China; the high rates of cancer of the mouth in India; the high rates of urinary bladder cancer in certain parts of Africa and of cancer of the esophagus in other parts of Africa; the low rates of breast cancer in Japan and in parts of Africa, and the higher rates of breast cancer in unmarried women and in married women who have not nursed their children; the low rates of cancer of the cervix and the body of the uterus in Israel and in Jewish women of other countries; the high degree of association between cigarette smoking and cancer of the lungs; the rarity of cancer of the penis in males who have been circumcised; the thirteenfold greater frequency of cancer of the prostate in American men than in Japanese men; the relation, in Caucasians, of cancer of the skin to exposure to sunlight and the very rare occurrence of this type of cancer among Negroes; the higher cancer rates in persons who are overweight; the inverse relationship of cancer to socioeconomic class; and the relation of leukemia and of cancer of bones and of lymphoid tissues to excessive exposure to radiation.

Studies which reveal so many different and apparently unrelated facts concerning cancer may seem to confuse rather than to clarify the problem of causation. On the other hand, each additional piece of reliable information contributes something more toward an understanding of this disease.

THE CAUSES OF CANCER

Since there are many different types of cancer, most students of the problem believe that there are multiple causes, rather than a single cause, of cancer. Some eminent scientists think that certain human cancers will eventually be proved to be due to or initiated by viruses, as is already known to be true for some cancers of animals and of birds, and for warts in man.

Whatever the cause or causes of cancer, the basic process is a change in the DNA or RNA, i.e., in the reproductive mechanism—or genes—of a cell, as a result of which the cell loses its normal reproductive restraint and so reproduces without limit. (See page 339).

The cancer cell tends to be larger than the normal cell, and its nucleus disproportionately large in relation to total cell size. In dividing, it may produce three or more new cells instead of two, as in normal cell division. The cancer cell is less adhesive to adjacent cells than normal cells are.

If a virus is the cause, it probably combines with and alters the genes of the cells, which become cancerous. If chemical or metabolic disturbances are the cause, they act through their effect upon the genes.

If viruses cause cancer, one naturally wonders whether cancers are communicable. If so, this communicability is not obvious. The probable answer is that the cancer virus, like certain other viruses, may be present in our bodies from birth, living in equilibrium with our body cells; and that only when this balance is disturbed does the virus cause disease. This possibility is not without precedent, because this is what happens with herpes labialis, or cold sores. This condition is caused by a virus which is continuously present in the body but which causes disease only when there is irritation from a "cold," from tobacco, from exposure to sunlight, or from other stimuli, most of them unknown. A possible exception is Burkitt's lymphoma in Africa. Studies of this form of cancer strongly suggest that it is caused by a virus and transmitted by a mosquito. If this is proved to be true, the implications will be tremendously significant.

Even though the fundamental cause of cancer is a disturbance in the genes of cells, contributory factors are also commonly spoken of as causes of cancer. Prominent among these are cigarette smoke in lung cancer; sunlight, soot, or other irritating substances in skin cancer; and radiation in leukemia and in cancer of the bones. Such contributory factors may be trigger mechanisms that upset the balance between cancer viruses and body cells, or they may disturb the chemical processes' of the cell in a manner that causes a similar result.

Heredity is frequently suggested as a cause of cancer, but in general this view is not supported by scientific evidence. A notable exception is retinoblastoma, a rare tumor of the eye which occurs in about one person in 10,000 in the general population but is frequently found in several children in a family or in a parent and child. This cancer has recently been shown to be transmitted by a dominant gene. Certain tumors of the blood vessels are also hereditary. Furthermore, the unusual prevalence of specific types of cancer in certain families suggests a familiar susceptibility. Close female relatives of women with breast cancer develop the disease about three times as frequently as women in the general population. Likewise cancer of the stomach, colon, and rectum occurs with unusual frequency in certain families.

In view of these facts, it is natural that members of families in which cancer occurs should have a special concern about the disease. They should, therefore, inform themselves about the particular type of cancer involved and its warning signals. They should also consult with their physicians and have regular, complete physical examinations, which will detect many cancers in an early and usually curable stage.

TYPES OF CANCER

Although cancer may develop anywhere in the body, it rarely originates in certain tissues and organs, such as muscle, fat, bones, small intestine, and spleen. Most cancers arise in the digestive system. Next in frequency among men are cancers of the respiratory system, genital organs, and skin; and among women, cancers of the breast, genital organs, and skin. (Figure 5.6a shows the most common sites of fatal cancers.)

We will consider a few of these cancers, selected on the basis of prevalence, seriousness, and the availability of control measures.

Cancer of the lung Cancer of the lung, the leading cause of cancer deaths in this country, has increased with such rapidity in recent years that it is sometimes referred to as an *epidemic*. In 1940, cancer of the lung caused 7,121 deaths in the United States; in 1950, 18,313 deaths; in 1960, 36,420 deaths, and in 1970, 61,700 deaths—51,200 of men and 10,500 of women. Although lung cancer is much more common in men than in women, the rate of increase has been greater in recent years among women than among men.

By far the greatest cause of lung cancer is cigarette smoking, with the degree of risk related to the amount of smoking, the degree of inhalation, and the age at which smoking was begun. (See Figure 5.7.) Death rates from lung cancer among cigar and pipe smokers are much lower than among cigarette smokers, probably because cigar and pipe smokers rarely inhale. For further consideration of smoking and cancer, see Chapter 7.

Another suspected cause of lung cancer is general air pollution. Polluted air may contain various cancer-producing chemicals from motor car exhausts and from the burning of coal, oil, and other materials; and death rates from lung cancer show some increase with size of communities. On the other hand, studies in California show no difference in frequency of lung cancer among non-smoking men in the Los Angeles area, where the air is heavily polluted, and in areas of the state where there is little or no air pollution.

Lung cancer may be caused also by prolonged inhalation of several different substances, e.g., dust containing radioactive material, chromates, nickel, and asbestos. Exposure of the general population to these substances, however, is negligible, and precautionary measures have eliminated dangerous exposure of workers in industries in which such dusts occur. Cigarette smoking, however, multiplies the risk of lung cancer in at least two of these groups of workers: uranium miners and asbestos workers.

Symptoms of lung cancer are usually vague and frequently considered "only a cigarette cough." Chest pain may occur. Occasionally, blood-streaked sputum is the first recognized symptom. Unfortunately, when these symptoms occur, the cancer is frequently far advanced.

Diagnosis is most commonly made or at least confirmed by an x-ray. If such x-ray examinations are made routinely—at least every 6 months for regular cigarette smokers—the possibility of discovering the cancer at an early stage is vastly greater than if one waits until suggestive symptoms occur.

Treatment is surgical removal of the lung or lobe of the lung in which the cancer is located. X-ray treatment is frequently used following surgery or if removal is impossible. Only 3 to 5 percent of those in whom lung cancer is diagnosed are cured. If the cancer is discovered early, usually by routine x-ray examination before symptoms have appeared, and is promptly treated, the cure rate is increased to between 25 and 35 percent.

Fortunately, prevention of most of this prevalent and highly serious cancer is possible—first, by avoiding the cigarette habit, and, second, by giving up cigarettes if you are already a smoker. Various long-time studies show that the death rate from lung cancer among cigarette smokers who dis-

Figure 5.7 Lung cancer death rates for men and women, in relation to number of cigarettes smoked per day. Diagnoses are based on death certificates.

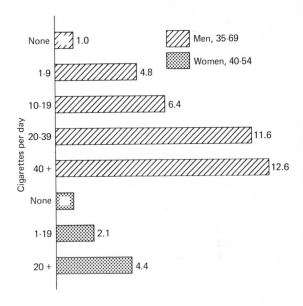

continue smoking, even though they have smoked heavily for many years, at the end of 5 years is only half as great as that for persons who continue to smoke; at the end of 10 years, it is not much greater than the rate for those who have never smoked.

Cancer of the breast With 69,000 new cases and 30,350 deaths—30,100 of them women and 250 men—in 1970, cancer of the breast continues to be the leading cause of cancer deaths among women in this country. About 6 of every 100 women will die of this disease.

Breast cancer is most likely to develop after the age of 45 but is not infrequent in women in their thirties and occurs even in college women. Early it is usually a painless lump, but as it progresses it may cause changes in the shape of the breast and retraction of or bleeding from the nipple. If untreated, it may result in large, ulcerating masses. Breast cancer may spread through the lymphatic system or the bloodstream to other parts of the body, there to grow and spread still further, eventually destroying life. Some breast cancers grow very slowly; others grow rapidly and metastasize early.

At least 90 percent of breast cancers are first noted as lumps in the breast by women themselves. Women can learn to look for and find these lumps when they are very small, less than 1/2 inch across. The American Cancer Society has published a pamphlet called *Breast Self-examination* (available from local units) and has produced a motion picture on the same subject. Many millions of women have learned how to examine their breasts through these media. The society recommends that girls of high school and college age be instructed in the technique of breast self-examination and encouraged to make this lifesaving procedure a regular lifetime habit.

A simple method by which girls can begin breast self-examination is to feel the breast gently while bathing. The water and the soap make it easy to do this. The examination should be done with the flat of the hand, fingers together, using a circular motion, starting at the breastbone and going outward, upward, inward, and downward in smaller circles until the entire breast, including the nipple area, has been examined. The right hand should be used to examine the left breast and the left hand the right breast. (See Figure 5.8.) If any

bump or unusual condition is found, a physician should be consulted without delay.

Not all lumps in the breast are cancers. Some are cysts, some are masses of fat, some are fibrous changes that occur with age, and some are benign tumors, i.e., new growths which develop for a time but then cease growing and do not spread to other parts of the body. All lumps, or suspected lumps, however, should be examined by a physician. Frequently, it is necessary to do a biopsy, i.e., to remove the lump through a small incision for microscopic examination to determine whether it is a cancer or a benign tumor.

The cause of breast cancer is unknown, although there is much interesting and significant information about the disease. For example, breast cancer is six times as frequent among American women as among Japanese women; it is more frequent in unmarried women than in married women, and more frequent in mothers who have not nursed their children than in mothers who have successfully done so. It is more frequent in women whose mothers, sisters, or grandmothers have had breast cancer; and it is less frequent in women who have had their ovaries removed.

The diagnosis of breast cancer is made by careful examination of the lumps which a woman or

Figure 5.8   How a woman should examine her breasts.

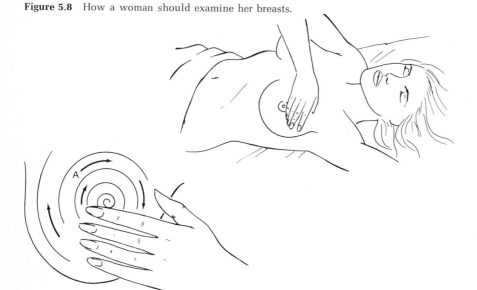

her physician has discovered. At times taking an x-ray of the breast, called *mammography*, is helpful in making an early diagnosis, as is a new procedure called *thermography*, which measures differences in skin temperature, slightly higher temperature being produced by the increased blood flow in malignant tissue.

All single lumps in the breast should be removed. Multiple small lumps throughout the breasts are often due to a relatively unimportant disease known as chronic cystic mastitis. If the physician makes this diagnosis, he may decide that only regular examinations are necessary.

In operations upon the breast it is the responsibility of the surgeon to decide how much surgery is necessary. This frequently cannot be determined until a piece of the tissue taken during the operation is examined microscopically by a pathologist. On the basis of that report plus his own clinical judgment, the surgeon must decide the extent of surgery which is necessary to eliminate the disease. If the tumor is benign—and between 65 and 80 percent of tumors of the breast examined by biopsy are found to be benign—removal of the tumor is all that is required. On the other hand, if it is malignant, it may be necessary to remove not only the breast but also the surrounding tissue and adjacent lymph nodes, up into the armpit. This operation is called a *radical mastectomy*. With more advanced cancers, treatments may vary; again, the decision is based on the experience and judgment of the surgeon and of consulting radiologists and other specialists. It is estimated that 300,000 women now living in the United States have had operations for breast cancer.

Even advanced breast cancer is not necessarily hopeless. Much can be done by treatments with x-rays, hormones, certain drugs, and special surgical techniques to control the growth of the cancer, to relieve pain, and in some instances to cause regressions for long periods of time.

Nationally, the frequency and the death rates of breast cancer have remained essentially unchanged for the past 30 years. However, in many clinics and in the experience of many surgeons, it has been found that the cure rate for patients with breast cancer has improved significantly during the past decade, primarily because of earlier diagnosis and treatment. In fact, the cure rate for patients whose disease is discovered early and treated promptly and properly is almost double that for those whose cancer is not discovered until it becomes advanced. The University of Minnesota reports that 31 out of 34 women (91 percent) were alive and well 5 years after operations for breast cancer which had been discovered on routine cancer-detection examinations and which had not spread to local lymph nodes; 16 out of 21 (76 percent) were well 10 years after operations under similar conditions. These survival rates of 5 and 10 years are the same as for women of corresponding ages without breast cancer. The general 5-year cure rate after surgery, as determined by a nationwide survey, is 83 percent. This series, however, includes women who did not consult physicians until after the appearance of signs or symptoms and in whom the disease was more advanced than in the University of Minnesota group. If the cancer has spread to adjacent lymph nodes, the 5-year cure rate is substantially reduced, but even then the situation is still far from hopeless: 80 percent for the Minnesota series and 52 percent for the general average.

The major reason why the general death rate for breast cancer has not declined more significantly is that not enough breast cancers are discovered early. The responsibility for this rests primarily with the patients themselves. Although most breast cancers are found by patients, many are discovered too late, or women wait too long to bring the symptoms, usually a painless lump, to the attention of their doctors.

In addition to examining their breasts, women should have a careful examination of their breasts as part of a regular annual physical examination. Many lives can be saved and much suffering and disability prevented if women will learn how to examine their breasts, will do so regularly and conscientiously, and will report promptly to their physicians and cooperate with them in the investigation of any suspected abnormalities.

Cancer of the uterus Cancer of the uterus attacks about 44,000 women and causes the death of 13,000 women each year in this country; most of these deaths are unnecessary. Of these fatal uterine cancers, about 3,500 arise in the body of the uterus and 9,500 in the cervix, i.e., in the lower necklike portion of the uterus which extends into the upper end of the vagina.

This type of cancer is less frequent in single women, notably nuns, than in married women, and its occurrence seems to be related to early sexual activity, early pregnancy, low socioeconomic status, and sexual promiscuity.

It is infrequent among Jewish women and among women of certain other religious groups in which the males are all circumcised. This probably is because circumcision prevents the accumulation and thus the introduction into the vagina of secretions which may contain irritating and carcinogenic substances. It appears also that cleanliness of the sex organs of males and females reduces the likelihood of cervical cancer. This is the probable reason that although American Indian women generally have a high rate of cervical cancer, this disease is rare among the Navajos, who have exceptionally high standards of personal hygiene.

The most common symptom of cancer of the uterus is abnormal bleeding or discharge, either between menstrual periods or after the menopause. Any evidence of such bleeding or discharge should be investigated by a physician without delay.

Far better, however, than to await the appearance of symptoms is for every adult woman to have a "Pap test" or a "Pap smear" each year, preferably as part of a regular pelvic and general physical examination. This test, or rather examination, is named for Dr. George Papanicolau, who developed it after years of dedicated, painstaking research. The test consists of a microscopic examination of cells which have been shed from the cervix of the uterus. There are several simple, painless procedures for obtaining these cells, which are smeared on a glass slide, stained, and examined under a microscope. If abnormal cells suggestive of cancer are present, a further examination is essential. This usually includes a biopsy, i.e., a microscopic examination of a piece of tissue from the area from which the cells have come. By this examination beginning cancers can be discovered; they can then be completely removed, frequently by means of a relatively minor operation.

The development of the Pap test has been a real breakthrough in the control of cancer of the uterus. If women would utilize it regularly and follow through on any suspicious findings, the suffering and the deaths caused by cancer of the cervix could be completely eliminated and many other cancers of the uterus could be diagnosed while still curable. Progress in this direction is substantial and heartening, for the age-adjusted death rate from uterine cancer declined from 27 per 100,000 women in 1930 to 18 in 1950 and to 10 in 1970. Yet only about half the women in this country have ever had a Pap test and many of those who have had one or two tests do not have them regularly.

Since some women are unable to have a physician make this test in connection with a pelvic examination, a special kit has been developed with which a woman can herself obtain by vaginal irrigation a specimen for examination. Information concerning the availability of these kits can be obtained from one's physician or from the American Cancer Society.

Cancers of the digestive organs Approximately 100,000 cancer deaths in this country each year—one-third of the total—are from cancers which develop in organs or tissues associated with the digestive processes. The following are the most common of these cancers:

Cancer of the tissues of the mouth, including the pharynx, are responsible for 6,950 deaths each year in this country: 5,100 in men and 1,850 in women. Most of these cancers are due to chronic irritation from snuff, tobacco chewing, or smoking; to unhygienic mouths; or to jagged teeth or ill-fitting dentures. These cancers, therefore, are clearly preventable. Persistent sores, crusts, growths, or white spots on tongue, lips, or cheek are danger signals and should be investigated promptly and treated properly.

Cancer of the esophagus causes about 4,600 deaths of men and 1,500 of women each year. Major identifiable causes are heavy drinking of "hard liquor" and heavy smoking. A common early symptom is difficulty in swallowing. Cure rates are low.

Cancer of the stomach, which for some years has been decreasing, still causes about 15,600 deaths each year (9,300 in men and 6,300 in women), and *cancer of the colon and rectum* causes about 45,800 deaths a year, approximately equally divided among men and women.

Cancer of the urinary bladder This causes about 6,100 deaths of men and 2,800 deaths of women each year, has been shown by many studies to occur more frequently in cigarette smokers than in nonsmokers. Common symptoms of cancer of the bladder are difficulty of urination and blood in the urine.

Leukemia *Leukemia,* which literally means "white blood," is the name of a malignant disease in which white blood corpuscles are produced in overwhelming numbers. In 1970 leukemia caused the death of about 8,400 males and 6,300 females in the United States. Of these about 1 in 7 were children under the age of 15. The leukemia death rate has increased by 50 percent over the past 20 years, with the greatest increase among adults. Childhood leukemia is most frequent at 3 or 4 years of age, with a gradual decrease to 9 or 10. In adults leukemia begins to appear more frequently at about 35 years of age and becomes increasingly frequent through later life. It is more common in males than in females and more common in whites than in blacks.

The cause of human leukemia is unknown, although in mice excessive exposure to x-rays will produce leukemia, as will the injection of a mouse leukemia virus. Some investigators believe that viruses may cause leukemia in man; although this is still unproved, research on this possibility is being greatly intensified. In human being it is estimated that 5 to 10 percent of leukemia cases are due to radiation, about half of the radiation being from the environment and half from exposure for medical purposes. According to an extensive 3-year study, leukemia is more common among children whose mothers received x-rays before the children were conceived or during pregnancy, and among children who received x-ray treatments themselves, than among other children. This risk, however, is very small and does not warrant the avoidance of necessary radiation for either treatment or diagnostic purposes.

Early symptoms of leukemia in children may simulate a respiratory infection or rheumatic fever, with fever, sore throat, and migrating aches and pains. In the early stage it is most often detected during a routine laboratory examination of the blood before the patient has symptoms. Leukemia should be suspected when a patient is anemic, pale, easily fatigued, or has a tendency to hemorrhages.

Ten years ago only about 5 percent of children with acute leukemia survived a year. Today approximately 50 percent survive for more than a year, and some continue in good health for a number of years. Patients with chronic leukemia, which usually occurs after the age of 35, survive much longer.

The treatment of leukemia is one of the most active and important areas of cancer research. Several drugs or certain combinations of drugs result in the complete disappearance of symptoms in up to 90 percent of patients who have been critically ill with this disease; and in centers with specialized staff and facilities, 25 to 30 percent are now surviving 5 years or more and half of these have been free from symptoms for 10 to 15 years. Some seem to be cured. Unfortunately, in most patients, this improvement is only temporary; after a time the leukemia becomes resistant to the drugs and symptoms recur.

Cancer of the skin Currently, about 110,000 cases of skin cancer, with 5,000 deaths, occur annually in the United States. Skin cancer develops more frequently in persons with light or ruddy skins than in persons with dark skins. It is rare in Negroes. Most cancers of the skin are preventable or curable. (See page 232.)

THE CONTROL OF CANCER

PREVENTION OF CANCER

The prevention of cancer depends primarily on the avoidance of exposure to substances or conditions that cause cancer. This was first demonstrated in 1775 by Sir Percival Pott, a British physician, who noted that cancers of the scrotum occurred with great frequency among chimney sweeps and then proved that these cancers could be prevented by regular washing after exposure to soot.

The most important environmental cause of cancer is cigarette smoking; also incriminated, though to a less extent, is the use of tobacco in other forms, such as cigars, pipes, snuff, and chewing tobacco. The avoidance of excessive exposure to sunlight, particularly by blond persons, will prevent many cases of cancer of the skin. And the reduction of exposure to cancer-producing substances has virtually eliminated the cancers associated with certain occupations, such as bladder tumors in the aniline dye and the rubber industries; skin cancers from pitch, coal tar, paraffin, and certain plastics and lacquers; and lung cancer among arsenic, beryllium chromate, and nonsmoking asbestos workers and uranium miners.

Cleanliness reduces the frequency of cancer of the penis in men and of cancer of the genital organs in women. Cancer of the penis practically never occurs in men who have been circumcised, and cancer of the cervix is infrequent among women whose husbands have been circumcised.

TREATMENT OF CANCER

A prime requisite for the successful treatment of cancer is its discovery while it is still localized, i.e., before it has spread to adjacent tissues or to other parts of the body. For some cancers, early diagnosis is not difficult. This is particularly true of cancers on the surface of the body or in body orifices that can be easily examined, and of cancers from which abnormal cells are given off in a manner that permits their collection and examination.

To obtain such early diagnosis, regular physical examinations, as advised by one's physician, are most important. Important also is alertness to the development of signs and symptoms which may be due to cancer. The American Cancer Society has listed these as the Seven Warning signals:

1 Unusual bleeding or discharge
2 A lump or thickening in the breast or elsewhere
3 A sore that does not heal
4 Change in bowel or bladder habits
5 Hoarseness or cough
6 Indigestion or difficulty in swallowing
7 Change in a wart or mole

Such signs or symptoms are usually due to conditions other than cancer. Their nature, however, should always be investigated by a physician to determine the cause and to obtain proper care.

The objective of treatment of cancer is to remove or destroy the cancer cells without serious damage to other body cells and tissues. This is accomplished primarily by surgery or radiation.

When the cancer is localized, complete removal or destruction is usually possible, but when cancer cells have invaded surrounding tissues or have spread through blood or lymph vessels to other parts of the body, complete removal or destruction is impossible.

Radiation for the treatment of cancer is usually provided by x-ray machines, "cobalt bombs," or some other high-voltage apparatus. To be successful, radiotherapy requires precise techniques as well as proper and adequate sources of radiation.

Radiation is sometimes used in conjunction with surgery to destroy cancer cells that may have been left after an operation. It is useful also to retard the growth and decrease the size of cancers that cannot be removed, thereby relieving pain and giving the patient added months or years of life. In some instances, extremely high-voltage radiation causes some advanced cancers, even of the lung, to regress and in a few instances to disappear.

Certain drugs, antibiotics, chemicals, and hormones are also utilized for the treatment of cancer, particularly for cancers such as leukemia which affect the body as a whole, or those which have spread from their original source throughout the body. One of these drugs, called *methotrexate*, has cured a considerable number of patients with choriocarcinoma, a rare (but uniformly fatal if untreated) cancer that occasionally follows childbirth. This same drug is now resulting in the apparent cure of a considerable proportion of patients with Burkitt's lymphoma—a highly fatal type of cancer that is found primarily in children in tropical Africa.

In the treatment of certain types of cancer, drugs or hormones sometimes give dramatic results. Patients who are incapacitated, and even near death, regain their health. Unfortunately, after varying intervals of weeks, months, or years, the disease usually recurs and progresses. In some instances cancers which have become resistant to one drug will respond favorably to another drug— but again only temporarily.

The chemotherapy (drug treatment) of cancer is under extensive and intensive investigation. Each year brings some progress, and it is hoped that increasingly effective drugs will be developed. This hope, however, must be tempered by caution against unjustified claims for drugs or preparations that are promoted for the treatment of cancer without adequate testing and evaluation.

CANCER QUACKERY

The cancer quack is the most despicable of all the vultures who prey upon human misery. He alleges that he cures cancer without surgery, using electrical treatments, salves, light, diet, injections, pills, etc. His treatment is worthless; but worse still, while the patient relies on his treatment, the cancer progresses until even the best of medical care is unavailing.

The reasons why some people believe that irregular forms of treatment have been helpful are: (1) cancer is a capricious disease; it has many forms; it does not always run a predictable course; (2) cancer can be accurately diagnosed only by a biopsy, but this procedure is not always followed and people may be told that they have cancer when they do not have it at all; (3) the recognized treatments—radiation and surgery—do not always yield immediate results on which their ultimate success can be evaluated; and (4) patients with cancer occasionally, though very rarely, recover from the disease spontaneously. In these cases, the immune mechanism of the body apparently destroys the cancer.

PRESENT OPPORTUNITIES

Research on cancer is being accelerated, with practically every branch of medical science participating. Although the ultimate cure or prevention of cancer must await new research discoveries, there is much that can be done to protect oneself and one's family from this disease. For example, the 75,000 cancer deaths a year—200 a day—due to cigarette smoking are clearly preventable; also, at least 8,000 deaths a year from cancer of the cervix could be prevented if women would have regular Pap smear examinations with proper follow-up when indicated. If people would be alert for the warning signals of cancer, many cancers would be discovered early, when the possibilities of cure are vastly greater than after they have become advanced. Thus there is a tremendous opportunity for the saving of lives that might be lost to cancer, probably greater than that which exists for any other disease in this country.

To achieve this and to dispel the devastating fear which the possibility of cancer carries for most persons, the public needs to understand more about cancer and to cooperate with physicians in its prevention and in its early detection. As the astronaut Colonel John Glenn said in reply to a question about fear in connection with his flight into orbit, "You fear the least what you know the most about!!"

QUESTIONS FOR DISCUSSION AND SELF-EXAMINATION

1 Why are heart disease, stroke, and cancer discussed in one chapter? Do you consider the authors' decision justified and why?

2 Explain the relationships between events and processes represented by the following terms: coronary thrombosis, cerebral thrombosis, cerebral hemorrhage, arteriosclerosis, atherosclerosis, hypertension, myocardial infarction, heart attack, angina pectoris.

3 For what types of heart disease have death rates increased and for what types have they decreased in the recent past?

4 In what ways is timing important in heart massage ("closed-chest cardiac massage")? When should it be performed?

5 What relation does blood clotting have to different diseases of the heart and blood vessels?

6 Which cancers have been increasing in frequency and which decreasing? What explanations are available?

7 What is the relationship between the terms *tumor* and *cancer*?

8 Which malignant disease is most common among young people and which among old people?

9 How can the chances of extended survival from cancer be predicted? Which facts make short survival likely and which make long survival likely?

10 Which cancers are related to cigarette smoking?

REFERENCES AND READING SUGGESTIONS

BOOKS

Briney, Kenneth L.: *Cardiovascular Disease—A Matter of Prevention*, Wadsworth Publishing Company, Inc., Belmont, Calif., 1970.

A 75-page paperback which splendidly summarizes the significant information concerning the major diseases of the heart and circulatory system, with special emphasis upon reducing the risk of heart disease.

Blakeslee, Alton, and Jeremiah Stamler: *Your Heart Has Nine Lives: Nine Steps to Heart Health*, Prentice-Hall, Inc., Englewood Cliffs, N.J., 1963.

An interesting and scientifically sound book about the various types of heart disease, their causes, and what can be done to prevent them.

Cameron, Charles S.: *The Truth about Cancer* (paperback), Collier Books, The Macmillan Company, New York, 1967.

A readable, informative, and fascinating book by the former medical and scientific director of the American Cancer Society about this dread disease and man's efforts to understand, prevent, and cure it. The information presented can save many lives now needlessly sacrificed to cancer.

Glemser, Bernard: *Man against Cancer*, Funk & Wagnalls, a division of Reader's Digest Books, Inc., New York, 1969.

A readable, popular account of some important recent efforts in cancer research: geographic incidence of different cancers, Burkitt's tumor, the promise of immunology, and so forth.

Sarno, John E., M.D., and Sarno, Martha T.: *Stroke, The Condition and the Patient*, McGraw-Hill Book Company, New York, 1970.

A sound and interesting consideration of the causes and consequences of strokes: physical, emotional, and intellectual.

Shimkin, Michael B.: *Science and Cancer*, rev. ed., U.S. Department of Health, Education, and Welfare, 1970.

This splendid, nontechnical paperback of 159 pages, like the first edition, presents a fascinating story of current knowledge about the nature of cancer, its cause, prevention, diagnosis, and treatment. The author, a former associate director of the National Cancer Institute, is a distinguished scientist, teacher, and writer, who has the courage to conclude that "victory is a reasonable expectation."

PAMPHLETS AND PERIODICALS

The American Cancer Society and The American Heart Association have folders and pamphlets on all aspects of cancer and of heart disease. These are available from local and national offices.

Answers to 101 Questions about Cancer, American Cancer Society, New York.

Concise and authoritative answers to the questions that people ask about cancer.

Blakeslee, Alton L: *How to Live with Heart Trouble*, Public Affairs Pamphlet, New York.

Cancer Facts and Figures, published annually by the American Cancer Society, New York.

A compilation of the latest data and significant information concerning cancer.

Cardiovascular Diseases in the U.S.: Facts and Figures, published annually by the American Heart Association, New York, and the National Heart Institute, Bethesda, Md.

Heart Facts, American Heart Association, New York.

An annual report on the situation relative to heart disease in the United States and the changes which have occurred during the past year.

Stare, Frederick J.: *Nutritional Suggestions for the Primary Prevention of Coronary Heart Disease*, American Dietetic Association, Chicago, 1966.

A lucid presentation of this important subject by a recognized authority.

Viruses as a Cause of Cancer: A Report on Research, American Cancer Society, New York, 1969.

A small, readable booklet which gives an overview of this important area of cancer research.

6

ACCIDENTS, ARTHRITIS, AND REHABILITATION

A 47-year-old woman who has had unusually severe rheumatoid arthritis in her hands for more than a decade has had surgery to straighten fingers made crooked by her disease. She is now spending 2 weeks in a hospital on a rehabilitation service while physiotherapists work with her to improve the strength and coordination of the wasted arms and hands, and occupational therapists work with her to help her learn to hold spoons and forks and combs again. She will go home able to care for herself and her house once more.

A powerfully built 240-pound football end sits on a table in the training room lifting a 20-pound sandbag attached to his right foot until his lower leg stands straight out from the table. If you look at his right leg carefully, you will see the scar where the cartilage has been removed from his right knee and you will notice that his right thigh is 2 inches smaller than his left because of atrophy of his muscles. The victim of a football accident, he is also benefiting from rehabilitation.

These two disparate human beings represent the more than a quarter million Americans who each year become disabled enough to need rehabilitation services. Our rehabilitation facilities are still insufficient to help all of them properly. This chapter discusses the most common problems which lead to the need for rehabilitation, as well as lesser disabilities, and also describes the nature of rehabilitation itself.

ACCIDENTS

For persons of college age, accidents far exceed any other condition or disease as a cause of death and disability. In this country approximately 114,000 people die from accidents each year. Of these, approximately 10,000 are of college age. Automobiles are involved in most of these accidents.

Table 6.1 Accidental deaths in the United States in 1970, compared with fatalities in United States wars

	Total no. of fatalities
Accidental deaths	114,000
Motor vehicle deaths	54,800
Revolutionary War	4,044
War of 1812	1,956
War with Mexico	1,549
Civil War,	114,757 (North)
	95,000 (South)
Spanish-American War	1,443
World War I	51,259
World War II,	237,049
Korean conflict	33,660

Progress has been made in reducing the *rates* of some accidents, but the *number* of serious accidents for the population as a whole is still alarming. In 1970, one person in the United States was disabled every 3 seconds—over 11 million persons in all who were disabled, meaning that they could not engage in their usual activities for at least 1 day. An accidental death occurred about every 10 minutes. The total cost of all accidents in 1970 was over $27 billion in property damages, medical expenses, wage losses, and other losses.

Accidental deaths in each recent year have exceeded the combat deaths of the United States Armed Forces in any war except the Civil War and World War II; Table 6.1 shows the figures. In an average 10-day period in any recent year more Americans were killed on our highways than in the carnage of the first 10 days of the Normandy invasion of the continent of Europe in 1944. In any given recent year, accidental deaths have numbered about three times the total United States combat deaths in Vietnam for the first 5 years of major American involvement there.

Not only are accidents the fourth cause of death in the United States generally, but they are the leading cause of death in all age brackets from 1 year to 44 years of age. In the age bracket from 15 to 24, accidents cause more than six times as many deaths as the second and third causes (homicide and cancer) lumped together.

Accidents vary by age, and they also vary by geography. Wyoming has the highest death rate from accidents (109.5 deaths per 100,000 population in 1970), and Connecticut has the lowest rate (37.0), followed closely by Hawaii (37.7) and Rhode Island (39.0). Wyoming's high rate is due to the rural environment, in which motorists drive long distances at high rates of speed, causing high accident rates, and to the association of mining and farming with high accident rates. Connecticut, Hawaii, and Rhode Island are smaller and more densely populated, and the inhabitants drive shorter distances and work at less hazardous occupations; in addition, like many heavily populated states, these states have had active and successful highway safety programs.

For purposes of classification and prevention, accidents are divided into four principal groups: home, work, other public, and motor-vehicle accidents. (Motor-vehicle accidents are discussed more fully in Chapter 2.) (See also Table 6.2.)

HOME ACCIDENTS

Although the home is usually thought of as a place of safety and even refuge from the world, 26,000 deaths occurred in American homes during 1970 from accidents. Such deaths are most common in the very young and the very old; combinations of feebleness and carelessness are particularly hazardous for these age groups. Falls claim a large number of the elderly, accounting for more than three-quarters of the accidental deaths in the home among those over 75 years of age. Not only stairs and ladders, but such items as scatter rugs and small obstructions on the floor lead to these dangerous falls. For the very young (under 5 years old) the most hazardous types of accidents are fires,

Table 6.2 Transportation accident death rates in the United States, 1965

Kind of transportation	Passenger deaths	Rate per 100,000,000 passenger miles
Passenger automobiles and taxis	32,700	2.4
Passenger automobiles on turnpikes	400	1.1
Airplanes, scheduled	205	0.38
Buses	110	0.18
Railroad trains	12	0.07

SOURCE: From *Accident Facts*, National Safety Council, Chicago, Ill., 1966.

choking on food or some other swallowed object, and suffocating in plastic bags, bedclothes, or other materials.

Although poisoning causes fewer deaths than the above types of accidents, it deserves stress because it is highly preventable. Each year more than 500,000 children swallow poisons accidentally. In 1968, 250 children under 4 died. Nearly half of these deaths were caused by drugs, which toddlers frequently find within reach and ingest in their innocent ignorance. Aspirin, the drug most commonly involved, is responsible for about half the poisonings and 25 percent of the deaths from poisonings among children under 5. The aspirin hazard is accentuated by the facts that adults regard aspirin as innocuous and are also less susceptible to overdosage. Some parents administer flavored "children's aspirin" to their children and tell them that it is candy. Naturally, when the children find it later, they are tempted to take as many tablets as they can swallow, sometimes with fatal results. Chemicals such as cleaning agents, insecticides, and lye, which an adult would not think of placing in his mouth, are taken by children without thought when they are left accessible. Therefore all potentially dangerous substances must be kept well out of the reach of small children, even for brief periods.

A common cause of childhood poisoning, particularly in the ghettos and other slums of our cities, is lead. The origin of this lead is paint. Lead-free paints have been available for years, but landlords, anxious to economize, have failed to remove lead paints from pre-World War II housing and to substitute leadfree paint. Toddlers who gnaw on this paint can develop lead poisoning. The poisoning may come on gradually and without clear evidence of the nature of the illness; later, the children develop severe symptoms. Or if the dose they have received is large, they may become ill suddenly. The symptoms of severe lead poisoning include abdominal pain, forceful vomiting, tremors, convulsions, muscle cramps and weakness, fatigue, and peculiar behavior. Death sometimes results.

Several states have enacted legislation to reduce the chance of lead poisoning's occurring. In 1970, for example, New York prohibited lead paint on inside surfaces, windows, porches, or toys.

Lead poisoning can also occur from use of lead in industrial processes, notably the manufacture of automobile batteries. Leaded gasoline has caused contamination of urban atmosphere, and city dwellers often have low levels of body lead to start with; if they are exposed to further lead, they develop lead poisoning easily.

Appliances play their part in causing injury and even death at home. Cuts and penetrating wounds from objects thrown by rotary lawn mowers, electrocution by faulty electrical circuits, burns from faulty heating and cooking equipment, and even radiation from color television sets are hazards. To investigate the extent of these hazards and to develop pretesting programs to eliminate them, the Ninetieth Congress established the National Commission of Product Safety. The commission is investigating some 200 different categories of household products.

Most of the more than 4 million annual home accidents can be prevented by simple precautions such as the following:

1 Prevent home fires by not smoking in bed or on upholstered furniture, by keeping electric cords and equipment in good repair, by disposing of inflammable trash, rags, and grease promptly, and by using fire screens in front of fireplaces.

2 Provide adequate lighting and handrails for stairways; use firm stepladders, not chairs, for reaching objects beyond grasp.

3 Do not store objects on stairs or near common pathways in the house; prevent the accumulation of ice and snow on porches and stairs.

4 Scatter rugs must be skidproof. Do not have slippery floors, and do not leave loose objects lying around on floors.

5 Do not use inflammable cleaning fluids indoors, do not use any cleaning fluids without excellent ventilation.

6 Keep knives, garden tools, broken glass, boiling water, open fires, matches, chemicals, and all drugs out of the reach of children.

7 Never leave preschool children to play alone.

8 Keep all poisonous substances in clearly

marked containers, out of the reach of children and preferably locked.

9   Keep drugs and medicines in locked cabinets. Throw all leftover medicines and drugs away; do not throw them into wastebaskets, garbage cans, or trash piles where children may find them, but flush them down the toilet.

10   Be careful of doors that stand ajar and of blind swinging doors.

11   Provide handholds in bathtubs and showers, and use nonskid mats in tubs when showering.

12   Guard against leaky or rubber tubing on gas stoves.

13   Do not start automobiles in garages with the garage doors closed.

To attain safety,all members of a family must recognize and understand safety rules and the concept of safety. Such measures as family fire drills contribute to the protection of the family in case of emergency.

Increasing recognition of the importance of safety has led to a gradual decline in the rate of home accidents. Thus nearly as many Americans died in home accidents in 1912 as today, despite the large increase in population. The death rate in home accidents reached a peak of about 30 deaths in each 100,000 people in 1936, but by 1970 had declined to about 13 in 100,000. The credit for this improvement belongs to increasing individual awareness of the importance of safety and to improved methods of building, safer methods of installing electricity and gas, and better building codes.

ACCIDENTS AT WORK

Workers have more deaths and injuries off the job than on the job, but the total of work injuries is still large: 2,200,000 disabling injuries in 1970, of which 14,200 were fatal and 80,000 resulted in some permanent disability. The frequency of accidents varies widely by industry. Mining leads the list of hazardous industries, followed by marine transportation and by construction.

Fortunately, increased attention to safety on the job has led to a steady decline in death rates from work accidents; the peak came in 1937, when 19,000 American workers died in such accidents— 43 out of every 100,000 workers. The rate is now less than half the 1937 rate, so that roughly 15,000 workers finish each year alive who would have died had the 1937 rates persisted.

Injuries to the trunk are the most frequent work accidents, with injuries to the thumbs and fingers following next. (Much time is lost from work because of inflammations of the skin from chemical irritations and sensitivities, but these do not count as accidents).

Passage by the states of industrial compensation laws and other legislation requiring safety measures also has given effective impetus to the prevention of industrial accidents. In almost all states, any worker, including a student working part time for his college or university is covered by workmen's compensation liability. If a worker is injured in his work, say by cutting his hand, both his medical expenses and any time lost from the job will be compensable, which means that the employer must pay these costs or hold an insurance contract which will cover them. This requirement adds to the motivation which an employer feels to provide safe working conditions.

As a result of improved safety, workers suffer more accidental deaths and injuries off the job than they do on the job. In recent years, three times more workers have died from off-the-job accidents than from on-the-job accidents.

OTHER PUBLIC ACCIDENTS

This category includes deaths in public places or places used in a public way, but not involving motor vehicles. Most deaths in sports and recreation are included, with drownings providing the largest single category (Figure 6.1 illustrates artificial respiration.)

Athletic injuries are a common form of public accident familiar to college students. Most of the deaths in organized sports come in football, but the majority of football deaths come in unsupervised events, particularly sandlot. The tremendous potential for damage to the human musculoskeletal system appears in the fact that a fullback hitting another player can generate a force which has been measured at 3,660 times the force of gravity on the surface of the helmet.

To protect the athlete, the American Medical Association urges a bill of rights for all those who play team contact sports, covering the rights to safe equipment, to good coaching, and to good

Figure 6.1   Artificial respiration by the mouth-to-mouth method. Source: Department of Defense, Office of Civil Defense; and Department of Health, Education, and Welfare.

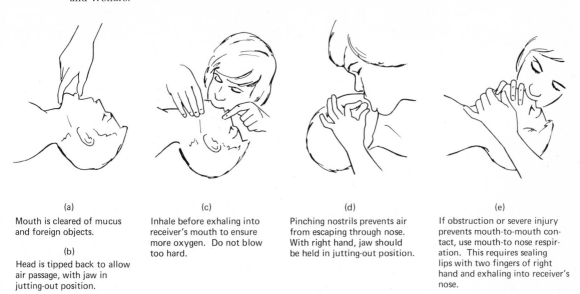

(a)
Mouth is cleared of mucus and foreign objects.

(b)
Head is tipped back to allow air passage, with jaw in jutting-out position.

(c)
Inhale before exhaling into receiver's mouth to ensure more oxygen. Do not blow too hard.

(d)
Pinching nostrils prevents air from escaping through nose. With right hand, jaw should be held in jutting-out position.

(e)
If obstruction or severe injury prevents mouth-to-mouth contact, use mouth-to-nose respiration. This requires sealing lips with two fingers of right hand and exhaling into receiver's nose.

medical attention at all contests, by a doctor whose word is law about whether or not the injured athlete can continue to compete.

FARM ACCIDENTS

Although only about 5 percent of the American population still lives on the farm, accidents to this group are a significant national problem. In 1970, 6,700 farm residents died accidentally, for a death rate of 69.0 for each 100,000 farm residents. In agricultural work, there were 1,700 deaths. Farmers work long hours and use much dangerous equipment, which they are sometimes not well trained to handle.

ARTHRITIS

Arthritis (see also Chapter 23) is many diseases, which have the common property of afflicting the joints of the body. Literally, *arthritis* means "inflammation of joints." The range of disease is from the mild, if bothersome, fibrositis, which causes aching and stiffness but no crippling, to the crippling of severe forms of rheumatoid arthritis.

In 1966, 17 million Americans had arthritis, and the numbers have increased each year since. Arthritis claims a quarter million new victims each year, and causes 3.4 million people to be disabled at any one time. The costs to the national economy from lost wages, medical costs, and other factors are at least $3,645 million a year, according to the Arthritis Foundation. Compared with an average of 27 days lost for each disabling work injury, arthritis patients lose an average of 80 days a year. (See Table 6.3.)

JOINT PAINS

Many people have joint pains for either a short or a long period without having arthritis. One or more joints ache, but no objective changes are present. Sometimes pain is the remnant of injury. Sprains of joints and strains of adjacent muscles may have caused temporary swelling and deformity, and the pain may persist long after the appearance of the joint has returned to normal. Especially when a joint is in constant use, aching following a sprain can persist for weeks or months.

Pain in joints, or "arthralgia," can occur in many diseases. Notably, any fever is likely to cause

Table 6.3 Estimated average number of persons with arthritis or rheumatism in the United States

Age	Total, both sexes		Males		Females	
	Number, thousands	Rate per 1,000	Number, thousands	Rate per 1,000	Number, thousands	Rate per 1,000
Total, all ages	10,845	63.9	3,806	46.1	7,039	80.7
—17	42	0.7	18	0.6	24	0.8
17–24	145	8.3	51	5.9	94	10.7
25–34	533	23.6	177	16.3	356	30.2
35–44	1,204	52.3	412	37.2	792	66.3
45–54	2,253	113.6	808	83.5	1,445	142.3
55–64	2,770	185.5	998	138.9	1,772	228.6
65–74	2,477	255.4	898	198.2	1,579	305.6
75+	1,421	286.0	444	205.8	977	347.4

SOURCE: *Satistical Review*, National Foundation, New York, New York.

aching in joints. This aching does not mean that the joints are involved in any specific way by the infection which causes the fever, *unless* one or more joints are definitely enlarged, hot, or red, in which case they should be brought to the attention of a physician.

OSTEOARTHRITIS

Also called *degenerative arthritis*, osteoarthritis occurs with increasing frequency as age progresses. Wear and tear is one of its major causes, but it occurs prematurely in the thirties and forties in a few families. Osteoarthritis can be detected in 97 percent of people over the age of 60, according to some x-ray studies.

Most osteoarthritis is relatively mild. It causes pain in the joints involved. In the typical case, the end joints of the fingers become deformed, the knees ache and creak, and the back loses its mobility and is painful from time to time. More severe cases damage the hips, making walking progressively difficult. When the hips are disabled the entire joints, or parts of them, can be replaced by artificial joints through modern surgical techniques. Because motion is uncomfortable, victims of osteoarthritis are tempted to remain inactive or at least limit their activities. Such inactivity contributes to increasing disability, however. Keeping active is an important part of treatment, as it preserves the ability to use the joints affected.

Currently, there is no cure for this disease and it is difficult to prevent it from progressing. Fortunately, it rarely confines the patient to bed. Aspirin and other medications help control pain,

physiotherapy is helpful, and occasionally surgery (particularly for osteoarthritis of the hip) relieves pain and greatly improves the patient's ability to move around. Osteoarthritis is made worse by obesity and by injury.

RHEUMATOID ARTHRITIS

Second in frequency to osteoarthritis among the froms of arthritis is rheumatoid arthritis, a painful joint disease which can cripple joints permanently. Rheumatoid arthritis afflicts at least 5 million Americans.

Rheumatoid arthritis may occur at any age. Children or old people may develop it, but most frequently it starts in the thirties or the forties. It afflicts women more often than men. At its start, one or more joints become not only painful, but swollen, red, and hot. The swelling is not just a sensation of enlargement, but is easily demonstrable; a joint swollen by rheumatoid arthritis is usually 50 percent larger than it was before its involvement, or than a similar joint elsewhere which is uninvolved (more often than not, however, corresponding joints on opposite sides of the body are both involved to some extent).

The pain of rheumatoid arthritis can be moderate or severe. Stiffness is bothersome. It is most noticeable early in the morning, and the typical patient with active rheumatoid arthritis takes from half an hour to 2 hours in the morning before he can move with relative freedom from stiffness.

The pain and swelling of rheumatoid arthritis represents actual inflammation (but not infection with bacteria) within the joints and specifically of the lining, called the *synovia*. This inflammation can progress and, as it does so, damage—even destroy—joints. In this severe type, the joints become progressively enlarged and deformed, with the range of motion and the strength becoming less and less. Fortunately, with modern treatment, such crippling need take place in no more than 15 percent of cases. Fortunately, too, in some cases the signs and symptoms of the disease disappear entirely, either permanently or temporarily. Since the disease can recur it is correct to speak of such a time as a remission rather than a cure.

The cause or causes of rheumatoid arthritis are unknown. Much attention has focused on events within the cells of the synovia. There is evidence of general reaction to some component of these cells. It is also possible that these cells are affected by a very slow-growing virus. In 1969 a group of investigators from UCLA reported that they had successfully transmitted an "active agent" from the tissues of patients with rheumatoid arthritis to mice, where it was passed from generation to generation. They hypothesized that this might be a "slow virus," one whose effects are manifested only slowly and over a long period of time.

Whatever the fundamental cause or causes, it is clear that mental and physical strain, infections, operations, trauma, and excessive exposure to cold can make arthritis worse. Such factors even seem to precipitate the onset of the disease in a few people.

The treatment of rheumatoid arthritis is much more satisfactory now than it once was. Aspirin in large doses is the most important treatment, according to all experts in the disease. Not only does this relieve pain, but it suppresses the inflammatory process in the joints. Many physicians have the patient take enough aspirin that his ears ring slightly most of the time; if this dose causes distress in the abdomen, the distress can be treated or prevented with antacids. During the 1950s, ACTH, cortisone, and the cortisone relatives seemed to hold great promise, but their side effects proved so great and their long-term curative powers so limited that they are used now only for short periods or for special reasons.

Several other drugs are also useful in helping to control this serious disease: aralen phosphate and other antimalarial drugs, indomethacin, and gold salts. Heat in varied forms is important in the treatment and control of symptoms.

When rheumatoid arthritis progresses to crippling, rehabilitation services become important. patients must learn to compensate for functions lost by one or more joints. Surgery can reconstruct some of these joints, however, and restore some function.

ANKYLOZING SPONDYLITIS
Formerly classified with rheumatoid arthritis, ankylozing spondylitis affects the spine but rarely the joints of the rest of the body. It causes pain and loss of mobility of the spine, with the spine eventually becoming entirely fixed in one position. Unlike rheumatoid arthritis, it afflicts primarily men.

GOUT
Although the usual estimates are that 5 percent of all cases of arthritis are caused by gout, some experts think it much more common. Gout is actually a disease of the body's ability to metabolize a protein breakdown product called *uric acid*. The uric acid in the body increases and crystals of uric acid precipitate in the joints, causing attacks of painful inflammation. It can afflict just one joint (usually at the base of the great toe) or several joints at once. Any patient with arthritis should have the amount of uric acid in his blood measured to determine whether his arthritis is or is not due to gout. Gout is a very treatable disease, but if untreated because of failure to diagnose, it can progress to crippling and even death by injury to the kidneys. An acute attack of gout can be helped by colchicine, by cortisone derivatives, and by other agents; but more important, there are several drugs which help the body to get rid of its excess uric acid and thus keep the disease under control, as insulin keeps diabetes under control.

OTHER CAUSES OF ARTHRITIS AND THE TREATMENT OF ARTHRITIS
Various other diseases can cause either mild or severe arthritis. Their occurrence makes it even more important that a patient with arthritis be thoroughly investigated by a competent physician and be observed over a period of time. Both the skin disease psoriasis and ulcerative colitis are

associated with an arthritis which is usually mild to moderate. The arthritis of lupus erythematosis is not severe in itself, but is a manifestation of a disease which is potentially fatal and needs the most careful medical management. A few types of bacteria, notably the bacteria which cause gonorrhea, can invade joints and cause acute arthritis; these cases of arthritis need prompt treatment in order to prevent permanent damage to the joints involved.

Patients with arthritis have long maintained that they "can feel it in their joints" when the weather is going to change. Scientists have confirmed that this power is not imaginery; a carefully controlled study showed that weather does affect the joints of victims of arthritis. Patients with arthritis lived for a time in a chamber in which the temperature, air flow, electrical charge, humidity, and pressure could be controlled. When the humidity was increased and the barometric pressure decreased (with the temperature constant), three out of four patients with either rheumatoid arthritis or osteoarthritis developed increased pain, stiffness, and tenderness of joints. The worsening of symptoms was more severe in patients with rheumatoid arthritis than in those with osteoarthritis.

Arthritis provides a favorite ground on which irregular medical practitioners and "healers" attempt to exploit the sick. Since most cases of arthritis are chronic and take months or even years to run their course, patients may become discouraged with sound but unspectacular treatment and resort to illusory promises. The false methods employed are legion and include various kinds of baths, manipulations, electrical treatments, diets, foot twisting, and mental healing. Each method claims its cures, and some number their adherents by the thousands.

Apparent "cures" of arthritis by quack methods are possible because arthritis normally goes through cycles of improvement. A considerable nervous element exists in many cases of arthritis, the pain causing psychological upset and the psychological upset aggravating the pain. Sometimes deeper psychological problems are important also. Any treatment in which the patient has confidence may be of some benefit, apparent or real; any treatment applied when improvement is about to occur will appear to produce a "specific" cure, sometimes felt to be a "miraculous result."

Unfortunately there is no cure for arthritis. Intelligent, individualized, and patient treatment will give considerable relief in most cases and permanent improvement in some. Resorting to unproved and unscientific treatments may allow crippling to proceed to an irreversible point, while proper treatment could have prevented it (particularly in rheumatoid arthritis).

OTHER NEEDS FOR REHABILITATION

Although the majority of cases for which rehabilitation services are needed are caused by accidents and arthritis, any disease which distorts or destroys an important function of the body may make rehabilitation necessary. Chronic lung disease, particularly emphysema, calls for the patient to engage in breathing exercises which may restore some of his breathing function; it also calls for him to adjust his living to a less physically active pace. The patient with cancer of the larynx loses his vocal cords if his larynx is removed; however, he can be taught to speak with the aid of a mechanical vibrator held to the side of his throat. Rehabilitation services can teach many of these people to take care of themselves and communicate effectively with others.

Two neurological diseases are common causes of disability. One is multiple sclerosis, a disease which affects the fibers of the long nerve tracts by a process known as *demyelinization*, and which often strikes young or middle-aged people. Multiple sclerosis is a disease of very varied manifestations; a frequent symptom, however, is lack of coordination, eventually progressing to loss of ability to move a limb. Fortunately the progress of the disease to such a point is usually slow and often punctuated with periods of remission. Fortunately, too, modern treatment is often effective in slowing the progress of the disease. But as function is gradually lost, rehabilitation services are needed.

The other neurological disease causing a frequent need for rehabilitation services is Parkinsonism. Most commonly a disease of older people, its most prominent feature is a severe tremor.

Patients also lose control of purposeful motion, lose facial expression, have back pains, and sweat excessively. In the late 1960s, a drug called L-Dopa was developed which has had considerable success in controlling the symptoms of this debilitating disease. The disease still limits the function of many patients, however. Rehabilitation services are frequently helpful.

REHABILITATION OF PERSONS WITH DISABLING CONDITIONS

As the above discussion makes clear, one of our major health problems is the large number of persons disabled by accidents, war injuries, birth injuries, congenital disabilities, arthritis, strokes, and other neurological diseases. The problem exists among all age groups—among small children, students in school, working-age adults, and people in their advanced years.

World Wars I and II focused the attention of the country on the size of the disability problem. At the same time, it gave special impetus to rehabilitation programs designed to overcome disability, not only for war casualties, but for the population generally.

Estimates by the Office of Vocational Rehabilitation (U.S. Department of Health, Education, and Welfare) and the Bureau of the Census indicate that there are about 2 million disabled persons in this country who could earn their own living if vocational rehabilitation services were provided for them. Each year about 250,000 persons become so disabled that they need vocational rehabilitation services to become employable, but only about half of these are rehabilitated.

In addition, there are many thousands of disabled people who need rehabilitation services to carry out their normal pursuits. Among children, for example, the natural goal of rehabilitation is to enable the child to attend school and enjoy the many activities of a normal growing child. For thousands of adults with extremely severe disabilities, the goal is to recover enough function to be able to care for their own personal needs and to be as fully active as possible.

In the present-day concept and practice of rehabilitation, the skills of several professions are merged into a concentrated program to deal with the disability. Effective rehabilitation begins with a thorough evaluation by medical and other ex-

perts to get a complete picture of the nature of the disability. When the evaluation is completed, the rehabilitation needs can be identified and a program of therapy developed, utilizing medical and surgical services, physical therapy, occupational therapy, and a variety of other services to meet the educational, vocational, and social needs of the patient.

Thus a complete rehabilitation program involves teamwork on the part of personnel in many specialties. These include psychiatrists, internists, orthopedic surgeons, neurologists, physical therapists, occupational therapists, psychologists, rehabilitation counselors, teachers, and social workers. When the disability is severe, rehabilitation is involved and time-consuming process, requiring skill and patience of the highest order. The results, however, more than justify the expense and effort.

At the Minneapolis Veterans Hospital some years ago, one building was devoted to the care of 80 patients who were expected to spend the rest of their lives in bed. For the patients, this meant a seemingly hopeless existence. For the Veterans Administration, it meant many years of medical, nursing, and other hospital care.

An active rehabilitation program was started. By the end of the first year, half these men had gone back to their homes. Of these, half had taken some type of remunerative employment. The others who left the hospital were able to care for themselves in their homes and enjoy other activities. Of those who remained in the hospital, half were able to be up and about and take care of themselves for most purposes. Of the total group, only 20 were still bed patients at the end of the year—and some of these were making progress toward self-care. In the space of one year, this rehabilitation program saved the taxpayers millions of dollars and made life worth living again for these veterans and their families.

A study by the United States Office of Vocational Rehabilitation and the cooperating state rehabilitation agencies has demonstrated the purely economic gains of rehabilitation. Of the 92,500 persons rehabilitated in their programs during a recent fiscal year, almost 65,000 had been unemployed when accepted for rehabilitation services. Nearly one out of five (about 18,500) had been dependent on public assistance at an annual cost to the taxpayers of $18 million. The total cost of rehabilitating these persons was $18 million, so that it cost no more to restore them to a lifetime of useful work than it would have cost to continue them on public welfare for just 1 year. Before rehabilitation, the group's total yearly earnings were $70 million; after completion of rehabilitation, their earnings jumped to $180 million. In the 3 years following rehabilitation, the federal income taxes paid by the group more than repaid the entire federal investment in their rehabilitation, and it was estimated that in their lifetimes these persons would return more than $10 in federal income taxes for every dollar of federal funds spent on their rehabilitation.

This state-federal program of vocational rehabilitation is financed by both state and federal funds. It provides medical and other evaluation, hospitalization, medical and surgical services, vocational counseling, artificial limbs and other prosthetic devices, and job training and placement as well as other services, depending on the disabled individual's requirements. Each state makes its own vocational rehabilitation program available to its citizens, with the federal government sharing in the financing.

In addition, many nongovernmental organizations are helping with this work. The National Foundation for Infantile Paralysis (now the National Foundation) made an invaluable contribution to the better care of poliomyelitis victims in this country and now helps many persons disabled by other illnesses. The foundation has financed extensive medical care and rehabilitation services; it has provided funds for a large-scale program of specialized training for physicians, therapists, medical social workers, and others. It has launched a program of financial support for better under-graduate and graduate training in the health services. Similarly, the National Society for Crippled Children and Adults, with its state and local affiliates, conducts an important nationwide program of services. The "Shrine" builds and operates hospitals throughout the nation for the care of crippled children. The American Cancer Society assists in the provision of rehabilitation services for persons who have had major surgical operations for cancer. Among these are the 10,000 to 15,000 persons who have had their larynxes removed because of cancer; to many of these patients rehabilitation services restore the priceless gift of speech. Still other national and local charitable organizations operate clinics for the physically handicapped and furnish various types of rehabilitation services.

Frequently, people with handicaps take jobs in which the handicap actually eliminates the problems that ordinarily plague able-bodied workers. The deaf, for instance, fill many jobs in noisy industrial operations, where other workers find the noise intolerable. An unusual example is the employment of two young deaf girls as board markers in a busy brokerage firm. The constant hubbub, as sales are made and prices change, had caused previous employees to quit, but the two deaf girls do a fine job and enjoy their work.

Throughout the country, general hospitals, nursing homes, and other institutions are providing custodial care for thousands of persons, many of them mothers and fathers of young children, who could be home with their families; many could be productive members of society if adequate rehabilitation services were available to them. To provide these services requires more personnel trained in rehabilitation and a high degree of community interest and support for the conduct of these programs.

QUESTIONS FOR DISCUSSION AND SELF-EXAMINATION

1 Why are accidents, arthritis, and rehabilitation discussed in the same chapter? Do you consider the authors' decision justified and why?
2 What events are classified as accidents? In what ways do the literal and functional meanings of the word *accident* differ? What are the most common types of accidental death?
3 What is the most common cause of death and disability among college-age people in the United States?
4 What do you consider the three most important measures for a family to take to prevent accidents in the home? Justify your answer.
5 What changes have occurred in the rates of work accidents in the past 30 years? To what are these changes attributable?

6　What types of problems can cause joint pains? How many of these are properly classified as arthritis? Defend your answer.

7　What types of arthritis are likely to lead to crippling (in the sense of being unable to use the joint for ordinary purposes), and how can such crippling be prevented?

8　Which type of arthritis is actually a disease of the body's metabolism? Describe it and its origin.

9　What human and economic benefits result from rehabilitation?

10　What are the principal diseases and conditions which call for rehabilitation services?

REFERENCES AND READING SUGGESTIONS

BOOKS

American Red Cross: *Textbook in First Aid*, 4th ed. rev., Doubleday & Company, Inc., Garden City, N.Y., 1957.

Rusk, Howard A.: *New Hope for the Handicapped*, Harper & Row, Publishers, Incorporated, New York, 1959.

　Developments and discoveries of help to disabled persons; numerous illustrations.

PAMPHLETS AND PERIODICALS

50 Years of Vocational Rehabilitation in the U.S.A., U.S. Department of Health, Education, and Welfare, 1970.

　For many years the Office of Vocational Rehabilitation was little known, but its current programs to salvage human resources are among the most worthwhile and least expensive programs of our government: more than 2½ million dependent handicapped men, women, and teenagers have been placed in useful jobs. This booklet tells the story of this great achievement.

Accident Facts, National Safety Council, Chicago, published yearly.

　A gold mine of information concerning all types of accidents and their prevention.

The Arthritis Hoax: A Research Study, Public Affairs Pamphlet, New York.

　Information concerning the ways in which arthritis sufferers are swindled.

Switzer, Mary E., and Howard A. Rusk: *Doing Something for the Disabled*, Public Affairs Pamphlet 197, New York.

7

TOBACCO

In 1964 for the first time in history the number of cigarettes smoked by the average American was less than the year before. This chapter will consider the reasons for this change in an old, firmly established, socially acceptable, and widespread habit.

Tobacco was colonial America's most valuable export and helped to finance the Revolutionary War. Tobacco was smoked in pipes, in cigars, and in crude cigarettes; powered tobacco was used as snuff or mixed with molasses and chewed. Smoking, however, did not become widespread until machines were developed for the mass production of cigarettes, so that cigarettes became easily available, neatly packaged, and suitable for promotion by advertising techniques.

During World War I cigarettes were provided, mostly free, to United States soldiers. The result was a tremendous increase in cigarette smoking. A second increase in smokers followed the advertising and other promotional campaigns that led to the acceptance of smoking by women.

Greatly increased advertising which associates smoking with health, vigor, romance, success, and the good life has presented an almost irresistible appeal to youth to take up the habit. The result was a phenomenal annual increase in the number of cigarettes sold and in per-capita consumption. In 1963 a peak of 4,345 cigarettes per year per person 18 years of age and older was reached. In 1964 a drop followed the release of the *Surgeon General's Report on Smoking and Health*. In 1965 and 1966 new increases occurred. In 1967, however, a downward trend began which has continued since then. As a result, in 1970 there were 10 million fewer cigarette smokers in the United States than in 1966, despite a population increase during this period.

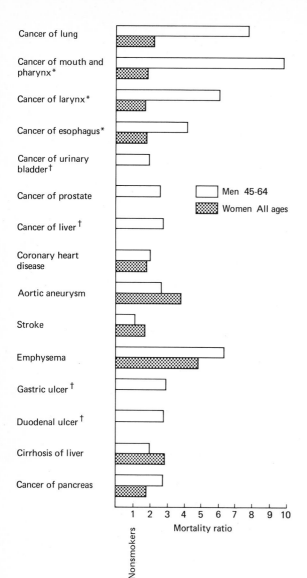

Cancer of lung

Cancer of mouth and pharynx*

Cancer of larynx*

Cancer of esophagus*

Cancer of urinary bladder†

Cancer of prostate

Cancer of liver †

Coronary heart disease

Aortic aneurysm

Stroke

Emphysema

Gastric ulcer †

Duodenal ulcer †

Cirrhosis of liver

Cancer of pancreas

☐ Men 45-64
▨ Women All ages

1 2 3 4 5 6 7 8 9 10
Nonsmokers   Mortality ratio

*Because of small numbers of these cancers in group of women studied, these cancers were combined in computing mortality ratios.

†Because of small numbers of deaths from these causes among women studied, mortality rates were not computed.

Figure 7.1   Major causes of death among cigarette smokers as compared with nonsmokers, by sex. Mortality ratio for nonsmokers in all cases = 1. Source: American Cancer Society.

WHY THE CHANGE

The basic reason for the change in public attitude about cigarette smoking is the vast accumulation of medical and scientific evidence concerning the serious damage that the use of tobacco, particularly cigarettes, does to health. There had long been suspicion of this, and from time to time significant medical reports were published. However, it is only during the past 25 years that the really conclusive studies of this subject have been conducted.

A major reason that the effects of cigarette smoking were not discovered earlier is that the disabling and fatal diseases caused by smoking develop slowly, with 20, 30, or even more years elapsing before the disease is recognized. Unfortunately, by the time the smoking-related diseases are diagnosed, they frequently have advanced to a point that a cure is difficult if not impossible. Only within the past quarter century have vast numbers of people smoked cigarettes long enough to have the effects become apparent in mortality statistics.

The studies upon which the effects of smoking are based are of three types: (1) epidemiological: a comparison of the rates of illness and death of smokers and of nonsmokers; (2) pathological: the microscopic examination of tissues from smokers and from nonsmokers; and (3) experimental: the effects upon laboratory animals of exposure to tobacco smoke and its products.

The Suregon General has estimated that cigarette smoking is responsible for at least 300,000 deaths each year in the United States—more than 800 a day. Approximately half of those are due to cardiovascular diseases, about one-fourth to cancer, and about one-fourth to other diseases. (See Figure 7.1.)

HARMFUL COMPONENTS OF TOBACCO

Tobacco smoke is a mixture of gases, vapors, and chemical compounds. The relative amount of each depends upon the type of tobacco used, the way it is smoked, and the temperature at which it is burned. The higher the temperature, the greater the amount of these substances produced. While air is being drawn through a cigarette, the temperature of the burning zone reaches approximately 880°C, a temperature hot enough to melt sodium chloride and to cause many chemical substances to decompose

The potentially harmful gases in cigarette

smoke include carbon monoxide in a concentration 400 times the amount considered safe in industrial exposure and hydrogen cyanide in a concentration 160 times that considered safe in industry. Hydrogen cyanide is a powerful poison.

Carbon monoxide, the deadly gas from automobile exhausts, combines with hemoglobin in red blood cells, thereby reducing the oxygen-carrying capacity of the blood. In the blood of an average smoker 2 to 6 percent of the hemoglobin is inactivated by carbon monoxide, and in a heavy smoker up to 10 percent is inactivated. Since carbon monoxide has a much greater affinity for hemoglobin than does oxygen, it drives oxygen from the blood. This reduction of available oxygen decreases ability to perform strenuous activity and makes smokers "short of breath" upon exertion. Carbon monoxide also decreases tolerance to high altitudes and has an effect upon the sensitivity of the eye, particularly at night. There is scientific evidence also that increased amounts of carbon monoxide in the blood contribute to the development of arteriosclerosis. In fact, of 520 patients who had symptoms of obstruction of the arterial circulation for more than 5 years, none who quit smoking needed amputation of the toes or legs because of gangrene, but of those who continued smoking 11 percent required an amputation. If carbon monoxide levels in the blood reach 30 percent, serious acute illness results. At levels above 60 percent death occurs.

TOBACCO TAR

Several hundred different chemicals make up the particulate matter in tobacco smoke. There are millions or even billions of these particles per cubic centimeter of smoke. This particulate matter condenses to form brown, sticky tar. It can be seen around the exhausts of the ventilating systems of airplanes or by blowing smoke through a handkerchief. Cigarette smoke also contains a radioactive compound, plutonium 210. If a dilute solution of tar, from just a few packages of cigarettes, is painted repeatedly on the skin of laboratory animals, 60 percent of the animals will develop cancers of the skin within a year.

Nicotine is a colorless, oily compound found in tobacco. In concentrated form it is one of the most powerful poisons known. It has no medical use but until recently it was marketed as an insecticide. Because it is so dangerous if misused, this insecticide is no longer commercially available. The injection of one drop, 70 milligrams, will cause the death of a man of average weight within a few minutes. The same amount placed on the gum of a dog will kill the dog. The nicotine content of cigarettes sold in this country ranges from 0.5 milligrams per cigarette in some brands to 2 milligrams in others.

Certain chemicals in tobacco tar, called *cocarcinogens*, do not produce cancers themselves but act with other chemicals to stimulate the growth of certain cancers. Other compounds, called *phenols*, first stop and then destroy the protective action of the cilia that line the respiratory tract. Still others are irritants which cause cigarette cough and probably are responsible for the gradual destruction of lung tissue that results in emphysema. Every smoker absorbs some of the nicotine and the tars in cigarette smoke. Those who inhale retain most of these substances in the body. Because the tobacco acts to filter out some of the tar and nicotine in the smoke, the amount of tar taken into the body in smoking the last third of a cigarette is several times the amount in the first third, and therefore several times as injurious.

IMMEDIATE EFFECTS OF SMOKING

The beginning smoker often has symptoms of mild nicotine poisoning. Even habitual smokers sometimes show the same effects. These symptoms include dizziness, faintness, rapid pulse, cold, clammy skin, and sometimes nausea, vomiting, and diarrhea. In most people, smoking reduces the appetite and dulls the senses of taste and smell. The brown stains left on the teeth and fingers of cigarette smokers are caused by tobacco tars. The tars are responsible for the loss of the sense of smell, for unpleasant mouth conditions, and for the malodorous breath of smokers.

DIGESTION

A cigar, a cigarette, or a pipe after meals may give the habitual smoker a certain comfortable and satisfied feeling. On the other hand, the use of tobacco may give rise to various chronic digestive disturbances. Several studies have shown that ulcers of the stomach are five times as frequent and ulcers of the duodenum twice as frequent in cigarette smokers as in nonsmokers and that cancer of the stomach is 40 percent more likely to develop in smokers than in nonsmokers.

THE NERVOUS SYSTEM

The most notable effect of nicotine is a transient stimulation followed by depression of both the sympathetic and the central nervous systems. Nicotine also causes a discharge of epinephrine from the adrenal glands. This in turn stimulates the nervous system and other endocrine glands and causes the release of glycogen (sugar) from the liver. The result is a feeling of stimulation or "kick" and relief of fatigue. This, however, is transient and is followed by depression and further fatigue. Nicotine is believed to be the addictive ingredient of tobacco.

THE RESPIRATORY SYSTEM

Tobacco smoke contains substances which irritate the mucous membrane of the respiratory tract; excessive smoking causes cough, hoarseness, bronchitis, and other related conditions. "Smoker's throat," "smoker's larynx," "smoker's cough," and "smoker's bronchitis" have for years been common terms. These symptoms usually disappear when one stops smoking.

The bronchial tubes of the lungs have a remarkable protective mechanism. The cells lining these tubes and tubules secrete mucus, a sticky fluid which collects particles of soot, dust, and other substances in inhaled air. This mucus is carried up through the bronchial tubes and the trachea by the action of the cilia and is either swallowed or expectorated. The cilia are little hairlike structures which protrude from the inner surface of the respiratory passages and maintain a continuous whiplike motion of about 900 beats a minute. Particles of inhaled dust and other substances trapped in the mucus are forced up and out, keeping the lungs clean and protecting the bronchial tubes from damage. If the pollution of the inhaled air is more than this system can remove, or if the cilia are destroyed or fail to work, this protection is lost. Cigarette smoke first slows ciliary action, then stops it, and eventually destroys the cilia.

An analysis of respiratory diseases among 179 boys 14 to 19 years of age in a New Jersey school showed that severe respiratory illnesses were 9 times as frequent among regular smokers as among nonsmokers, and 2.6 times as common among occasional smokers as among nonsmokers.

These findings are consistent with the statement by nose and throat specialists that they can easily identify a smoker by the irritated, inflamed appearance of the mucous membranes of the nose and pharynx. The relationship of smoking to bronchitis and emphysema is discussed further in Chapter 18 and also later in this chapter.

CIRCULATION

The heart rate increases when smoking. In one group of young people studied, the average increase after a single cigarette was 21 beats per minute. Occasionally, the heartbeat becomes irregular and there is pain in the chest. Blood pressure usually rises and may remain elevated for some time.

Smoking causes the small arteries to contract—that is, to become smaller. This cuts down the flow of blood through these vessels and results in a lowering of the temperature of the skin.

FATIGUE

Some people think that tobacco relieves fatigue. This may be because nicotine causes a temporary increase of sugar in the blood, and more sugar means more fuel for the muscles. After a brief time, however, the fuel is used up and the feeling of fatigue is greater than before. It is also said that smoking relaxes nervous tension. This is doubtless true for habituated smokers whose craving for a smoke is relieved by a cigarette. There is no evidence that cigarette smoking has any other tranquilizing effects.

THE ENDOCRINE SYSTEM

Cigarette smoking or the injection of nicotine stimulates the adrenal gland to produce increased amounts of hormones which affect the action of other organs and other glands of internal secretion. In a recent study, nine cigarette smokers smoked cigarettes in the normal manner for 30 minutes. The average rise of adrenal hormones in the blood was 47 percent. By contrast a group of control subjects who had not smoked showed a decline in these hormones, which normally vary according to the time of day. The one subject who smoked cigars and a pipe instead of cigarettes showed no rise in hormone level.

The physicians who made this study did not suggest what effects, if any, the smoking-hormone link might have on health. However, excessive adrenal hormones have long been thought to be a factor in human diseases such as hypertension.

TOBACCO AND CANCER

The disease which people most frequently associate with smoking is cancer, particularly cancer of the lungs. Lung cancer causes more deaths than any other type of cancer, rarely occurs in nonsmokers, and is usually rapidly fatal.

The relation of cigarette smoking to cancer of the lungs was proved beyond reasonable doubt in the 1950s. It was reported that 2,357 deaths in the United States were due to lung cancer in 1930, 7,121 in 1940, 18,313 in 1950, 36,340 in 1960, and 61,700 in 1970. If these trends continue until the year 2000, there will be 125,000 deaths annually in the United States from lung cancer. Of deaths from lung cancer, about 90 percent are attributable to cigarette smoking. Death rates from lung cancer increase in proportion to the following factors[1]:

1 *The number of cigarettes smoked:* The risk of dying from lung cancer for men aged 35 to 84 who smoke less than one pack of cigarettes a day is six times as great, and for men who smoke two or more packs a day sixteen times as great, as for nonsmokers; for women who smoke a pack or more a day the risk of dying from lung cancer is more than four times as great as for women who do not smoke.
2 *Inhalation:* If one inhales, about 90 percent of the particulate matter (tar and nicotine) in the smoke is retained in the body; if one does not inhale, only about 10 percent. Everyone who smokes inhales some of the smoke.
3 *Age of beginning to smoke:* Men who started smoking before 15 years of age run nearly five times as much risk of dying from lung cancer as men who started smoking after the age of 25; women who started smoking before age 25 run twice as much risk of dying from lung cancer as women

who did not start smoking until after 25. Two reasons for the greater risk for persons who start to smoke early in life are that the lungs are exposed to cigarette smoke for more years and that those who start smoking early in life generally inhale more and smoke more heavily than those who start smoking later in life. It is also possible that the lung tissue is particularly susceptible to the effects of cigarette smoke in early life.

Recent research indicates that if one stops smoking before cancer has actually started, lung tissue tends to repair itself, even if so-called *precancerous* changes are present. The beneficial effects of giving up smoking even for those who have smoked for years are obvious from these facts. Beginning 1 year after the cessation of smoking, the risk of lung cancer decreases progressively, until after 10 years it is only slightly higher than for those who have never been regular smokers.

AIR POLLUTION AND LUNG CANCER

Tobacco smoke is the most intensely polluted air anyone breathes. If the general atmosphere were as heavily polluted as tobacco smoke, it would be impossible to see across the street. Furthermore, the smoke from a cigarette, pipe, or cigar is taken directly into the mouth, throat, and respitory tract, thereby bypassing the filtration mechanism of the nose which normally removes at least 75 percent of the foreign matter from the air.

The air we breathe normally is polluted by smoke, soot, chemicals, and the fumes from the combustion of gasoline and fuel oil. These air pollutants contain substances known to be carcinogenic, or cancer-producing, as well as substances that cause chronic bronchitis and emphysema.

Statistics indicate that the incidence of lung cancer among nonsmokers has remained constant while that among smokers has increased logarithmically. Many experts believe that environmental

[1]E. C. Hammond, *Smoking in Relation to the Death Rates of One Million Men and Women,* National Cancer Institute, Monograph 19, January, 1966, pp. 127–204.

air pollution in conjunction with inhalation of tars and nicotine has caused the increase.

ORAL CANCER

Cancers of the lip, tongue, pharynx, and other tissues inside the mouth occur with greatly increased frequency in persons who smoke, chew tobacco, or use snuff. The death rate from cancers of the oral cavity is ten times as high for cigarette smokers and five times as high for pipe and cigar smokers as it is for people who do not smoke at all.

OTHER CANCERS ASSOCIATED WITH SMOKING

Cancer of the larynx is 6 times more frequent and cancer of the esophagus 4 times more frequent in male cigarette smokers 45 to 64 years of age than in nonsmokers. Similar rates for other cancers are as follows: cancer of the pancreas 2.7 times as high in cigarette smokers as in nonsmokers; cancer of the liver and biliary passages 2.8 times higher; cancer of the urinary bladder 2 times higher; cancer of the stomach and the kidney 1.4 times higher; and leukemia 1.4 times higher.

Women smokers have death rates 2.2 times as high as nonsmokers for lung cancer; and 1.8 times as high for cancer of the mouth, larynx, esophagus, and pancreas. The rate of increase of these cancers among women, however, has become as rapid as among men. And in view of the great increase in smoking by women in recent years, future death rates among women for cancers associated with smoking may well catch up with the rates for men.

EVIDENCE FROM
THE LABORATORY

The production of lung cancer in animals by exposing them to cigarette smoke is difficult because most animals forced to breathe cigarette smoke die from respiratory diseases before sufficient time elapses for them to develop cancer.

At the meeting of the American Cancer Society in January 1970, a study was reported in which lung cancer was demonstrated in dogs trained to smoke through a tube implanted in the neck so that when a lighted cigarette was inserted into this tube and the dog breathed in, the smoke entered the trachea. After becoming used to "smoking," these dogs whined for cigarettes, and wagged their tails when they were provided. In this experiment, which lasted about 4 years, 8 dogs, which served as "controls," had tubes inserted but were not given cigarettes. Of the others, 24 were put on a regimen of "heavy smoking" of nonfilter cigarettes (7 per day); 12 on a "light schedule" of nonfilter smoking; and 12 on a regimen of filter-tip smoking.[2]

After more than 2 years none of the control dogs had died, but half of the heavy smokers, 1/6 of the light nonfilter smokers, and 1/6 of the filter smokers had died. The remaining dogs were then put to death and their lungs examined. Tumors were found in 25 percent of the controls (2 out of 8); 33 percent of those on "effective" filter-tip cigarettes (4 out of 12); 58 percent of those on a light schedule of nonfilter cigarettes (7 out of 12); and 79 percent of the heavy smokers of nonfilters (19 out of 24). Virtually all the heavy smokers showed evidence of emphysema as well. The death rates and the tumors produced were in direct relation to the amount of tar and nicotine in the smoke inhaled.

These results show beyond question that cigarette smoking will produce cancer in laboratory animals as well as in man; that the number of tumors is directly related to the amount of smoking; and that "effective filters" reduce but do not eliminate the hazard.[3]

Briefly summarized, the evidence that cigarette smoking causes lung cancer is as follows: (1) Cigarette smoke contains substances that produce lung cancer in animals. (2) Lung cancer and several other cancers are many times more frequent among cigarette smokers than among nonsmokers. (3) The incidence of these cancers increases with the amount of smoking, the duration of smoking, and the degree of inhalation, and decreases with the cessation of smoking.

[2]The smoke of these filter-tip cigarettes contained less tar and 37 percent less nicotine than smoke from cigarettes from the same package with the filter removed.
[3]E. C. Hammond, Oscar Auerbach, David Kirman, and Lawerence Garfinkel, "Effects of Cigarette Smoking on Dogs," *Ca—A Journal for Clinicians*, American Cancer Society, New York, March-April 1971.

CARDIOVASCULAR DISEASES[4] AND SMOKING

CORONARY HEART DISEASE

In 1940 a study of 2,400 electrocardiograms of apparently healthy men showed 50 percent more abnormal electrocardiograms of smokers than of nonsmokers. This was suggestive of heart damage, but the association of cigarette smoking and coronary heart disease was first convincingly demonstrated by long-time studies of smokers and nonsmokers in England, in Albany, New York, in Framingham, Massachusetts, and nationwide in the American Cancer Society study of a million men and women.[5] The conclusions of all these studies are essentially the same.

1 Death rates from coronary heart disease for men and women 45 to 54 years of age are 2.8 times as high for men and 2 times as high for women who smoke a package or more of cigarettes a day as for nonsmokers.
2 Death rates increase with the number of cigarettes smoked per day, with the degree of inhalation, and with the age at which smoking was begun—it is one-third higher for those who started to smoke before age 15 than for those who started after age 25.
3 The greatest relative risk of death from heart disease among smokers as compared with nonsmokers is in the age group 40 to 49, with less difference in each succeeding decade.
4 Coronary death rates are little higher for pipe and cigar smokers than for nonsmokers.
5 Death rates decrease with the cessation of smoking.
6 Microscopic examinations of the hearts of persons who are killed or who die from diseases other than coronary heart disease show that there are more plaques—that is, raised, roughened spots upon which thrombi tend to develop—and much more extensive artherosclerosis in the coronary arteries of smokers than in those of nonsmokers.

A study by the Health Insurance Plan of Greater New York involving some 110,000 adult men and women reveals that male smokers as a whole are twice as likely to suffer heart attacks as nonsmokers and that smokers who are physically inactive are three times as likely to suffer attacks as smokers who have been physically active. Also, if a smoker has a heart attack, his chances of surviving are twice as good if he has been physically active. The study concludes that to avoid heart attacks it is best to be a nonsmoker who is at least moderately active. Such an individual is nine times less likely to have a fatal heart attack than his inactive smoking counterpart.

CESSATION OF SMOKING AND HEART DISEASE

Some people who stop smoking gain weight. Overweight is associated with an increased risk of heart disease. Therefore, it is argued—particularly by smokers who want an excuse to continue smoking—that any reduction in risk of coronary heart disease from giving up smoking is offset by the increased risk from overweight. That this is not true is evident from the fact that overall death rates of smokers from coronary heart disease decrease rapidly with the cessation of smoking. Thus the increased risk of coronary disease from the gain in weight that some smokers experience when they stop smoking is small in comparison with the reduced risk which results from stopping smoking. In fact, it has been calculated that a man of average weight who smoked two packs of cigarettes a day would have to gain at least 75 pounds to offset the improvement in his life expectancy from stopping smoking.

Buerger's disease, a rare but serious disease of the blood vessels, has long been recognized as due primarily to the use of tobacco. In this disease, which is also called *thromboangiitis obliterans*, blood flow to the extremities is progressively reduced. In advanced cases, gangrene, particularly of the lower extremities, frequently occurs and amputation of the affected part—toes, fingers, legs, or arms—becomes necessary. Patients with Buerger's disease must discontinue completely the use of tobacco in any form. If this is not done or if smoking is resumed, the disease is reactivated and may result in further gangrene and amputations.

[4]See also Chapter 5.
[5]Hammond, *op. cit.*

That this sometimes occurs is convincing evidence of the addictive power of tobacco.

STROKE
Stroke is another serious and frequently tragic disease associated with smoking (see page 67 for a description of strokes). The American Cancer Society study found that death rates from strokes are 74 percent higher among women and 38 percent higher among men who smoke cigarettes than among nonsmokers; the greatest relative risk of death from strokes in people who smoke is in the surprisingly young age group 45 to 54.

AORTIC ANEURYSM
Another disease of the circulatory system significantly related to smoking is aortic aneurysm—a ballooning of the aorta due to a weakening of its walls. When this condition develops, death usually follows rupture of the aneurysm. Why this disease occurs with increased frequency in cigarette smokers is unknown. Yet all studies confirm this relationship.

CHRONIC BRONCHITIS AND EMPHYSEMA[6]
Although not so lethal as cancer and heart disease, chronic bronchitis and emphysema are debilitating diseases which result directly from cigarette smoking. The most frequent symptoms that cause persons with chronic bronchitis or emphysema to seek medical care are cough, fatigue, and shortness of breath. Unfortunately, by the time these patients see a physician more than half of the lung tissue may have been destroyed. Many of these patients therefore have to live the rest of their lives as partial or complete pulmonary cripples.

Chronic bronchitis has long been associated with smoking but by most people it is not taken seriously and is commonly referred to as "merely a cigarette cough."

According to a study of the University of Colorado, 95 percent of emphysema patients with a loss of 50 percent or more of their lung function are heavy cigarette smokers. Emphysema is a disease in which the lungs lose their elasticity and cannot expand and contract normally to draw in and force out air. Heart failure is a common immediate cause of death from emphysema. In patients with emphysema the lung tissue which has been destroyed cannot be replaced, but cessation of smoking is usually followed by a decrease of symptoms and an arrest in the progress of the disease.

Deaths from chronic bronchitis and emphysema increased more than tenfold in the 20-year period between 1945 and 1965—from 2,038 to 22,686. If this rate of increase continues, 100,000 persons in the United States will die from these diseases in 1975.

OTHER CONDITIONS ASSOCIATED WITH CIGARETTE SMOKING

PEPTIC ULCER
The term *peptic ulcer* includes ulcers of the stomach and the duodenum. Deaths from ulcers of the stomach are four times as frequent in smokers as in nonsmokers, and deaths from ulcers of the duodenum are three times as frequent.

CIRRHOSIS OF THE LIVER
Cirrhosis of the liver is shown by several studies to be about twice as frequent a cause of death in cigarette smokers as in nonsmokers. However, since excessive use of alcohol contributes to cirrhosis of the liver and since most heavy drinkers are also heavy smokers, it is not clear that cigarette smoking is independently related to cirrhosis of the liver.

LOSS OF TEETH
Periodontal disease, particularly inflammation of the gums, destruction of supporting bony tissue, and loss of teeth, is much more frequent among smokers than among nonsmokers. Women smokers between 20 and 39 years of age have twice as great a chance of developing advanced periodontal disease, and of losing some or all of their teeth, as have nonsmoking women in that age group. Furthermore, the study indicates that men of any given age who smoke cigarettes develop as much

periodontal disease as do nonsmoking men 15 years older; and that the chances of being toothless between 30 and 59 years of age are twice as great for men who smoke as for those who do not.[6]

ACCIDENTS

Smoking contributes directly to accidents by causing fires. In 1965, 163,000 fires resulting in a property loss of $80 million were linked to smoking or to matches used in smoking. Although no complete record is available, it is estimated that about 1,800 people a year die from fires caused by smoking.

Several studies indicate a relation between smoking and traffic accidents (see page 15). An insurance company in the state of Washington is offering a "package automobile-insurance policy" which is expected to result in average savings of $40 a year to persons who have not smoked cigarettes for 2 years or more.

SMOKING DURING PREGNANCY

In a study of 7,500 patients, the incidence of spontaneous abortion and premature births was nearly twice as great for smoking mothers as for nonsmoking mothers; and the average weight of newborn infants of mothers who smoked regularly

[6]Harold A. Solomon, Roger Priore, and Irving Bross, "Cigarette Smoking and Periodontal Disease," *Journal of the American Dental Association*, vol. 77, p. 1081, November 1968.

throughout pregnancy was 170 grams less than the weight of infants of mothers who never smoked. It is possible also that nursing infants may be affected by the traces of nicotine which have been found in the milk of mothers who smoke.

Using a technique that makes possible the visualization of blood flow through organs and tissues of the body, several investigators in this country have shown that smoking cigarettes substantially reduces blood flow through the placenta from which the developing baby obtains its oxygen and its food.

A 10-year study in Britain concludes that "regular smoking during pregnancy retards growth of the fetus, and may cause stillbirth and abortion; the retarding effect is a direct one. One in five of unsuccessful pregnancies in women who smoke regularly might have been successful if the mother did not smoke."

The 1971 United States Surgeon General's report to Congress on the health consequences of smoking stated that there is now a substantial body of evidence which clearly supports the view that maternal smoking during pregnancy harms the unborn child by exerting a retarding influence on fetal growth. It also says that one-third of all women of childbearing age are smokers and that the numbers are building up as more and more teenage girls get started on the smoking habit.

ILLNESS AND DISABILITY

Another effect of smoking that has long been recognized by physicians but only recently extensively measured is its relation to illness and disability. Such measurement has been taken annually since 1964 as part of the National Health Survey conducted by the U.S. Public Health Service. Among the conclusions of this survey relative to smoking are the following:

1 Days lost from work by men who smoke two or more packs of cigarettes a day are 65 percent higher and by women 75 percent higher than by nonsmokers.

2 Days spent in bed because of illness are 72 percent higher for men and 132 percent

higher for women who smoke two or more packs a day than for nonsmokers.

3 Hospitalization rates are 50 percent higher for heavy smokers than for nonsmokers.

4 For the nation as a whole, there are now 77 million "excess" lost workdays (days lost which would not have been lost if cigarette smokers had the same rates as people who have never smoked regularly) associated with smoking each year. The excess loss of 77 million workdays represents almost 20 percent of the entire annual work loss from illness in the United States.

5 Incidence rates (that is, frequency) for a number of illnesses are much higher for

smokers than for nonsmokers. Among these are chronic bronchitis, emphysema, sinusitis, peptic ulcer, and heart conditions.

6 There are over a million more cases of chronic bronchitis and emphysema in the nation than there would be if all people had the same rate as those who never smoked.

7 Sinusitis is 75 percent more frequent in heavy smokers than in people who have never smoked regularly. And there are 1.8 million more cases of sinusitis in this country every year than there would be if all people had the same rate as those who never smoked.

8 Peptic ulcers (that is, ulcers of the stomach or duodenum) were reported in the survey as almost 100 percent higher for male smokers and 50 percent higher for female smokers than for male and female non-smokers. There are 1 million more cases of peptic ulcer each year in this country than there would be if all people had the same

rate as those who have never smoked regularly.

CIGAR AND PIPE SMOKING

Pipe and cigar smokers have rates for cancer of the lung 2 times as high as nonsmokers; for cancer of the buccal cavity 4.9 times as high; for cancer of the esophagus and cancer of the larynx 3 to 4 times as high. Studies also show some relationship of cigar and pipe smoking to coronary heart disease, peripheral vascular disease, and emphysema. However, these diseases are much less closely related to cigar and pipe smoking than to cigarette smoking.

The overall death rate is also much less affected by cigar and pipe smoking than by cigarette smoking. For men who smoke only cigars the death rate is 22 percent higher than for nonsmokers between the ages of 45 and 64, and 5 percent higher for men over 65. For pipe smokers, the mortality rate is 11 percent higher than for nonsmokers between 45 and 64, and 2 percent higher for those over 65.

SMOKING AND THE LENGTH OF LIFE

At the World Conference on Smoking and Health in 1967 a group of distinguished biostatisticians presented a report which shows the life expectancy at various ages of nonsmokers and of cigarette smokers, and the life expectancy of smokers in relation to the number of cigarettes smoked per day. The study shows that the life expectancy of a man 25 years of age is reduced by 4.6 years if he smokes less than a half a pack of cigarettes a day; by 5.5 years if he smokes ½ to 1 pack a day; by 6.2 years if he smokes 1 to 2 packs a day; and by 8.3 years if he smokes 2 or more packs a day. Comparable data covering smoking habits and death rates for women were not adequate to prepare similar life-expectancy tables.

The chances that a 25-year-old man will die before 65—during the peak years of his family and professional or business responsibilities—are 50 percent greater for one who smokes less than half a pack of cigarettes a day than for a nonsmoker; 70

percent greater for one who smokes one-half to one pack a day; 77 percent greater for one who smokes one to two packs a day; and 109 percent greater (more than twice as great) for one who smokes two or more packs a day.

That heavy smoking almost doubles the risk of dying during what should be the most active and productive years of life is not recognized by most young smokers. They may not be concerned whether they live to be 70, 75, or older but they are concerned about death or disability during their forties, fifties, or sixties.

A computation of "working years" lost in relation to cigarette smoking—that is, the years of life lost between 25 and 65—shows that men who smoke fewer than ten cigarettes a day lose on the average of 1.8 more working years and that men who smoke two or more packs a day lose 4.9 more working years of life than nonsmokers. Similar data for women are not available.

WHO SMOKES?

Until 30 or 40 years ago smoking was limited almost exclusively to men. Boys and occasionally girls experimented with cigarettes but few smoked regularly. The few women who smoked did so mostly in the privacy of their homes.

Today the situation is vastly different, with girls smoking almost as much as boys. The tobacco industry is promoting this with appealing advertisements "just for women." In the past 7 years there has been a substantial drop in smoking among men but no similar drop among women.

The American Cancer Society study of a million men and women shows that in males the lowest percentage of smokers is among college graduates, the highest among high school dropouts. In females, college graduates and women with no high school education have a smaller percentage of smokers than other groups. Also a larger proportion of college graduates have given up smoking and a larger proportion of college graduates smoke low-tar, low-nicotine cigarettes.

Other studies show that the greatest amount of smoking is by men in lower socioeconomic groups. In other words, those who smoke most are the ones who can least afford either the cost of cigarettes, for which the average smoker spends $150 to $300 a year, or—and this is vastly more important—the cost of the illnesses and the disabilities that result from smoking. Dr. Philippe Shubik, a committee chairman of the International Union against Cancer, noting the decrease in smoking among the better-educated, said: "It seems that the more intelligent people have decided to preserve themselves and the more stupid to eliminate themselves."

SMOKING BY PHYSICIANS

Of very special interest and significance are reports that relatively few physicians now smoke cigarettes. It is notable also that the greatest decreases in smoking by physicians have occurred among chest surgeons, pathologists, and radiologists—the physicians who specialize in the diagnosis and care of patients who suffer from diseases attributable to smoking. Nationwide it is estimated that 100,000 physicians have stopped smoking. Concerning this the U.S. Public Health Service says: "Maybe they know something you don't."

WHY PEOPLE SMOKE

The reasons people smoke are varied and complex. Learning to smoke is unpleasant for everyone and intolerable for many. It is only after one has developed a tolerance for tobacco that smoking ceases to be distressing, and it is not until one becomes habituated that smoking seems pleasurable.

Many boys and girls start smoking to show their independence, as a symbol of revolt against authority, to feel sophisticated and grown-up, to be "one of the crowd," to gain social status, to have something to do. A junior high school paper of Queens, New York, put it this way: "Kids start smoking 'to be in'—the great urge of every teenager. Start smoking; after all, it looks real hip and adult." The advertisers of cigarettes exploit this urge by creating an image of the smoker as an outstanding athlete; a handsome, virile outdoor man; a nonchalant campus leader; a man who succeeds; or a sophisticated, charming young woman.

Dr. Daniel Horn, director of the National Clearinghouse for Smoking and Health, says that people smoke cigarettes for one or more of the following reasons: (1) for stimulation—such as to get started in the morning; (2) because of addiction—such a smoker "must have" a cigarette after a certain amount of time has elapsed; (3) to reduce negative feelings, such as distress, anger, or fear; (4) out of habit—a behavior pattern followed almost involuntarily; (5) for oral gratification—the satisfaction derived from having something in the mouth; (6) for pleasurable relaxation—to enhance positive feelings, as after a good dinner.

EFFECTS OF SMOKING UPON NONSMOKERS

Physicians have long known that some people are made uncomfortable or acutely ill by exposure to tobacco smoke. A clinical study of this phenomenon, made by the Pediatric Allergy Service of the University of Kansas Medical Center, concludes that intolerance to tobacco smoke is common in both allergic and nonallergic patients, and that the most common complaints are eye irritation, nasal symptoms (sneezing, blocking, discharge, itching, and dryness), headache, and cough. It also concludes that the effects of tobacco smoke appear to be of an irritative rather than an allergic character: "The many individuals who develop symptoms from tobacco smoke need the understanding and support of their physician in helping them to avoid its noxious effects."

A different type of study, dealing with the effects of exposure of children to tobacco smoke, has been reported by a team of investigators at Wayne State University in Detroit. In this study the number of acute illnesses among children under 16 years of age in homes in which there is parental smoking is compared with the number of illnesses of children in homes in which parents do not smoke. The results show that rates of acute illnesses (mostly respiratory) are approximately twice as high among smokers' children as among nonsmokers' children. There is also some evidence that the amount of smoke in the home environment may be related to the chance of illness in adults. This study confirms the results of a similar study made in Denver and reported in 1967.

Irrespective of such possible serious long-time effects of smoking upon others, an increasing number of nonsmokers are beginning to insist upon their right to breathe air unpolluted by tobacco smoke. The extent and the increase of such sentiments is indicated by the results of questionnaire surveys of passengers on commuter trains in the New York City area about whether they prefer to ride in smoking or in no-smoking cars. Five years ago 66 percent said that they preferred no-smoking cars. The railroad therefore increased the proportion of no-smoking cars. Then in 1969, noting that the no-smoking cars were still crowded while there were vacant seats in the smoking cars, the railroad conducted another survey. The results of this survey indicated that 78 percent of passengers preferred to ride in no-smoking cars. Most airlines are now providing no-smoking areas on their airplanes.

And the United States Surgeon General in a press conference in January 1971 stated,

Evidence is accumulating that the non-smoker may have untoward effects from the air pollution his neighbor forces upon him. Non-smokers have as much right to clean and wholesome air as smokers have their so-called "right to pollute." It is high time to bar smoking from all confined public places, such as theatres, airplanes, trains, buses, and restaurants. We should interpret the Bill of Rights for the non-smokers as well as for the smoker.

IF YOU MUST SMOKE

The best health advice for those who do not smoke is "Never start the habit"; and for those who do smoke, "Stop completely." However, for those who are unable or unwilling to stop, the U.S. Public Health Service has prepared a pamphlet which says that by following a few simple rules, one can reduce the hazard.

1   Switch to pipes or cigars.
2   Smoke cigarettes with less tar and nicotine.
3   Do not smoke cigarettes all the way down: the last third of a cigarette yields twice as much tar and nicotine as the first third, be-

cause tobacco itself is a good filter. (An easy way to do this is to mark the cigarettes from each new package with a red ring around the middle of the tobacco-filled portion of the cigarette and then smoke each cigarette only to this ring.)
4   Take fewer draws on each cigarette. The "extra puffs" in longer cigarettes are extra perils for you.
5   Reduce inhaling: do not consciously inhale.
6   Smoke fewer cigarettes each day.

LESS HARMFUL CIGARETTES

The demand for filter-tip cigarettes is clear evidence that most smokers are anxious to reduce the hazard of their smoking. In 1952 filter-tip cigarettes made up only 1 percent of sales; 20 years later they accounted for 90 percent. The increase is doubtless because the public believes that filters provide at least some protection against the harmful substances in the smoke. For some filters this is true, for others untrue. Mentholated cigarettes also have been popular, but although the addition of menthol to tobacco gives the smoke a medicated taste, it does not affect the tar and nicotine content or in any way reduce the harmful effects of smoking.

The amounts of harmful substances in tobacco smoke—tars, nicotine, and certain gases—are dependent primarily upon the type and the amount of tobacco used, the process of "curing," the addition of certain chemicals to the tobacco, the temperature of burning, the way a cigarette is smoked, and the effectiveness of filtration. By altering these factors, cigarette manufacturers can control most of the ingredients of the smoke.

Considerable improvement in this regard was made about 10 years ago. Between 1957 and 1961, the tar content of all major brands and the nicotine content of most major brands were reduced; and in most filter-tip cigarettes the reduction was substantial. Since 1961 about half of comparable types of major-brand cigarettes have shown further though small reductions; the others have shown small increases of tar and nicotine content.

Why, with these possibilities of producing less harmful cigarettes, do tobacco companies not do so? And why do some of them object to giving the public information about the tar and nicotine content of the various brands of cigarettes? Certainly the tobacco companies do not wish to harm people. They do, however, wish to sell cigarettes. Since tar provides "flavor" in cigarette smoke, they fear that if the tar content of a cigarette is too low, people may not smoke it. Also, if the nicotine content is too low, the cigarettes may not give the "kick" of satisfaction to which a regular smoker is accustomed. Furthermore, since nicotine is believed to be the addictive constituent of the smoke, if the nicotine content is reduced it may be easier for the smoker to stop altogether—an effect that tobacco companies would regret.

New brands with low tar and low nicotine content have been marketed recently, and several have become quite popular. Unfortunately for the public, the increased margin of safety provided by many filters has been more than offset by the introduction and intensive promotion of extra-long 100-millimeter cigarettes, some of which, in spite of filters, are very high in both tar and nicotine.

It has been suggested that if smokers switch to low-tar, low-nicotine cigarettes they will smoke proportionately more in their desire for the same effects. Experience has shown that this does not happen, but that those who do change generally smoke the same amount as previously. In fact, the switch to low-tar, low-nicotine cigarettes may be a first step toward quitting.

Much research is in progress by tobacco companies, the government, and independent investigators to find a way to make cigarette smoking less harmful and still acceptable to the smoker. Some progress has been made in this direction, but a cigarette that can be *demonstrated* to be "safe" and still acceptable to smokers is not in sight.

Cigarette smokers who are unwilling or unable to give up the habit should seek information from the U.S. Public Health Service, the Federal Trade Commission, or a local health department or health agency about the results of the most recent Federal Trade Commission tests relative to the tar and nicotine content of the smoke of cigarettes on the American market.

GIVING UP SMOKING

The U.S. Public Health Services estimates that 29 million Americans have given up cigarette smoking. Surveys indicate that most smokers—up to 86 percent in one survey—say that they would like to break the habit; and practically all say that they hope their children will not smoke. Why do so many people want to stop smoking? Many have symptoms of diseases associated with smoking and have been ordered by their doctors to stop. Some want to stop because of the influence that their smoking has upon others, particularly children. Still others, although in good health, have decided that the health hazards and the costs of smoking are too great.

What are the rewards of stopping? Those who give up smoking have less illness, less hospitalization, less time lost from work. Unless cancer has already started, discontinuance of cigarette smoking can mean longer life. Death rates of those who stop smoking decrease sharply as compared with those who continue smoking. Ten years after a person has given up cigarette smoking, his life expectancy is almost the same as that of someone who has never smoked regularly. Convincing evidence of the value of giving up smoking is that over a 10-year period the death rate from lung cancer among British physicians, a substantial portion of whom had stopped smoking, *decreased* by 30 percent while the death rate from lung cancer among British men in general *increased* by 25 percent.

There are long-range benefits, but there are immediate rewards also, including reduction and early disappearance of cough, nasal stuffiness, and discharge. Food tastes better, tensions decrease, and sleep is sounder. Fatigue, shortness of breath, and that "dark brown" taste and "fuzzy feeling" in the mouth disappear.

TYPES OF SMOKERS

Many smokers find it relatively easy to stop smoking if they *really* want to. Others find it difficult or almost unbearable for days, weeks, or even longer. To find the reasons for such difference psychologists have been studying the characteristics of smokers and have concluded that there are several types of smokers who may be classified somewhat as follows: stimulation smokers, handling smokers, relaxation smokers, crutch smokers, craving smokers, and habit smokers. While the reasons given by people for smoking may in many cases include several of these classifications, one reason tends to be more prominent than the others for each person. Psychologists believe that analysis of one's smoking habits—even self-analysis—is helpful in understanding the reasons for smoking and in breaking the habit.[7]

Some smokers, often people who are successful in other aspects of living, find that willpower does not enable them to give up cigarettes. They try to stop; they do not succeed; and they feel guilty about their failure. But failure does not indicate that they are weak, merely that they are different. To achieve success, their approach must be less through determination and more through perseverence. A good book or pamphlet on the subject may help.[8]

Placing cigarettes in unaccustomed places or pockets and putting matches, lighters, and ashtrays out of reach help to break the unconscious routine.

Drinking frequent glasses of water; changing from coffee to tea if coffee has been a signal for a cigarette; nibbling fruit, crackers, or cookies; sucking hard candies; and chewing gum or bits of ginger are helpful to many.

Keeping away for a few days from friends who are smokers, or working in the library or other rooms where smoking is forbidden may reduce the temptation to smoke.

Deep breathing, a walk around the block, or other, more strenuous exercise relieves tension.

Bantron or Nikoban tablets are recommended by some doctors, not by others. One should check with his physician to make sure there is no medical reason for not using them.

Most persons select a day on which they will quit absolutely; others find it easier to reduce gradually. To reduce gradually one must formulate a definite schedule: for example, decide not to smoke between nine and ten, eleven and twelve, or one and two o'clock, and later increase the no-smoking periods from 1 hour to 1½ hours, then to 2 hours; smoke only after meals; smoke only in the evening. Or it may help to give up smoking first at the times that smoking means least to you, i.e., during relatively low-tension, low-pressure periods, and gradually extend this to other times of the day.

In gradual withdrawal you can wrap your cigarettes in many sheets of paper; strive to use only the left hand if you normally hold cigarettes in your right hand; or hold the cigarette in a different corner of your mouth. You can smoke only half of each cigarette, or can make it a point not to

---

[7]Copies of *Smoker's Self-Testing Kit* are available from the National Clearinghouse for Smoking and Health, U.S. Public Health Service, Washington, D.C.

[8]Recommended is a pocket-size pamphlet entitled, *If You Want to Give Up Cigarettes*. This interesting readable pamphlet contains helpful suggestions for those who would like to stop smoking. It is available without charge from the American Cancer Society: local units, state divisions, or the national office.

have the change necessary to purchase cigarettes from a machine.

Many people decide to stop for only 1 day at a time. They promise themselves 24 hours of freedom from cigarettes. Then when the day is over they make a pledge to desist for another day; then another, and another. At the end of any 24-hour period they can go back to cigarettes without betraying themselves—but they usually do not.

Dr. Donald T. Fredrickson, formerly director of the Smoking Control Program of New York City, says,

To think of giving up cigarettes as a denial is a mistake. The smoker should not feel that he is giving up something of value. If he does, he will feel sorry for himself; he will brood on his sufferings, which will become increasingly severe and possibly unendurable. Instead he should feel that he is adding something to his life—a new dimension of self-control. He is teaching himself a more positive, constructive, self-fulfilling way to behave. There is evidence that the development of control over cigarette smoking, for some at least, tends to influence other areas of behavior, bringing a renewed sense of one's capacity to deal more constructively with other "problems of living." When experienced, this can serve as a powerful incentive reinforcing nonsmoking behavior.

Programs to aid people who really want to give up smoking are of several types: (1) quitting on your own: programs of self-help based upon books, pamphlets, magazine articles, radio or television programs, lectures, etc.; (2) group sessions, often called *withdrawal programs* or *clinics*; (3) actual clinics operated by hospitals or medical or health organizations; (4) individual medical care provided by a physician in a doctor-patient relationship.

Self-help or do-it-yourself programs are all that many smokers need. Sufficiently motivated people are convinced that they can manage their own lives. They enjoy challenging themselves; with the exercise of willpower they break the habit. The ex-smoker teaches himself a more positive, more constructive, more rewarding behavior, and feels better physically.

Increasingly, health departments, health centers, hospitals, and individual physicians are offering special programs of group sessions, withdrawal clinics, or individual medical counseling.

At the World Conference on Smoking and Health, Sir George Godber said: "It is never *too late* to stop smoking for the benefit of one's health; and it is never *too early* to stop for the benefit of those—particularly children—who will be influenced by your example."

A PERSONAL DECISION

The conclusion that cigarette smoking is a serious health hazard is inescapable. The scientific data, some of which are presented in this book, as well as the statements of responsible medical and health authorities in this country and abroad, leave no doubt about this. Yet cigarette smoking is widespread and socially acceptable, and to many smokers it provides certain satisfactions. Most of these appear to be psychological, although the drug effect of nicotine is probably an important factor in the strongly addicted smoker.

Smoking also is big business, promoted by extensive, attractive, and persuasive advertising and by the ablest public relations that an $8 billion business can provide. Its effective political lobbies try to guard against legislative actions or ad-

ministrative controls that may interfere with this business.

Government regulation of the labeling, advertising, and other types of promotion of cigarettes is important, but cigarettes will always be available. The decision about what to do about smoking is therefore up to the individual. As a behavioral phenomenon and a psychological habit it can be understood and changed. With adequate information and strong motivation—and in some cases with support and guidance—smoking can be avoided or controlled as one wishes. The individual, however, must initiate his own self-help program or must himself decide to seek professional help when he is unable to break the habit on his own.

QUESTIONS FOR DISCUSSION AND SELF-EXAMINATION

1   Describe and comment on the changes in the amount of cigarette smoking in the past 50 years.
2   Detail the harmful effects of the various toxic substances in cigarette smoke.
3   Compare the short-term effects of cigarettes with their long-term effects.
4   What is the relation of cigarette smoking to general air pollution in causing lung cancer?
5   How are (a) number of cigarettes smoked, (b) inhalation of cigarette smoke, and (c) age of beginning to smoke related to the likelihood of developing lung cancer? Give details.
6   How does the relation of cigarette smoking to lung cancer correspond to the relation of cigarette smoking to heart disease? Describe the similarities and differences.
7   What is the effect of cigarette smoking on total deaths in the United States? How does this compare with other causes of death, such as traffic accidents?
8   How much and what kind of disability does cigarette smoking contribute to?
9   How can dangers of cigarette smoking be reduced?
10 What factors affect the success of individuals in stopping smoking?

REFERENCES AND READING SUGGESTIONS

BOOKS

Diehl, Harold S.: *Tobacco and Your Health—The Smoking Controversy,* McGraw-Hill Book Company, New York, 1969.

A comprehensive consideration of all aspects of the smoking problem: the effects upon health, the costs, why there is a controversy, the reasons people smoke, how one can stop, and the basis for decision.

The Health Consequences of Smoking, a report of the Surgeon General, U.S. Department of Health, Education, and Welfare, 1971.

This report to Congress is the most comprehensive review of the evidence regarding the health consequences of smoking since the first Surgeon General's report in 1964. It summarizes more than 20 years of smoking and health research, and presents new evidence on the relationship of smoking to cardiovascular diseases, to chronic obstructive bronchopulmonary diseases, to cancers of many types, and to pregnancy. (Also annual reports in 1972, etc.)

Royal College of Physicians of London: *Smoking and Health Now: A New Report and Summary on Smoking and Its Effects on Health,* Pitman Periodical and Scientific Publishing Co., Landau, West Germany, and New York, 1971.

Smoking and Health, U.S. Public Service Report, Department of Health, Education, and Welfare, 1964.

The most comprehensive and authoritative report ever made of the scientific work on this important health problem. It presents a scientific analysis of thousands of epidemiological, biological, pharmacological, pathological, and other studies of the subject. The study was directed by an advisory committee of ten distinguished physicians and scientists, appointed by the Surgeon General, with the approval not only of medical and health organizations concerned with this problem but also of the tobacco industry. It has had a tremendous influence upon the world's thinking about this health issue.

PAMPHLETS AND PERIODICALS

A Summary of Proceedings of the National Conference on Smoking and Health, Sept. 9–11, 1970, sponsored by National Interagency Council on Smoking and Health, 419 Park Avenue South, New York, New York 10016.

This is a splendid summary of the formal presentations and the short discussions of this 3-day conference on all aspects of the smoking problem, participated in by 300 representatives of concerned organizations from nearly every state in this country, from Canada, and from England.

Brody, Jane E., and Engquist, Richard: *Women and Smoking*, Public Affairs Pamphlet No. 475, New York, 1972.

A comprehensive, interesting, and medically sound summary of this subject by Jane Brody, distinguished science writer of *The New York Times*, and by her colleague Richard Engquist.

Corwin, Emil: *Smoking: A World Problem*, Health Services, Mental Health Administration, U.S. Department of Health, Education, and Welfare, June 1971.

A splendid overview of the health problem which smoking presents throughout the world and what various countries are doing about it.

Elliott, Lawrence: "Still Dying for a Smoke?" *Reader's Digest*, July, 1971.

Eye-opening new evidence from recent British and American studies proves more conclusively than ever that tobacco road is indeed a dead end.

Ross, Walter S.: "The High Cost of Smoking," *Reader's Digest*, p. 105, March 1972.

A realistic analysis of what cigarette smoking costs in hard cash, not including its effects on health and in shortening life.

8

ALCOHOL AND OTHER MIND-ALTERING DRUGS

Chemical agents which alter consciousness have been widely used in many different societies throughout man's history. They have served sometimes to facilitate socializing or celebration among members of the community, other times as an acceptable means of relaxation or "escape" for the individual from the problems and anxieties of his daily existence. In addition, some religions have used certain drugs as a means of achieving "transcendence" or a closer union with God in their rituals. It is not difficult to see these three aspects of drug use reflected in American society today. There is an important difference, however. In simpler cultures, drugs had a well-defined place, and there was little or no abuse; drugs were used with care, within the limits imposed and universally accepted by the society. In the United States today, however, there is great confusion about the legitimate place of drugs in everyday life, ignorance of the real affects of these drugs, and inconsistency of attitude.

Many questions are being asked today in an attempt to establish some consistent rules for our society. What is more important, the right of the individual to personal experience with drugs or the right of society, through use of the law, to protect its members, particularly its children, from possibly harmful experimentation? Why is "getting stoned" any more immoral than "having a couple of drinks to relax" before dinner? How much is advertising responsible for the "take-a-pill" syndrome of so many Americans?

The drive to make all drugs legal is not surprising in a country where drug use and abuse are already so great. Millions of Americans have a serious problem with alcohol, 3 million abuse barbiturate sleeping pills, 1 million overuse amphetamine stimulants, 50 percent or more of college students on the East and West Coasts have used marijuana at least once, there may be 600,000 heroin addicts in the United States, and the average adult American smokes more than 4,000 cigarettes each year. An article in the October 18, 1971, issue of *The New York Times* revealed widespread drug use among athletes in every sport. Some of the drugs (barbiturates and amphetamines) most widely used by athletes can be addicting; others, such as male hormones, can cause profound bodily changes, making it very possible that the benefits of athletic participation may be offset by the harm done by the drugs used to increase the chances of competing successfully. The introduction of drug use into an area where the emphasis was once on individual achievement raises serious questions about how values in our society have changed.

TERMINOLOGY IN DRUG USE

The term "drugs" has had changing connotations. Forty years ago it meant "medicine" and evoked an image of the corner drugstore. Later it referred particularly to narcotic drugs (defined below). And now the word "drugs" in a newspaper headline usually refers to any of the drugs which are used illegally and which alter mood, consciousness, or perception.

The word *addiction* indicates a strong physical dependence on a drug; *habituation* indicates a strong but strictly psychological need for a drug. Although at one time these terms were frequently used by many authorities, they are being replaced more and more by *drug dependence*, a term which suggests correctly that any type of dependence usually harms the individual, his community, or both. It also suggests correctly that distinguishing between addiction and habituation is often difficult. The habit of cigarette smoking, for example, is strong in many people; authorities disagree about whether there is a physical dependence.

Nevertheless, addiction is a definite phenomenon. The physical need of the addict's body for the addicting drug does exist. The process of addiction has three components: first, the compulsion to take the drug, to continue to take it, and to obtain it by any means necessary; second, increasing tolerance to the drug, so that larger and larger doses are necessary to obtain the same physical and psychic effects; and third, physical and psychological dependence, so that illness follows withdrawal.

Habituation in some people may become as powerful as an addiction, compelling the victims to center their lives on obtaining and using the drug. A habituated person may behave much the same as someone addicted to a narcotic. If he cannot get his drug, he becomes anxious, restless, and unable to concentrate on anything else, though he does not become physically ill. Medical journals record a few people who have even been habituated to water (needing a container of water with them at all times) or to nose drops.

Coffee, tea, and cola beverages occasionally may be habit-forming. Tobacco causes very severe habituation, with extreme discomfort when the drug is discontinued, so that some authorities call it *addicting*. Alcohol in moderation is merely habit-forming for persons, but addiction occurs commonly and severely; the withdrawal symptoms for an alcoholic are called *delirium tremens*, or *the DTs*, and result in a high mortality rate. The most overpowering addictions, however, are to cocaine, opium, heroin, and morphine, and to synthetic substitutes for morphine such as demerol and methadone.

ALCOHOL

Picture a pharmaceutical manufacturer petitioning the Food and Drug Administration for permission to manufacture and sell, without prescription, a new drug, using the following arguments:

"I have a magnificent new drug to promote. Used properly, it will relax people, make them more sociable, and make their troubles more bearable. It is a liquid which can be made palatable in many ways. It is sure to attain great popularity."

"Can it do any harm?" the FDA would ask.

"Oh yes. Even in small doses it interferes with fine, skilled movements of the fingers and other parts of the body, and in larger doses marked uncoordination occurs. It is an anesthetic, though not a very safe one, and in very large doses can kill. Used regularly over a long period of time it can damage the brain and liver, unless unusual dietary precautions are taken."

"Does it cause drug dependency?"

"Oh, yes. Many people, though perhaps only a minority, become habituated to it rather easily, and a few of these develop complete addiction. The habituation should help sales, and the production, processing, distribution, and sales of this product should give work to millions of Americans."

Obviously, the Food and Drug Administration would not even consider the application to manufacture such a drug. Agents which do much less harm have been severely criticized and removed from the market in the past. And yet such a product is readily available in the United States today: alcohol, scientifically known as *ethyl alcohol* or *ethanol.*

Alcohol is here to stay, at least for the predictable future. The attempt to eliminate alcohol from the American scene in the 1920s, known as *Prohibition,* was accompanied by widespread bootlegging and manipulation by the underworld of crime. In 1932 national Prohibition was repealed and in most states liquor was soon legal again. Neither Prohibition nor repeal solved the many problems which may result from the use of alcohol. These must be combated by individuals and society—and the fight will not be a short one.

THE EFFECTS OF ALCOHOL

Alcohol has many effects on the human organism. Some of these were mentioned above: its effect on coordination, its ability to damage the brain and liver, and its capacity to habituate and addict.

Fundamentally, alcohol depresses parts of the nervous system. In addition to the effects on coordination, which start even with very small doses, it depresses the higher brain centers which provide judgment, restraint, and inhibition to human thought. In the early stages of drinking, the depression of these brain centers usually causes pleasant sensations, even though efficiency is lessened. Indeed, along with the impairment of judgment, self-confidence often increases and one may actually have the illusion of increased skill, even to the point of omnipotence.

Among the other physiological effects of al-

cohol there is a dilation of the blood vessels, resulting in a flushing of the skin and a sensation of warmth. The increased flow of blood to the skin is dangerous if the drinker is exposed to severe cold, for his body then loses heat very readily. (Normally in severe cold the blood vessels near the skin are constricted and the blood flow is small, thus causing a sensation of cold but at the same time conserving body heat.) The increased perspiration which may result from drinking alcohol enhances the loss of heat.

Heavier doses of alcohol have additional hazards. Alcohol is absorbed into the body very quickly from the stomach and small intestine, the process being completed in about 2½ hours. Although small amounts are eliminated intact by kidneys and lungs, the body oxidizes most of the alcohol to carbon dioxide and water, chiefly in the liver. Since the oxidation proceeds slowly, the effects of alcohol last far longer than the period during which it is being absorbed. Many factors, such as the amount of food already in the stomach, influence the absorption of alcohol; there is even evidence that chronic alcoholics burn alcohol more rapidly than others and tolerate large doses more readily. Nevertheless, by drinking alcohol rapidly and in large enough quantities, any person may depress his brain progressively into incoherency of thought and action, then coma, and finally death. Fortunately a potential fatal dose in the stomach is usually vomited.

DISEASES OF ALCOHOL USE

Numerous diseases afflict alcoholics, and new conditions are occasionally discovered (in 1970 an unusual type of anemia due to alcoholism was reported). Two of the most severe are cirrhosis of the liver, the tenth leading cause of death in the United States, and a psychotic state (insanity) known as *Korsakoff's syndrome.* Alcohol is not the only cause of cirrhosis, but it is involved in the development of the great majority of cases. In cirrhosis, the combination of excess alcohol and insufficient protein and vitamins in the diet causes the destruction of large numbers of liver cells and the growth of broad bands of scar tissue through the liver. The liver is increasingly prevented from doing its essential tasks of breaking down some chemicals and building up others. As a result, the cirrhotic patient develops weakness, debility, jaundice, swelling of the abdomen, bleeding from the upper part of the intestinal tract, and finally coma and death.

In Korsakoff's syndrome there is damage to cells of the cerebral cortex, which controls thinking; persons suffering from Korsakoff's syndrome lose their memories and regress into a childlike state which can deteriorate into incoherence. There is some evidence that alcohol, at least in the doses received from three drinks or more, causes clumping of the oxygen-carrying red blood cells in the blood vessels. This in turn causes a lack of oxygen supply to the brain, producing not only anoxia (which may feel pleasant) but also damage to hundreds or thousands of brain cells.

A third common alcoholic disease was referred to above: delerium tremens. This is the withdrawal disease for alcoholics. A person who has been drinking heavily for either a long period (months) or a short period (weeks) decides to stop or is forced to stop for one reason or another. Within a few days he becomes tremulous and increasingly shaky. He cannot sleep for long. He begins to see people or things which are not there, and is usually confused about time and about where he is. Although more easily treated today than it used to be, this condition still deserves its other nickname: "the shakes and the horrors." It causes many deaths through its own debilitating effects and through the severe infections by which it is frequently complicated.

THE COSTS OF ALCOHOL

What does alcohol cost the United States? Conservatively, 60,000 lives and $25 to $50 billion each year. Cirrhosis, chiefly a disease of alcoholism, takes roughly 26,000 lives each year, and alcohol is heavily involved in 25,000 highway deaths each year (see Figure 8.1). Other accidents and other alcoholic diseases account for 10,000 deaths, and there are probably more from infections and injuries which would not have happened except for alcohol. This yearly cost in lives is substantially greater than the 49,024 American servicemen dead in Vietnam during the first 6 years of major American involvement.

The economic costs start with the $15 billion spent yearly for alcoholic beverages by American citizens (1968 figure); then there is the property damage incurred in automobile accidents, fires, and other disasters to which alcohol contributes; and last there are the "social costs" of income lost when people are incapacitated or die prematurely from alcohol.

Cirrhosis has been increasing in frequency.

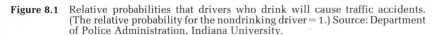

Figure 8.1 Relative probabilities that drivers who drink will cause traffic accidents. (The relative probability for the nondrinking driver = 1.) Source: Department of Police Administration, Indiana University.

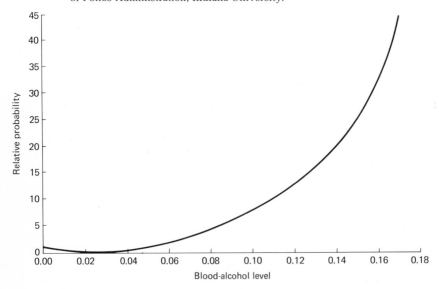

Figure 8.2   Abuse of alcohol is on the increase in the United States. Source: *Medical World News*, March 17, 1972, p. 6.

	Population	Alcoholics	Percent of alcoholics	Loss in wages and productivity
1958	174,640,000	5,000,000	2.0%	Not available
1966	195,384,000	6,500,000	3.3%	$2.43 billion
1971	205,914,000	9,600,000	4.6%	$10 billion

Nationally, the death rate has been about 15 for each 100,000 people, but in New York City, the mortality rate increased from 18 in 1948 to 34.7 in 1967. In Baltimore in some recent years, cirrhosis has been the leading cause of sudden nonviolent death in the age group from 25 to 44. For other alcoholic diseases (not including motor-vehicle deaths caused by alcohol), the death rate in recent years has been 10 per 100,000.

The number of alcoholics in the United States is a heavily debated figure. Conservative estimates have put the figure at 5 to 6 million, but many people working closely with problems of alcohol and with heavy drinkers feel that the number is very much greater. Large corporations which have instituted programs to help alcoholics among their employees have often found that up to 5 percent of their workers have major problems with alcohol; this would make the estimate 5 million alcoholics in the United States too small. Not only do those who drink heavily usually try to hide their drinking habits, but close friends and relatives usually help them do so. A severe hangover which prevents John from going to work is reported by John's wife on the telephone as an attack of "the flu." If John has "a breath on him" when he comes to the office another morning, or if he doesn't get anything done for 2 or 3 hours, his closest associates may try to do his work for him and not let anyone in a superior position know about his situation. This "covering up" means that official figures of alcoholics tend to be too low. (Fig. 8.2)

A careful analysis of the drinking patterns of American adults was carried out in the late 1960s by a group from Washington University in St. Louis.[1] Interviewing a scientifically chosen sample of over 2,700 adults across the country, they found the following proportions of alcohol users:

Abstainers—32 percent. Drink not at all or less than once a year.

Infrequent drinkers—15 percent. Drink less than once a month, but at least once a year.

Light drinkers—28 percent. Drink at least once a month, usually only once or a few times each month, occasionally nearly every day but only one or two drinks on each occasion.

Moderate drinkers—13 percent. Drink either heavily at least once a month, or several drinks each day.

Heavy drinkers—12 percent. Predominantly follow one of two patterns: daily drinking with at least five drinks occasionally, or heavy drinking (five, six, or more drinks) once or twice a week.

Nearly half the adults in the country, then, drink less frequently than once a month, or not at all. Of the abstainers, 31 percent say they do not drink because of religious or moral reasons, 26 percent say that they just do not like to drink, and 26 percent more say that they have no need or desire for alcohol. Twenty percent find that drinking is bad for the health, and 20 percent report being exposed to bad examples of drinking in the past (the figures add to more than 100 percent because

[1]Don Caholan and others. *American Drinking Practices*, Rutgers Center of Alcohol Studies, New Brunswick, N.J., 1969.

many reported more than one reason for not drinking). Older people are less likely to drink than younger, and many of them have given up drinking; women are more likely to be abstainers than men. In a society where alcohol is widely used and advertised, it is impressive that so many choose not to drink.

On the other hand, the number of heavy drinkers among middle-aged men is impressive, even frightening. Thirty percent of all men between 45 and 49 and 40 percent of all men *drinkers* of 45 to 49 are heavy drinkers. Metropolitan areas have many more heavy drinkers, proportionally, than rural areas, and the center cities and larger suburbs have the greatest incidence of heavy drinkers in the metropolitan areas.

CHRONIC ALCOHOLISM: ITS PATTERNS AND DEVELOPMENT

College students are rarely alcoholics, but alcoholic drinking patterns may develop in college students and can lead to the full-blown disease later on in life. Unfortunately, in either early or late stages, people often deny that they have a drinking problem. Many people take pride in how much they can drink and how well they "hold their liquor." This is intimately related to their self-image or the image they want to convey to others. If persuading the true alcoholic that he has a problem and must do something about it is difficult, convincing a young person that some of his habits have serious implications for the future is well-nigh impossible.

The road to alcoholism from beginning to end is usually 7 to 12 years long; women traverse it more rapidly than men. The road varies both in time and in details; not everyone who starts on it will necessarily follow it to its end. In particular, at various points along the way the more intelligent and psychologically sound people will realize that they are losing their usual rapport with their human environment; then and there they will "go on the wagon." But once a person has gone substatinally further in his drinking habits than have others in his own social group, there is a strong chance that he will go down the whole road and become a chronic alcoholic.

When severe chronic alcoholism is established, the alcoholic's physical condition usually deteriorates. His average length of life is about 10 years less than that of his nonalcoholic contemporaries. Cirrhosis or brain damage kills some chronic alcoholics, and others meet violent deaths, while others die prematurely of infections or other intercurrent ailments that would not threaten the life of a healthy person.

CAUSES OF ALCOHOLISM

Strong suspicion persists that some biological defect or abnormality predisposes some people to alcoholism. So far, however, no change in body structure or function has been found which can be proved to cause alcoholism. Nothing accounts for the development of alcoholism in some and not in others with similar social and psychological backgrounds. The search for biological cause goes on.

One observation that points to a biological predisposition for alcoholism is that rats exposed to alcohol behave just as humans do: some become chronic alcoholics, some become teetotalers, and others are like social drinkers, taking some amounts of alcohol but preferring other fluids to drink as a rule. Two observations on rats *may* have importance for human society: some rats which initially refused alcohol consumed it in large quantities after a period of forced intake; and rats take increased amounts of alcohol following a period of stress.

Even though biological cause(s) for alcoholism may exist, it is clear that there are important psychological and sociological causes. Studies at the Massachusetts General Hospital have identified five personality characteristics of chronic alcoholics.[2] The most common of these is low frustration tolerance. For example, a student with an alcoholic personality has an appointment at the health service or with his adviser. When he arrives for the appointment, the doctor or the adviser is still busy and must keep him waiting. The student expostulates or waits in silence, and leaves in a few minutes rather than waiting for the doctor or adviser as most other students would do.

The second common trait is superficial sociability. When sober, alcoholics are usually agreeable, affable, even garrulous. Often they have a good sense of humor and tell stories well. But when they try to become close to anyone else, the relationship tends to break down with expressions

[2]Morris E. Chafetz, H. T. Blane, and M. J. Hill, *Frontiers of Alcoholism;* Science House, 1970.

of hostility, guilt, and recrimination. The college student who drinks more heavily than his friends, and who is universally known as a "good guy" but has few or no really close friends, is a very serious candidate for chronic alcoholism within a few years.

Third, the alcoholic has deep feelings of inferiority which he often tries to hide with attitudes and expressions of superiority. When they speak frankly, alcoholics often express feelings of being "just plain no good," accept failure as their obvious due, and belittle their own abilities. At the same time, they may insist on preferential treatment; they tend to be "name droppers" who often mention the important people that they know; and they can exaggerate past accomplishments.

Fourth, most alcoholics are fearful, particularly of anything which poses a real challenge to them. They are afraid of testing themselves and their capabilities. This characteristic is related to their feelings of inferiority.

Finally, alcoholics have a strong need to be dependent on some dominant person. This need may be openly expressed; the alcoholic functions at his best, and perhaps functions only, when under firm and close direct guidance. Others deny the need, boasting of their independence and independent strength; only careful observation will show them to be dependent on repeated expressions of support and friendship, and perhaps indirectly on the guidance of some other person. Sometimes, however—and this can be very difficult for those around them—they fluctuate widely between desperate requests for help and support on the one hand and vigorous proclamations of self-reliance and independence on the other. Because of the strain involved in maintaining these two contradictory roles, such alcoholics are often depressed, and suicide can become a real danger.

Alcoholics tend to have typical family backgrounds. The mother of an alcoholic has most often been domineering or overprotective or both; the father very likely was absent much or all of the time; if present, the father tended to be ineffective and distant in manner (perhaps as a result of alcohol).

The attitudes of one's culture toward alcohol are significant. Such groups as the Jews and the Italians, which approve the use of restricted amounts of alcohol on family and social occasions but which strongly disapprove of the excessive use of alcohol and the use of alcohol to deal with psychological tension, have a low incidence of alcoholism among their members. Families of other groups can well adopt this approach for their own children, teaching them that small amounts of alcohol for convivial or ceremonious purposes are permissible but that large doses are unacceptable.

Certain religious groups, such as the Mormons and Baptists, teach that drinking is sinful and do not tolerate any use of alcohol among their members. Alcoholism is therefore virtually absent in these groups. It is understandably easier to practice total abstention in a social environment where alcohol is rare or absent than where it is accepted; and in deciding their own policy, parents must consider that a child may grow up to live in an environment in which drinking is accepted and even encouraged. Ultimately, however, parents must decide on the basis of their own beliefs what they will teach their children about drinking, and then teach these standards not by being overly authoritarian but by expressing their convictions plainly and firmly, and by acting on their convictions, realizing that their values are conveyed most clearly by the example they set in their own lives.

PREVENTION AND TREATMENT OF ALCOHOLISM

As in the prevention of other emotional ills, a warm, loving relationship with both parents who simultaneously make clear their definite expectations about the child's conduct, is important to prevent alcoholism from developing later in life. However, a person cannot change the parents he is born with, or the factors that have influenced and shaped him in his early life. The practical problem then, is to recognize a tendency to alcoholism as early as possible and take effective steps against it. In any college class, at least one person in twenty is a potential alcoholic. The psychological and social factors which predispose to chronic alcoholism were described above. If they will, individuals can recognize the danger signs in themselves and in their friends.

When childhood and adolescence give way to adulthood, parental influence is often minimal in matters such as drinking. It is difficult to prevent or cure alcoholism in a society in which drinking is an important part of the social pattern. Too often those who ask for help really want to be told that they can continue drinking while their alcoholism is treated. Nevertheless, many individuals come to the realization that their drinking is getting out of control and then succeed in stopping or (more rarely) controlling their alcoholic intake. Relatives and friends can often be helpful in this process— when they are understanding and empathetic as well as realistic, rather than exhortative, critical, and punitive.

Treatment of the early stages of alcoholism is the best way to prevent the later ones from developing. This is the approach taken by most programs to combat, prevent, cope with, or treat alcoholism, the most successful and important of which is Alcoholics Anonymous (AA). Founded in 1934 by a few persons who had succeed in controlling their alcoholism, AA is now international, with over 6,000 chapters in the United States alone. AA's primary requirement is that the person requesting help recognize and admit that he has a problem with alcohol, and agree that the disease of alcoholism responds only to stopping all alcoholic intake. The members of the organization spare virtually no effort at any time of day or night to provide help for those who ask help in overcoming their strong urge to drink. AA recognizes that those who succeed in stopping alcohol intake are controlled, not cured, alcoholics. Members who are successful cannot return to "moderate" or even "light" drinking. Many of them stay in the organization for continued moral support, and help others who have drinking problems.

The success AA has experienced in this field does not mean that other approaches and treatments for alcoholism are not worthwhile. Medical treatment of its complications is essential. Psychiatric treatment of underlying emotional problems is helpful, often in collaboration with membership in AA. Recent studies suggest that group therapy is more effective than individual treatment in many cases. A drug, disulfiram, is available for selected cases; it makes the taker ill, even seriously ill, if he drinks alcohol while taking it, thus providing an additional motivation for abstinence.

THE LAW AND ALCOHOLISM

Approximately half of the arrests made by police in the United States are for drunkenness or for some offense associated with drunkenness. The cost in time and effort diverted from more important tasks of law enforcement is enormous. And yet, society usually makes no other provision for the individual whose behavior appears to be out of control because of alcohol.

In 1968, in the Powell case, the Supreme Court of the United States refused to declare imprisonment for public drunkenness unconstitutional as a "cruel and unusual punishment." If the court had decided the other way, drunkenness would have ceased to be illegal, and society would have been obligated to create more hospitals and other treatment facilities for alcoholics.

Despite the Powell case, the Minnesota Supreme Court ruled in 1969 that Bernard Charles Ferron, who stated that he had been drunk at least 50 percent of the time in the previous 20 years, could not be convicted under Minnesota's public drunkenness law. The court held that Ferron's drinking was beyond his control. The Minnesota Legislature had previously provided for the "commitment, care and treatment of inebriate persons."

THE PSYCHEDELICS

Psychedelic drugs alter perception of the environment and of the self. The activity of some, such as marijuana, which also has sedative properties, is comparatively mild, while others, like LSD, have more powerful effects.

All the psychedelic drugs are currently illegal in the United States. Not only does this add the danger of arrest and criminal conviction to whatever health hazards exist, but it means that the drugs must be bought on the black market. Drugs bought on the black market vary widely in their strength (dose) and even in their identity. At the end of the sixties and beginning of the seventies, for example, most of the "mescaline" sold on the East Coast was actually LSD. The narcotic bought "on the street" can be either very weak or very strong, though the latter is unlikely. When someone who has been getting weak doses of a drug suddenly receives a strong dose, he is likely to have a vigorous reaction; in the case of heroin, the reaction is often fatal. The psychedelics are often adulterated with other agents; strychnine is one drug which has been added to mescaline, "speed," DMT, LSD, and other agents. Strychnine is a stimulant for the nervous system and mind which can be fatal in comparatively small doses.

Marijuana is the most commonly used product prepared from the hemp plant, *Cannabis*. Marijuana, commonly referred to as *grass* or *pot*, can be smoked in home-rolled cigarettes or in pipes. The flowering tops of the plant are the parts richest in the active ingredients of marijuana. Plants grown close to the equator have more of the active ingredients than plants grown well North or South of the equator, and it was recently discovered that both male and female plants contain the active ingredients.

The effects of one or two cigarettes ("joints") of marijuana are usually mild, although on rare occasions there may be strong unpleasant effects. Relaxation, often a passive and contemplative mood, a mild feeling of well-being, and accentuation of sounds and sights are usually defined as a mild high. Time often seems to pass more slowly or more rapidly than normally, which may be the reason for its use by some musicians. Although musicians often have the sense of playing more expertly, their performance is likely to suffer by objective standards. Similarly, although one may feel that his control of muscular skills is increased, in fact the distortions of sensations (especially loss of depth perception) may damage performance.

Smoking more joints, smoking stronger forms of marijuana or the concentrated resin—hashish or "hash"—or being particularly susceptible to the drug may produce stronger effects. There may be serious distortions of sound, sight, and time; hallucinations; panic; and on rare occasions, acute psychoses (episodes of insanity). A dozen acute psychoses were reported in 1969 among United States armed forces in Vietnam, and in two of them, the patient murdered another solider. The type of marijuana available in Vietnam is known to be strong, and the social climate for taking the drug there is not conducive to a calm experience. In 1971, a report from Philadelphia described six severe psychoses due to marijuana, but some authorities believed that these might have been due to other causes.

There are other dangers associated with use of marijuana. First, frequent use of marijuana or other drugs by children or young adults removes them from the realities of daily life, and delays or perhaps prevents them from growing up. The young person who often uses marijuana choses to restrict his experiences to pleasurable, passive ones, and thus does not permit his relationships with others or his ability to deal with success and failure to develop. Second, the escalation phenomenon is real. There is no evidence that those going from marijuana to harder drugs, whether "acid" (LSD), "speed" (methamphetamine), or heroin, do so because of the chemical nature of marijuana. However, of the few who use marijuana regularly and frequently (daily), between 20 and 40 percent also use stronger drugs, with their added hazards. This statistical relationship between use of marijuana and use of hard drugs is probably the result of several factors: marijuana users as compared with nonusers are more likely to be curious about stronger drugs, more sympathetic to people who use them, more aware of where to obtain them and through friends who use them, more likely to be able to observe their effects—and thus less afraid to experiment. The progression to harder drugs, however, is not a sinking into the "irresistable whirlpool of addiction," leading to actual habituation or addiction, but rather a series of choices made by each individual.

Third, there appears to be an "amotivational syndrome" which afflicts some drug users, even those who use only marijuana. In this syndrome, students and others lose all interest in their usual activities, particularly studies. They devote themselves primarily to smoking grass and using other drugs. There have always been students who have lost motivation, but some physicians who have worked closely with student drug users believe that the loss of motivation is sometimes a specific result of the drug use. Some students are not happy with their loss of motivation; they wish to be as they were before, and seek help from doctors and others to get off drugs.

The fourth danger associated with the use of marijuana is that its long-term effects are uncertain. Some writers and artists testify that they are not productive when on drugs, and there is a small amount of evidence that regular users of marijuana and other psychedelics have some loss of memory and impaired ability to concentrate.

Of the other psychedelic drugs, LSD (lysergic acid diethylamide, or acid) is the most commonly used. Its effects can be mimicked by other psychedelics like mescaline and psilocybin if the dose is high enough. It regularly produces hallucinations, sometimes in a rapid, haphazard fashion that is frightening. The boundaries of the self seem vague or formless, which is frightening to some people but leaves others feeling mystically enriched. For some introspection may be enhanced.

However, it is impossible to know beforehand what a "trip" will be like, even based on one's own previous experience. While LSD sometimes produces profound, intensely beautiful experiences, it also leaves the user open to loss of control of his thoughts and feelings. Many people cannot cope with a release of repressed thoughts and emotions, loss of logical (even verbal) thought processes, inexplicable fear and panic, and the feelings of helplessness and vulnerability that may accompany this. Because a person usually does not know the exact composition and potency of the drug he is taking, he is placing himself at its mercy. It is easy to dismiss the reports of hallucinogen-induced psychosis by saying that those so affected are already in psychological trouble. It is important to remember, however, that a trip is not "all in the mind" but a direct result of flooding the brain with powerful chemicals whose effect on the processes of the mind are only slightly understood. Of course, much of an individual's drug experience is a product of his personality, but even the most stable person can be given a temporary psychosis by a sufficiently large overdose of LSD. And few people are able to judge how much inner strength they have for coping with a drug experience.

Substantial publicity and concern have centered on the possibility that LSD can cause disease and congenital deformities through its ability to split chromosomes. This ability to damage chromosomes was noted several years ago, but its significance was uncertain because other chemicals also damage chromosomes. As further scientific investigations have been completed, however, it has seemed more and more probable that LSD can cause and has caused serious congenital malformations, particularly of the brain and nervous system, in the children of women who have used LSD during the first few months of pregnancy.

Anyone who is familiar with drugs knows that it is especially dangerous to take psychedelics when alone. The presence of a familiar and trusted friend is important during any trip and particularly so during a bad trip, to help the victim through a difficult period. Patient, gentle friends are often successful in helping trippers recover from panic, but if the response is not prompt, the help of a doctor familiar with drugs should be obtained. If a "bad trip" involves prolonged hallucinations and disorientation, then early medical care is important. Proper medication and supportive care may prevent prolonged hospitalization.

SEDATIVES AND STIMULANTS

In the late 1960s it was estimated that there were 3,000 deaths yearly in the United States from barbiturates and amphetamines, and that there were 20 million barbiturate users and 10 million amphetamine users in the country. Barbiturates, referred to as *goofballs* when obtained illegally, are commonly used for sleeping medication, while amphetamines are the most commonly used types of stimulants, aside from the caffeine found in coffee, for example, and in over-the-counter preparations available in pharmacies.

Sedatives make people sleepy. In large doses, they produce coma, so that the individual cannot be awakened and finally death may result. All the sedatives have the same effect, although barbiturates are probably the most dangerous of the sedatives. (Most drugs which are sold without prescription in pharmacies to produce sleep are actually antihistamines, or combinations of an antihistamine and other ingredients.)

The barbiturates can cause drug dependency. When used regularly over a period of time, people develop a tolerance for them and have to take larger doses to produce the same effect. It is possible to build up to very large doses, which then have no more effect (or even less) than small doses in nonregular users. When an addicted person tries to stop taking these large doses suddenly, he becomes violently ill; the withdrawal symptoms are often more uncomfortable and more likely to end in death than those resulting from withdrawal from heroin or other narcotics. Fortunately, very few people become addicted to barbiturates.

The amphetamine stimulants have been

abused by millions of people who start taking them in order to lose weight or stay awake for a long period of time. Finding that after a short period of use, the same dose is no longer effective, they take larger amounts and become dependent on the drugs. As with the barbiturates, it is possible to build up the dosage and become addicted to truly huge amounts which would kill the normal person.

Amphetamines stimulate all the body cells, but they stimulate the brain and nervous system more than other tissues. They produce wakefulness, and give an illusion of increased efficiency. This illusion sometimes masks inefficiency or marked disorganization of the mind; there are examples of students who took amphetamines before examinations and thought that they had produced superior examinations, but who later found that their examination papers consisted of their name written over and over and over again on page after page, or of other meaningless "answers." The amphetamines also diminish appetite, a property which has led to their use as diet pills (see Chapter 12).

The most commonly used amphetamine in the drug culture has been methamphetamine, also known as *methedrine* or *speed*. Speed kills. The large doses used by drug users are most often "mainlined," injected into a vein. The "speed freak" loses appetite and loses weight, often develops hepatitis, an inflammatory disease of the liver, and is susceptible to other infections. He is aggressive, even violent, and often paranoid. His "highs" are followed by profound lows, for which he must take more amphetamines; and the highs are so uncomfortable that he tries to assuage them with drugs that produce "lows," such as heroin or barbiturates. The mortality rate from this practice is high.

Because amphetamines and sedatives are legally prescribed but are haphazardly distributed from one user to another, there has been considera-

tion of restricting even their legal use. In 1971, the American Medical Association warned physicians to restrict their prescriptions for amphetamines. Sweden has led the way in such control. After a period of serious abuse when amphetamines were freely available, Sweden made all use of amphetamines illegal and successfully cut down on the amount making its way into illegal channels. Then in 1969, physicians in Uppsala, Sweden, started a 1-year trial period during which all sedatives, sleeping pills, and habit-forming drugs were issued only in very small quantities. The program was aimed at reducing the amounts of such drugs to be found in home medicine cabinets. If the program proved successful, it was to be made nationwide.

COCAINE

Perhaps one of the most widely used stimulants is cocaine. Cocaine is a derivative of the coca plant that grows in the highland regions of South America and the Pacific. For centuries, the natives of these areas have chewed the leaves of this plant to relieve fatigue and to depress the appetite. The cocaine extracted from the leaves is far more potent than the leaves alone. In addition, cocaine users generally sniff or mainline the drug, which makes the effects far more intense than ingestion by mouth.

Henri Charriere describes a fellow convict, a user of cocaine, in a recent novel, *Papillon*: "Some days he was nervous and excitable. I began to realize that he was calm when he'd had a visitor and was chewing the leaves he was brought. One day he gave me half a leaf and I understood. My tongue, palate, and lips lost all feeling."

The abuse of cocaine is widespread. There is a dangerous dependency that develops as the user finds he has a tolerance and thus gets less effect from a small amount of the drug. Continual use of cocaine results in digestive disorders, nausea, insomnia, delusions and hallucinations, and finally convulsions.

THE NARCOTICS

Throughout the centuries one of mankind's greatest drug problems has been the use of narcotics. The term *narcotic*, derived from the Greek word for "making numb," has been applied to various drug groups. Medically it refers to the drugs derived from the opium poppy and their synthetic equiv-

alents; these drugs kill pain, relieve anxiety, depress brain function, and in larger doses, lead to coma and death. They have the properties common to all addicting drugs: the user develops tolerance for increasing doses and has withdrawal symptoms after the drug is stopped abruptly. With chronic addiction, debility, malnutrition, loss of appetite for sex and food, and social disorganization usually occur. Since these drugs are usually mainlined, hepatitis and other infections are common. The mortality rate is high from these complications and from the overdose and toxic reactions to the drugs: about 1 percent of heroin addicts in New York City die this way each year. (See Figure 8.3.)

Heroin gives more relief of anxiety and causes addiction more rapidly than other narcotics. The length of time taken to addict varies from person to person; it is not true that a single injection will addict. On the other hand, people usually pass the point of no return before they reach the point of physical addiction. A study in St. Louis showed that in one group there, any man who had taken heroin as many as six times inevitably went on to become addicted. Because of the high cost of heroin, most male addicts in American cities ob-

tain their funds from theft and most female addicts from prostitution.

The treatment of heroin addiction has been unsatisfactory. The two federal hospitals for the treatment of narcotic addiction, at Lexington, Kentucky, and at Fort Worth, Texas, have never had substantial success in "curing" addicts and are being converted to rehabilitation institutes. The increased number of addicts, particularly in the metropolitan areas, has required more effective and more local methods of treatment than are available in distant hospitals. Mere legal pressure is generally not enough to convince addicts to give up their habit.

Two approaches have shown limited promise. Numerous communities of ex-addicts (Synanon, Daytop, Gaudenzia, and so forth) have been set up on the principles of strict renunciation of drugs by residents of the community, strict self-government by the residents, and strict adherence to giving up

Figure 8.3 The trend of narcotics-related deaths in New York City, 1960 to 1971. Source: Metropolitan Life Insurance Company, New York, Statistical Bulletin, February 1972.

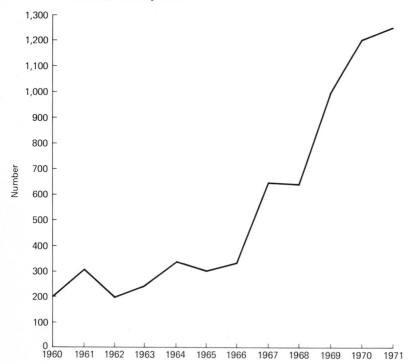

drugs as the highest goal in life. Making heavy demands on their participants and relying on voluntary participation, these programs have been "the answer" for a limited number of addicts.

The second approach which has shown definite but limited value has been methadone maintenance. Pioneered by Dr. Vincent Dole and Dr. Marie Nyswander in New York City, the methadone treatment relies on substituting a relatively benign narcotic, methadone, for the much more dangerous and disrupting heroin. Subjects who take methadone regularly get little or no "high" if they take heroin; they are blocked. On methadone they usually can work and live relatively normal lives. The methadone program has converted many debilitated, socially useless addicts living by crime into stronger, useful citizens who have self-respect, satisfaction in life, and the ability to earn their own living. The methadone program, however, is far from universally successful, requires that addicts be given careful counseling and rehabilitation, has had some deaths, and has been criticized for leaving addicts as addicts. Methadone itself can be dangerous; to those unaccustomed to its use, large doses can kill, just as an "OD" (overdose) of heroin can kill.

THE LAW AND DRUGS

In the United States, the traditional assumption has been that society through its laws has a right to regulate private use of drugs. In 1919, under the Eighteenth Amendment to the Constitution and the Volstead Act, alcoholic beverages of all sorts became illegal in the United States; the Eighteenth Amendment was repealed in 1933. By the Harrison Narcotic Act of 1914 the use of narcotic drugs was made illegal throughout the country. In the 1930s marijuana was added to the list of narcotic drugs, and it was not until 1970 that this medically unsound classification was changed legally. In 1970, the former Bureau of Narcotics became the Bureau of Narcotics and Dangerous Drugs, with authority over narcotics, sedatives, stimulants, and psychedelic drugs. By all these laws and regulatory bodies, the United States as a society has attempted to prohibit or restrict not only traffic in but use of drugs considered dangerous. This attempt has had only limited success. With the exception of some success in confining the use of narcotics until the 1960s, it is questionable whether the law has had more than superficial effects on drug use. Similarly, during Prohibition, only moderate restriction of actual use of alcohol occurred, and illegal traffic prospered, with great spurs to organized crime.

At the present time the country is engaged in a great debate on whether to "legalize" marijuana. A poll of college students in New York indicated that almost nine out of ten opposed legal penalties for the use or possession of marijuana (and for the use or possession of other mind-affecting drugs, even though the respondents in general felt that they would never use the drugs themselves). After appointing the Marijuana Commission in 1971, however, President Richard M. Nixon announced that even if the commission recommended "legalization" of marijuana, he would reject the recommendation. Most legislators have been cautious about supporting the idea of legalization because of the active opposition of some parts of the population.

However, the term *legalization* has acquired highly emotional overtones and oversimplified the issues. There are actually several questions being raised. First, should there be legal penalties against the use or possession of marijuana (or other drugs)? Second, should there be legal penalties against the sale or distribution of marijuana (or any other drug)? If penalties are appropriate, what penalties are effective in stopping use or distribution? If penalties are not appropriate for either possession or distribution, what controls should be placed on material distributed? Should a government monopoly be instituted, for example, similar to the state liquor stores that exist in some states?

Behind the questions above are some deeper questions, which have not been adequately answered by either experts or public opinion. Should the law discriminate among different dangerous drugs (alcohol, marijuana, heroin)? In what ways? On what basis? Is law effective in altering private behavior at all, and if so under what circumstances? What are society's obligations to provide deterrents, alternate interests, treatment facilities, and rehabilitation facilities for different kinds of drug abusers? What kinds of drug abusers desire, need, and will accept help? And finally, what is the relationship between legal coercion and effective treatment?

TEA, COFFEE, COCOA, AND COLA BEVERAGES

Widespread use of tea, coffee, cocoa, and cola beverages is common among people in many different parts of the world. The use of coffee, which comes from the seeds of *Coffea arabica* and other species of *Coffea*, is said to have originated in Arabia; tea, which consists of the dried leaves of *Thea sinensis*, is associated with China; cocoa, obtained from the seeds of *Theobroma cacao*, had its early use in Brazil and Central America; kola, the brown bitter nut of the tropical *Cola acuminata*, has been chewed for years in India and Africa. There is a Chinese legend that tea leaves were first eaten by a Buddhist ascetic who noted their stimulating effect and used them to help him stay awake for 9 years and contemplate Buddha. A legend about the use of coffee states that Arabian shepherds noticed that goats which ate coffee berries were stimulated and did not rest; this observation led to the making of a beverage from coffee berries to ward off sleep.

For our purposes tea and coffee may be considered together because the important constituent of each is caffeine. Although tea leaves contain more caffeine than coffee beans, an ordinary cup of coffee or a strong cup of tea contains approximately 1½ grains of caffeine. Cocoa contains theobromine, which is similar to caffeine both in chemical structure and in physiological effects except that it is less stimulating to the brain. Tea and coffee have no food value, and the food value of cocoa without milk or sugar is negligible. In cola drinks the flavoring is principally an extract of the kola nut which contains both caffeine and theobromine. It is believed that the caffeine is the more important of the two. The amount of caffeine found in cola beverages is approximately one-third the amount contained in an equivalent volume of coffee.

Caffeine has a stimulating effect on the brain; it promotes a sense of well-being and reduces fatigue and drowsiness. Although the speed of reaction to many stimuli is increased by caffeine, the accuracy of response is reduced. Caffeine in large amounts may lead to nervousness, wakefulness, and other manifestations, such as headaches and dizziness. Respiration and circulation are moderately stimulated by caffeine; premature heartbeats often occur. One of the most obvious effects of caffeine is to increase the output of urine.

The most common cause for restricting the use of tea or coffee is the stimulating effect of caffeine on the nervous system. Insomnia, nervousness, and headaches occasionally result from even the moderate use of tea or coffee. Many people find that caffeine causes "heartburn" and other gastric discomfort.

There is considerable difference of opinion about whether the habitual use of caffeine beverages is beneficial, harmful, or has no effect. Continuous use undoubtedly results in the development of some tolerance, but this disappears rather promptly when caffeine is discontinued. People who are particularly susceptible to caffeine or are afflicted with nervousness or certain other diseases, however, undoubtedly would do better to forego tea and coffee entirely. The effect of caffeine on children has not been shown to be different from that on adults, but any drug stimulation of children, who are normally highly active, is clearly undesirable. Furthermore, the use of tea, coffee, and cola drinks by children tends to crowd milk and fruit juices, with their essential food elements, out of the diet.

QUESTIONS FOR DISCUSSION AND SELF-EXAMINATION

1 Describe the various uses and meanings of the words *drug*, *addiction*, and *habituation*. How are the three terms related to each other?

2 Describe the effects of alcohol on (a) the brain and (b) the circulatory system.

3 Describe the contribution that alcohol makes

to the development of (a) cirrhosis of the liver, (b) Korsakoff's syndrome, and (c) delirium tremens. Describe each condition briefly.

4 Both drinking alcohol and smoking cigarettes can be habituating and perhaps addicting. Compare and contrast patterns of use of the two agents, and the development of habituation.

5 Describe the effects of social attitudes toward alcohol and toward other mind-altering drugs on the development of patterns of abuse.

6 Compare the short-term and long-term effects of marijuana and LSD.

7 Under what circumstances and influences do some people increase their drug use of marijuana to "stronger" drugs such as LSD, amphetamines, and heroin?

8 Describe and compare the adverse psychological states sometimes produced by (a) LSD, (b) marijuana, (c) amphetamines, and (d) heroin.

9 Describe the possible advantages and disadvantages (to individuals and to society) of "legalizing" (a) marijuana, (b) LSD, and (c) heroin.

10 What is the common ingredient of tea, coffee, and cola, and what is its effect?

REFERENCES AND READING SUGGESTIONS

BOOKS

Bloomquist, Edward R.: *Marijuana, The Second Trip,* Glencoe Press, The Macmillan Company, New York, 1971.

Thorough and well documented, but conservative.

Blum, Richard H., et al.: *Society and Drugs,* vol. 1, *Students and Drugs,* vol. 2, Jeffrey Bass, San Francisco, 1969.

Fascinating social science studies and approaches to drugs.

Brill, Leen, and Louis Lieberman, *Authority and Addiction,* Little Brown and Company, Boston, 1969.

Describes a program of investigation and management in Washington Heights, New York City. Interesting statistics, and good insights.

Grinspoon, Lester, M.D., and Peter Hedblom: "Amphetamines Reconsidered," *Saturday Review,* July 8, 1972, pp. 33–46.

An amazing story of the development of amphetamines, their medical use, and their current widespread illicit use. The authors find that the addictive potential of amphetamines may exceed that of heroin. There are more amphetamine addicts than heroin addicts—perhaps by a ratio of ten to one.

Marty Mann's New Primer on Alcoholism, National Council on Alcoholism, New York, 1963.

A useful and authoritative book about alcoholism, its nature, its symptoms, and the latest proven methods of treatment.

Masters, R. E. L., and Jean Houston: *The Varieties of Psychedelic Experience,* Holt, Rinehart and Winston, Inc., New York, 1966.

A discerning consideration of the effects of the new mind-influencing drugs—the hallucinogens or psychedelic drugs—on normal people, including observations at drug sessions and reports by persons who have undergone the drug experience.

PAMPHLETS AND PERIODICALS

Alcoholism—Activities of the U.S. Department of Health, Education, and Welfare, Government Printing Office, 1966.

Analysis of the problem, its causes, and what can be done about it.

Answers to the Most Frequently Asked Questions about Drug Abuse, National Clearinghouse for Drug Abuse Information, Chevy Chase, Md.

The Attack on Narcotics, New York State Narcotic Addiction Control Commission, Albany, N.Y., 1966.

A splendid analysis of the problem of narcotic addiction and report of New York State's comprehensive and bold new program for its control.

Block, Marvin A.: *Alcoholism Is a Disease,* American Medical Association, Chicago.

A realistic discussion and practical approach to this problem by the chairman of the AMA Committee on Alcoholism.

"The Drug Takers," *Life-Time* Special Report, New York, 1965.

Fine, absorbing, significant articles concerning the illicit traffic in drugs and the personal and social aspects of addiction to narcotics and "mind-meddling drugs."

9

MENTAL HEALTH

When Sigmund Freud was asked about the characteristics of a mentally healthy person, he replied, briefly, "Love and work." Today our best descriptions of mental health are in similar terms of successful and appropriate function. Freud's mention of love can be enlarged to include various types of appropriate and mature emotional relationships. His mention of work can be expanded to include successful performance of the various intellectual and physical tasks of life, whether or not they include conventional jobs.

Mental health is far more than the absence of mental illness. Happiness, peace of mind, satisfaction in achievement, and the enjoyment of life are all aspects of mental health. A person who possesses good mental health gets along well with himself and with most others. He meets the numerous small irritations of every day, along with the occasional major problems, with courage and poise. He grows from these experiences and increases in maturity thereby. He is able to pursue realistic goals effectively, to live comfortably with others and to achieve satisfaction in doing a part of the work of the world.

THE "NORMAL" PERSON

Is there such a thing as a mentally "normal" person? If "normality" means conformity, or an unwillingness to protest injustice, or having a socially determined pattern of interests, abilities, or values, then "normality" exists but would not seem desirable to most educated people. But if "normality" means self-fulfillment, self-comfort, and related achievements, then it both exists and seems desirable. In this sense, *normal* means "mentally healthy" and *normality* means "positive mental health"; both these terms are in current use.

A publication of the Joint Commission on Mental Illness and Health views mental health under six headings:

1 Attitudes toward the self: The mentally healthy person is comfortable with himself but also realistic about his own strengths and weaknesses.
2 Self-fulfillment: He is able to grow and develop until his potential is reached in the areas which interest him and which are important to his self-interest and personal goals.
3 Integration: His personality is consistent, and he does not hamper his relations with others or his efforts in practical affairs by bizarre attitudes or behavior.
4 Autonomy: He does not depend on others' opinions of him and his work in order to be happy and satisfied. Warm relations with other human beings are usually meaningful and important to him, and he appreciates proper recognition, but he takes satisfaction from knowing himself that he has done a good job or lived up to his own values.
5 Perception of reality: He knows what the facts are and does not badly misinterpret his environment (including the attitudes of others).
6 Relationship to the environment: Not only is he realistic in his view of the environment, but he uses it appropriately and, if possible, does not allow himself to be driven by it from his goals and self-interests.

Much learning of social patterns is accomplished through *reinforcement* of the proper responses. For example, the child is helpful to his mother; the mother reinforces the child with a smile and with praise. After this has happened a few times, it is "natural" for the child to be helpful. Conversely, if no reinforcement takes place, the response of helpfulness is gradually *extinguished*.

The traditional view has been that a warm, strong family is the most important ingredient in creating a healthy adult. The danger in recognizing an unhappy childhood as predisposing to poor mental health is that the person who has had such a childhood may use it as an excuse for not trying to achieve maturity and health. An important study of sixty-five members of student councils at three liberal arts colleges, conducted while the students were in college and 10 years later, has confirmed that a good family life contributes importantly to future mental health; nevertheless a few people with apparently good family lives as children develop into adults with impaired function in their mental health, and some with poor family lives as children develop into adults with superior function in their mental health. In this group, among 45 people with good mental health 10 years out of college, 27 had come from homes with good emotional climates, 22 from homes with fair emotional climates, and 6 from homes with questionable or poor emotional climate. Of the 18 with impaired mental health, 2 came from homes with excellent emotional climates and 4 from homes with fair emotional climates, the other 12 from homes with impaired emotional climate.[1]

For some people, perhaps most, once a good mental health foundation is established, adversities, defeats, and frustrations often result in *improved* ability to handle difficult situations. Even when adversity exists in childhood, adults may overcome that adversity to reach uncommon heights of happiness, partly through recognition of their accomplishment. In the student-council study, there were a few people whose families had been unhappy in childhood who had happy marriages; Cox describes a "rare kind of happiness in their marriages," with a "sort of enduring surprise" at the existence of this happiness.

[1] Rachel Dunaway Cox, *Youth into Maturity*, Mental Health Materials Center, New York, 1970.

THE ANATOMY OF THE PERSONALITY

The ability to deal with adversity and the ability to postpone immediate gratifications in favor of more important long-term goals are important for maturity and mental health. These abilities are first among the ego strengths. The ego is the conscious, organized, structured part of the personality which enables one to deal affectively with the realities of life. It also helps in handling the often imperious, though unconscious, drives of the id and the sometimes domineering controls of the superego. This division of the personality into ego, id, and superego originated with Sigmund Freud's work; although the definitions and the nature of the three divisions are still debated, the classification is still valid and useful, though some psychologists reject it.

The *ego* defends a person and his mental health in adversity; it allows him to set realistic, long-term goals; it allows him to be aware of himself as a unique human being with his own characteristics which he can cherish or try to change as he sees fit.

The *id*, a term not always used by psychologists who dislike Freud's hypotheses, includes the instinctive and impulsive forces in man's nature. All the immutable, fixed, instinctive drives in mankind are included within the id. Sexual drives are probably the most familiar part of the id, but drives for self-expression of all sorts, for curiosity, and perhaps for some anger properly are classified within the id. By definition, these drives are not rational and are not aware of contradictions. In any society where there are two or more human beings, the id must have control and direction by the ego in order for the society to continue to exist.

The *superego*, roughly comparable to the term *conscience*, develops out of the ego (or, according to some, is part of the ego). Parents and other authorities guide the behavior of children and tell them what is right and wrong. As they grow older, they "internalize" these standards of right and wrong, sometimes in identical form to those that their parents had, sometimes adapting them or choosing from among them. Then, if they choose to ignore these standards, the resulting conflict makes them uncomfortable. Thus it has been said about the early New England Puritans that their religious code could not keep them from sinning but that it kept them from enjoying it.

Many observers believe that the superego in American society is weaker than it used to be. Perhaps because many parents spend less time with their children than did parents of previous generations, perhaps because of the omnipresent television set with its emphasis on violence, perhaps because of the growing importance and strength of the youth culture which stimulates the development of independent standards at an early age, strong internal controls and strong convictions about personal standards seem less common. "Everyone's doing it" and a tendency to downgrade both law and custom are prevailing attitudes in many groups of varying ages. It is not that older customs and rules are being supplanted by new customs and rules; there are just fewer customs and rules and they are less strong.

Yet many people are left with their own inhibitions and internal controls; the surrounding culture often pressures them to try to abandon these controls, which is psychologically difficult or sometimes impossible. If they do "knuckle under" to these pressures, they feel unhappy and in conflict. Take, for example, cheating. A student may find himself in a group that pays little attention to rules against cheating, whose members think they can cheat and get away with it. Not only will a student with strong internal standards disapprove of such behavior and consider it damaging to the community, but if he succumbs to the temptation of an offer of illegal help from a friend, he will feel guilty and uncomfortable. He may even develop somatic symptoms such as the overbreathing, heart pounding, and panic of an anxiety attack. It takes maturity to have a normally developed superego and to feel comfortable with its action, disregarding the contrary activities of others.

The entire id and parts of the superego and ego lie within the unconscious mind. This means that thoughts and feelings in the unconscious are hidden from the conscious mind and can be brought out only by deliberate effort, or perhaps not at all. The existence of the unconscious is normal, and every adult human being has one. It is only when major conflicts occur within the unconscious that disability, unhappiness, and other adverse symptoms occur.

BODY AND MIND

The close, inseparable connection of body and mind causes bodily symptoms to result from psychological conflict and tension. Figure 9.1 shows some of these symptoms, commonly called *psychosomatic* and *psychogenic* symptoms.

On the one hand, the condition of the body influences and affects the mind and the emotions. Loss of vision or of hearing, for example, may lead to feelings of depression or to more severe psychiatric disorders. At times everyone experiences the feelings of discouragement and depression which accompany excessive fatigue or unrelenting pain. Everything looks dismal; it is difficult to concentrate on jobs to be done or to be pleasant or even civil to others. To minimize or to be resistant to such feelings, it is important to have good physical health and adequate nutrition, rest, exercise, and recreation.

Conversely, the mind affects the body in many ways, unconsciously as well as consciously. We blush with embarrassment, we flush with anger, we pale and may become weak and faint with fright. These are easily observable effects of emotional responses, exerted usually through the autonomic (involuntary) nervous system and certain of the endocrine glands. (See Chapter 19.)

Fear and anger activate the autonomic nervous system and stimulate the adrenal glands to produce increased amounts of epinephrine (adrenaline).

Epinephrine has many effects on the body, including increases in the heart rate and the blood pressure, and the release from the liver of glycogen, a highly concentrated form of food which the muscles utilize to produce energy. All this prepares the body for supreme effort. The epinephrine-stimulated person becomes capable of physical or mental achievements far in excess of what he normally could do.

For example, four men were driving along a narrow mountain highway when a rockslide blocked the road and threatened to sweep them over a precipice. They lifted the car and turned it around, then drove back to safety. Later, they attempted to repeat their feat of strength, but were unable to lift the car an inch off the ground.

Strong emotions, however, may seriously impair judgment and control. Recognizing this, people should not drive when angry, depressed, or preoccupied.

The immediate physiological effects of sudden

Figure 9.1   Some disturbances which may be psychosomatic (or emotional) in nature.

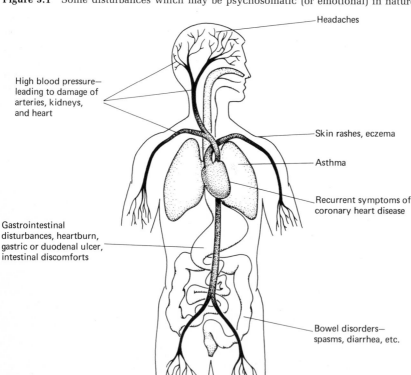

Headaches

High blood pressure—leading to damage of arteries, kidneys, and heart

Skin rashes, eczema

Asthma

Recurrent symptoms of coronary heart disease

Gastrointestinal disturbances, heartburn, gastric or duodenal ulcer, intestinal discomforts

Bowel disorders—spasms, diarrhea, etc.

strong emotions, even including the vomiting and diarrhea which sometimes occur, are usually of short duration and produce no lasting ill effects. But if emotional responses of this kind are frequent or persistent, physical illnesses such as high blood pressure, ulcers of the stomach or duodenum, or spastic bowel may develop.

Among other illnesses which may be attributable at least in part to "nervous" or emotional causes are headaches, fatigue, arthritis, allergies, and certain skin disorders. In fact, it is estimated that at least half the patients who visit physicians do so because of complaints which are primarily nervous in origin and that, in addition, many physical illnesses have nervous components which contribute to the patient's symptoms.

That an illness is nervous or "functional" in nature does not mean that it is unreal. The pain suffered by patients with such conditions is just as real as the pain from serious organic diseases, and may be even more severe and demoralizing. Examples of this type of illness are legion. Every physician encounters them daily in his practice. Furthermore, some psychologically based illnesses such as peptic ulcer or ulcerative colitis may, if severe, cause death.

Illustrative of how potent the effect of the mind on bodily processes can be are reports such as the following: A certain woman had never liked milk but had not noticed any special sensitivity to it until after the birth of her first child at age 23. By age 35, she had become so sensitive to milk that she vomited if she drank milk or ate any food that was made with milk. In the course of an examination her physician introduced some liquids into her stomach by means of a stomach tube. Among these liquids, without her realizing it, was some milk. No nausea or vomiting occurred. Later the physician introduced some water into her stomach by the same method but led her to believe that it was milk. This time immediate vomiting followed. Experiments with similar results have been reported on patients suffering from asthma, migraine, and other psychosomatic diseases.

In demonstrations of the relationship of mind and body, subjects can deliberately affect body processes which had been thought to be beyond deliberate control. Blood pressure, pulse rate, intestinal function, and skin temperature have been controlled by changes in the nervous system. In an intriguing experiment, a group of Harvard researchers demonstrated that normal young men could be taught to lower their own blood pressures merely by giving them a simple reward. Whenever their blood pressure became lower, the reward was given. Various wires were attached to the subjects, and they did not know what bodily functions were being monitored. With the flashing of a light and a brief glimpse of a pin-up girl as the reward, their blood pressures quickly fell and stayed low for an extended period after the mind-body unit had learned that a pleasant reward accompanied lower blood pressure.

BASIC EMOTIONAL NEEDS

The technical facts about personality and about the relationship between mind and body lead to a recognition of basic emotional needs. These include love and warm personal relationships; independence and individual autonomy; security and freedom from unusually frequent or unusually severe uncertainty; achievement and success, with appropriate recognition and approval; faith and the ability to identify with ideals greater than the self; sex and creativeness; guidance and examples in living; and contact with other human beings.

Love is an essential need of every human being. Children need the love of parents and of brothers and sisters; parents need the love of each other and of their children. We all need the love of associates and friends. Love, however, is unselfish. It requires giving as much as receiving. It is nurtured by kindness, sympathy, tenderness, helpfulness, and tolerance. Happiness is a major by-product of such love. (Figure 9.2.)

Emotions and actions that are inherently selfish are sometimes proclaimed as love. The father who rules the family sternly but unfeelingly and insists that he does so because of love, and the demanding mother who insists upon more time, attention, and devotion from her children than they can possibly give, are examples of selfishness masquerading in the guise of love. True and re-

Figure 9.2   Loneliness is frightening to a child. (Photograph by B. Cole.)

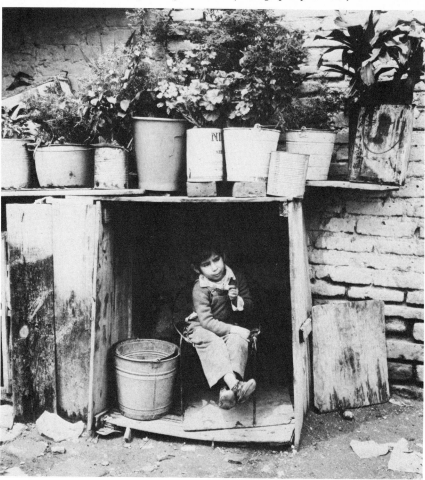

warding love thinks of others rather than of self.

Independence or individual autonomy is both an emotional need and a right of every individual in a free society. Everyone wants the right to develop and utilize his abilities; the right to choose and obtain appropriate work and an appropriate place to live; the right to marry on the basis of love and to establish a home; the right of free speech; the right to worship according to the practices of the religious group to which he belongs; the right to participate in the society and the government of which he is a part. Independence is both a right and a privilege which an individual should earn and merit.

With independence and freedom comes responsibility. Sons and daughters who wish to drive the family car should demonstrate not only their ability to drive, but also their readiness to accept the responsibilities for safe driving that go along with operating an automobile. Individuals should strive for the independence which is necessary for the development and satisfaction of their personalities, but in so doing, they must realize that they merit freedom and independence only as they recognize and respect the rights and freedoms of others.

Security provided by a good home and loving parents is needed by infants and children. Even young adults excited by new-found independence have greater peace of mind if they know that the doors of warm, accepting, parental homes are still open to them. Responsible adults also need a feeling of security against the misfortunes that may befall them: want, illness, failure, loneliness. On the other hand, too much emphasis on security may result in mediocrity. The men and women who blaze the trails of human progress, who attain positions of distinction in life, who rise above the crowd, are the ones who have had sufficient confidence in themselves to be willing to sacrifice a certain amount of security in the hope of greater achievements in the future. This applies to many young men and women who, in order to attend college, give up employment opportunities and borrow money. It is important to strive to satisfy the need for security; but one must realize that security is relative, that nothing in life is entirely secure, and that many feelings of insecurity are fanciful and not really based on fact.

Achievement, accompanied by a sense of personal worth, is another basic emotional need. In college, this need may be satisfied by doing well scholastically; by playing on an athletic team; by participating in other extracurricular activities; by joining a fraternity, sorority, or club; by making friends. In later life, the need for achievement may be satisfied by doing a job well, whatever the job may be; by establishing a good home for the family; by rendering worthwhile service to others; by participating in community and group activities; by improving one's education through learning a new language or studying art, literature, music, nature, or another subject.

Faith in some power or force outside and greater than ourselves is important to healthful living. It shows an ability to identify with some important ideal or ideals. Many people find this need fulfilled in their belief in God, whether or not within a formal religion. Others may speak of the power of nature or of the laws of the universe. Many have strongly held convictions about the

organization of society and what they believe in for their country, their community, or their ethnic group. The recognition and acceptance of faith can be an important element in maintaining emotional security and a sense of direction in life.

Sex is a powerful drive with profound influence on behavior and feelings. Mature satisfaction of sex impulses, through the relationship of marriage, gratifies physical needs in conjunction with other needs such as establishing a home, bringing up a family, and considering and being responsible for others. It is important to satisfy sexual needs, but actions which are morally and socially unacceptable or destructive to the individuals involved produce unhappiness and conflict. Promiscuity is often evidence of a psychiatric character disorder.

Guidance or examples in living largely determine habits and patterns of behavior. Early home influences are most important in the development of emotional patterns, habits of behavior, and standards of values. On the whole, children tend to be like their parents in a wide range of characteristics. Boys usually identify with their fathers, and girls with their mothers. When parents are emotionally mature, effective, and understanding, their children have a good opportunity to develop sound emotional health; when parents lack maturity, effectiveness, and understanding, their children are handicapped by an unhealthy environment, although some other guidance or example in living can compensate for the lack.

Companionship is a basic emotional need of both children and adults. Prolonged isolation can produce mental abnormality. Examples are the psychoses developed by prisoners in solitary confinement, by refugees deprived of communication by language barriers, and by the hard of hearing. People satisfy many of their emotional needs through companionship. The most rewarding companionships are with persons one admires and respects, for whom he feels affection, and with whom he can be himself.

REACTIONS TO PSYCHOLOGICAL CONFLICTS

It is impossible to satisfy emotional needs at all times. If one person tried to do so, he would soon interfere with the rights and emotional needs of

others. Many people are denied rights because of color, creed, or social or economic postion. Some are unable to satisfy emotional needs because of situations or people in the family, college, or job. Still others have emotional and psychological defects which block the way to satisfying emotional needs.

Sometimes, the inadequately met emotional need can be put off until later, and one may adjust well for the time being. At other times, he may *sublimate* his needs and goals into other directions. Althea Gibson, who in 1958 won the world's major tennis championship for women, suffered many frustrations as a black girl in Harlem. However, concentrating on activities in which she had special abilities, she achieved great personal satisfactions, including winning the coveted Wimbledon Championship Tennis Cup.

When the adjustment to delay or frustration is inadequate, however, or when no sublimation of a drive takes place, various mechanisms and reactions come into existence. Some of the more common types are discussed below.

SUPPRESSION

When we deliberately put a thought or feeling "out of mind" we are suppressing it. We can call it back at any time we choose, in contrast to a repressed thought which has never reached consciousness and cannot be called up voluntarily. Suppression is necessary. Everyone has occasional thoughts or fantasies which, if put into action, would bring him into conflict with personal conviction, with parental teaching, with religious or other moral codes, or with the law. Some conscious suppression of such thoughts is necessary, but suppression used too frequently may contribute to feelings of failure, insecurity, tension, and depression and to other symptoms of mental ill health.

Psychiatrically, thoughts, impulses, ideas, fantasies, wishes, and dreams are not real issues of right or wrong, are not moral issues, and are not against behavioral codes. What really counts is not what people think about doing, but what they actually do. Yet, the burden of guilt that people carry because of thought or impulses may be enormous and can be very self-destructive. It is important for good mental health that people understand this so that they may try not to be unduly disturbed about their inappropriate impulses. Only when such impulses become so strong that they are almost irresistible is it important to receive psychiatric or psychological help.

REPRESSION

When a feeling, thought, or impulse becomes active in the unconscious mind but is unacceptable to the values and standards which dominate the person's mind, a kind of censorship prevents it from becoming conscious. In most societies, for example, it is unacceptable to have sexual interest in certain close relatives. Thoughts of such sexual interest never enter the conscious minds of most people in those societies. This type of repression causes no trouble under most circumstances. Only when inner conflicts result in the repression of *all* impulses in a given area, such as sex or competitiveness, do symptoms result. If an individual is unable to accept *any* thoughts about sex in his conscious mind, or if he is unable to express *any* feelings of competition with others, then he is in trouble.

FEELINGS OF INFERIORITY

Every intelligent person experiences feelings of inferiority at some times. Such feelings are not abnormal and need not be disturbing. No one can excel in everything, and few reach their full ambitions. Yet some persons concentrate so much attention on their inadequacies or supposed inadequacies, constantly comparing themselves unfavorably with others, that they are unhappy and handicapped in their human relations. One should recognize his handicaps or limitations but consider them in relation to abilities and capacities. On the basis of such an appraisal, he can turn to fields in which the possibilities of achieving satisfaction are greatest. When feelings of inadequacy persist despite clear evidence that the person is able to hold his own in the world, then the feelings are likely to be due to a depression, a specific psychiatric illness (perhaps with few other manifestations) needing specific care.

DAYDREAMING

It is out of dreams that ambition, inventions, scientific discoveries, and social movements are born. He who does not "dream dreams" is dull and unimaginative. Yet exaggerated daydreaming which becomes a preoccupation may be a substitute for real experience and accomplishment. Although achieving success and escaping unpleasant situations is less satisfying in a world of make-believe than in a world of reality, it is easier. For this reason excessive daydreaming is likely to occur in neurotic individuals.

WORRY

Worry is an ineffectual expenditure of time and nervous energy on uncertainties or situations often beyond one's control. Some worry is natural and inevitable, as when a major problem confronts a person; but most worry is over trivialities and is out of proportion to the importance of the problems at hand. Its result is often confused and disorganized thinking, which interferes with both accomplishment and peace of mind.

Worry is easy, though useless. It saps energy from other interests and tasks. Worry can often be controlled by concentrating on work or hobbies, or on physical exercise. Worry often needs to be shared with a trusted friend or friendly group who can help to dissipate the excess emotion involved and to place the worry in perspective.

Closely related to worry is fear, which, if justified, may prevent injury or death.

ANXIETY

Related to worry and fear, but different from them, is anxiety, a feeling of foreboding or concern about the present or future. Most often the anxious person is partly or completely unaware of what makes him anxious; or to put it another way, his feeling of discomfort is much greater than the problem in his mind would justify. Many psychiatrists feel that most human anxiety harks back to fears which existed in childhood: fear of punishment, of not being loved, or of deeper psychological threats. Many psychological problems of adult life are believed to be intimately related to the ways in which people ward off anxiety. All people have psychological defenses against anxiety, often called *ego defenses*; repression, denial, sublimation, rationalization, and reaction formation are ego defenses discussed in this section.

INSECURITY

Closely related to worry, fear, and anxiety are feelings of insecurity. These feelings may be related to a person's health or to his ability to succeed in college, make the athletic team, make and hold friends, make a place for himself socially, support his family, or succeed in his business or profession. If such feelings are unjustified, then he should seek to banish them. On the other hand, if there are elements of insecurity in his real situation, they should be appraised and faced realistically; steps should be taken to overcome them or to view them in proper perspective.

ANGER, HOSTILITY, AND REBELLION

Negative feelings toward other human beings are part of everyone's life. When someone else hurts you by stealing your boy friend or girl friend, you feel annoyed, at the very least. But often negative feelings are not justified by the outside events, or are based on a misinterpretation of the events (perhaps the boy friend just became disenchanted with you and did not become interested in another girl until later). Then angry or hostile feelings are merely a way to avoid facing your own problems— a way which can disturb people around you.

Some people are often or always hostile, usually as a result, at least in part, of unsatisfied emotional needs earlier in their lives. These hostile people can become involved in fights, mob violence, sexual promiscuity, alcoholism, hostile domination of a family, or other asocial behavior.

Rebellion is a special kind of hostility. Unsatisfied emotional needs, especially the need for independence, frequently lead to rebellion in adolescence. This rebellion, manifested by excessive opposition to suggestions and direction from parents and others in authority, does not necessarily predict a continuing hostile attitude toward life or a continuing social difficulty.

Violent and aggressive behavior may be influenced by brain dysfunction. Stimulation of a certain part of the brain near its center, the amygdala, in both animals and man has produced aggressive behavior. A mild-mannered lady when so stimulated became angry and hostile, threatening to strike the person controlling the stimulus. These symptoms disappeared when the stimulus ceased, and she apologized. The practical importance of this function is uncertain. In some people, aggressive behavior has been correlated with unusual patterns of brain waves. Hormones, too, have some correlation with aggression. Of crimes of violence performed by women, 62 percent occurred in the week just before the onset of their menstrual period, but only 2 percent at the end of the menstrual period. In children, a condition of uncertain origin, called a *hyperkinetic state* and often partially controllable by drugs, includes aggressive and uncooperative behavior. (See also Chapter 10, page 147, for the effect of genetics on criminal behavior.)

WITHDRAWAL

When faced with difficult or unpleasant situations, most people have an urge to escape, to withdraw into themselves or their homes where during infancy and childhood they felt security and love. Illness frequently provides the excuse or justification for such withdrawal. The child who is having a difficult time at school with teachers or associates may remember a time when he was ill and did not have to go to school. He may therefore begin to wonder whether or not he really feels well and actually may develop symptoms of headache, beginning cold, or upset stomach. In the comfort and security of his home he receives the loving attention and care which he missed at school. As a result of this he feels better.

Among adults, illnesses of various types develop on a similar basis. The illness unconsciously provides the justification for escaping from unsatisfactory life situations and thus a temporary solution to existing difficulties. It is not, however, a solution and, if continued, is likely to result in chronic invalidism or other disabling behavior. Psychiatric aid may be necessary to enable such a person to discover the reasons that lead him to frequent illness and to help him to face the problems directly.

DENIAL

Denial is somewhat similar to suppression. Instead of putting a thought aside, one insists that something never happened, or that it was not significant. Denial can be a useful mechanism when it does not involve basic or important needs, drives, or facts. In an amusing (and self-aware) example, an expectant father wrote the following three notes in the father's book outside the delivery room at a hospital where his wife was in labor: First, "Nine A.M. I declare here and now that my wife, Barbara, will give birth to a beautiful girl whom we shall name Nicolle." Second, "One P.M. Nicolle, come on, dammit." And finally, "Five P.M. Just got the word. It's a boy. Just exactly what I wanted. Who'd want a girl with a dumb name like Nicolle." On the other hand, when an industrial plant announces that it will have to close in 6 months, but one of the

workers says that it will never happen or that he will be transferred, he is using a denial which is dangerous to his welfare.

SEX CONFLICTS

For most people, the sex emotion is most completely satisfied when an enduring, loving relationship with someone else has been established. The psychological and emotional responses associated with sex are strong and complicated. They require open discussion and understanding to prevent excessive conflict and disability. Many of the emotional conflicts related to sex stem from ignorance and misinformation. Chapters 20 and 21 are devoted to a discussion of physical, psychological, and social aspects of human sexuality.

RATIONALIZATION

Rationalization is a type of mental self-deception. It consists in excusing or justifying failures, shortcomings, or other events by explanations which seem to relieve the individual of responsibility or blame. This is not a satisfactory way of dealing with problems, but it may enable a person to live with his inadequacies, at least for a limited period of time. Far better than rationalization, however, is a frank recognition of shortcomings, combined with the formulation of a plan to overcome them or to live peacefully with them.

REACTION FORMATION

Unknown to most people, but very common in life, reaction formation is a way of protecting the self against anxiety by adopting the very opposite of an uncomfortable urge which has been strong in one's personality. For example, it is not unusual to find men who had some scrapes with the law as teen-agers overcome these unnacceptable urges and become policemen, lawyers, or clergymen as adults. Some people who have strong homosexual facets to their personalities, perhaps unknown to themselves, undergo reaction formation and become aggressively heterosexual; perhaps they are promiscuous, or talk much of the time about sexual subjects, or have intercourse with a husband or wife unusually frequently and in a compulsive manner.

SUBLIMATION

All of us must channel some of our drives into more acceptable forms. For example, a boy who had set three or four fires in his home joined the Boy Scouts and became known as the boy who could get a fire started under *any* circumstances. Sexual drives are often partially sublimated into creative or artistic activities. Physical exercise, especially in contact sport, often serves as sublimation for angry or hostile feelings.

Reaction formation and sublimation have highly desirable social results. They should be welcomed by both individual and society.

MAINTAINING MENTAL HEALTH

At times, everyone develops fears, anxieties, and tensions that must be released if mental and emotional disturbances are to be avoided. In many instances frank discussion with an understanding friend, teacher, religious counselor, or physician is helpful. In others, the expert and experienced help of a psychiatrist is necessary. Discussing—and facing—problems helps to dispel conflicts and permit the direction of energies into healthful and satisfying channels.

OPPORTUNITIES FOR THE INDIVIDUAL

Mental health is more readily attained through experience, and by living with other people, than by intellectual exercise and self-will. Specific rules and directions cannot guarantee that mental health will be maintained and emotional disorders avoided. An understanding of the discussions above may help many people adjust to and control their environments, and the following general guides will promote happiness and mental health for most people:

1 Believe in yourself. Ralph Waldo Emerson, in his famous essay "Trust Thyself," says, "Self trust (without conceit) is the first secret of success. Cast out fear; rely on your own inner resources; trust life and it will repay your trust. . . . Trust thyself and trust the wisdom and integrity of others. . . . Nothing is at last sacred but the integrity of your own mind. . . ."

2 Retain or develop some impelling interest or interests, in which you can lose and forget yourself. These may be your job or profession, your family, your home, nature, sports, hobbies, music, literature, art, etc. Helping some other person or people can be an impelling interest in itself.

3 Set goals for yourself that are reasonably attainable. A long step toward good mental health is accepting oneself and one's limitations. Thales, a Greek sage and philosopher, when asked what was difficult replied, "To know oneself." Difficult of attainment as it may be, such knowledge is of utmost value. On the other hand, it is dangerous to use handicaps as an excuse for not attempting some useful and satisfactory work. Everyone has capacities as well as limitations. A person should take stock of his assets so as to direct his efforts along lines in which he may expect the greatest degree of continuing accomplishment and lasting personal satisfaction.

4 Live one day at a time. Most of the things we worry about never happen or are beyond our control. St. Francis of Assisi, when asked while hoeing his garden what he would do if he knew that this were his last day on earth, replied that he would continue hoeing his garden. Such a reply reflects a mind that is at peace with itself and with the world.

5 Realize that your conflicts and weaknesses are not unique but are shared by many others. Most people have mixed feelings toward others in general and toward members of their own families.

6 Remember that when your burdens seem heaviest and your problems insurmountable, you can always lighten someone else's burden a little, thereby helping yourself as well.

7 Understand that personal tensions may show up in many unexpected ways and that their true meaning may not be readily discernible. Such tensions may give rise to bodily symptoms. They may be the sole cause or a contributing cause of many types of sickness.

8 Find some person or persons—a professional person or a mature friend—with whom you can talk out problems in a

confidential relationship. Confused attitudes and feelings are often clarified by putting them into words spoken to someone who will not tell you what to do but will be a good listener and help you to recognize your own feelings and wants.

9 Healthy individuals have a sense of integrity. The continuing development of conscience is an important part of attaining mental health.

10 A sense of right and wrong and a feeling of moral responsibility for one's behavior are most important. However, it is also important to try to free oneself from feelings of unnecessary guilt and from the inevitable sense of failure which is certain to result from a belief that one must avoid having thoughts, feelings, and impulses upon which it would be wrong or unacceptable to act.

11 Be slow to criticize, quick to sympathize. Be generous in offering encouragement and commendation. To do so is helpful to those who give as well as to those who receive.

12 Appreciate mental health not as something to be practiced at specified intervals, but as a way of living and meeting the normal adjustments of life. The mentally healthy person constantly seeks to develop the ability to face frustrations realistically rather than to run from them.

OPPORTUNITIES FOR THE PROFESSIONAL

Professional workers in the field of mental health are interested in promoting and preserving mental health as well as in treating mental illness. A major recent movement in psychiatry is known as *community psychiatry*. By its principles, psychiatrists and other mental-health professionals (psychologists, psychiatric social workers, nurses) move out of hospitals and consulting rooms to deal with people and groups in their home environments. If the police have arrested a local citizen, and his neighbors feel that he has been arrested unjustly, the community worker will help the neighbors talk with the police so that there can be some mutual understanding. If a community feels that its school system is giving inappropriate education, the community worker will help the two communicate. If

drugs are a problem in the community, the community worker can help many people and groups find some common interest or goal and advise them in directing their actions constructively rather than wasting their energies in accusing each other of lack of understanding and evil intentions.

More technically, preventive medicine has a subdivision called *preventive psychiatry*, which has received increasing attention. Preventive medicine as applied in psychiatry can be divided into three phases:

1 Primary prevention, which eliminates the source of illness. For example, eradication of syphilis in the community by education, prophylaxis, and early treatment prevents damage to the brain by the syphilis spirochete, a process which used to cause thousands of cases each year of general paresis, a serious mental disease. Elimination of both complete suppression and complete permissiveness of hostile and sexual impulses in childhood will prevent some of the problems that children might later have in control and expression.

2 Secondary prevention is the *early* detection, treatment, and cure of an illness so that no dysfunction exists or remains. Two good examples are the early treatment of cretinism (the thyroid deficiency of infancy and childhood) with thyroid hormone (see Chapter 19, Hormones), and the early detection (shortly after birth) of the metabolic disease phenylpyruvic oligophrenia, so that mental retardation can be prevented by proper diet. In another sphere, a mental health professional may help a family and a school understand that the apparently unorthodox behavior of a sixth-grade boy merely represents a moderate degree of hyperactiveness, a need to engage in frequent movement and activity. By allowing him to satisfy this need instead of conforming to the strict rules imposed on other children, parents and school can engage his cooperation, release his real abilities, and prevent him from sliding gradually into juvenile delinquency.

3 Tertiary prevention modifies an ailment to allow the afflicted person to function as

well as possible. In this sense, the modern treatments of schizophrenia and depres- sion described in Chapter 10 contribute to mental health.

QUESTIONS FOR DISCUSSION AND SELF-EXAMINATION

1 Discuss in specific terms the relation between "normality" and "mental health."
2 What are the similarities and differences, in training and in function, among the psychiatrist, the clinical psychologist, and the psychiatric social worker?
3 What factors are important in the development of good adult mental health?
4 What is meant by *reinforcement* and by *extinguishment* in psychology? How do these processes contribute to maturation?
5 Describe the differences and the relationships among id, ego, and superego.
6 Discuss the effects which the mind may have on the body.
7 How are reactions to psychological conflicts related to basic emotional needs?
8 What do you regard as the three most important of the basic emotional needs? Defend your answer.
9 How does suppression differ from repression? How are the two related to other responses to psychological conflicts?
10 Discuss the role of conscious planning as compared with the role of the unconscious mechanisms in mental health.

REFERENCES AND READING SUGGESTIONS

BOOKS

Spock, Benjamin: *Problems of Parents*, Houghton-Mifflin Company, Boston, 1962.

Advice to parents on how to ease family tensions and cope with various specific problems.

Strecker, Edward A., and Kenneth A. Appel: *Discovering Ourselves*, The Macmillan Company, New York, 1962.

Two distinguished psychiatrists discuss in nontechnical language emotional development and disturbances which trouble many people.

PAMPHLETS AND PERIODICALS

Blanton, Smiley: "The Best Prescription I Know," *Reader's Digest*, December 1962, p. 64.

A distinguished psychiatrist discusses the role of the unconscious in coping with emotional problems.

Boehn, George A. W.: "That Wonderful Machine, the Brain," *Fortune*, February 1963, p. 125.

An excellent report on the fascinating research concerning the many vital and complex functions of the brain.

Cooley, Donald G.: "Cells That Communicate," *Today's Health*, May 1963, p. 20.

A splendid article on the miracles of cellular communication that are carried out in the brain and nervous system.

Mental Health Is: 1-2-3, National Association for Mental Health, New York.

Important characteristics of people with good mental health.

Pratt, Dallas, and Jack Neher: *Mental Health Is a Family Affair*, Public Affairs Pamphlet, New York.

Saunders, David S.: "A Bookshelf on Mental Health," *American Journal of Public Health*, vol. 55, p. 502, April 1965.

An overview of the mental health picture, 1955–1965.

Thorman, George: *Toward Mental Health*, Public Affairs Pamphlet, New York.

What Every Child Needs, National Association for Mental Health, New York.

The emotional needs of children that should be recognized and satisfied.

10

MENTAL DISTURBANCES

In earlier times and in different cultures people with mental disturbances have been considered to be either possessed by evil spirits or especially gifted by the gods. What does the term *mental disturbances* mean to Americans in the 1970s? It means, for example, a college student who spends 2 months in a mental hospital and 6 months in convalescence before he can return to college. It means a 50-year-old man with schizophrenia who has spent the last 31 years of his life on the "back ward" of a state hospital. It means a woman, formerly cheerful and bright, who has become gloomy, despondent, lacking in self-confidence—in short, depressed—and who will commit suicide next week if her family do not get her into a hospital. It means a successful 42-year-old doctor who has almost bled to death from his psychologically caused duodenal ulcer. It means a young woman incapacitated by tension headaches, a child in an institution for the mentally retarded, a boy under

treatment for epilepsy, a drug addict, a chronic alcoholic, a habitual criminal, and many other people. Mental illness is not something remote from ordinary human experience, kept locked away in a hospital ward, but a condition often touching our own friends and relatives, and even ourselves. The problems connected with mental disturbances were dramatized in 1972 by the controversy surrounding the nomination of Senator Thomas Eagleton as the Democratic vice-presidential candidate. When it was revealed that Eagleton had been treated for mental disturbance, the issue grew so heated that he was forced to withdraw his candidacy.

Throughout the United States and the world, mental illnesses are a major cause of disability. The mentally ill constitute almost half of all the patients in the hospitals of the United States. Federal and state governments of the United States maintain almost half a million hospital beds for patients with mental illnesses. Of all rejections for and separations from military service, more than half are based on mental defects, failure to attain intellectual standards, and psychological difficulties. If past experience continues to hold true, about one in every twelve children born this year in the United States will suffer a mental illness sometime in his life severe enough to cause hospitalization.

Reasonable estimates of the number of mentally ill run as high as 17 million, and even this may be a low figure. A study of residents of mid-Manhattan, New York City, showed that only 18.5 percent were free of symptoms of mental illness. In this study, a group of trained investigators carefully interviewed the adult residents of a large area. Just over half had mild to moderately severe symptoms, such as bothersome tension, undue nervousness, or other definite psychological disturbances, which did not prevent them, however, from leading their daily lives. Almost a quarter of the residents had severe and at least partially incapacitating mental and emotional illnesses, leaving just under one in five well.

Also included in the "reasonable estimates" of 17 million mentally ill are the 5 or 6 million alcoholics in the country, the 500,000 to 700,000 narcotic addicts, and the 300,000 to 500,000 juvenile delinquents. Some experts put the numbers higher. Mental illness also accounts for a substantial number of divorces, crimes, work absenteeism, unemployment, and other personal troubles.

THE PSYCHOSES

The mention of "mental illness" often brings to mind a patient confined to a mental hospital, someone who is "crazy." Although many people with mental illness are not in hospitals, most psychotic patients—those suffering from the psychoses—cannot cope with the world and must be confined. These patients have great difficulty in making correct interpretations of themselves and the world around them. Their difficulty has nothing to do with whether or not they accept the traditional political and cultural wisdom; it has to do with whether they see themselves realistically, whether they see their neighbors realistically, and whether they see the physical environment realistically. Although there are cases in which mental illness is difficult to establish, it is clear that the following mental patients have serious malfunction of their minds: a person who has had a brilliant career but who suddenly begins to feel that he is worthless and is tempted to commit suicide; a person who believes that he is a prominent historical or religious figure from the past; and a person who sees or hears things that no one else can see or hear.

SCHIZOPHRENIA

Schizophrenia, the most common type of psychosis, is characterized by delusions, hallucinations, abnormal suspicions (paranoid thinking), disorientation and other loss of contact with reality, bizarre actions, and senseless talk and laughter. Few, if any, patients have all these symptoms and some have only one or two.

Delusions are mistaken ideas about reality or identity: the patient, for example, may think he is Julius Caesar. Hallucinations consist of seeing or hearing sights or sounds which do not exist. These symptoms can be very frightening; a person may hear menacing or accusing voices, or believe that he is being ordered to do something wrong. Paranoid thoughts in patients with schizophrenia attribute to other people purposes or powers which they do not possess and which are usually malevolently directed against the patient. This is more than a simple misunderstanding or misinpretation of actual events: it may reach the point of completely groundless belief. Someone may be convinced that the police are persecuting him, that his bank is trying to ruin him, that others are plotting to kill him or can control his mind. The term *paranoid* is too widely and inaccurately used today, often to attack a person with whom one disagrees on a political or other emotionally charged issue.

Disorientation means that the patient is unreasonably confused about the day, the year, or the place. Many people wake up and take a few moments to remember just where they are; they are disoriented for those few minutes, but they do not remain disoriented for days or weeks at a time, as some schizophrenics do.

Schizophrenia most commonly begins during adolescence or early adulthood, although the disordered thoughts may not be obvious for months or years to those around the patient. In many such cases, a young man or woman, perhaps previously bright and attractive, gradually undergoes a personality change, becoming more and more listless, eccentric, and preoccupied; he avoids friends and it is difficult to hold general conversations with him, although he may be able to talk at length on some subject of interest to him. In some people, the onset of the illness is sudden instead of gradual, in which case the prognosis for rapid recovery is usually better.

In some cases of schizophrenia, the patient complains of peculiar physical symptoms and may even feel that his body is rotting away. If he has paranoid schizophrenia he becomes suspicious and distrustful, and his suspicions eventually center on one person or group of people who, often unknown to themselves, he believes influencing him or plotting against him in some way.

Schizophrenia may be associated with furtive glances and smiles, smirking looks, bizarre posturing or facemaking, mute and trancelike withdrawal (catatonic schizophrenia), or shuffling automation. In its worst stages all contact with the world seems to have been lost. People in this condition are often placed on the back wards of mental hospitals, where they stay for months or years. Rarely do schizophrenics harm others, although their language may be full of violence; they are more likely to turn the violence against themselves and commit suicide.

Schizophrenia is a disease of major importance, with some 60,000 new cases diagnosed each year in the United States. Approximately half of all hospitalized mentally ill patients have this disease; thus one-fourth of all the hospital beds in the country are occupied by patients with this one illness.

The cause (or causes) of schizophrenia is unknown, but some doctors believe that there may be a chemical component. Over the last two decades in particular there has been intensive search for a substance or substances in the body specifically correlated with schizophrenia. This substance or substances might be either causative, producing symptoms by its toxic action on the brain, or diagnostic, a by-product of the disease whose detection would allow early and definitive diagnosis. The search has been discouraging. Demonstration of abnormal proteins, abnormal protein derivatives, or abnormal distribution of biochemical componets have not proved to be consistent in schizophrenia, and have not been well correlated with symptoms and abnormalities. The search continues.

On the other hand, heredity appears to be one of the factors which cause people to become schizophrenic. Although heredity by itself does not cause schizophrenia, a person who is predisposed to the disease by heredity is more likely to become schizophrenic when subjected to certain kinds of social and psychological pressures than is a person who does not have such a hereditary background.

The evidence is clear. Identical twins whose heredity includes schizophrenia and who are raised apart from each other frequently both develop schizophrenia, as do identical twins with similar hereditary backgrounds who are raised together. In general, blood relatives of schizophrenics have a high incidence not only of schizophrenia but also of "schizoid" (schizophrenialike) states such as excess suspiciousness, peculiar personality patterns, and so forth. Even mental retardation is slightly more frequent among the relatives of schizophrenics than in the general population. Schizophrenia also occurs more frequently in patients with celiac disease (a hereditary disease whose major symptom is poor absorption of certain foods from the intestinal tract) and in the relatives of these patients than in the population as a whole.

Progress in treating schizophrenia has been encouraging. In 1930 three out of every ten schizophrenics under the age of 35 in hospitals died each year. Now the mortality is only a fifth of that. Between 1938 and 1948 one out of every three schizophrenics admitted to a hospital for the first time remained in the hospital for 10 years or more. By 1968, that figure had fallen to one out of twenty and was still falling. In recent years, the absolute number of schizophrenics in United States hospitals has decreased 3 percent each year, despite a rising national population.

Various treatment methods have contributed to this decline. The neuroleptics or major tranquilizers have been of the greatest importance in treating schizophrenia. (See the box on page 142.)

MIND-AFFECTING DRUGS

Many drugs are available to modify the processes of the mind for therapeutic or other purposes. The first of these developed were the sedatives—the barbiturates—and the stimulants—the mild caffeine and the more powerful amphetamines. Then tranquilizers were developed. Drugs which can cause hallucinations were put into a separate class. In 1966, a World Health Organization Committee approved a new classification:

1 Neuroleptics, also known as *major tranquilizers*, which have therapeutic effects on psychoses. The phenothiazines, such as Thorazine, are the best known. Many of them also have side effects on the nervous system.
2 Anxiolytic sedatives. Agents which promote sleep, help combat convulsions, and allay anxiety. They include the barbiturates and meprobamate ("Miltown," "Equanil").
3 Antidepressants, also called *psychic energizers*. They combat depression, but do not stimulate as the amphetamines do.
4 Psychostimulants. Drugs which increase the level of alertness and/or motivation. They include caffeine and the amphetamines.
5 Psycholeptics, also called *hallucinogens* and *psychedelics*. They produce abnormal cognitive and perceptual mental effects, and include LSD, the *Cannabis* products (marijuana, hashish, etc.), DMT, and mescaline.

It has also been very helpful to have hospital patients spend part of each day outside the hospital when they are able to do so. Some patients can be treated entirely on an out-patient basis. In 1967 and 1968, the Emergency Treatment unit at the Connecticut Mental Health Center in New Haven treated 500 persons, mostly acutely ill psychotic or depressed patients. More than 80 percent returned to their homes and jobs after only 3 days of hospitalization, with a 30-day period of ambulatory treatment following. Fewer than one out of three had to return to the emergency unit. Women responded to treatment somewhat better than men. Emphasis in treatment was on working out immediate problems, with tranquilizers used as needed.

DEPRESSION AND THE MANIC-DEPRESSIVE DISORDERS

Depression in all its forms is even more common than schizophrenia. Most people have times when they feel discouraged or sad. Real-life disasters, such as the death of a close relative, normally cause feelings of depression; we must grieve at such times, but we know that the grief will pass if we carry on with our usual activities.

Depression becomes abnormal and passes into psychosis when the victim's feelings become extremely unrelated to reality. Severely depressed people feel alone, without friends, love, status, or esteem. Nothing excites them any more, their usual pastimes are uninteresting, and life has lost its meaning. They are chronically tired, with their fatigue usually worse in the morning, and often complain of aches, pains, poor digestion, poor bowel function, loss of sleep (most typically with early-morning awakening), loss of appetite, loss of weight, menstrual disturbances, and loss of sexual interests. They tend to be irritable, quarrelsome, and negligent of schoolwork, household responsibilites, and business. Escape may be sought in alcohol, drugs, social withdrawal, or suicide.

Although rare in childhood, depression may appear at any time from adolescence onward. It is particularly common in women about the time of the menopause, when it is often referred to as *menopausal depression* or *involutional melancholia.* This is an unusually severe type of depression, but readily treatable.

Sometimes, depression appears as part of a cycle alternating between elation and sadness. Elation, like depression, is an expected feeling, and most welcome, especially when it accompanies a joyful event or personal success. But when it is unrelated to reality and is accompanied by great overactivity of mind and body, then it represents illness. At such times, patients neglect sleep, often exhausting those around them, and show poor judgment, taking on many more tasks and much more difficult tasks than they are equipped to handle. This is the manic phase of manic-depressive disorders, and is usually followed by a depression.

An association between manic-depressive psychosis and color blindness points to another possible hereditary influence on mental illness. Although the chances are small that any one colorblind person will develop a manic-depressive psychosis, more people who have manic-depressive disorders are color-blind than would be predicted statistically.

Many famous people have suffered from depression. Abraham Lincoln as a young man had recurrent depressions and had repeated difficulties in many of his endeavors: storekeeping, the law, politics, and love. Then, after a year of unusually deep depression, he was able to turn his thoughts and energies outward instead of inward, was able to rise to the challenges presented to him, and became the resolute, purposeful man we know of. William James, the famous psychologist, could accomplish almost nothing as a young man, and was almost a recluse in his early twenties. Then, apparently as a result of being inspired by an essay on the meaning of personal liberty, he reorganized his thinking and his life, becoming a famous and productive man.

In combating depression, it is important to be able to draw on personal resources, as did Lincoln and James. Concentration on achievement rather than failure, attempts to turn outward to other people and their needs instead of inward to personal problems, growth of a religious or philosophical faith, and the support of friends are all important. But when depression is severe or when it does not yield readily to personal effort, today's citizens can count on more effective help than was available in an earlier day. The professional help offered by a psychiatrist is often beneficial. Modern antidepressant drugs sometimes help, and electroshock treatment will dramatically cut short many severe depressions, particularly those of middle life. In many cases, particularly of mild depression, the illness comes from an abnormal turning-in of anger at the outside world; psychotherapy can help the individual to accept his feelings and express them openly, rather than in the form of mental illness.

Suicide   An end result of some severe depressions is attempted or successful suicide. Suicide may be impetuous, but usually has been talked about and planned for days, months, or even years. About 75 percent of people who successfully commit suicide have attempted it before.

Approximately 20,000 deaths by suicide are reported in the United States each year. This number, however, is probably less than half the actual total, for many deaths by suicide are reported as due to other causes because of the social stigma attached in this country to suicide. For the country as a whole, suicide ranks tenth as a cause of death, but it ranks fourth among persons between 15 and 34 years of age (and second among college students); fifth, between 35 and 44; sixth, between 45 and 54; and seventh, between 55 and 64. Deaths from suicide are higher among whites than among nonwhites, and higher among males than among females, although suicide attempts are more frequent among females than among males. (See Figure 10.1.)

A recent study of 225 suicides among former students of the University of Pennsylvania and Harvard University showed that suicide is more likely to occur if the parents are separated; if the father is dead; if the father is a professional man with a college education; if the suicide victim was a cigarette smoker as a student, had attended a secondary boarding school, had not participated in extracurricular activites including athletics, had failed to be graduated from college, had been underweight, had had allergies, had considered himself in ill health, or had been inclined to insomnia, worry, self-consciousness, feelings of persecution, secretiveness or seclusiveness, anxiety, and depression.

Many would-be suicides wish to be saved;

Figure 10.1 Suicide in the United States: rates per 100,000 by age, color, and sex.

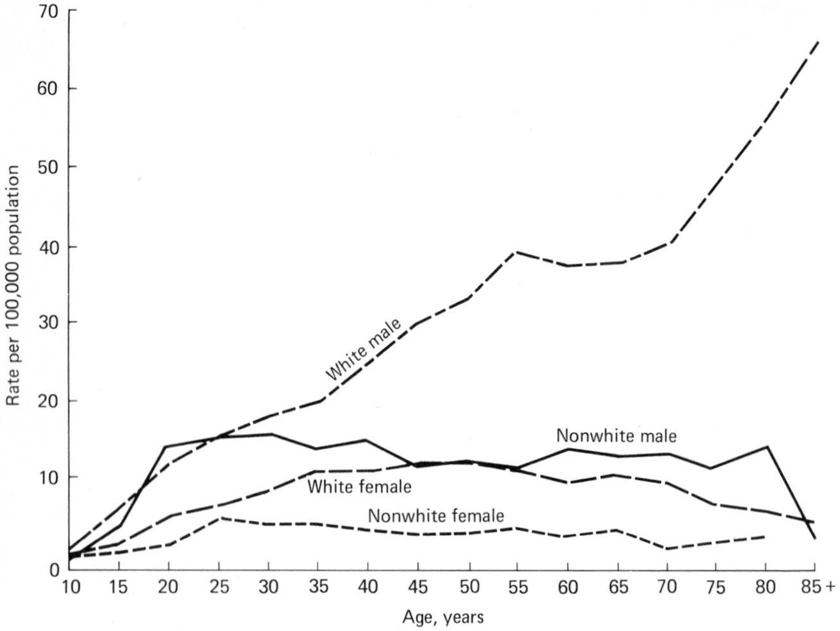

hence a threat of suicide or an attempt at suicide should be considered a cry for help. In such situations, psychiatric or other professional help may save a life and alleviate the basic condition responsible for the depression. To provide such aid several cities have established "suicide centers." Suicide is more preventable than many other causes of death, and most patients can be shown better ways than suicide to resolve their problems, conflicts, and crises.

When someone talks of suicide Talk of suicide should never be ignored. People who talk about suicide are much more likely to attempt it than those who do not. If a friend or relative mentions that he is considering suicide, take him seriously. Encourage him to tell you all about his feelings and thoughts. Don't try to argue about intellectual matters, such as why life is worthwhile. Do assure him that feelings of depression and unworthiness, feelings that life is not worth while, and so forth, can be temporary. Try to persuade him to seek psychiatric help; offer to go with him to a doctor's office. If there are others who are close to him, particularly a relative, spouse, or girl or boy friend, try to involve them. You may save a life.

OTHER PSYCHOSES

Many processes which damage the brain can cause a secondary psychosis, mimicking schizophrenia or depression in some cases. Syphilis of the brain was one of the most common types of psychosis until modern treatment, particularly penicillin, almost eliminated it in this country. The degenerative processes of old age are extremely common causes of psychosis. Hardening of the arteries (arteriosclerosis), which causes small areas of scarlike tissue to form in the brain, is thought to cause many cases of senile psychosis. However, the mechanism or mechanisms by which senile psychosis occurs are largely unknown.

Senile psychosis differs from many other mental illnesses in that there is damage to the normal functions of the brain. Thus, the intellectual and memory functions are affected, in contrast to other disorders such as schizophrenia, in which normal (or often superior) intellect is manifested along with the symptoms of the illness. Senile psychosis may show the same symptoms as other mental illness, however.

Only a minority of people beyond the age of 70 develop senile psychosis. Senile patients tend to do better at home than in institutions, when their behavior permits such care. Unfamiliar surroundings and people tend to confuse them and to increase their symptoms. Unfortunately, however, their illnesses often progress to the point where they may need more care and restriction of their aimless wandering than they can normally receive at home.

THE NEUROSES

More common than the psychoses are the neuroses. This large group of psychological problems includes tension headaches, "nervous stomachs," "irritable colons," minor depressions, anxieties, obsessions, compulsions, insomnias, and fatigue unexplained by physical disease. Careful interviewing of people leading normal lives will usually reveal some of these symptoms, often very minor ones. People with neurotic problems have relatively good insights into reality and are usually responsible and useful citizens. They are able to carry on their daily tasks, although sometimes with less efficiency and less personal satisfaction than if they had no neurotic symptoms.

Many times the cause of such problems appears to be something in the patient's life. A housewife with three small, boisterous children and a salesman husband who spends long periods away from home "has a right" to tension headaches and insomnia. A graduate student who has failed his general examinations once and is studying 16 hours a day at the present time "has a right" to have nausea and slight diarrhea. A premedical student who is studying for a final examination in organic chemistry which he believes, perhaps falsely, will determine whether or not he will be admitted to medical school "has a right" to have insomnia. But these explanations are inadequate; the reason for this inadequacy is that there are other people in similar circumstances under identical or very similar stresses who are *not* having symptoms. It is therefore clear that there has to be something *within* the person himself which predisposes him to develop symptoms under stress. Furthermore, there are others who have symptoms most of the time in the midst of lives of average stress.

The reason for neurotic symptoms is unclear. Perhaps heredity contributes, though there are no

Other brain-damaging causes of psychosis include injury, brain tumor, nutritional deficiencies (particularly pellegra, as described on page 165), and certain drugs. In severe infections, with high fever or circulating toxins or both, an acute confused state often occurs which is called a *toxic psychosis* and is temporary.

statistics similar to those for schizophrenia quoted above. The traditional psychiatric opinion describes a neurotic symptom as a defense used against anxiety. If a person did not have the symptom, he would have to face the anxiety directly, and that would be too painful. Symptoms may have a "language" of their own; for example, a person with intestinal cramps may be "griped" at the world, his boss, or his wife. Emotional fatigue often results from being trapped in a situation chosen by the patient himself. College professors often have such fatigue when they have chosen to write on a dull subject. They cannot gracefully withdraw from writing; their only defense is fatigue, which calls for rest (away from the dull topic).

In some cases, however, there are biochemical changes which are involved in neurotic symptoms, not necessarily as the primary cause. Infusions of sodium lactate into patients with anxiety neurosis recreates in them such symptoms as palpitation, dyspnea and breathlessness, sighing, tiredness, tightness in the throat, and apprehension; these effects of sodium lactate can be blocked by injections of calcium.

A common mistake attributes neurotic symptoms to "imagination." Nothing could be further from the truth. These emotionally caused symptoms are as real as a broken leg or a heart attack. Often they are more uncomfortable, because they are less responsive to treatment. To be sure, they are less dangerous, and in addition, the average life expectancy of people with neurotic symptoms is reported to be longer than that of people without them.

Sedatives and tranquilizers may give temporary relief to neurotic symptoms, but they solve neither the problems within the individual nor the problems in his environment. Planning life to avoid stressful situations is useful but may restrict opportunity. At the present time only psycho-

therapy offers the hope of lasting relief for chronic or recurrent symptoms.

PSYCHOSOMATIC DISORDERS

Psychosomatic disorders are illnesses in which a structural change in the body takes place partly or wholly as a result of psychological stimuli, conflicts, and problems. While the term *psychosomatic* means literally "mind-body," illnesses such as nervous stomach which involve no structural change in the body are usually not included in the category.

The effect of mind on body is great, as the following story indicates. For 13 years Charlie and Josephine had been inseparable. One day, as Josephine watched in terror, policemen shot Charlie dead. Josephine drew near Charlie's lifeless form. Sinking to her knees, she quietly laid her head on his bloody body. The policemen let Josephine express her grief in the hope she would gain relief. But, although she had been healthy until the shooting, Josephine died 15 minutes later, never having raised her head from Charlie's body. Josephine and Charlie are not characters from an opera or a movie, but from real life. But they were llamas escaped from a zoo, not human beings.

Dr. George L. Engel of the University of Rochester has studied the psychological states that precede sudden shifts from good health to severe, even fatal, illness in humans, and finds that "giving up" frequently does precede the decline. After the death of a spouse, for example, men and women die with more than statistically predicted frequency in the next few months. However, most of the relationships between the mind and illness of the body are not so dramatic as that of Josephine, and are related to specific diseases.

The illnesses which are strongly psychosomatic (at least in some cases) are peptic ulcer of the stomach and duodenum, ulcerative colitis, hypertension, and bronchial asthma. Some physicians also include eczema, rheumatoid arthritis, and other diseases. In each of these diseases, specific emotional problems have been linked with the bodily changes, and sometimes dramatic improvements in the illness take place with simple changes in internal or external emotional stimuli. For example, an underworld character with high blood pressure was admitted to the hospital for study. Not only was his blood pressure very high (220/140) but there were signs of damage to his heart and his kidneys. He was under constant strain not only because of his occupation but because his girl friend, whom he insisted on visiting regularly, lived in a district controlled by a rival underworld figure. His visits to her were at some risk to his life. When he entered the hospital, ceasing his occupation for the time being and, more important, ceasing visits to his girl friend, his blood pressure returned to normal without any medicine and his electrocardiogram became normal.

Psychosomatic illnesses can be fatal, and the medical treatment must often include psychological help as well as medicine, diet, and other supportive measures.

CHARACTER DISORDERS

Another major group of illnesses is the character disorders, which are responsible for many criminals, delinquents, alcoholics, drug addicts, and sexual deviants. The most characteristic example is the "con man": a person who is charming, intelligent, and winning but who is insincere and has a long series of ingenious tricks for separating people from their money. Such people lack a mature conscience and are given to antisocial behavior.

They do not appear insane or unable to take responsibility for their conduct, and yet they often behave as if they were unable to control themselves. They are usually able to interpret their environment accurately; the problem is that there is something "missing" in their personalities.

A psychiatric term now often used for people with character disorders is *sociopathic personality*; *psychopathic personality* is an older variant. People with character disorders often seem to suffer little and to have little motivation to change their behavior and orientation toward life, making this disorder almost totally unresponsive to psychiatric treatment, but they often cause considerable suffering for their close relatives and friends.

An inherited disorder has been discovered as a possible contributing factor in criminal behavior.

Men with an XYY chromosomal pattern (an extra Y sex chromosome) engage in violent and criminal behavior more often than people with normal chromosomal patterns. Relatively few such men actually commit crimes, but the predisposition seems to have been clearly established. So far no successful treatment for this condition has been discovered.

EMOTIONALLY SICK CHILDREN

Emotionally sick children are a special category, since their symptoms and problems do not align themselves clearly with any of the above groups. They suffer from the early stages of all or many of the conditions referred to above, as well as from many problems which will disappear before they grow to adulthood. School problems, discipline problems, bed-wetting, childhood delinquency, some psychosomatic disorders, and nervousness are all indicators of emotional disturbance. Whenever possible, the causes of such symptoms should be investigated; often corrective action at this early point can avoid a life of unhappiness, physical illness, psychological disturbance, or antisocial behavior.

One group of emotionally ill children has received special attention recently: children with hyperkinesis. Intelligent and quick, they lack patience and the ability to sustain interest over a period of time. In the classroom, their attention wanders, they make noise and commotion, and they may appear to be ringleaders in troublemaking. They push in lines, and are disorderly. It has been reported that medication, particularly the amphetamines and some of the mood elevators, has been successful in increasing their span of interest and their cooperation in class.

THE TREATMENT OF PSYCHOLOGICAL DISORDERS

The treatment of schizophrenia and depression was briefly discussed above. This section will discuss the different types of treatment which are available to those who may need help for any of the psychological illnesses.

To start with, there is no mental illness known today which can be "cured" by some particular treatment, as, for example, strep throat or tonsillitis can be cured by penicillin. There is not even any treatment, or group of treatments, which will control the harmful processes of mental illness in a predictable, effective manner, similar to the way the modern drugs for the treatment of hypertension control high blood pressure. The processes of the mind are more complicated, and specific treatments have not yet been developed for the various mental illnesses.

What does exist, however, is a range of treatment methods which can be used in varied combinations and which are often, but not consistently, successful. They have greatest success when the patient himself is able to cooperate and is anxious for an improvement in his condition. Almost all treatment of mental illness today includes some psychotherapy, which proceeds through the use of talk. Since these disorders involve disturbed thought, it is not surprising that one of the most effective therapies involves words, the only universal way of expressing thought, and also involves the relationships between human beings, the most important subject on which to expend words.

Some drugs are useful in treating psychological disorders. As previously mentioned, the major tranquillizers seem to help control the abnormal thought processes of schizophrenia. Tranquillizers and sedatives are useful in relieving the anxiety and tension of many neurotic problems, and may also relieve some of the bodily symptoms, such as abdominal cramps and diarrhea, which sometimes accompany neuroses. But since they do not help the patient work through the underlying conflicts which are producing his anxiety (and may actually be a substitute for honestly facing up to his problems) they are usually used as a supplement to psychotherapy. The box on page 142 describes the various drugs which affect mood and thinking.

In recent years, huge doses of vitamins, particulary niacin (vitamin B²) have been suggested as a method of treating schizophrenia and other psychological disorders. This "megavitamin" therapy is alleged to actually cure schizophrenia by directly altering the harmful process in the brain (although the exact nature of this harmful process has never been established). One group of scientists has published statistics which indicate that megavitamin therapy is better than any other type of therapy, but others have been unable to reproduce their results. Therefore, the majority of psychiatrists remain skeptical about the value of this method of treatment.

When a person experiences severe difficulties in coping with reality, the question usually arises whether he should be urged or compelled to enter a hospital. When the person is a threat to others or to himself, there is usually no doubt about the answer: the people around him want him in the hospital, the law gives physicians and police the ability to confine him, and he is often unable to maintain himself in a free community. There are other occasions, however, when a person's thinking is clearly deranged and his ability to carry on his usual activities is impaired, but he is not dangerous to himself or to other people. Some people in this condition feel frightened at being "out of control" and welcome the protection of a psychiatric hospital or hospital division. Others do not recognize that their thinking is unusual or that they are suffering from a mental illness. In this situation, the patient's relatives, along with his physician or physicians, must decide whether the benefits of the treatment that he will receive in the hospital will outweigh the resentment he may feel at being confined.

In psychiatric hospitals or hospital divisions, drugs, psychotherapy, and careful supervision are supplemented by occupational therapy—working at tasks for diversion, for practice in controlling thoughts, or for vocational training. Group therapy may also be offered, and in some "therapeutic communities" patients join with staff in setting rules for the communities and helping to decide when other patients are ready for given privileges, such as weekend leaves at home. Shock treatment may be another valuable part of the hospital regime. There are various ways of giving shock, but electroshock is the most commonly used at the present time. Shock is most useful in cases of severe depression, or when feelings of depression are part of the illness. When used to excess it can destroy memory and even reduce the mental capacity of the patient, but when used with caution it is a safe and valuable treatment.

The treatment most familiar to college students is psychotherapy. Psychotherapy works by providing the patient with both catharsis and support. In *catharsis*, the patient pours out his feelings and problems to a good listener, who may not even be a mental health professional. Most people who try to be good human beings perform this function from time to time. It is a temptation to the lay person, however, to take too much responsibility for someone who wants to confide. Although such a person may enjoy pouring out his soul to a friend or relative, he may *need* some further therapy. Furthermore, the lay person may be tempted to give explanations for the abnormal psychological processes at hand, perhaps on the basis of a course in psychology or some reading in the field. As many experienced psychiatrists and psychologists (but unfortunately not many laymen) know well, a correct diagnosis of a mental illness can often be made only after much careful observation, and therapy must be conducted with equal care. It is easy for an ill-informed layman to do more harm than good if he tries to "help" friends and family members who have serious emotional disturbances.

Support is important to everyone; a person who has support knows that a significant other person cares about him and what happens to him. This is one of the most important things people receive from their friends and family. It should also be possible to feel this type of support in the "cinical" relationship with a therapist; and in fact much of the success of psychotherapy comes from a patient's feeling the acceptance, respect, and sympathy of the therapist, not merely from the therapist's application of whatever theories he holds.

Much of modern psychotherapy aims at giving the patient *insight* into his conflicts and problems so that he can face them directly, and not have to create inefficient and uncomfortable symptoms to protect himself against the anxiety they produce. But he himself must choose to seek insight and must choose to confront his conflicts and problems directly, no matter how painful and distressing this process may be. Psychotherapy, in addition, makes use of the feelings the patient develops about his therapist, called the *transference* in Freudian terminology. If the patient is able to admit these feelings, with the help of his therapist, and to recognize how they spring from parts of his past experience, especially from his childhood, then he may be able to gain insight much more rapidly.

Another type of psychotherapy is *behavior therapy*, which may be used by itself or in combination with insight therapy. It works by a method akin to conditioning. If someone has a phobia about flying, for example, he is gradually accommodated to the idea of flying by talk, pictures, and stories, all in a very pleasant and reassuring setting. The approximation to actual flying gradually increases; toward the end of therapy he may be taken to see airplanes taking off and landing, while enjoying some favorite snack. In other words, his reaction to flying as a pleasurable experience is gradually reinforced, while his reaction to flying as an anxiety-producing experience is gradually extinguished. Eventually the person is able to fly with little or no anxiety. Another variant of behavior therapy works by the association of an undesirable thought or behavior with a painful experience. A patient who has a sexual fetish (say a man who derives sexual excitement from a woman's stocking) may be given gradually increasing electric shocks while looking at or feeling his fetish object. Eventually it will no longer give him any pleasure. This is desirable because the fetish often interferes with full sexual satisfaction or prevents the development of a good relationship with a partner.

Group therapy has become increasingly important in recent years. Often carried out in conjunction with individual therapy, group therapy is particularly useful when a major aspect of a person's problem is unsatisfactory relationships with others. Usually a group of between seven and twelve members meets with its leader once or twice a week. If this leader is a competent mental health professional, group sessions can give the participants much insight into their relationships with others and a greater sensitivity to other people's feelings. The group member may become better able to see others as people like himself, with the same thoughts, feelings, and fears, and through the support and acceptance he receives from the group he may be able to see himself as a worthwhile human being, capable of feeling real love and closeness to others.

Unfortunately, group therapy—under such names as *T groups*, *encounter groups*, and *sensitivity training sessions*—has become something of a fad in this country. This has led to the abuse of a legitimate method of psychotherapy. Groups are often led by untrained people, who lack the knowledge, experience, and skill to direct the group along the path most beneficial to each of its members. Consequently there may be destructive criticism heaped upon one member, or strong group pressure on a person to do things he may find embarrassing or frightening; or problems the group is not qualified to handle may be uncovered. Occasionally patients who have been rather disturbed before the group meeting are thrown into severe confusion or even psychosis by experiences at the meeting, and even those with more mental stability are not benefited by "therapy" given by ignorant and unqualified people. A good (i.e., psychiatrically or psychologically trained) group leader is necessary for a good group—a leader who will carefully screen the applicants before the group starts and make sure that no one is exposed to situations he is not strong enough to face.

THE RESULTS OF THERAPY

Although some studies in the past have indicated little benefit from psychotherapy, investigations in recent years have shown that psychotherapy of various types frequently does make a difference in the outcome of mental disturbance. A review by Dr. Julian Meltzoff and Dr. Melvin Kornreich[1] reports on more than 100 studies which compared treated patients with controls (people with similar symptoms who were not treated). In 80 percent of these studies, the treated patients improved more than did the untreated ones. The range of different types of disorders in these studies is impressive: they include alcoholics, psychotic hospitalized women, juvenile delinquents, and people with

[1]*Psychology* Today, vol. V, no. 2, July 1971.

ulcerative colitis, as well as people with more common anxieties, phobias, and other neurotic problems. In a study of particular interest to college students, 40 students at Ohio State University who had severe personal problems and were doing poor work were divided at random into a group given immediate therapy and a group who were promised therapy 90 days later. With progress assessed by a variety of ratings and tests, the treated students showed more improvement than the nontreated.

For therapy to be successful, however, not only a competent therapist but a willing and eager patient is necessary. The patient who is genuinely anxious not only to get rid of his symptoms but to delve into the origins of his conflicts is much more likely to improve than the patient who enters therapy reluctantly, perhaps only because he has been requested to do so by someone else. The person who wishes help should inquire about the different therapists and types of therapies available. He should try to find someone who not only has a reputation for competence but with whom he feels comfortable talking, although he must realize that if he has trouble talking with each of several therapists, the fault probably lies within himself. He must also prepare to give the therapy a major investment of effort, time, and perhaps money.

PSYCHOTHERAPISTS

Many different types of personnel supply the various therapies for psychological disorders. In addition to psychiatrists, psychologists, and social workers, nurses and nonprofessional aides are important in different settings. Workers from communities are now being trained and used in community mental health programs. Another recent development is the use of college students to answer telephone hot lines which other students or people from the community can call to ask questions or express their worries about drugs, sex, suicide, or any other subjects which may be troubling them.

A psychiatrist is a physician who has a regular M.D. degree and who has had in addition special training and experience in the diagnosis and treatment of mental and emotional illnesses. He is interested also in the processes of thinking, feeling, and behaving in normal people. A clinical psychologist has had advanced training, usually leading to a doctor of philosophy degree, with special emphasis on normal and abnormal functions of the mind. Psychologists also receive special training in testing techniques used in the study of the personality in health and illness. A social worker has had advanced training, usually leading to a master's degree, concerning the social, economic, and family forces which influence human adjustment in health and illness.

Mental health services are found in both academic and nonacademic communities, and may be either associated with hospitals or independent. At their best, these services are able to deal with the full range of problems which occur in their community.

MENTAL RETARDATION

Mental retardation—formerly called *feeblemindedness*—is a condition characterized by subnormal intellectual functioning that originates during the developmental period and is associated with impairment of adaptive behavior. It is not a disease or an illness. Mentally retarded persons learn at a slower rate than normal persons and usually have difficulty in making satisfactory social adjustments.

It is estimated that 5½ million Americans are mentally retarded—most of them slightly—and that about 126,000 retarded children are born each year.

Degrees of retardation are now classified as mild, moderate, severe, or profound. Table 10.1 shows the number of retarded persons in the United States by age and degree of retardation.

The majority of the mildly retarded can be self-sufficient and even self-maintaining in adult life, particularly in situations in which the emotional and intellectual demands are not too great. Many

Table 10.1 Estimated distribution of retardates in the United States by age and degree of retardation

Degree of retardation	All ages		Age by years	
	Number	Percent	Under 20	20 and over
Total	5,635,000	100.0	2,300,000	3,335,000
Profound (IQ 20 or below)	85,000	1.5	50,000	35,000
Severe (IQ 20–35)	200,000	3.5	100,000	100,000
Moderate (IQ 36–51)	350,000	6.0	150,000	200,000
Mild (IQ 52–67)	5,000,000	89.0	2,000,000	3,000,000

SOURCE: From An Introduction to Mental Retardation, The Secretary's Committee on Mental Retardation, U.S. Department of Health, Education, and Welfare.

of the moderately retarded show surprising capacity to achieve in special schools or classes, in vocational training, and in work in sheltered environments. The profoundly retarded need constand care; most of them are in special institutions.

There are numerous causes of mental retardation. Some cases are due to diseases of the mother during pregnancy, such as German measles (page 268); some to x-rays of the uterine area or to drugs, e.g., thalidomide, taken during pregnancy. Some follow brain damage at birth. Some are due to nutritional deficiencies; some to disorders of metabolism; some to malfunction of endocrine glands. By far the greatest causative factor, however, is heredity: either the direct inheritance of mental deficiency or the inheritance of some condition, such as mongolism or phenylketonuria, which may produce mental retardation.

Treatment seeks to improve physical health, to cure contributory diseases or conditions, and to alleviate the handicap of limited intellectual capacity through special education, training, and rehabilitation. For treatment to be effective, the condition must be promptly recognized and measures instituted early in life. Although treatment has limited capacity to increase intellectual capacity, it has marked capacity to increase social functioning. Parents of a retarded child suffer great emotional distress, and society has the obligation to help them with their child by supporting the public and private institutions that work with retarded youngsters.

EPILEPSY

Epilepsy is a disorder of the nervous system characterized by "fits," or seizures, which occur with or without convulsive movements and with or without loss of consciousness. Attacks of epilepsy are produced by brief, recurrent episodes of abnormal energy released by injured or functionally impaired brain cells.

It is estimated that about 1 person in 100 has had epileptic seizures—this is a total of 2 million Americans. About 75 percent of these seizures originate in persons under 20 years of age, with the highest incidence in children under 5 years old.

In the severe form of epilepsy, known as *grand mal*, a person may fall to the ground and become unconscious, with foaming at the mouth and violent muscular movements. Another form, known as *petit mal*, is very mild and lasts only a second or two. Such attacks may occur several times a day, with the person going into a silent stare or having a mild seizure with hallucinations, temper tantrums, or outbursts of temper. Sometimes premonitory symptoms warn the patient of an impending seizure; on the other hand, attacks may occur without any warning. Less common types of epilepsy include psychomotor epilepsy, in which the person goes through some repetitive act, such as undressing, in a purposeless way, or narcolepsy, in which the person suddenly falls asleep, especially in response to coughing or laughing.

In most patients it is impossible to discover the cause of epilepsy. In others it may be due to faulty development of the brain, complications or injuries during birth, certain infectious diseases of early childhood accompanied by high fever, tumors of the brain or acute head injuries, certain vascular or blood disturbances, metabolic and endocrine disorders; or chemical poisonings.

During a grand-mal convulsion, the patient should be prevented from injuring himself by falling against or striking nearby objects and from biting his tongue. A wad of paper or a stick should be placed between his teeth. After the attack is over, the patient should be permitted to rest and sleep. He can then usually return to normal activity, without impairment and with little memory of the attack.

Epilepsy does not impair intelligence or cause insanity, although some cases of mental retardation are associated with convulsions. Heredity contributes to a minority of cases of epilepsy; the identical twin of a person with epilepsy has a 60 percent chance of having epilepsy, but a brother or sister has only a 10 percent chance. About 80 percent of cases of epileptic seizures are controllable by drugs, or occasionally by surgery. Under good medical supervision and treatment, most epileptics can attend regular schools and colleges, are employable, can drive, and are able to lead normal lives.

QUESTIONS FOR DISCUSSION AND SELF-EXAMINATION

1 What justifications are there for saying that over half the population of the United States has symptoms of emotional disturbance?
2 What are the similarities and the differences between psychosis and neurosis?
3 What are proper and incorrect uses of the term *paranoid*? In what disease or diseases does paranoia appear?
4 In what way has progress been made in the treatment of schizophrenia?
5 Discuss what is known about biological (as opposed to psychosocial) causes of schizophrenia.
6 What feelings and symptoms are frequently found in depressed people?
7 In what respect is the old saying "Someone who talks about suicide probably will never do it" wrong? Discuss the implications of the facts.
8 Discuss the different types of psychotherapy and drug therapy to mental disorders, and the relation of the two approaches to each other.
9 Discuss the causes and treatment of mental retardation.
10 To what mental disturbances are college students vulnerable? (See also Chapter 2.)

REFERENCES AND READING SUGGESTIONS

BOOKS

Martin, Lealon E., *Mental Health—Mental Illness: Revolution in Progress*, McGraw-Hill Book Company, New York, 1970.

A readable, brief, yet comprehensive book about the current status of mental illness and the new and more effective ways of preventing and treating it.

Jacobs, Jerry: *Adolescent Suicide.* John Wiley & Sons, Inc., New York, 1971.

A work which is heavy on sociology and on prevention; technical at points. Several interesting studies are reported.

Reed, Sheldon and Elizabeth: *Mental Retardation —A Family Study*, W. B. Saunders Company, Philadelphia, 1965.

An intensive study by two distinguished geneticists of the influence of genetic factors on mental retardation.

Srole, Leo, Thomas S. Langner, Stanley T. Michael, Marvin K. Opler, and Thomas A. Rennie: *Mental Health in the Metropolis: The Midtown Manhattan Study*, McGraw-Hill Book Company, New

York, 1962.

This is a monumental report of a psychiatric and sociological survey of a residential area of 175,000 in New York City. Persons interviewed lived in homes which ranged from "Gold Coast" apartments to congested slum tenements. The relationship of mental illness to various sociological factors was examined.

Varah, Chad (Ed.): *The Samaritans: To Help Those Tempted to Suicide or Despair,* The Macmillan Company, New York, 1966.

Twelve splendid papers given at conferences of an organization that sprang up when a London clergyman announced that he was available by telephone at any hour to persons who felt driven to self-destruction.

PAMPHLETS AND PERIODICALS

Blanton, Smiley: "The Bible's Timeless—and Timely—Insights," *Reader's Digest,* August 1966, p. 93.

A well-known psychiatrist demonstrates the extraordinary wisdom of the Bible in dealing with emotional problems that have haunted the human race from the beginning—and are more than ever with us today.

"Disturbed Americans," Special Supplement of *The Atlantic,* July 1964, pp. 72–119.

A series of splendid articles with the following titles: "The Meaning of Mental Illnesses"; "The Uncommitted Cortex—The Child's Changing Brain"; "State Care"; "Psychiatric Treatment"; "College Students in Trouble"; "Psychiatrists and the Poor"; "Mental Disease and the Urban Hospital"; "The Help We Need"; "Institutional Peonage."

Herzog, Arthur: "Suicide Can't Be Eliminated," *The New York Times Magazine,* Mar. 20, 1966, p. 32.

A comprehensive and searching survey of this serious and complicated problem.

"Inside a Modern Psychiatric Hospital," *World Health,* April 1966.

An enlightening and encouraging report of patients' experiences in a modern psychiatric hospital.

Stern, Edith M.: *Mental Illness: A Guide for the Family,* National Association for Mental Health, New York, 1966.

A helpful consideration of the problems involved in the care of and association with those who are mentally or emotionally disturbed.

11

FOOD FOR THE WORLD'S HEALTH AND YOURS

Today there is an increasing emphasis on diet. The amount of literature published on this subject in the last few years is a direct result of this concern for better nutrition. Many Americans no longer take their diet lightly but have become concerned about the effects of the foods they eat on the functions of the body. Some carry this interest further than others, eating foods that coincide with certain philosophies. One thing is sure: People have become more aware of the fact that nutrition plays an important part in the life of the whole man, influencing many different aspects of his being—health and life span being two of the most important factors influenced by diet.

In recent years, Americans have also become aware of the presence of malnutrition among American families living in poverty. Malnutrition is not a problem affecting only the underdeveloped nations of the world. The United States, one of the world's most prosperous nations, must come to terms with the problem of malnutrition which exists among its own poor.

ENERGY, LIFE, AND NUTRITION

Every living thing, from the simplest form of plant life to the most complex animal, must have food for growth, food for energy, food to regulate body processes, and food to replace worn-out tissues. The choice of foods eaten—nutrition—is so instinctive that few people give it the thought necessary to assure the best of health.

The chemical components of food are numerous and complex; the needs of the body are far from simple. In many underdeveloped countries, supplies of food are so limited and the public knowledge of nutrition is so scanty that diseases due to malnutrition are common. In most areas of the United States, food supplies are ample, and only economic want and ignorance cause undernutrition.

The nutrients which human beings need fall into six groups based on chemical structure: proteins, carbohydrates, fats, vitamins, minerals, and water. No one nutrient can be eliminated from the diet without severe damage to the body. Some cells need more of certain nutrients than others. The total needs of all cells make up the nutritional requirement of the whole body.

DIGESTION

Most foods enter the mouth in a highly organized form which cannot be absorbed by the body or used by the cells. The purpose of digestion is to break down these foods into chemical units simple and small enough to be absorbed and utilized. Digestion results from at least four types of action in the intestinal tract: first, the mechanical squeezing and liquefying actions of the intestinal tract; second, the chemical action of the hydrochloric acid in the stomach; third, the action of myriad bacteria which live in the intestinal tract; and fourth and most important, the chemical action of the many enzymes contained in the digestive juices which are mixed with the food in the intestinal tract. The products of digestion are absorbed through the intestinal tract into the blood, a multipurpose liquid which carries food, water, and oxygen to the cells and also carries the waste products of cell activity (see Figure 11.1) to the kidneys and elsewhere to be excreted or decomposed.

Figure 11.1   Alimentary canal with digestive glands.

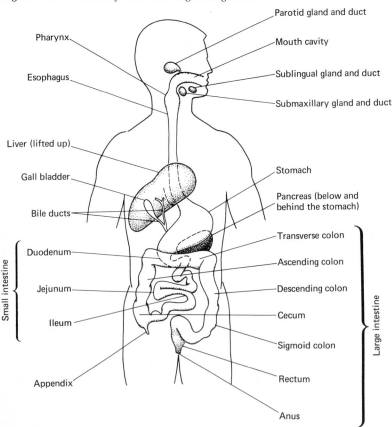

Figure 11.2 Photosynthesis and the nitrogen cycle.

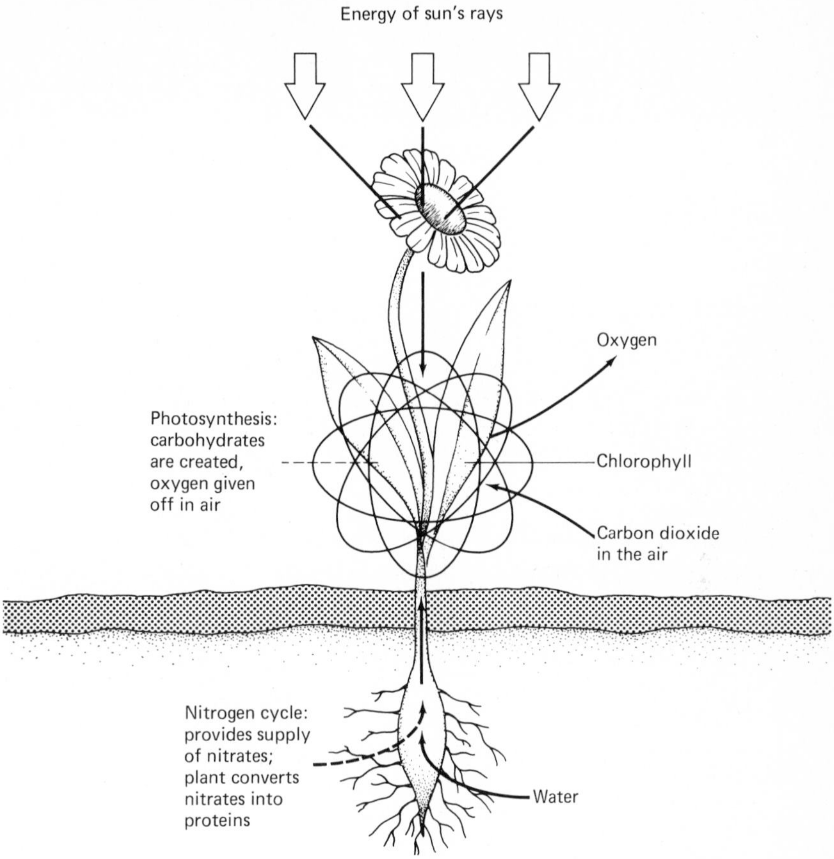

Energy of sun's rays

Oxygen

Photosynthesis:
carbohydrates
are created,
oxygen given
off in air

Chlorophyll

Carbon dioxide
in the air

Nitrogen cycle:
provides supply
of nitrates;
plant converts
nitrates into
proteins

Water

PLANTS AND MAN'S FOOD

The basic source of man's food supply—except for water and certain minerals—is the plant kingdom. Sunlight shining on the plant leaves activates a chemical called *chlorophyll* which triggers the metabolic cycle in plants. Plants utilize oxygen, carbon dioxide, nitrogen, water, and mineral salts from the soil and air. From these they manufacture within their own cells the proteins, carbohydrates, fats, and vitamins which serve as food for man and other animals. (See Figure 11.2.) All forms of life need carbon and nitrogen, but animals are unable to utilize these elements unless they are combined with hydrogen and oxygen to form the organic chemical compounds called *proteins, carbohydrates, fats,* and *vitamins.*

When eaten by human beings and other animals, the proteins, fats, and carbohydrates of the plants are broken down into simple chemical units, absorbed into the bloodstream, carried throughout the body, and then either reconstructed to form tissues in the animal or "burned" to supply energy to cells throughout the body. Food consisting of animal meat breaks down in the same way, with the main components being protein and fat.

The food cycle is completed when bacteria in the ground and in the bodies of animals (these are not disease-producing bacteria) break down dead parts of plants, animals, and animal excreta into chemicals that can again be utilized by growing plants, which in turn may be used by animals as food. The *nitrogen-fixing* bacteria, found chiefly around the nodules or roots of legumes such as peas and beans, are able to take nitrogen from the air and combine it with other chemical elements to form nitrogen-containing compounds needed for the growth of plants and animals.

Different plants have different chemical constituents and therefore have different values as food. Most grains and some vegetables are rich in carbohydrates and are thus high-energy foods. Other plants such as soybeans and peanuts are excellent sources of protein.

THE NEED FOR PROTEINS

Protein, one of the three sources of energy in the diet, is essential primarily for growth and cell regeneration. Except for water, protein is the chief constituent of all muscle, gland, and nerve tissue, of many hormones and enzymes, and of blood. The body needs new protein daily to build new tissue and to replace tissues that constantly wear out. Without it, children develop kwashiorkor, and adults develop cirrhosis of the liver and other debilitating or fatal diseases. Abundant in meat, eggs, milk, and cheese, protein also occurs moderately in beans and to lesser extents in other vegetables. All proteins contain nitrogen in addition to carbon, hydrogen, and oxygen. Proteins may also contain sulfur, phosphorus, iron, and other minerals, all built into complex molecules of large size.

These complex protein molecules are formed of small and simpler nitrogenous compounds called *amino acids.* Approximately twenty-one different amino acids occur in practically all common proteins. Eight of these cannot be manufactured by the human body and therefore must come directly from some food source.

Proteins which include all eight of these—the *essential amino acids*—are called *complete proteins;* those which lack some of the essential amino acids are called *incomplete proteins.* Meat and fish are the most reliable sources of complete proteins. Other animal sources, such as egg whites, milk, and other dairy products, provide complete proteins in lower concentrations. A few plants, notably nuts, soybeans, and other members of the bean family, contain complete proteins in smaller amounts. By eating a large quantity of these plant products, supplemented by milk, cheese, and eggs, a vegetarian can maintain an adequate supply of proteins for good health.

The protein requirements of the body vary with the rate of growth. During childhood, pregnancy, and lactation large intakes are needed—at least 1½ grams of protein daily per kilogram of body weight. Adults need 1 gram of protein per kilogram of body weight each day; an intake the equivalent of about 0.5 gram per pound, or about 2 ounces of meat daily for an adult of 150 pounds. Most Americans who eat meat or fish daily exceed the recommended minimum.

Adults should obtain at least half of their minimum protein requirement from foods which contain complete proteins: growing children should obtain three-fourths of their protein from complete proteins. Drinking additional milk is an easy way to obtain extra proteins along with calcium.

"Filled" and "imitation" milks and cream have appeared on the market in recent years. Filled milks use milk solids, especially proteins, to which other nonmilk fats are added. Filled milks are reliable sources of protein and calcium, therefore. Imitation milk, however, contains no milk products. Each type varies substantially from brand to brand. Both filled and imitation milks often use coconut oil fats, which are high in saturated fatty acids and may raise blood cholesterol.

CARBOHYDRATES FOR ENERGY

The expenditure of energy is basic to life itself. Even in sleep the body is expending energy in the beating of the heart, the maintenance of muscle tone, breathing, the digestive processes, the secretion by glands, and the myriad chemical activities within each body cell. To support these basic functions the body must have energy. The source of this energy is the foods we eat, particularly the carbohydrates—sugars and starches.

Energy is measured in calories. (See Figure 11.3). A calorie is the amount of heat necessary to raise the temperature of 1 liter of water 1°C or 1 quart of water 1⅝°F. One gram (1/30 ounce) of protein or carbohydrate will provide 4 calories of heat whereas 1 gram of fat will provide 9 calories. At a basal, resting state the body needs 11 calories for each pound of body weight for a 24-hour period. For example, a person weighing 120 pounds has a basal energy requirement of about 1320 calories. As the metabolism of the body increases, the body expends more calories.

The best way of determining the adequacy of the energy intake in food is to compare one's weight with the ideal weight for one's age, sex, and height. (See Table 12.1.) If it is not caused by disease, excessive underweight or a continuing loss of weight indicates that the person has not been eating sufficient calories. Similarly, overweight or a continuing gain in weight indicates that the person has been taking in too many calories. Maintenance of the ideal body weight over a period of time indicates that caloric intake and caloric expenditure of energy by the body are in proper balance. The body gets its energy from proteins, fats, or carbohydrates. If energy is not readily available from food, the body utilizes its stored fats.

American diets vary widely, from area to area and among those on differing financial levels. However, in this country fats form a much higher proportion of total calories eaten than they do in underdeveloped countries. A typical distribution in the United States would be 15 percent of calories from proteins, 40 percent from fats, and 45 percent from carbohydrates. In underdeveloped countries as much as 80 to 90 percent, or even more, of the calories may come from carbohydrates.

Carbohydrates are one of the staples of all diets. Containing carbon, hydrogen, and oxygen, carbohydrates always have 2 hydrogen atoms for every oxygen atom. Multiple units of simple sugars combine to form starches such as dextrose or glucose, which must be broken down by digestion before they can be used by the body.

The chief sources of carbohydrates are cereals —in the form of breads as well as breakfast cereals —sugars, vegetables, and fruits. Among the vegetables, potatoes, rice, corn, and peas provide the highest concentration of carbohydrates. Most carbohydrates are relatively inexpensive foods. As a result, individuals or communities with little money to spend on food are likely to satisfy their hunger with a high-carbohydrate diet.

Some of the carbohydrate foods are also important sources of vitamins; examples are vitamin C in citrus fruits, thiamine (vitamin B[1]) in whole

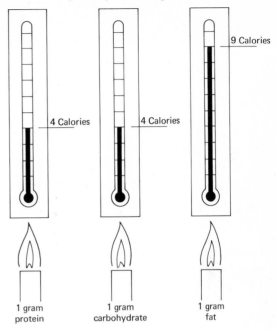

Figure 11.3 Calories (units of heat) released when proteins, carbohydrates, and fats are oxidized (burned) in the body.

9 Calories

4 Calories   4 Calories

1 gram   1 gram   1 gram
protein   carbohydrate   fat

grains, and vitamin A in yellow vegetables.

The digestion of starches begins in the mouth. As food is chewed, it is mixed with saliva, which contains an enzyme, *ptyalin*. Ptyalin starts unlinking the sugar molecules that are combined in the starch structure. In the small intestine, enzymes from the pancreas and from glands in the intestinal wall complete the breakdown into simple sugars. These simple sugars are adsorbed through the intestinal wall into the bloodstream and carried throughout the body, where tissue cells withdraw them according to their needs. (See Figure 11.4.) Sugars not burned for energy form glycogen—a complex carbohydrate similar to starch—which is stored in the liver and muscles; some sugars are broken down still further and then recombined into fats which are stored throughout the body. When food does not supply enough calories to meet energy needs, the body draws upon and utilizes these deposits of glycogen and fat.

The regulation of the amount of sugar in the blood and body tissues and the mechanism of its use are complicated. *Insulin*, the hormone circulating chemical secreted by the pancreas directly into the bloodstream, plays an essential role, al-

Figure 11.4 The oxidization (burning) of carbohydrates (sugars) in the muscle cell releases heat.

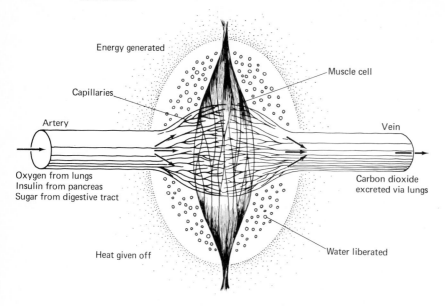

Energy generated

Muscle cell

Capillaries

Artery

Vein

Oxygen from lungs
Insulin from pancreas
Sugar from digestive tract

Carbon dioxide
excreted via lungs

Heat given off

Water liberated

though the exact mechanism of its action is not known. It is clear, however, that insulin makes it possible for the tissues to burn sugars efficiently. Insulin and cell enzymes allow sugars to burn by combining with oxygen within body cells to produce carbon dioxide and water. The carbon dioxide, a gas, is removed by the blood. As the blood passes through the lungs, excess carbon dioxide is released into the air. Without insulin, the cells of the body are unable to burn sugar, and thus the amount of sugar in the blood and in the tissues of the body increases. This occurrence, together with other disturbances in the body chemistry, constitutes the disease *diabetes*. (Diabetes is discussed in Chapter 19.)

Too low a level of blood sugar may also occur; this condition is called *hypoglycemia*. This usually mild condition is due to an excess secretion of insulin caused by eating a meal composed of too high a proportion of carbohydrates. Excess fatigue, faintness, and sweating may result from an inadequate amount of sugar in the blood. In time, the blood-sugar level will increase normally, or it can be boosted by eating a small quantity of sugar-rich food.

When hypoglycemic (low-blood-sugar) symptons occur, they can be corrected by a diet that includes more protein than carbohydrate. The immediate symptoms, however, if really due to hypoglycemia, will *always* respond to intake of sugar or starch, which will increase the blood sugar. Hypoglycemia can also be prevented and even reversed, by exercise, which causes secretion of epinephrine and an increase in the blood sugar.

FATS: NEEDS AND CONTROLS

Fats, like carbohydrates, are composed of carbon, hydrogen, and oxygen, but the proportions are different in fats. Fats have two components: glycerol, a small molecule with three carbon atoms linked to one another, and fatty acids, with larger numbers of carbon atoms linked to form chains of varying lengths. In the so-called *saturated* fatty acids, the carbon atoms have all the hydrogen atoms that they can hold; in the *unsaturated* fatty acids, the carbon atoms have the potential for bonding with more hydrogen. Recent investigations of the relationship of fat to heart disease have called attention to the fact that it is the fats that contain saturated rather than unsaturated fatty acids that are related to arteriosclerosis. As a result, some margarines label the proportion of unsaturated fatty acids contained. In general, the fats from animals are saturated and those from vegetables, seafoods, and poultry are unsaturated. In the table of the nutritive values of foods, Appendix, page 423, unsaturated fats in various foods are divided into two groups: the oleic acid or moderately unsaturated group and the linoleic or highly unsaturated group, also called *polyunsaturated*.

Oils consist of predominately unsaturated fatty acids, and, in general, the greater the degree of unsaturation, the softer or more liquid the substance. Through hydrogenation, unsaturated fatty acids take on additional hydrogen atoms. As a result, the fats become firm or solid. Commercially this extensively used process converts naturally occurring oils into the solid forms. Dietary fats occur not only in obvious foods such as butter, margarine, and the visible fat around meats, but also in homogenized milk, in all other dairy products except skim milk and skim milk products, in the graining and between the muscle fibers of meats, in the yolks of eggs, in nuts, and even, to a minor extent, in some vegetables.

In addition to providing calories for energy, fats diminish the contractions of the stomach and the rate at which the glands of the stomach secrete acid and enzymes. This slows down the digestive process, causes the stomach to empty less rapidly, and delays hunger pains. This characteristic has been used in the treatment of peptic ulcer.

Digestion of fats occurs in the small intestine. Bile, secreted by the liver and concentrated by the gallbladder, emulsifies fats as they pass through the first portion of the small intestine: i.e., bile breaks up the fat globules into tiny particles. Enzymes then go to work on these tiny fat particles and split off the fatty acids, which are readily absorbed into the blood and circulated throughout the body. Like sugars, fatty acids may be burned for energy, or they may be stored in the fat cells throughout the body.

Fatty acids are essential to health, but there is an overabundance of fats in almost all diets in the United States. Fat is fattening. Since fat produces a little more than twice as many calories as the same unit of weight of carbohydrates or protein, fat is literally more than twice as fattening as the other two types of energy foods.

Recently, attention has focused on the possible role of fat in causing atherosclerosis and arteriosclerosis. These conditions affecting the coronary arteries which supply blood to the heart muscle, give rise to coronary heart disease—the leading cause of death in this country. Considerable evidence has demonstrated that those who eat a great deal of fat are more likely to have atherosclerosis and heart attacks than those whose diets contain little fat. The fats that consist primarily of saturated fatty acids appear to be the most dangerous. In fact polyunsaturated fatty acids may reduce the amount of cholesterol in the blood. Among the foods which contain significant amounts of polyunsaturated fatty acids are corn oil, cottonseed oil, most nuts, fish oils, fish, and seafood. When tests show that the cholesterol in the blood is above average levels, other blood tests are conducted, and special diets and medications are utilized to reduce the level of fat in the blood.

Contrary to earlier opinion, the amount of cholesterol eaten as food has little influence on the amount of cholesterol in the body. The reason is that the liver manufactures cholesterol out of foods, primarily saturated fats, in vastly greater amounts than are ever taken into the body as food. Keeping dietary saturated fatty acids to a minimum, however, diminishes the production of cholesterol by the liver.

There are many other factors in the production of atherosclerosis and heart attacks. High levels of sugars and other carbohydrates in the diet raise the blood fats in some people. As discussed in Chapter 5, factors such as smoking, lack of exercise, psychological stress, and heredity are important in the causation of coronary artery disease.

THE NEED FOR WATER

Water is the most important single constituent of the living organism. A man may survive a month or longer without food, but death will occur within a few days if he is deprived of water. About two-thirds of the weight of an adult is water. The important sources of body fluids are water taken as drink, water contained in food, and water formed in the oxidation, or burning, of foods in the body.

Water is lost from the body in the urine, in the feces, in perspiration, and through evaporation from the skin and lungs. In solutions that are primarily water, foods are digested, the products of digestion are carried to the tissue cells, and the waste products are taken away. Under average conditions an adult requires approximately 3 quarts of water per day. An ordinary diet provides two-thirds of this amount in food. The rest needs to be taken as drink.

Practical generalizations concerning the body's needs for fluids are that thirst is usually a safe and reliable criterion of the amount of water which is needed. There is a greater likelihood of taking too little than too much fluid; 6 glasses of liquid a day, in addition to that contained in food, is a reasonable estimate of the average desirable intake. Unfortunately, some people dislike water and learn to ignore the existence of thirst. Such people may need to pay conscious attention to their fluid intake in order to make sure that it is adequate. The easiest guide to adequate fluid is in noting the amount of urine passed each day. If you are urinating every two or three hours, you can be sure your fluid intake is sufficient for health under ordinary circumstances.

THE NEED FOR MINERALS

The minerals known to be essential to the body include calcium, phosphorus, iron, iodine, copper, chlorine, cobalt, fluorine, magnesium, manganese, molybdenum, potassium, selenium, sodium, sulfur, and zinc. Despite their importance, the absolute amounts of minerals in the body are small. In fact, only traces of most minerals are needed by the body.

CALCIUM AND PHOSPHORUS

These two minerals give strength and hardness to bones and teeth. A proper concentration of calcium in the blood and body fluids is necessary also to prevent irritability of the nervous system and muscles. Lack of calcium may result in cramps, twitching, and possibly even convulsions and death. Even the heart cannot function properly unless there is an adequate amount of calcium in the blood.

Growing children and pregnant and lactating mothers need more calcium and phosphorus than other people; an amount equal to that supplied in an extra quart of milk daily is usually sufficient. Older children and adults usually drink less milk than they need. Hence, their diet needs to contain other foods rich in these elements, such as cheese, green leafy vegetables, broccoli, and nuts. If the diet does not provide sufficient calcium to meet the needs of the body, calcium may be withdrawn from the bones and teeth. This occasionally occurs in pregnancy when calcium from the bones and teeth of the mother is utilized to meet the needs of the developing child. In such a situation the bones serve as the reservoir of calcium within the body.

IRON

The body must have iron to form hemoglobin, the chemical compound which gives blood its red color and transports oxygen from the lungs to the tissues. In general, a well-balanced diet will provide all the iron that a healthy person needs. However, for infants and for women during the years of menstruation, physicians frequently prescribe preparations which provide additional amounts of iron.

Foods rich in iron include meat (especially liver), eggs, green leafy vegetables, and whole-grain or enriched bread and other cereal products. The absorption of iron from the intestinal tract varies with the need of the body, and for example, someone who has lost blood will absorb iron more readily than someone who has not. Usually, only 10 to 20 percent of the iron in the diet is absorbed; ascorbic acid, or vitamin C, increases the rate of absorption.

IODINE

Iodine is needed by the thyroid gland to manufacture its thyroid hormone, which regulates cell activity. In areas of the world where idoine does not occur in the water and soil, nor in the plants and animals, an enlargement of the thyroid gland (called *goiter*) is common. The amount of iodine needed to prevent this condition is tiny, no more than 100 milligrams (0.003 ounce) a year. In this country, it has been possible to eliminate this type of goiter by using iodized salt. (See also page 296.)

SODIUM AND POTASSIUM

Sodium is an important constituent of the blood and other body fluids. Fortunately, salt (sodium chloride) deficiency rarely occurs except in very hot weather. Even then, it is rarely necessary to take salt tablets and it is safer and more comfortable merely to add extra salt to food. For those who day after day must do heavy work or exercise in the heat, the most satisfactory way of obtaining extra salt is to drink lightly salted water at frequent intervals in small amounts. A level teaspoon of salt to a quart of water, which is about half the concentration of the salt in the body fluids, is sufficient. A thirsty person who drinks such water replenishes his salt in an adequate and safe amount as he replenishes his body water. In addition, special solutions which supply the chief minerals necessary to the body in carefully balanced proportions (sodium chloride, potassium, phosphorus) are absorbed through the intestinal wall very quickly. Potassium and sodium chloride are supplied in adequate amounts in most diets, and under normal conditions no special source is needed.

A comparison of two Japanese villages led to some interesting observations. One village had an unusually large number of strokes (cerebral hemorrhages and other cerebral vascular accidents); the other village had only the expected number of strokes. The village with many strokes had a very high-salt diet in comparison to the other village. The implications are not that all those who take much salt develop hypertension, but only an excess number.

ZINC

Zinc is a mineral needed in only trace amounts, but it is essential to health. In parts of the world where little meat is available in the diet, zinc deficiencies occur. In children, growth and sexual maturation are retarded when there is a zinc deficiency, but the retardation can be overcome quickly when zinc is added to the diet. If the diet of a pregnant woman is severely deficient in zinc, congenital malformations of various sorts are more likely to occur in her child. Body zinc is diminished in kwashiorkor, the protein deficiency disease described below.

FLUORIDE

Fluoride in tiny amounts is essential to the development of caries-resistant teeth. In older people, fluorides appear to improve the crystalline structure of bones, making them more sturdy and less susceptible to the thinning process called osteoporosis and to the many fractures resulting therefrom. Many communities now add fluorides to their water supplies in amounts that will provide the ideal proportion of 1 part per million. Fluoride is found in most drinking water, but in only a few parts of the United States is it found in the ideal proportion. For a discussion of this subject, see pages 221–224.

TRACE MINERALS

Many other minerals are necessary in trace amounts for the successful completion of chemical reactions in the cells: for example, a small amount of copper is necessary if iron is to be utilized. However, these trace minerals are needed only in amounts which are supplied by virtually any diet.

THE NEED FOR VITAMINS

Vitamins are chemical compounds which facilitate or make possible chemical reactions in cells throughout the body. They produce no heat, no energy, and no major material for tissue building. The body's daily need for vitamins is exceedingly small and is measured in milligrams. Vitamins are, however, essential to growth and to health, for without them the chemical processes of the body could not continue.

Diseases due to deficiencies of vitamins have been known for a long time and still are prevalent where people are unable to get sufficient and proper foods. In healthy people vitamin supplements produce no benefits that a well-balanced diet will not provide. In fact, most of the vitamins that are taken as pills are excreted rapidly in the urine or otherwise eliminated or destroyed without benefit to the taker—thus providing support for the comment that Americans have the most expensive urine in the world.

The desirable daily intake of certain vitamins is published from time to time by the Food and Nutrition Board of the National Research Council. These recommendations apply to the fat-soluble vitamins A and D and to the water-soluble vitamins thiamine, riboflavin, niacin, and ascorbic acid. Diets based on the four food groups described on page 168 will under almost all circumstances supply adequate amounts of these and other vitamins.

VITAMIN A

Vitamin A, which is fat-soluble and is often called the *growth vitamin* or the *anti-infective vitamin*, is necessary for the formation and maintenance of normal epithelial tissues, such as the skin and the mucous membranes lining the respiratory passages. Deficiency of this viatmin may cause irritation of the skin and mucous membranes, and a disease of the eye called *xerophthalmia*. Night blindness may also result from vitamin A deficiency, since proper functioning of the retina of the eye, which detects light, depends on vitamin A.

The body can obtain vitamin A from fish-liver oils, liver, cream, and whole milk. It also manufactures vitamin A from carotene, the yellow pigment of certain vegetables and plants. Reliable vegetable sources for carotene include the yellow vegetables —carrots, sweet potatoes, and squash; green leafy vegetables such as spinach and lettuce; and some fruits such as tomatoes, apricots, cantaloupes, peaches, and prunes. A human diet should contain at least one of these foods at least every other day. The body can store considerable vitamin A except in infancy and childhood. Regular supplies of the vitamin are therefore particularly important in youth.

VITAMIN D

The other principal fat-soluble vitamin, vitamin D, is needed for the absorption of calcium from the intestinal tract. The adult needs only minimal amounts of vitamin D, but children who are forming their skeletal systems need at least 400 units of vitamin D daily. Insufficient vitamin D over a period of time causes development of rickets, the symptoms of which are deformities of the bones, particularly knobby ribs and bowed legs. A child with rickets is also irritable, weak, restless, anemic, flabby, and susceptible to infections.

The richest sources of vitamin D are fish oils, particularly cod-liver oil and halibut-liver oil, which used to be given to children routinely. Now vitamin D is included in the vitamin supplements given by pediatricians to all infants and many children. In addition, most milk, regular, skimmed, and powdered, sold commercially in the United States is fortified with 400 units of vitamin D per quart, so that the child who drinks a quart a day, the recommended quantity, obtains sufficient vitamin D. The human body can also manufacture vitamin D in the skin through the action of sunlight, so that in warm sunny climates where children play outdoors most of the time with at least arms and legs exposed to the sunlight, rickets is not a problem.

Vitamin D in excessive amounts causes calcium to be precipitated in the kidneys and elsewhere.

OTHER FAT-SOLUBLE VITAMINS

Vitamin K, essential for blood clotting in wounds, is supplied in adequate amounts by a well-balanced diet and by the action of intestinal bacteria. Supplementary amounts are given, usually by injection, to pregnant women just before delivery and to newborn infants, in order to minimize the chance of excessive bleeding due to an undetected deficiency of this vitamin.

Vitamin E is related to muscular function and to normal function of the reproductive system, but is so abundant in foods that deficiency rarely occurs in human beings. However, premature babies have been known to develop an anemia which can be corrected by vitamin E. Because the body stores vitamin E, it is virtually impossible to create a vitamin E deficiency in older children or adults.

THE VITAMIN B GROUP

This large group of water-soluble vitamins acts within the cells of the body to promote chemical processes essential to life. The diseases beriberi and pellagra are due to deficiencies of two members of the vitamin B group, thiamine and niacin, and pernicious anemia is due to a deficiency of vitamin B^{12}. Pernicious anemia is usually caused by the inability of the stomach to absorb the vitamin from the diet.

Thiamine, vitamin B^1, is necessary for the integration by the body cells of sugar and other carbohydrates. The most reliable sources of this vitamin are grains and their products. Whole rice is an excellent source of thiamine. The major cause of its deficiency disease, beriberi, is "polishing" of rice, a process which most populations prefer for taste but which removes the thiamine contained in the outer coating of the rice. In this country, thiamine is lost when wheat is ground and bleached to make white flour, but most white breads sold commercially are "enriched" by the addition of thiamine. Beriberi causes serious weakness of the heart, damage to the nervous system, general weakness, loss of appetite, and failure of growth. Minor degrees of thiamine deficiency may also impair health.

The discovery of the relationship between thiamine deficiency and disease dates to 1897, when a Dutch physician produced in pigeons a disease which resembled beriberi, and then cured it by feeding the birds whole-grain cereals, milk, and other substances. In 1936, the chemical synthesis of pure thiamine made large-scale production of this vitamin possible.

In addition to whole grains such as wheat and rice, foods which are excellent sources of thiamine are pork, liver, sweetbreads, kidney, and legumes; smaller amounts are found in other fruits and vegetables. Although the body stores of thiamine are limited, it takes 2 or 3 months of deprivation to produce a serious deficiency.

Riboflavin, vitamin B^2, is essential for processes which add oxygen to several compounds within cells. Without it, growth ceases and the skin and mucous membranes begin to break down. A person with a severe deficiency of riboflavin has cracked lips, a sore tongue with a peculiar magenta color, and burning, itching eyes. The best sources of riboflavin are milk and meat. A pint of milk and one serving of meat daily will prevent deficiency. Other sources include eggs, green leafy vegetables, legumes, and whole-grain products.

Niacin, the third important B vitamin, is needed for the body's carbohydrate chemistry. Niacin deficiency causes pellagra, whose characteristic symptoms are often referred to as the "three D's": dermatitis (inflammation of the skin), diarrhea (frequent loose bowel movements), and dementia (loss of intellectual function). A fourth D, death, can occur. The body is able to synthesize niacin from the amino acid tryptophan. Diets therefore must be deficient in both niacin and tryptophan to produce niacin deficiency. A diet of

corn meal, salt pork, and molasses produces pellagra with great regularity. Since in the southeastern United States this was a common diet through the early years of this century, pellagra was prevalent. Milk, eggs, beef, wheat, whole corn, and peanuts are the best sources of niacin, and a diet which includes these foods effectively prevents pellagra.

Vitamin B^{12} is essential for the synthesis of hemoglobin. Since there are ample sources of this vitamin in foods, especially in meat, a deficiency rarely occurs except when the stomach fails to secrete acid and enzymes, or in vegetarians. Since the vitamin is also necessary for the proper functioning of the nervous system, patients with pernicious anemia often have damage to the nervous system, including loss of intellectual function. Neither vitamin B^{12} nor any other vitamin is useful in the treatment of general fatigue, frequent colds, or other symptoms not related to vitamin deficiency. Vitamins used in an attempt to treat such conditions are wasted and may even do harm if their use prevents or delays a thorough search for health problems underlying the symptoms.

Deficiency of vitamin B^6, or pyridoxine, can lead to convulsions, anemia, and the excretion of abnormal compounds in the urine. Common in animals fed restricted diets, vitamin B^6 deficiency is rare in human beings.

Other B vitamins include pantothenic acid, inositol, folic acid, choline, and biotin. These substances are amply supplied in well-balanced diets which meet other nutritional requirements. Deficiencies are rare, but may occur under unusual circumstances: for example, a deficiency of folic acid contributes to an anemia that sometimes occurs in pregnancy.

ASCORBIC ACID (VITAMIN C)

Ascorbic acid is essential for the chemical processes which transfer hydrogen ions from one molecule to another; it is important also in the formation of intercellular substance, a sort of "cement" that holds body cells together.

The disease caused by its lack, scurvy, has been known for hundreds of years as a particular scourge of sailors and explorers who were unable to get the fresh, raw fruits and vegetables which contain vitamin C. The common symptoms are bleeding from the gums and elsewhere, loss of the teeth, and bone pain. In milder forms of vitamin C deficiency, delay of wound healing may be the only symptom. Vitamin C deficiency may not be obvious until a wound, perhaps following surgery, fails to heal properly. Ten milligrams of vitamin C a day will prevent scurvy, but the recommended amount for good health is 60 to 100 mg daily.

Citrus fruits and their juices are the standard sources of vitamin C, but many other fresh fruits and vegetables contain this vitamin. Long cooking or exposure to air causes vitamin C to decompose. Although the body stores it for long periods, daily intake of foods containing vitamin C is desirable. (See Chapter 18 for a discussion of vitamin C and colds.)

DIET AND HEALTH

Dietary customs vary with economic situations and with local traditions. One of the greatest differences in human diets lies in the comparative amounts of starch (especially of cereal or root origin) and protein in the diet. The people of the world can be divided into three main groups according to their nutrition:

1 Over 1 billion people in industrialized nations who have diets with large amounts of good-quality protein, mostly of animal origin. (The quality of protein depends on its amino-acid content.)
2 Between 1.5 and 2.0 billion people whose diets are mostly cereal grains.
3 About 100 million people whose diets are composed mostly of cassava and other roots. This is the group whose diet has the least protein of all; less than 2 percent of such a diet is protein.

The diets of groups 2 and 3 are badly deficient in protein, but they are also deficient in seven vitamins (vitamin A, thiamine, riboflavin, niacin, vitamin B^{12}, vitamin D, and ascorbic acid) and in three minerals (calcium, iron, and iodine). With the expansion of the world's population, an even higher percentage of people will have to depend on starches unless an alternative source of protein is found. It is for this reason that nutritionists have started to focus so much attention on plants as

OTHER DISEASES OF MALNUTRITION

Kwashiorkor occurs when the protein in the diet of a child is badly deficient, but the total calories (mainly from starches) are more nearly adequate. The belly becomes bloated and the arms and legs pipestem thin. Afflicted children are listless, weak, debilitated, and subject to infections. Death is common, but the disease responds promptly to protein supplements in the diet.

In contrast, when both protein and total calories are severely deficient, the child is shrunken and wrinkled, looking like an aged person or a mummy. Weakness, listlessness, and susceptibility to infection occur, and death is common. This disease is called *marasmus*.

sources of protein. Other plans have been proposed. One, already in operation in a few areas with moderate success, is the use of fish meal to supplement ordinary cereal flour. In the world's fish catch, there are huge amounts of fish not ordinarily suitable for eating because of an undesirable taste. These fish contain good protein which until recently was wasted. Through special processes the fish taste is removed and the fish is ground into meal.

Another proposal is to add individual amino acids to the cereals eaten by protein-starved populations. Some experts estimate that for less than $2 a year per child, sufficient amino acids to meet minimal requirements for growing children could be added to cereal diets.

Americans often think of malnutrition as something that happens to foreigners, unfortunate people who live in undeveloped countries. However, hunger occurs at home, too. One estimate is that 10 million Americans are undernourished. Most of them are in the quarter of the population with the lowest income. The national nutrition survey of 1968 documented the existence of malnutrition in the United States. A sample of the areas where 75 to 80 percent of families live in poverty was studied. Among these families:

15 percent of children were retarded in growth, some of them as much as 2 years behind well-nourished children by age 6.

35 to 55 percent of all people suffered one or more nutrient deficiencies.

33 percent of children were significantly anemic, and in need of immediate therapy.

4 percent of children under 6 had rickets.

4 to 5 percent of children had some form of kwashiokor.

5 percent of all people had goiter, due to low iodine content in their diet.

Vitamin deficiency diseases, kwashiorkor, anemia, and growth retardation are unquestionable evidence of undernutrition and inadequate distribution of food. Of equal or greater importance, however, is the effect of undernutrition on the human mind. Nutrition just before and just after birth is of crucial importance to the development of the brain. In man, the most rapid period of brain growth occurs in the last few weeks before birth, and the second most rapid period occurs in the few weeks just after birth. In rats, even mild undernutrition at the time of fastest brain growth brings a lasting deficit in brain size and in the number of brain cells. This deficit cannot be corrected by improved feeding at a later time.

The human brain reaches 80 percent of its adult weight by the age of 3. Undernourished children have smaller head circumferences than do children with adequate diets; this deficit is known to persist through the tenth year of life and presumably is permanent. In addition, and more generally, it has been known for many years that children born to mothers with specific vitamin deficiencies have more than the usual number of congenital anomalies.

When pregnant women and their newborn offspring receive inadequate nourishment, the resulting children and adults are not able to reach the full intellectual growth available to other children born at the same time but given the best nutrition available. The nation in which such children grow up will make restricted progress towards a higher standard of living and better health. When racial discrimination and economic relations limit the nutrition of certain groups of people, the children born into these groups have inadequate nutrition for maximum intellectual development. These children can hardly hope to compete successfully with fully nourished, well-developed children, and later, as adults, they will still be at a disadvantage.

Poverty begets poor sanitation, poor sanitation begets intestinal parasites, poverty plus intestinal parasites beget poor nutrition, and poor nutrition begets poverty. The cycle is self-sustaining and only massive help from outside forces can break it.

CHOOSING A SENSIBLE DIET

No food contains all the nutrients in the amounts needed. All foods contain more than one nutrient, and as discussed earlier in this chapter, some foods are particularly rich in one or more nutrients. Choosing a diet wisely means eating foods which provide adequate daily amounts of the necessary nutrients. "Empty calories," such as are supplied in soft drinks, can tend to make a diet less than optimal—particularly among children, college students, and other young people.

The familiar "daily food guide" of four food groups provides an excellent and simple guide to a well-balanced diet which will supply all essential nutrients. (See Table 11.1.) Separately, each group contributes in special ways: enriched milk provides calcium, vitamin D, vitamin A, niacin, and some protein; meats provide protein, some fat, niacin, and riboflavin; vegetables and fruits provide carbohydrates and many of the vitamins; and so on.

In time of chronic illness a person may need a special diet because of the increased breakdown of tissue or the difficulty of the intestinal tract in absorbing nutrients; he may also need vitamins and other supplements. The needs of any special diet must be determined by a doctor.

Athletes often receive special diets. People who engage in vigorous physical activity need added calories in their diet in order to maintain weight. If they are gaining muscle size, they may need more protein than the standard allowance, although the diets of most college students regularly contain more than the standard allowance. However, the large steak which used to be served

Table 11.1 A daily food guide (four food groups)

Milk group (calcium):

Children	3 to 4 cups
Teenagers	4 or more cups
Adults	2 cups
Pregnant women	4 cups
Nursing mothers	6 cups

Meat group (protein):

Two or more servings of meat, fish, poultry, or eggs, with dry beans and peas and nuts as alternates

Vegetable and fruit group:

Four or more servings, including:

One dark green or deep yellow (for vitamin A) every other day

One citrus (for vitamin C)

Two others, including potatoes

Bread and cereal group:

Four or more servings of whole-grain, enriched, or restored bread or cereal

to athletes before athletic events is more likely to do harm than good. Before the game, an athlete needs a meal high in carbohydrates, which will be readily absorbed and utilized, but low in fat, which may delay emptying of the stomach, and low in protein, which is not digested so quickly as carbohydrate.

THE DANGERS OF UNUSUAL DIETS

Unusual diets are forced on many people in the world by social, racial, and economic factors. In America, some unusual and unhealthy diets are chosen voluntarily. Not all popularly promoted diets are unusual or unhealthy, of course. You can check their virtues easily. Do they contain foods from each of the basic four food groups? If not, forget them; they are more likely to harm than to help you.

VEGETARIANISM

The disciples of vegetarianism usually follow it either because they consider meat or fish deleterious to health or because they object to the destruction of animals to supply food for man. Most vegetarians use milk, butter, eggs, cheese, and other dairy products, all derived from animals, so that they really abstain only from meat.

Many health diets are based on a certain amount of truth. The virtue of vegetarianism, as far as health is concerned, derives from the excellent supply of vitamins, minerals, and carbohydrates in fruits and vegetables. The argument for vegetarianism from this standpoint, however, assumes that if enough vitamins are good, more must be better. This is not true. Furthermore, although it is possible to obtain adequate protein on a vegetarian diet by eating large amounts of soybeans and other legumes, or by supplementing these vegetables with dairy products, the danger of protein deficiency is real. Vitamin B[12] deficiency also may occur in vegetarians, causing damage to the nervous system and anemia.

VEGANISM

Those who adhere to veganism eat no food of animal origin, even milk, eggs, or cheese. The danger of developing protein malnutrition is even greater than with vegetarianism.

People who are convinced that they must adhere to vegetarianism or veganism should study foods and diet very carefully. By careful study, it is possible to plan a diet which can maintain health. One study of 26 people who had practiced veganism with great care showed no deleterious effects, even over 15 to 20 years.

DIETING AND SNACKING

Too often college students—and others—give a healthy, balanced diet a low priority. By trying to lose weight without considering nutrition, or giving other activities a high priority at the expense of the balanced diet, one may sacrifice his health. Attempting to lose weight by omitting breakfast or some other meal which is needed to provide a regular source of nutritional energy may lead to nutritional deficiencies. Snacks too can contribute to nutritional deficiencies, as they are often largely carbohydrate, "empty calories" from carbonated beverages, pastries, and the like.

FOOD QUACKERY

Many people waste money on food fads, and some thereby endanger their health. Promoters of nutritional products or dietary preparations have claimed to cure almost any disease, even cancer. The greatest danger comes when sick people abandon accepted treatment to experiment with food fads or when they attempt to treat serious symptoms with nutritional products of unknown reliability instead of going to their physicians for an examination.

Dietary supplements or miracle foods are promoted, usually in what sounds like a scientific presentation, by the exaggerated myths of nutrition: that most diseases are due to faulty diet; that soil depletion causes malnutrition and disease; that many foods are of little or no value because of overprocessing; that only "natural, organic" foods are good; and that mild, unrecognized deficiency diseases are common among the population, accounting for "that tired feeling," for aches or pains in almost any part of the body, for rashes and unsightly skin, and for other disabilities and disfigurements.

The American Medical Association estimates that over half a billion dollars are spent on unnecessary food supplements or miracle foods each year.

ORGANIC FOODS

A recent interest in organically grown food has caused the opening of health-food stores all over the country. Foods are organic if they are grown without the use of pesticides, herbicides, or chemical fertilizers. Many people who are concerned about pollution have turned to "health foods" generally, meaning organically grown or prepared foods. Unfortunately, these foods require special care during cultivation and are often more expensive than mass-produced foods.

QUESTIONS FOR DISCUSSION AND SELF-EXAMINATION

1 Give two examples of each of the six essential classifications of ingredients for human diets.
2 In what way is man's food supply dependent on the plant kingdom?
3 Describe three ways in which bacteria contribute to the production of food or nutrition.
4 Describe and discuss the similar and differing properties of carbohydrates, fat, and protein.
5 From what sources do human beings get most of their fat-soluble vitamins? Most of their water-soluble vitamins? What would be the consequences of chronic absence of each of these sources from the diet?

6 How widespread in the world are diets with inadequate protein? What is the implication of this and what are possible consequences? Be specific.
7 What are the nature and significance of "essential amino acids" and "nonessential amino acids"?
8 How is the level of sugar in blood controlled? What happens when control is defective?
9 What are the implications of unsaturated fats, saturated fats, and total fats in the diet?
10 Which minerals are most likely to be missing from an American diet and why?

REFERENCES AND READING SUGGESTIONS

BOOKS

Keys, Ancel, and Margaret Keys: *Eat Well and Stay Well*, 2d ed., Doubleday & Company, Inc., Garden City, N.Y., 1963.

An interesting and practical guide to good eating and good nutrition.

Robinson, C.H.: *Basic Nutrition and Diet Therapy*, The Macmillan Company, New York, 1965.

The principles of good nutrition and their application to the improvement of health.

Stare, Frederick: *Eating for Good Health*, Doubleday & Company, Inc., Garden City, N.Y., 1964.

This recognized authority on nutrition writes well for the public.

PAMPHLETS AND PERIODICALS

Bulletins on nutrition, infant feeding, and food preservation, U.S. Public Health Service, Department of Agriculture and Children's Bureau, Washington.

Dietary Fat and Human Health, Food and Nutrition Board of National Academy of Sciences, Washington.

A critical review and analysis of the role of dietary fats in human nutrition and of their role in atherosclerosis.

"The Energy Factory: How Food Finally Produces Power," *Life*, Mar. 29, 1963, p. 48.

A scientific, yet understandable, presentation of the chemical processes within cells which convert foods into energy and materials for growth. Excellent illustrations.

Grollman, Arthur: "A Common-sense Guide to Cholesterol," *Today's Health*, August 1966, p. 3.

An interview with a distinguished professor of experimental medicine.

"High-protein Biscuit for Asian Children," *Science News*, June 25, 1966, p. 514.

Mayer, Jean: "Massive Dose Vitamins—the Newest Craze," *Family Health*, February 1972, p. 25.

This distinguished professor of Nutrition at Harvard and Chairman of the White House Conference on Food, Nutrition, and Health discusses the risks incurred in taking large doses of vitamins.

Ratcliff, J. D.: "Do Traces of Metals Decide Our Fate?" *Today's Health*, March, 1966, p. 34.

A fascinating story of current research concerning minerals which in minute amounts are essential to health but which in excess are exceedingly toxic.

Recommended Dietary Allowances, 6th ed. rev., National Research Council, National Academy of Sciences, publication 1146, Washington. 1966.

An authoritative considerations of all food groups in the human diet; recommended allowances for children and adults and an extensive bibliography.

"Vitamin Crackdown," *Time*, July 1, 1966, p. 48.

What Consumers Should Know about Food Standards, Food and Drug Administration Publication 8, U.S. Department of Health, Education, and Welfare.

Food shoppers who are interested in laws that protect their health and pocketbooks can get useful information from this pamphlet.

12

OBESITY AND DIGESTIVE DISORDERS AND DISEASES

We usually speak poetically of the heart as the seat of emotion, but in some cultures the seat of emotion is thought to be the liver, and in some the stomach. Perhaps the latter is not far wrong. Certainly the intestinal tract is more easily disturbed in function by outside stimuli than almost any other part of the body, and the effects of the emotions on the intestinal tract have long been observed in both man and animals. For instance, an ancient Hindu custom required a person suspected of a crime to chew a mouthful of rice and after a time to spit it out on a fig leaf. If the rice was dry, it was taken as proof that fear of discovery had prevented the secretion of saliva, and the suspect was adjudged guilty.

The digestive system can also be beset with disease, sometimes aggravated by emotional states, as in peptic ulcers, and sometimes not, as in food poisoning, cancer, and other diseases. One of the problems involving the digestive system that has grown increasingly troublesome in our affluent times is due to the unfortunate habit the intestinal tract has of absorbing more food than the body needs. The result is overweight, which causes illness and may cause death.

OVERWEIGHT

Obesity is one of the greatest controllable threats to the life and health of both men and women in this country: over 50 million Americans are obese. Weight above average is not dangerous when it is due to a massive skeleton or to heavy muscles, but most overweight is excess fat, or obesity.

A small amount of fat in the body is desirable and useful; up to 15 percent of the body should be fatty tissue. Such a proportion of fat provides normal and desirable body contour, padding for various organs, and a reservoir of energy for times of food shortage, protecting the protein supplies of the body. However, when fat increases beyond 15 percent it is harmful. An easy way to check for excess fat is to pick up a fold of skin on the abdomen; if a roll of fat can be gathered under the skin, the body has excess fat.

The health hazards of obesity have been described as the "five D's": disfigurement, discomfort, disability, disease, and death. Obesity disfigures; it is usually less than attractive, often ugly. Obesity causes discomfort: joints carry the greater burden; osteoarthritis develops more rapidly in obese than in thinner people; movement is more difficult, particularly as years advance. Obesity disables: osteoarthritis is not only painful but disabling; it can make walking and many other normal activities difficult. Moreover, in the later years of life, excessive weight by itself is enough to make moving around difficult. Obesity increases the incidence of many types of diseases: diabetes and high blood pressure are obvious examples, but even cancer is more common in obese people; gallstones, cirrhosis of the liver, strokes, and heart disease are other problems more common in the obese than in the thin. Obesity kills: the majority of the diseases which are prevalent among obese people have a high fatality rate.

AVERAGE AND IDEAL WEIGHTS

Life insurance companies have long known that obesity increases the benefits they must pay out. The payment of death benefits is expensive; therefore life insurance companies advise their policyholders to maintain ideal weights. When the policyholders follow the advice it means better health and longer life.

Life insurance researchers have amassed impressive data showing the high mortality in obese people. The massive and authoritative *Build and Blood Pressure Study*,[1] published a few years ago, showed that people over the age of 30 shorten their lives by being over the ideal weight. Among men over the age of 30, those who weight 10 to 15 pounds *under the average* for their height and age live the longest and are the healthiest. The mortality rate goes up at a very rapid rate when the

[1]Society of Actuaries, Chicago, 1959.

weight becomes 40 percent or more above average.

On the basis of these facts, the insurance actuaries have constructed tables of *ideal* weights. (See Table 12.1.) Tables of *average* weights, on the other hand, show weights that are excessive for optimal health, since the average person weighs too much. (See Table 12.2.)

Tables of average weights show different figures for different age groups, but tables of ideal

Table 12.1 Weight tables: desirable weights for men and women* of ages 25 and over

Height†		Weight, lb, according to frame (in indoor clothing)		
Feet	Inches	Small frame	Medium frame	Large frame
Men				
5	2	112–120	118–129	126–141
5	3	115–123	121–133	129–144
5	4	118–126	124–136	132–148
5	5	121–129	127–139	135–152
5	6	124–133	130–143	138–156
5	7	128–137	134–147	142–161
5	8	132–141	138–152	147–166
5	9	136–145	142–156	151–170
5	10	140–150	146–160	155–174
5	11	144–154	150–165	159–179
6	0	148–158	154–170	164–184
6	1	152–162	158–175	168–189
6	2	156–167	162–180	173–194
6	3	160–171	167–185	178–199
6	4	164–175	172–190	182–204
Women				
4	10	92– 98	96–107	104–119
4	11	94–101	98–110	106–122
5	0	96–104	101–113	109–125
5	1	99–107	104–116	112–128
5	2	102–110	107–119	115–131
5	3	105–113	110–122	118–134
5	4	108–116	113–126	121–138
5	5	111–119	116–130	125–142
5	6	114–123	120–135	129–146
5	7	118–127	124–139	133–150
5	8	122–131	128–143	137–154
5	9	126–135	132–147	141–158
5	10	130–140	136–151	145–163
5	11	134–144	140–155	149–168
6	0	138–148	144–159	153–173

*For girls between 18 and 25, subtract 1 pound for each year under 25.
†With shoes on: 1-inch heels for men; 2-inch heels for women.
SOURCE: Supplement to *How to Control Your Weight*, Metropolitan Life Booklet, New York, 1963.

Table 12.2 Mortality of men in different weight classes: in relation to that of persons insured at standard premium rates

| Weight class | Percentages of mortality among standard lives* | | | | | |
| | Ages under 40 | | | Ages 40 and over | | |
	Short	Medium	Tall	Short	Medium	Tall
Underweight:						
40 lb below average	115	115		120	100	100
20 lb below average	95	90	90	100	95	95
Average weight	100	100	100	100	100	100
Overweight:						
20 lb above average	115	110	110	120	120	110
40 lb above average	135	125	125	135	130	125
60 lb above average	190	145	145	160	150	145

*Figures indicate percentages of mortality as compared with those of average weight. Note that people of less than average weight have the lowest mortality.
SOURCE: Based on *Build and Blood Pressure Study*, Society of Actuaries, Chicago.

weights make no such allowance. It is unhealthy to put on weight as age advances, except when one is abnormally underweight to start with. On the contrary, optimal health requires the maintenance of college weight through the years, provided that that weight is in the ideal range. As age progresses, even with heavy manual labor or other physical exercise, some of the muscle which is characteristic of youth is replaced by fat. If additional pounds are added, the result is almost always too much body fat.

Comparison of the *Built and Blood Pressure Study* with earlier studies shows that the average weights of men had increased considerably in a generation but that the average weights of women had decreased. Increases in weight for short men and even for short women, however, were particularly large. Some of the decrease in women's weights was caused by the fact that it is fashionable for women to remain thin today. However, the women's weights reported in the study were not entirely reliable because they were recorded with heels higher than in the previous generation and because the study did not include a proportional number of women from poor social groups. A more recent study has shown that more poor women are obese than wealthy women.

In recent years American men and women have been increasing in height as well as in weight. During 40 years, the increase for men was approximately 1 inch and for women slightly less; the increase seems to have tapered off. This increase appears to be an economic phenomenon, presumably related to the more ample diets available to the American public. College men from the affluent parts of society had attained most of the gain in height by the 1930s, but by the 1960s most other college men had caught up with the affluent.

The ideal weights in Table 11.1 furnish a good guide for one who seeks optimal health. Allowing weight to rise significantly above these standards increases the chances of ill health and of dying prematurely. Nevertheless, individual variations do occur, so that what is true for a group is not necessarily true for every individual in the group. The individual may have a deformity, or he may have a highly developed, heavy muscle structure, or he may have a chronic disease. In such cases the ordinary standards of ideal weights may be inapplicable.

CAUSES OF OVERWEIGHT

Obesity occurs only when the food a person eats provides more calories than his body burns. Regulation of food intake is the most effective means of controlling body weight. When the energy value of the food eaten is less than the energy expenditure, the body burns stored body fat to compensate. If more calories are consumed than are needed for energy expenditure, the body stores the excess as fat, except during periods of growth. Therefore changes in either intake or expenditure of energy affect body weight.

This simple principle operates throughout life. The amount of body fat is visible evidence of the adequacy, deficiency, or excess of the caloric intake. As little as 100 extra calories—equal to 1 slice of bread and butter—eaten daily for a year causes a weight gain of 10 pounds; conversely, 100 calories subtracted from the daily diet causes a weight loss of 10 pounds.

EATING HABITS AS A CAUSE OF OBESITY

Very fat people are big eaters. Their habits may vary. Some eat a lot all the time, like the 300-pound man who lost 9 pounds in 3 days away from home because his refrigerator was not available for snacks. Others eat in "binges," like some alcoholics on "sprees."

The sensations of hunger, appetite, and satiety are important in controlling or expanding food intake. Hunger sensations are apparently due to contractions of the stomach, but satiety, the sensation of having had enough to eat or of being full, is regulated by the hypothalamus, a portion of the brain which lies just above the pituitary gland. In animals, destruction of small areas of the hypothalamus can cause overeating and obesity. Rarely, in a human being, damage to the hypothalamus by injury or by a ruptured or broken blood vessel may cause obesity.

In addition, the hypothalamus receives psychologically determined messages from the higher centers of the brain. These modify or dull the normal sensations of satiety, so that the person eats more than is necessary for his bodily needs. The pleasure derived from eating may provide satisfaction when other desires are not satisfied. Some people eat compulsively and may be unable to stop eating at an appropriate time, either at meals or between meals. Some compulsive eaters go on their eating binges when they are anxious or disturbed by inner emotions or by adverse circumstances in their lives.

UNDERACTIVITY AS A CAUSE OF OBESITY

Although virtually all very obese people and many people who have milder degrees of overweight eat more than thin people, underactivity is a major contributor to obesity. Physical activity requires energy and utilizes calories; inactivity allows fat to accumulate more readily. A study of high school girls showed that overweight girls in the group actually ate a little less than the thin girls, but were much less active. They walked less, they danced less, and they moved less in common daily routines as well as participating less in formal athletics. Another study involved two groups of men who weighed the same amount; one group ate more than the other, but walked *faster* than the other group that ate less. They were burning up the extra calories. (See Table 12.3.) Various other studies have confirmed that many people who say that they do not eat more than average are telling the truth; they eat an average amount (though it may be too much for them) but exercise too little. Even while sitting in a chair, one person may be moving his muscles frequently and thus burning calories while another is completely relaxed and burning few calories. Furthermore, an obese person frequently becomes less competent at and less comfortable in physical activities, so that he becomes still less active than he was before; the result is added weight. Once involved in this vicious circle, the fat person becomes increasingly obese.

INSULATION AS A FACTOR IN OBESITY

Another vicious circle, or feedback mechanism, which contributes to obesity is the insulation provided by fat. A layer of fat insulates the body so that an obese person loses heat more slowly than a thin person. Thus, in cold weather, a thin person has to burn more calories than a fat person just to stay warm. Consequently, if a thin person and a fat person take in equal amounts of calories and burn equal amounts of calories in activities, the fat person may gain weight while the thin person keeps the same weight or loses just because of the difference in amount of energy used to stay warm.

CARBOHYDRATES, INSULIN, AND OBESITY

Some doctors have suggested that carbohydrates (sugars and starches) "poison" some people, causing them to become obese. Though this seems an exaggeration, it is clear that some overweight people handle carbohydrates abnormally. Some obese people, for example, have been shown to secrete

Table 12.3 Effect of exercise in controlling weight

Calories	Food	Time required to burn, minutes*				
		Walking	Riding bicycle	Swimming	Running	Reclining
101	Apple, large	19	12	9	5	78
96	Bacon, 2 strips	18	12	9	5	74
114	Beer, 1 glass	22	14	10	6	88
78	Bread and butter	15	10	7	4	60
356	Cake, ½, 2-layer	68	43	32	18	274
27	Cheese, cottage, 1 tbsp	5	3	2	1	21
232	Chicken, fried, ½ breast	45	28	21	12	178
542	Chicken, TV dinner	104	66	48	28	417
15	Cookie, plain	3	2	1	1	12
151	Doughnut	29	18	13	8	116
110	Egg, fried	21	13	10	6	85
59	French dressing, 1 tbsp	11	7	5	3	45
167	Ham, 2 slices	32	20	15	9	128
350	Hamburger sandwich	67	43	31	18	269
193	Ice cream, ⅙ qt	37	24	17	10	148
502	Malted milk shake	97	61	45	26	386
166	Milk, 1 glass	32	20	15	9	128
120	Orange juice, 1 glass	23	15	11	6	92
124	Pancake with syrup	24	15	11	6	95
56	Peas, green, ½ cup	11	7	5	3	43
377	Pie, apple, ⅙	73	46	34	19	290
314	Pork chop, loin	60	38	28	16	242
108	Potato chips, 1 serving	21	13	10	6	83
180	Shrimp, French-fried	35	22	16	9	138
396	Spaghetti, 1 serving	76	48	35	20	305
400	Strawberry shortacke	77	49	36	21	308

*Calculated for person weighing 150-160 lb. at the following caloric expenditure per minute of activity: walking 5.2 cal (at 3½ mph); riding bicycle, 8.2 cal; swimming, 11.2 cal; running, 19.4 cal; reclining, 1.3 cal.

SOURCE: Adapted from R. Passmore and J.V.G.A. Durnin, *Physiologic Reviews*, vol. 35, no. 801, 1955.

too much insulin, the pancreatic hormone that controls blood sugar and other aspects of carbohydrate metabolism. One effect that insulin seems to have on the body is to promote transport of foodstuffs through the intestinal wall.

The anthropometrist and physician Edward Sheldon developed a method of classifying body build, known as "somatotyping," which has gained popularity and standing with both lay people and scientists. The three types of body build described by Sheldon are lifelong, probably determined by heredity or at least by very early developmental patterns, and are significant for weight patterns. The *mesomorph* is square and muscular, with broad shoulders and a heavyset chest. He often is heavy with muscle but not with fat. The *endomorph* is pudgy and rounded, with the abdomen predominating over the chest. He accumulates fat readily and must exert vigorous and continuing effort to avoid excess weight. The third type of body build is the *ectomorph*, slender and narrow; he is usually underweight and finds it difficult to gain weight. In his later years when his naturally restive activity diminishes he may begin to accumulate a little fat in the abdomen, a "pot" in common slang or an "ectomorphic derby hat" in anthropometric slang. Most people have combinations of these factors in their body build; pure mesomorphy, endomorphy, or ectomorphy is rare. A predominance of one over the other two is common, but a few people have almost an equal mixture of all three.

FACTORS THAT ARE NOT CAUSES OF OBESITY

Endocrine diseases are rare as causes of obesity. Rarely is thyroid underactivity a cause of being overweight, and moreover, not all hypothyroid people are overweight. Manipulation of the glands by medication or otherwise does not often help in the treatment of obesity.

Water retention also is not a cause of obesity. While people can retain fluid over a short period of time (notably women just before their menstrual periods), fluid never accounts for a significant proportion of overweight. Excess flesh is tissue made of fat with some carbohydrate, protein, and fluids.

Although earlier experiments had shown *no* difference in intestinal absorption between obese and normal individuals, several recent studies indicate the opposite: that obese individuals do take more foodstuffs than average through their intestinal walls into their bodies. Obese mice have been shown to absorb glucose more efficiently than normal mice, and another study showed that ten obese women absorbed the amino acid valine more readily than did fifteen women who were of normal weight.

One influence encouraging the production of too much insulin in the obese is the resistance of the overstuffed fat cells to insulin. A 70-kilogram (150-pound) man who becomes 20 percent overweight *doubles* the fatty tissue in his body, and is correspondingly resistant to the effect of insulin and encouraging of the secretion of insulin. Furthermore, a high-carbohydrate meal causes an outpouring of insulin. Not only does this insulin have its effects on the body metabolism, but the low blood sugar which may occur 3 hours later increases appetite and encourages food intake. Therefore the businessman (or student) who eats a high-carbohydrate meal and then sits quietly for several hours encourages the hypersecretion of insulin, the overabsorption of foodstuffs, the development of hypoglycemia, the underexpenditure of calories, an increase in appetite, and hence consumption of more carbohydrates—a feedback mechanism which results in obesity.

HOW TO LOSE WEIGHT

A successful campaign to lose weight can be planned easily from a study of the causes of obesity detailed above. The cardinal rules are: (1) eat less, (2) exercise more, and (3) stress proteins in the diet and eat fewer fats and carbohydrates.

When a large amount of weight is to be lost or when the person who must lose it is in middle age or beyond, the campaign to control weight should begin with a medical examination to determine fitness for the program and to plan the most effective ways to take weight off and to keep it off. In general it is easy to determine the caloric intake of any diet by use of standard tables. (See Appendix.) Use of such tables can also ensure that adequate vitamin and mineral nutrients are included in the diet. Many reducing diets do not make such provision and thus may cause undernutrition of essential nutrients, resulting in fatigue, nervousness, digestive disturbances, and irresistible craving for food. Occasionally, when a physician prescribes a very limited diet, he may also prescribe vitamins and other food supplements.

For small weight losses, simple, easy, and permanent weight reduction can also be achieved by using a little arithmetic to formulate a dietary program and then sticking to it. Reducing caloric intake by 50 calories per day—one slice of bread, one slice of bacon, or ½ tablespoon of butter or margarine—will cause the loss of 5 pounds in a year, if the degree of activity remains the same.

USEFUL PLANS FOR LOSING WEIGHT

A "social diet" consisting of regular curtailments of portions usually eaten is often an effective method of losing weight slowly over a period of time. Such a social diet avoids more than one slice of bread, or its equivalent, at a meal. Gravies and other cooked fats are avoided. Portions of everything are about one-fourth smaller than those previously taken; "seconds" and between-meal snacks or drinks other than water are forbidden.

On this regimen, almost every determined person will lose weight. One hundred patients in the New York City area succeeded in reducing their daily diets by 1400 calories through this plan. In many instances, the patient's friends—and sometimes even his family—did not know that he was on a diet.

Medicines have definite but limited value in aiding weight loss. During the early stages of weight reduction, physicians may prescribe amphetamines, which act on the nervous system, to depress appetite. Unfortunately, such drugs may lead to habituation in some patients if used for a long period of time. Furthermore, they tend to lose their effectiveness after a short period. Hence most physicians do not use them or limit their use to the early period of a weight-loss program, when getting used to smaller quantities of food is most difficult.

Group reinforcement and cooperation can be very helpful in programs of weight reduction. Some people who have worked with obese patients find them similar to those addicted to tobacco, alcohol, or drugs. The feeling of belonging to a group with common problems and common goals is essential to some of these people if they are to make real progress in controlling their weight. One organization with these characteristics is TOPS (for "Take off pounds"), which resembles Alcoholics Anonymous in its structure.

EXERCISE AS AN AID IN LOSING WEIGHT

Exercise is a valuable and important aid in losing weight. Young people in otherwise good health can exercise up to the point of discomfort without harm and in doing so use up many calories of energy. As a person gets older, however, he must be more cautious about the exercise that he takes. Persons over 40 should have annual physical examinations and ask advice about what exercise to take. Even in the decades past 40 people who are in good health may engage in vigorous exertion provided that they train for it conscientiously by exercising regularly and frequently.

Even mild exercise, performed daily, will result in significant weight loss. Twenty minutes of walking daily will bring the weight down 10 pounds in a year, provided that diet and other exercise remain the same. To put it another way, a doughnut contains about 150 calories, the amount that 18 minutes of bicycle riding or 8 minutes of

vigorous running will consume. Thus if one eats a doughnut, this amount of exercise will prevent the conversion of the calories into body fat. (See Table 12.3.) Regular, moderate exercise improves muscle tone and results in an increase in the oxidation (burning) of carbohydrates and fats of the body.

USELESS AND DANGEROUS APPROACHES TO WEIGHT LOSS

Losing fluid is a dramatic way to lower the reading on the scales temporarily, but it removes no flesh. Sweating—through exercise, through the old-fashioned sweatbox or steam room, or through the recently popular Finnish sauna—is one method of losing fluids; restricting the quantity of fluids drunk is another; and the use of diuretic pills or injections, which cause the kidneys to excrete more urine, is a third. These measures may have limited value for an athlete who must "make weight" to a certain level in order to compete in a given event, but the loss of fluids is of no value to the fat peson who has a long task of reducing flesh ahead of him. Dehydration can even damage health, for example by promoting the formation of kidney stones.

Most medical preparations for the reduction of weight are either worthless or dangerous. A few consist of cellulose or its derivatives, which swell in the stomach and may have limited usefulness in diminishing hunger, particularly between meals.

Finally, a useless and perhaps dangerous approach to losing weight may be called the "roller-coaster" method: taking off pounds through a "crash diet" and then abandoning dietary control so that the pounds gradually reappear in their old places. The obese person thus finishes with the same weight with which he started. Furthermore, during the period of weight gain, the amount of fat circulating in the bloodstream often increases to levels which are potentially dangerous. This may well be a time when fat is deposited in the walls of the coronary arteries, rendering the person susceptible to a later heart attack.

UNDERWEIGHT

The problems of thinness are more often esthetic than medical. As the discussion of ideal weight indicated, most people who weigh less than average are healthier and live longer than those who are

average or over average in weight. Anyone who wishes to gain weight should carefully examine his reasons to determine their validity.

Those who are excessively thin or who weigh

less than the ideal weight listed in Table 12.1 may find it difficult to gain weight. In order to gain weight the calorie intake must be raised so that it exceeds the energy expenditure. A moderately active person of average size uses up about 2500 calories per day, so that in order to gain weight significantly he would have to eat at least 3000 calories daily. It is necessary to provide additional calories in the most appetizing and digestible form. An extra meal at bedtime is often necessary to gain weight, because it increases food intake without impairing the appetite for the regular three meals. Between-meal feedings may provide extra calories but diminish appetite for the meals following. Many thin people are active physically; when they eat more they may unintentionally become still more active. Therefore increasing the hours of sleep at night and taking rest periods after lunch and supper may be valuable adjuncts to a weight-gaining diet.

INFECTIONS AND POISONINGS OF THE INTESTINAL TRACT

"Food poisoning," another health problem of the intestinal tract, includes all illnesses resulting from foods contaminated with disease-producing organisms or their products, from foods contaminated with chemical poisons, and from foods which contain poisons from plants and animals. Properly speaking, the term does not include "food idiosyncracies" or "food allergies" which cause unpleasant reactions in a few individuals but do not affect the vast majority of people.

Food poisonings most commonly result from contamination of food with bacteria or their products; less common is contamination with chemical poison. Bacteria account for about two-thirds of outbreaks of food poisoning, chemical poisons for under 10 percent, and viruses or unknown causes for the rest.

When one is afflicted by vomiting or diarrhea or both, it is tempting to attribute these symptoms to a particular food recently eaten or to a particular restaurant patronized. However, unless some others who ate the same meal also have been sick, and at approximately the same time, the chances are that food poisoning is not the cause of the illness. The majority of such isolated illnesses may be due to viruses acquired from other persons through the air or by personal contact. In the spring of 1971, for example, between 20,000 and 25,000 people in Morgantown, West Virginia, became ill with vomiting and diarrhea, but no bacterial or chemical cause could be found. It seemed likely that a virus infection had been passed from person to person.

Food poisoning is common, nevertheless. In 1968, 345 outbreaks, with 17,567 people afflicted, were reported in the United States (and many more were unreported).

BACTERIAL FOOD POISONING

1   Staphylococcal food poisoning   Probably the most common type of food poisoning, staphylococcal food poisoning, is due to a toxin formed by *Staphylococcus* bacteria in the contaminated food before it is served. Custards and pastries are particularly susceptible to contamination by these bacteria, and the toxin is formed in them by the bacteria when the food is not promptly refrigerated. Contamination occurs most often from a skin infection on the hands of a food handler.

The time between eating contaminated food and the appearance of symptoms of staphylococcal food poisoning is short—from 1 to 6 hours, usually from 2½ to 3 hours. The brief incubation period is a distinguishing characteristic. The onset is abrupt and sometimes violent. Vomiting is common, as is severe diarrhea, accompanied by abdominal pain and acute prostration. Fever may or may not be present. Deaths are very rare, and symptoms usually disappear in 5 or 6 hours, although they may last as long as 72 hours. Because of the short incubation and duration, many cases are never reported to the health department.

Prompt and adequate refrigeration of foods, especially of sliced and chopped meats and of custards and cream fillings, is very important in the control of staphylococcal food intoxication. These measures prevent the multipliction of organisms which may have been introduced into the foods. Food handlers should be educated to follow sanitary methods and should be excused from work temporarily if they have skin infections. Regulation of the sale of custard-filled products during summer months is another preventive measure which has proved of value.

2 Clostridial food poisoning Another group of bacteria, the *Clostridium* bacteria, cause illnesses almost identical to those caused by staphylococcal toxins, except that the incubation period between exposure and illness is longer, averaging 12 hours, and that the illness is usually milder. Clostridial food poisoning is less common than staphylococcal food poisoning.

3 Salmonella infections From 2 to 4 million Americans fall ill each year from salmonella infections acquired from their food. The *Salmonella* bacteria are common contaminants of various kinds of food, especially poultry. Flocks of poultry often harbor these bacteria without the infestation being readily detectable in either the live or the slaughtered birds. Even if recognized, the infection is difficult to eliminate except by sacrifice of the entire flock.

The first symptoms of salmonella infection usually appear about 12 hours (with a range of 6 to 48 hours) after one has eaten contaminated food. Severe diarrhea, vomiting, weakness, abdominal pain, and some fever at the onset are typical. Fatalities are uncommon except in the aged. Salmonella outbreaks often harm many people. A church supper in Shelby County, Tennessee, on October 16, 1968, was attended by 130 persons and contaminated turkey was served. Of 116 interviewed later, 98 had been ill with diarrhea, cramps, nausea, vomiting, or fever or some combination of these. At a nursing home in Baltimore in the last week of July 1970, a kitchen employee with diarrhea helped prepare the food for 136 patients. At least 62 of the patients developed the symptoms of salmonella infection, with 12 dying in the first few days and others remaining critically ill.

General measures for preventing salmonella infections call for the strictest possible attention to refrigeration and to the cleanliness of food-handling personnel, premises, and practices. Emphasis should be put on protection of food from vermin during processing and storage. Food handlers should not engage in their work while suffering from diarrhea.

At the beginning of this century, one of the major fatal diseases in the Western world was typhoid fever, a type of *Salmonella* which has since become rare. A severe epidemic, with a dozen deaths, in Aberdeen, Scotland, in 1964 serves as a reminder that laxity of sanitary standards can bring a resurgence of this most deadly of salmonella infections. Even more recently, in May and June of 1967, in a fraternity house at Stanford University, an epidemic of typhoid fever infected 31 people. Fortunately none was seriously ill and all responded promptly to treatment. A cook proved to have typhoid bacilli in the stool, but it was impossible to prove whether the cook was the source of the epidemic or had been infected at the same time as the fraternity brothers.

4 Botulism Though rare—causing only a few deaths each year—botulism is such a deadly disease that it deserves special attention. Its cause is a poison secreted by *clostridium botulinum* organisms as they grow in certain foods, usually home-canned vegetables.

Each year outbreaks of botulism continue to be reported. The organism multiplies only in the absence of air, but as it grows it liberates a powerful poison or toxin. This toxin rarely causes vomiting and diarrhea but is carried to the nervous system, where it causes paralysis. A guinea pig can be killed by 1/25,000,000 ounce of the toxin, and human beings have died from its effects after nibbling part of a pod of a spoiled string bean or after eating a small spoonful of affected corn.

Boiling destroys the toxin, and all home-canned vegetables should be thoroughly boiled to prevent botulism. Boiling does not kill the spores of the bacteria, but steam under pressure will kill them. The canning industry has instituted strict measures to ensure the safety of commercially canned goods. Nevertheless, in 1971 the toxin was discovered in a few cans of a nationally sold brand of soup after one death occurred.

Botulism is different from the other types of food poisoning in that its primary effects are on the nervous system, causing peculiar paralyses and then collapse of the circulation and breathing, leading to death. In only a fraction of cases does vomiting occur.

CHEMICALS IN FOOD

Many chemicals in food are useful and important and are deliberately added. Others are harmful, poisonous to some extent, whether added with intent or by mistake.

Various chemicals are added to many of the foods included in our daily menus. In fact, it would be difficult to put a whole meal together without them. They prevent rancidity, improve or change texture (as in homogenized milk and cheese), improve or preserve flavor and color, maintain quality between farm and table, help prevent spoilage, and prevent certain foods from breaking down, drying, and caking.

The harmlessness of such food additives is safeguarded by law and by the supervision of the United States Food and Drug Administration. Since 1959, food manufacturers have had to pre-test proposed food additives and submit their data to the Food and Drug Administration. The chemical additives must be safe in the amounts used in commercial foods and under the conditions of such use or they will not be permitted on the market.

Often chemicals are added to foods by mistake. A young mother making a birthday cake used a rat poison, barium carbonate, instead of flour because it was stored in the container which usually held flour; several children died. Another mother gave her children a dark liquid from the refrigerator, thinking it coffee. The liquid was actually an insecticide. The older child died in a few hours, while the younger, who spit out the liquid, was critically ill.

Safety requires, first, that no poisonous substance be stored in a container which is not clearly and prominently marked "poison"; second, that no materials not suitable for cooking be placed or stored with or even near cooking materials.

Occasionally, more gradual poisoning occurs because of food or drink. Small doses of arsenic can cause chronic poisoning, and in years gone by lead water pipes caused gradual lead poisoning. Antimony, cadmium, and zinc poisoning have occurred when foods have been cooked in utensils made of these materials; such utensils for the most part are not available for purchase today. Although in certain forms aluminum can be dangerous, aluminum cooking utensils are entirely safe. Storage of food in its original can is no more dangerous than storing it in a separate container; what produces spoilage in either container is bacterial growth introduced from the air, fingers, or a utensil and encouraged by time and suitable temperature.

Especially since the publication of Rachel Carson's *Silent Spring*[2] in 1962, increasing concern and attention have focused on the dangers of pesticides in foods and elsewhere. It has been estimated, for example, that 15 percent of the agricultural workers in California have suffered sickness from pesticides. The proper place of pesticides and the nature ot their many dangers are discussed in Chapter 3, human ecology.

Many plants and berries are poisonous to human beings. Some such materials contain chemicals which are useful in small quantities to treat human diseases but are dangerous in larger amounts. The foxglove plant is an example; it contains digitalis, which is a lifesaving drug in some cases of heart failure but which causes fatal irregularities of the heart in larger quantities.

Mushrooms are probably the most dangerous of plants in the United States, since many varieties are customarily eaten. Few of these are poisonous, but for the amateur there is no simple guide by which to tell the good from the bad. The only mushrooms which may be eaten safely are those which have been raised commercially or which can be positively identified by an expert. In 1965 mushrooms caused several deaths in New Jersey; in 1971, three deaths in California.

In recent years, many illnesses and a few deaths have been caused by hepatitis transmitted by clams, oysters, and other shellfish from contaminated waters. Sewage from cities and towns in an area carries the virus of infectious hepatitis, which is taken up by the shellfish and ingested by people. About 40 days later they develop the jaundice and other symptoms characteristic of hepatitis.

In some waters of the Pacific Ocean, mussels, clams, and other shellfish have proved acutely poisonous to human beings. The shellfish takes in certain forms of harmful but microscopic aquatic life as food, which becomes concentrated in the liver and poisons the people who eat the fish.

[2]See References and Reading Suggestions for Chapter 3.

SAFE FOOD HANDLING

Health departments in this country are assiduous in safeguarding the basic sources of food and drink from contamination. These efforts need constant reinforcement at the point of delivery to the ultimate consumer, the person who eats the food. Are those who prepare the food free of communicable disease? Are they clean in their personal habits? Are the methods they employ in serving foods sanitary?

Many cities and states require all food handlers in public eating places to have physical examinations before employment, and sometimes at yearly intervals. This offers some protection to the public, but more important by far is constant vigilance for daily high standards.

These high standards mean that each food handler and each supervisor of food handlers must take responsibility for personal and environmental standards. The food handler must wash his hands frequently and help keep the area where food is prepared immaculate. A cook could be a typhoid carrier all his life without ever infecting anyone if he always scrubbed his hands thoroughly after using the toilet and before handling foods. The food handler must be careful to report all skin infections and all intestinal infections in himself; the supervisor should keep him from handling food when he has such infections and should protect him from loss of wages so that he will not be tempted to conceal his illness. A food handler who has just had a physical examination could develop a skin infection the next day, conceal it, and introduce it into the food being prepared.

Adequate sanitary procedures should be part of the inital training of the food handler. It is important that this training be given as he begins his work. An important rule is: "Food sanitation habits are easier to form than to reform."

Anyone operating a food establishment must use the utmost care and observe many sanitary procedures if the health of his patrons is to be guarded. The most attractive surroundings are of little importance unless the food reaches the consumer free from contamination with disease agents.

MILK—A POTENTIALLY DANGEROUS FOOD

Milk is the only animal product extensively used in an uncooked state by Americans; since it is not cooked, it needs particular protection against contamination. Milk is difficult to obtain, transport, and deliver in a sanitary condition. Disease-producing organisms may get into the milk either from a diseased animal or from human beings who have contact with the milk. Diseases of animal origin which are transmissible through milk are tuberculosis, brucellosis, foot-and-mouth disease, and intestinal ailments resulting in diarrheal conditions, especially in children. In addition, milk handlers may introduce bacteria. A few bacteria accidentally added to milk at milking time may

Figure 12.1   Some parasitic infestations of man.

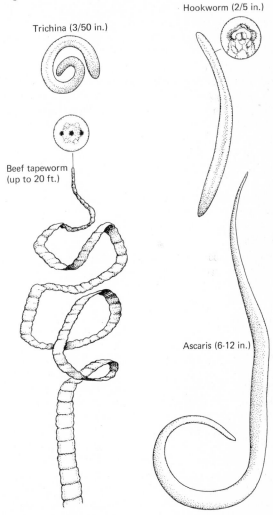

Trichina (3/50 in.)

Hookworm (2/5 in.)

Beef tapeworm (up to 20 ft.)

Ascaris (6-12 in.)

develop into many millions by the time the milk is used.

Fortunately, modern methods of dairying and pasteurization have eliminated most milk-borne disease in the United States. Almost all dairy herds are now free of both tuberculosis and brucellosis. Dairy barns are usually clean, milking is often done by machine rather than by human hands, the machines are kept clean, and transportation is rapid and carried out under refrigeration.

Most important, of course, is the process of pasteurization, which consists of heating milk according to careful standards. Like most important health advances, pasteurization was opposed at first by those who feared the loss of some ingredient or taste of the milk. In Chicago, officials were persuaded of the virtue of pasteurization when the health commissioner asked them to identify the unpasteurized milk among several unlabeled glasses of milk. One official was certain he had identified it, remarking. "That's real milk," but was then told that all the glasses contained pasteurized milk and that the glass of milk he had identified as unpasteurized merely had a drop of manure added to it.

Safe, healthful pasteurized milk will remain so only if kept refrigerated in the home and restaurant until used. In rural areas where family cows provide the milk supply, home pasteurization is very desirable; directions for carrying out pasteurization can be obtained from the U.S. Department of Agriculture.

OTHER DISEASES TRANSMITTED BY FOODS

In addition to the diseases discussed above, man may receive from his food tuberculosis, amebic and bacillary dysentery, infectious hepatitis, streptococcal infections, and various parasitic diseases, such as tapeworm and roundworm. Beef may transmit the beef tapeworm, pork the pork tapeworm and trichina, and fish the fish tapeworm.

The cysts of the tapeworm which occur in beef, pork, and fish are readily destroyed by heat, but drying and smoking will not destroy them. Thus in certain parts of the world where raw or dried fish is considered a delicacy, the fish tapeworm is very prevalent. Prevention of the disease consists of avoiding uncooked or inadequately cooked meat or fish. (See Figure 12.1.)

Trichinosis is an infestation of animals and man caused by a small worm, the *Trichinella spiralis*. (See Chapter 16.) Probably 25 million Americans have had trichinosis, most in a mild and unrecognized form, due to widespread use of pork products. Thorough cooking of all pork and pork products is an effective preventive measure which can be carried out by individual consumers.

HEALTH AND DISEASE IN THE DIGESTIVE SYSTEM

The intestinal tract is probably more easily disturbed in function by outside stimuli than any other part of the body. Fear and apprehension may produce diarrhea or constipation. Concern, worry, and annoyance frequently result in spasticity or crampiness of the muscles in the walls of the intestinal tract. This is usually accompanied by distension with gas and discomfort, frequently described by sufferers as a sensation of the intestines being "tied up in knots."

These effects of the emotions on the intestinal tract are produced by nervous stimuli, particularly those of the sympathetic and parasympathetic nervous system, which are not under control of the conscious mind. A person may or may not be able to express his emotion; sometimes he is unable even to recognize the presence of the emotion. But the nervous system can react to the emotion and transmit stimuli to the intestinal tract anyway. Unexpressed emotions may persist for days, weeks, or even years and thus produce chronic intestinal disorders as well as acute dysfunction. Good emotional health is therefore important to the health of the intestinal tract.

PSYCHOLOGICAL DISTURBANCES OF THE DIGESTIVE SYSTEM

From stimuli of the nervous system acting on the intestinal tract—and from other stimuli as well—come a variety of disorders which involve only the function of the intestinal tract, not its structure. Some of these functional disorders afflict primarily one part of the intestinal tract and have acquired names of their own. "Nervous indigestion," for example, is a disorder of the upper part of the intestinal tract characterized by discomfort or burning in the upper part of the abdomen; it is associated with excessive motility of the stomach, or excessive secretion of acid and other materials, or both.

Other functional disorders involve the large bowel, or colon, and are due to changes in the motility of that part of the intestinal tract. Varying combinations of crampy pain, constipation, diarrhea, bloating, and secretion of mucus lead to the names *mucous colitis, irritable colon,* and *spastic colitis.*

These functional disorders are uncomfortable and are often prolonged and difficult to relieve completely, but they do not shorten life or damage the patient's general health. Sometimes, however, the same symptoms may be a sign not of functional disorders but of more serious structural diseases. A physician may have to obtain x-rays, make other tests, and observe his patient over a period of time to arrive at a reliable diagnosis.

CONSTIPATION

Although apparently less common now than it was previously among the college generation, constipation is the most frequent of abdominal complaints. Constipation is not a specific disease which can be prevented or cured by any single form of treatment. Indeed, many cases of constipation occur only because of the worry that a person feels if he misses a bowel movement on a particular day. Some normal persons in good health have two or three bowel movements a day, while others who are equally well have only one bowel movement in 2 or 3 days. In general, bowels function best if they are left alone. Simple constipation, unrelated to structural disease, results from lack of tone in the abdominal and intestinal muscles, from lack of fluids and bulk in the diet, or from lack of exercise, as well as from psychological stimuli. The occurrence of constipation where regularity has been the previous habit calls for careful medical investigation for an underlying cause. If no underlying cause is present, simple measures such as increasing the amount of exercise taken, increasing bulk-producing fruits and vegetables in the diet, and drinking sufficient fluids are much preferable to the use of laxatives, which may make the bowel dependent on them.

PEPTIC ULCERS OF STOMACH AND DUODENUM

Burning sensations in the upper part of the abdomen, heartburn, and the need to take frequent milk or antacids often indicate a peptic ulcer in the stomach or duodenum. Peptic ulcers are often the result of stimuli from the central nervous system which increase the secretions of the stomach. They are a serious threat to health as well as a nuisance. About one person in ten will have an ulcer at some time in his life. It is now recognized that nervous

Figure 12.2 Factors in the development of peptic ulcers of stomach and duodenum.

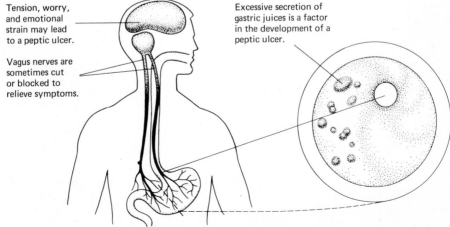

Tension, worry, and emotional strain may lead to a peptic ulcer.

Vagus nerves are sometimes cut or blocked to relieve symptoms.

Excessive secretion of gastric juices is a factor in the development of a peptic ulcer.

tension, worry, and emotional strain are prime causes of ulcer (See Figure 12.2.) The treatment therefore includes not only careful diet and medication to neutralize the stomach acid but also reduction of mental tension and turmoil.

Three complications may occur in ulcer: first, hemorrage, manifested by vomiting of blood or the passage of black or red stools; second, perforation of the ulcer through the wall of the intestinal tract into the abdominal cavity, causing very painful peritonitis; and third, obstruction at or near the pylorus (the exit from the stomach), causing repeated and prolonged vomiting.

An ulcer in the stomach itself may be or may become cancerous, but cancer of the duodenum is exceedingly rare.

CANCER OF THE INTESTINAL TRACT

Of all the diseases connected with the intestinal tract, cancers are obviously the most serious. Killing approximately 60,000 Americans each year, and causing great suffering and disibility, cancers of the intestinal tract are searched for carefully by physicians in patients past the age of 40. Cancers of the intestinal tract may occur in college-age people, although they rarely do.

Unfortunately the same symptoms that come from cancer, such as indigestion or constipation, often come from other diseases, many of them common functional, psychologically caused disorders. Even physicians may have trouble distinguishing one disease from another; the layman should not jump to the conclusion that a particular symptom is either serious or unimportant without careful evaluation by a physician.

CANCER OF THE COLON, RECTUM, AND STOMACH

About 70,000 new cases of cancer of the colon (large intestine) and rectum occur annually in this country. About 45,000 patients die, with the number of deaths of men and women approximately equal.

GALLSTONES, HEPATITIS, AND APPENDICITIS

Three other structural diseases of the intestinal tract deserve special attention because of their frequency and severity: gallstones, hepatitis, and appendicitis, all of which affect auxiliary parts of the intestinal tract.

Gallstones are rare in young people, but frequent in those in middle age and beyond. Formed by the precipitation of solids in the gallbladder (which temporarily stores most bile after it leaves the liver), these stones can cause pain, infection of the gallbladder, and jaundice in various combinations. Stones may remain in the gallbladder for months or years without causing trouble, but when a stone causes inflammation and infection in the wall of the gallbladder, with pain, fever, and increasing illness, an emergency operation is usually necessary. Because of this many physicians advise removal of gallbladders which contain stones before they become infected. At other times, a small stone may move from the gallbladder into the ducts leading from the liver and gallbladder to the intestinal tract. This movement is extremely painful, and the stone may become lodged at one point in the ducts, leading to progressive jaundice and damage to the liver. Sometimes merely the contractions of a gallbladder containing stones following a fatty meal are painful. The most serious (though rare) complication of gallstones is cancer of the gallbladder due to chronic irritation by the gallstones within it.

Another cause of jaundice is infectious hepatitis, a common virus infection of the liver. Contracted from infected water or food, or by personal contact with an infected person, hepatitis is an acute, uncomfortable illness which usually has associated fever and which takes weeks or months for recovery. Rarely the damage to the liver cells is so serious that the patient dies or develops permanent damage to the liver, with impairment of general health. Although there is no specific cure for hepatitis once it has developed, there is an excellent preventive: gamma globulin. Anyone who has been close to a person who becomes ill with infectious hepatitis should receive an injection of gamma globulin to protect himself against the disease. The Peace Corps routinely gives its volunteers injections of gamma globulin before they go to areas of the world where hepatitis is relatively common. People planning travel to tropical or semitropical countries should ask their physicians about the desirability of gamma globulin injections.

Appendicitis is familiar to almost everyone, but despite its frequency it is still a dangerous disease. Of the almost 2,000 annual American deaths from appendicitis, most can be explained by a single word: neglect. Proper attention to any persistent abdominal pain, early medical care, and immediate operation when indicated are the means of preventing deaths from appendicitis. The risk increases with each hour abdominal pain persists. When an operation is performed within 24 hours of the beginning of the attack, less than 1 percent of the patients die; but the risk is increased when the operation is delayed.

The use of cathartics (laxatives) during an attack of appendicitis greatly increases the risk. Many lives would be saved each year if all who develop a pain in the abdomen, particularly in the middle or lower right portion, consulted a physician immediately, if no one with abdominal pain received a laxative, and if operations were performed promptly in all cases of appendicitis.

QUESTIONS FOR DISCUSSION AND SELF-EXAMINATION

1 Describe the ways in which nutrition and disorders of the intestinal tract are affected by psychological and emotional factors.
2 Compare the effects of several bacterial, viral, and parasitic infections of the intestinal tract.
3 Discuss the relationship between weight and length of life.
4 What are the differences between ideal and average weights? Do these change after age 25? Why?
5 What is "somatotype" and what is its relationship to weight?

6 What factors which produce or increase obesity are under voluntary control and which are not?
7 What chemicals are placed on or otherwise are found in foods, and what is their effect?
8 What is the nature and function of foodhandler exams?
9 In what ways can cancer of the intestinal tract resemble other diseases?
10 What symptoms might initiate appendicitis and what factors might lead to perforation of the appendix with peritonitis?

REFERENCES AND READING SUGGESTIONS

BOOKS

Fishbein, Morris: *Your Weight and How to Control It*, Doubleday & Company, Inc., Garden City, N.Y., 1963.

A book by a distinguished medical author which physicians can and do recommend to their patients.

Maddox, Gaynor: *The Safe and Sure Way to Reduce*, Random House, Inc., New York, 1960.

One of the best popular books in this field. It should be useful to the general reader, parents, teachers, and others concerned with nutrition.

Obesity and Health, U.S. Public Health Service, 1966.

This small book is the report of a panel of nutrition experts, appointed by the National Heart Institute, to study the problem of obesity and to make recommendations about what can be done about it.

PAMPHLETS AND PERIODICALS

Haskim, S. D., and T. B. Van Ittalie: *Clinical and Physiological Aspects of Obesity*, American Dietetic Association, Chicago, 1965.

The important basic facts concerning this common condition.

Irwin, Michael H. K.: *Overweight—A Problem for Millions*, Public Affairs Pamphlet, New York.

The causes, results, prevention, and treatment of obesity.

Read, M. S., and F. P. Heald: *Adolescent Obesity*, American Dietetic Association, Chicago, 1965.

A summary of a symposium.

13

SOME HEALTH FACTORS IN DAILY LIFE

In the eighteenth century, windows in most bedrooms were nailed shut, for night air was believed to be a source of disease; early in the first half of the twentieth century, the usual health advice was to keep bedroom windows wide open at night no matter how cold the outside temperature.

The fashionable young lady of the nineteenth century never allowed the sun to affect her delicate complexion; in the twentieth century, increasing amounts of tan and increasing areas of tanned skin have been the predominating fashions.

In each case, there has been an implication that the current fashion has been a healthy one. But has it been? What do we know today of the best way to live day by day? Chapters 11 and 12 dealt with diet and its problems; this chapter will consider other aspects of daily life which affect health: fresh air, sunshine, exercise, rest, sleep, and recreation. How much of what many people believe and practice in regard to these health factors in our daily lives is based on fact, and how much on hearsay and advertising?

FRESH AIR

During the 16 to 20 breaths that the normal, resting person takes each minute, the human body takes in oxygen and discharges carbon dioxide into the outgoing air. This transfer takes place in the lungs across the microscopic membrane which separates the blood in its capillaries with their very thin walls from the air in the tiny alveoli (air sacs). Across that membrane gases pass rapidly.

Deprivation of oxygen for 4 to 6 minutes usually produces irreparable damage to the brain, and life ceases beyond hope of resuscitation within a few more minutes. These simple facts have been known, but the physical conditions of the air around us have been largely ignored.

The 1968 Olympic Games in Mexico City, nearly a mile and a half above sea level, focused attention on the effects of varying concentrations of gases on the body. Athletes not used to the higher altitude had difficulty performing well under reduced oxygen until they became used to it. Nearly everywhere on earth, the percentages of the different gases in the atmosphere remain remarkably constant: nitrogen, 78 percent; oxygen, 21 percent; carbon dioxide, only 0.04 percent (even in a closed, crowded room carbon dioxide rarely exceeds 0.2 percent); and other gases, a little less than 1 percent. But air pressure, the amount of air, and the amount of each constituent of air decrease with height above the earth. At the level of Mexico City—7,500 feet above sea level—there is about one-fourth less air in any given volume than at sea level. In the Chilean Andes and the Pamir Plain of the Himalayan Range people are living and working at 17,000 to 19,000 feet above sea level.

Fortunately, human beings have the capacity to adjust to these very different atmospheric conditions of life. Residents of places high above sea level have more hemoglobin and increased numbers of red blood cells in their bloodstreams to transport oxygen to their tissues. Heart rates and respiration rates increase in newcomers to high altitudes to compensate for the limited supply of oxygen available in each breath of air, but in the course of 2 or 3 weeks of acclimatization these effects wear off. Careful observations have been made on the performance of men at varying altitudes. Up to 10,000 feet, at least, the performance of excellent athletes from sea level who have become acclimatized can exceed that of good athletes from the higher level. For all, running performances at high altitude are slower than at sea level.

The diminished amount of oxygen at high altitudes became of immediate practical importance about the time of World War II when airplanes began to fly at high altitudes regularly. Then, and even now in some parts of the world, the lack of oxygen in planes at high altitudes was corrected by having personnel and passengers breathe pure oxygen through oxygen masks. Even though the gas pressure of this oxygen is less than at sea level, the fact that oxygen becomes close to 100 percent of the air breathed overcomes the "thinness" of the atmosphere. Today, modern airliners have pressurized cabins so that the amount of oxygen and other gases in a given volume of air remains close to what it is at sea level no matter how high the plane flies.

Lack of oxygen affects not only the cardiovascular system but also the brain; mental disturbances occur similar to those seen in alcoholic intoxication, especially false confidence.

Not only does diminished atmospheric pressure at high altitudes cause disturbances of human physiology; increased atmospheric pressure, experienced, for example, by divers or tunnel workers, also causes ill effects. If the pressure increases enough, it causes an intoxication; skin divers who venture too deep lose judgment because of the pressure and fail to return to the surface before they either run out of oxygen or lose consciousness. At lesser depths, difficulty occurs not with increasing pressure but with release of pressure, for with increased pressure larger quantities of nitrogen dissolve in the blood, and when the pressure is lowered rapidly in a quick return to the surface, the excess nitrogen forms tiny bubbles in the bloodstream. These bubbles block small blood vessels and prevent blood from reaching tissues, thus causing damage to many organs of the body. This condition is called the *bends* or *caisson disease*. (See page 369.)

OPEN WINDOWS?

Historically, the emphasis on "fresh air" in large quantities, regardless of comfort, dates back to its use in the treatment of tuberculosis. A famous physician of the nineteenth century, Dr. Edward Livingston Trudeau, made a spectacular and unexpected recovery from tuberculosis on a then-unorthodox regime of fresh air, rest, and nourishing food; he later founded a sanitarium to treat other patients with these methods. As time passed, however, it was realized that the fresh air was not significant in comparison with the other two elements of the treatment. A study made during the

First World War showed that pneumonia patients treated in chilly tents or sleeping porches had a mortality 4 times higher than those treated by otherwise identical methods in a warm environment.

In summary, mankind's need for fresh air turns out to be the need for clean air at comfortable temperature and humidity and at tolerable pressure. Open or closed windows are of minor importance, since the composition of air does not vary significantly from outdoors to indoors or from room to room. Whether to open or close windows should be determined by a person's comfort and sense of well-being, and by the purity and the temperature of the outdoor air.

AIR POLLUTION

A generation ago air pollution, although occasionally annoying, was not considered a health problem. Urbanization, industralization, and modern transportation have so completely changed this that smog and other pollution are major health problems. Federal, state, and local governments are enacting legislation and establishing commissions to control this and other pollution of the environment. (See pages 33–36.)

TEMPERATURE

Increased or decreased atmospheric pressures do not affect ordinary human life going on in the city and in the countryside at the elevations where people usually live. We must, however, cope with heat, cold, changes in humidity, storms, and in urban areas, smog and other forms of air pollution.

Human beings can tolerate marked changes in temperature without serious or lasting damage to their bodies. Extremes of temperature, however, do have their dangers. At low temperatures, the body loses heat rapidly when wind passes over the skin. Therefore bulky, loosely fitting clothes with wind-resistant coverings which provide the insulation of "dead space" around the body protect against cold most effectively. For example, when a 45-mile-per-hour wind is blowing at 30°F, exposed skin loses as much heat as it does at −40°F with no wind. (See Table 13.1.)

At very high temperatures, loss of body fluids by evaporation and difficulty in controlling body heat cause illness. The most serious heat illness is heat stroke, from which there is a high mortality. Each fall, a few football players practicing in temperatures above 100° Fahrenheit with too much clothing and too little opportunity to replace fluids die from heat stroke. The prevention of such unnecessary deaths takes careful planning by coach, doctor, and trainer working together.

Heat is produced constantly by the body; if excess heat is not eliminated, the body temperature rises; discomfort, inefficiency, and eventually death result. The chief methods by which the body disposes of excess body heat are direct transfer from the skin to the surrounding air, and the utilization of heat in evaporating sweat. When the temperature of the air is lower than the temperature of the body, heat loss is largely by direct transfer; but when the temperature of the air is higher than the temperature of the body, evaporation becomes the more important method. Both transfer and evaporation are influenced by the humidity and motion of the air.

As anyone who has sat quietly in hot, humid, still weather can testify, these conditions are most unpleasant. Because the air next to the skin is already saturated, or nearly so, if no new air replaces the saturated air sweat accumulates on the surface of the skin and the victim feels oppressed. (Humidity is measured as the percentage of moisture in the air in relation to the total amount of moisture which the air could hold at that temperature; 100 percent humidity means complete saturation.) The conditions which produce the greatest comfort for human beings are temperature about 70°F and humidity between 40 and 50 percent.

The apparent paradox that a humid day in the summer is oppressively hot and a damp day in the winter bitterly cold is due to two facts. In hot weather high humidity decreases heat loss by reducing evaporation, while in cold weather high humidity increases heat loss by facilitating the direct transfer of heat from the skin to the air.

Many of us spend most of our time during the

Table 13.1   Wind chill (equivalent temperatures on exposed flesh at varying wind velocity)

Instructions for use of the table:

1. First obtain the temperature and wind-velocity forecast data.
2. Locate the number at the top corresponding to the expected wind speed (or the number closest to this).
3. Read down this column until the number corresponding to the expected temperature (or the number closest to this) is reached.
4. From this point follow across to the right until the last number is reached under the column marked zero wind speed.
5. This is the equivalent temperature reading. Example: Weather information gives the expected temperature (at a given time, such as midnight) to be 35°F and the expected wind speed (at the same time, midnight) to be 20 miles per hour. Locate the 20 miles per hour column at the top, follow down this column to the number nearest to 35°F, which is 34°F. From this point, move all the way to the right on the same line and find the last number, which is −38°F. This means that with a temperature of 35°F and a wind of 20 miles per hour, the effect on all exposed flesh is the same as −38°F with no wind (the same as being in a deep freeze).

Wind velocity, miles per hour

Temperature, degrees Fahrenheit

45	35	25	20	15	10	5	3	2	1	0 — Equivalent temperature reading
90	89.5	89	88.5	88	87.75	87.5	87	86	84.5	83
82	81	80.5	80	79.5	78	76	74	72.5	70	60
72	71	69.5	68	67	65	60	57	53.5	47.5	23
63	61	59	57	55	52	44.5	39	34.5	20	11
51	49	47	45	42.5	38	28	18.5	11	0	−27
41	39	36	34	30.5	25	11	0	−9	−23.5	−38
									Below	Below
30	28	25	23	18	11	−5	−16.5	−40	−40	−40
								Below	Below	Below
20	18	14	11	6	−2	−19	−40	−40	−40	−40
							Below	Below	Below	Below
10	7.5	3	0	−6	−15	−35	−40	−40	−40	−40
						Below	Below	Below	Below	Below
0	−2.5	−8	−12	−18	−29	−40	−40	−40	−40	−40
					Below	Below	Below	Below	Below	Below
−11	−14	−18	−23	−30	−40	−40	−40	−40	−40	−40
				Below	Below	Below	Below	Below	Below	Below
−21	−24	−30	−35	−40	−40	−40	−40	−40	−40	−40
					Below	Below	Below	Below	Below	Below
−32	−35	−40	−40				−40	−40	−40	−40

SOURCE: Prepared by the Army Medical Research Laboratory, Fort Knox, Kentucky.

winter months in surroundings that are inadequately ventilated, excessively heated, and almost completely lacking in humidity. A major function of the membranes lining the nose is to warm inspired air if it is cold and to supply moisture to it so that it will have a humidity of 80 to 90 percent when it reaches the lungs. If the inspired air lacks reasonable humidity, breathing has an intense drying effect upon the membranes of the nose and throat.

SUNSHINE

In the health advice given early in this century sunshine was usually linked to fresh air as a major necessity. Scientifically, the sun's rays are electromagnetic waves traveling, like all light, at the rate of 186,000 miles per second. Only about 13 percent of these electromagnetic waves in sunshine are visible to the naked eye. With a prism the waves can be "sorted out" into a spectrum, or rainbow; the longest waves are red and the shortest violet. About 80 percent of the sun's rays lie in the invisible portion of the spectrum beyond the red, called *infrared;* infrared rays produce heat. Another 7 percent are shorter than the visible violet and are called *ultraviolet.*

The sun's rays are essential to man's existence on earth. Without the heat from the infrared end of the spectrum and the energy input which the ultraviolet end gives to the chlorophyll of plants, life would quickly halt. The direct contribution of sunlight to human biology is less important. Its action on the skin does make possible the manufacture of vitamin D. Before this was known and before vitamin D dietary supplements were used, deficiency of vitamin D during long winters led to frequent cases of rickets, a bone disease, in children. Since in the United States and other industrial countries most milk now is fortified with vitamin D and since most young children receive supplementary vitamins, the formation of vitamin D by the skin is no longer essential for health. Sunlight then becomes important not for its contribution to the biochemistry of the body but for its contribution to morale and to recreation, and because of the current aesthetic desirability of suntan.

On the other hand, sunlight has its deleterious effects. Chronic exposure to ultraviolet light produces more rapid aging of the skin and more frequent skin cancer than would occur ordinarily. A few people develop serious rashes on exposure to sun, and a few medications will render some others susceptible to such rashes. A rare disease, xeroderma pigmentosa, causes the appearance of brown, pigmented areas of the skin. These gradually develop into multiple skin cancers on exposure to light. (See page 233.)

A recent study[1] by the Department of Dermatology of the University of Pennsylvania School of Medicine concludes that sunlight, not aging, is responsible for the worst manifestations of senile skin. It is in a way unfortunate, the report states, that the damaging effects of sunlight upon the skin are not visible until decades after they have commenced. Nevertheless the medical facts of the advanced deterioration of the fibrous components of the skin in early adulthood demand that sun-

[1]Albert M. Klingman, "Early Destructive Effects of Sunlight on Human Skin," *Journal of the American Medical Association,* Dec. 29, 1969, p. 2377.

burn be identified as a health hazard. For those who insist upon sunbathing, the risk of serious skin damage can be reduced by avoiding exposure between 10 A.M. and 3 P.M. and by the frequent application of "sun screens," some of which give considerable protection. (See page 234.)

We have already mentioned the danger of sunstroke in those whose body heat is increased dangerously by the sun. The ability to withstand heat differs greatly among persons who are in normal health. Old persons, young children, the obese, patients with heart disease, and alcoholics are most easily affected by heat. Excessive exposure to heat may cause heat exhaustion, heat stroke (sunstroke), or heat cramps. Heat exhaustion is the most common of these conditions. In mild cases, fatigue, headache, and nausea occur; in severe cases, profuse perspiration, extreme weakness, and occasionally vomiting. Patients usually respond well to medical treatment; they should be given frequent small drinks of weak salt solution ($\frac{1}{2}$ teaspoon of salt in one-half glass of water every 5 minutes), should be removed from heat if possible, and should lie quietly in the shade with very few clothes on.

Heat cramps, often associated with heat exhaustion, are muscular cramps in the abdomen or extremities which follow the loss of sodium and other chemicals in profuse perspiration. Firm pressure on the afflicted muscle and drinking a weak salt solution usually control such cramps.

Heat stroke is by far the most dangerous of the three conditions, often proving fatal, particularly in the elderly. When an individual becomes very weak or unconscious in the heat and has a hot but dry skin with a rapid pulse, he probably has heat stroke, and a medical emergency exists. He should receive medical treatment, preferably in a hospital, as soon as possible. Until the medical supervision has been instituted, the treatment described under heat exhaustion should be followed; in addition the patient's body should be sponged with cold water or alcohol, or the patient should be placed in a tub of ice water.

EXERCISE AND PHYSICAL FITNESS

If the former insistence on plenty of fresh air and sunshine as essential to health must be modified, the need for regular exercise must stand unchal-

lenged. Indeed, many experts believe that urbanization, mechanization, and the general lack of physical exertion in daily life have contributed to poor health among the middle-aged and elderly of this country. Today a man seldom walks a few blocks to the drugstore or a woman to her neighbor's for coffee; instead they drive. Even golf is a seasonal sport, most often played on weekends. Indoors Americans can often even change the television channel without leaving their easy chairs.

The contributions of regular physical activity to health (aside from its contribution to athletic performance and to recreation) are four:

1 Muscles are kept developed and in tone ("hard and firm" as opposed to "soft and flabby"). Most people then feel more alert, comfortable, free of aches and pains, and ready to tackle both the intellectual and physical tasks of the day.

2 The cardiovascular system is kept in good tone, with the ability to respond easily to physical and emotional stresses.

3 Energy is burned, helping to keep weight under control.

4 The general metabolic processes of the body, particularly of the pituitary-adrenal glandular system, are stimulated, contributing to a general sense of well-being and probably also contributing to the body's ability to withstand the various kinds of stress which are inevitable accompaniments of life.

ATHLETIC PROGRAMS IN SCHOOL AND COLLEGE

Athletic programs are the most obvious examples of regular exercise. Virtually all colleges and an increasing number of elementary and secondary schools have good athletic programs for their students. These programs increase physical fitness and athletic skills and provide valuable recreation.

The superior athlete is the product of innate and developed talent and of carefully planned hard work. In performance, the qualities of the athlete are obvious: quick reflexes, rapid coordinations. Biochemically and physiologically, other qualities are important. Many athletes, particularly those in sports requiring endurance, have a greater than average lung capacity. Sir Roger Bannister, the first 4-minute-miler and now a phy-

sician, has demonstrated that gases can cross the thin barrier between lung and bloodstream more readily in the athlete than in the nonathlete. In vigorous exertion over a short period, the body is able to break down compounds to produce energy without using oxygen. For longer events, the athlete must assimilate and distribute large amounts of oxygen consistently.

The cardiovascular systems of athletes are particularly efficient. The athlete in top training usually has a pulse rate slower than the nontrained nonathlete and slower than he himself has when not in training. When he exercises his pulse does not rise to as rapid a rate as that of the nontrained man, and following exercise his pulse returns to normal more quickly. Many distance runners, crewmen, hockey players, and other endurance performers have resting pulses under 60 and a few under 40 (the average is 70). Vigorous exertion, which would drive the pulse of a nontrained man up to 200 or above, causes their pulses to rise only to 170 to 180. Athletes' pulses return to normal within a few minutes instead of in half an hour or more.

At all ages, programs of informal competition and of noncompetitive exercise are of greater importance to health than formal competitive athletics. These programs reach much larger groups of children and adults. Properly organized and conducted, they provide the physical and psychological benefits of exercise as well as improving motor skills and physical fitness generally. Many excellent secondary and college athletic programs aim at giving students skill in a team sport, skill in a racquet game, and if possible, some experience in a body-contact sport. These programs encourage participants to continue exercise throughout their lives.

School physical education programs should include girls as well as boys. The tendency to obesity is greater in females than in males, partly because women tend to be less active. Exercise contributes as much to the health of women as to that of men (with the minor proviso that heart disease is rare among women before the menopause, while men can reduce the likelihood of this common disaster of the thirties and forties by regular exercise). Women athletes appear to have less discomfort from menstruation than sedentary women. Better muscle tone improves posture;

muscular development and control of fat usually improve rather than detract from attractive body contours.

PHYSICAL FITNESS FOR ADULTS

Physical fitness programs require regular commitments of time, at least 4 times a week; at any age, physical conditioning is lost if regular exercise ceases for a short time, but the decline is much more rapid as age advances. Since the risks to the heart of sudden activity beyond the usual custom of the particular person increases as age advances, the physical fitness program of the man in his thirties, forties, and older should never begin with sudden bursts of activity, but rather with slow activity of gradually increasing duration and tempo. Few men (or women) above the age of 40 should exercise to their maximum effort for more than a second or two. Men and women past 30 who plan to start physical fitness programs should have careful examinations of their cardiovascular systems before they begin.

For some men and women, organized programs of squash, tennis, golf (*without* a golf cart), swimming, or some other sport carried on in a club or public facility best meets their need for continuing physical fitness. For others, an independent program is most useful. The most important point in a good exercise program is that it become as much a matter of routine as, say, brushing the teeth. (See Figure 13.1.)

EXERCISE AND ILLNESS

The current hospital practice of having most patients out of bed and moving about within a few days after surgery, even major surgery, would have been unthinkable a generation ago. However, experience, primarily during World War II, demonstrated that patients recover more rapidly if they are given as much physical activity as their conditions permit than if they are kept in bed for a period of convalescence. Their appetite is better, they sleep better, their body systems function better, they have fewer complications, their morale is better, and their recovery is accelerated. On the other hand, just keeping a well person in bed for a week or two is enough to reduce his vitality.

Today some mothers walk to and from the delivery room when having a baby. Even selected patients with coronary heart attacks and with strokes are reported to do better with early ambulation than with prolonged bed rest.

EXERCISE AND LENGTH OF LIFE

Two statements about exercise and length of life are valid. First, intercollegiate athletic competition in college neither increases nor decreases length of life. Several good studies show that college men and women live longer than noncollege citizens, but that athletes have no advantage over their nonathletic college peers.

The old idea that exercise damages the heart is false. Several years ago a rumor went about that all members of the Harvard championship crew of 1948 had died. The rumor was untrue; not only were all members of the 1948 crew alive and free of heart disease, but all members of the 1914 Harvard crew were also alive and were holding annual reunions at which they rowed a short distance in a shell.

Second, regular exercise throughout life helps to protect against heart disease. The best evidence for this comes from the ingenious observations of Morris and his associates in England. They studied the extensive records of the London Transport Authority and found that the active conductors (who have to climb the steps of the two-decker buses and are usually on the move) have much less coronary heart disease than the sedentary bus drivers. These findings have been supported by the work of several other investigators; for example, vigorous exercise helps control weight and concomitantly helps control the blood-cholesterol level of those eating high-calorie, high-fat diets.

An important addendum to these statements about length of life is that the physically active person has added vigor and mobility in old age.

EXERCISE AND POSTURE

Good posture (see Figure 13.2) is an asset to any man or woman, boy or girl. It prevents fatigue and backache. It improves personal appearance and suggests poise, self-confidence, and health. Many a job applicant makes an unfavorable first impression because of poor posture.

Poor posture may be related to body build and other hereditary factors, to habits, to fatigue, to poor development and use of the muscles of the back, abdomen, and legs, or to some combination of these factors. Good posture comes naturally to a

Figure 13.1 Helpful exercises for the whole family. Source: Adapted from Bonnie Pruden. "How to Get More Out of Life," *Reader's Digest*, March 1958. Reproduced by permission of the Reader's Digest Association, Inc., Pleasantville, N.Y.

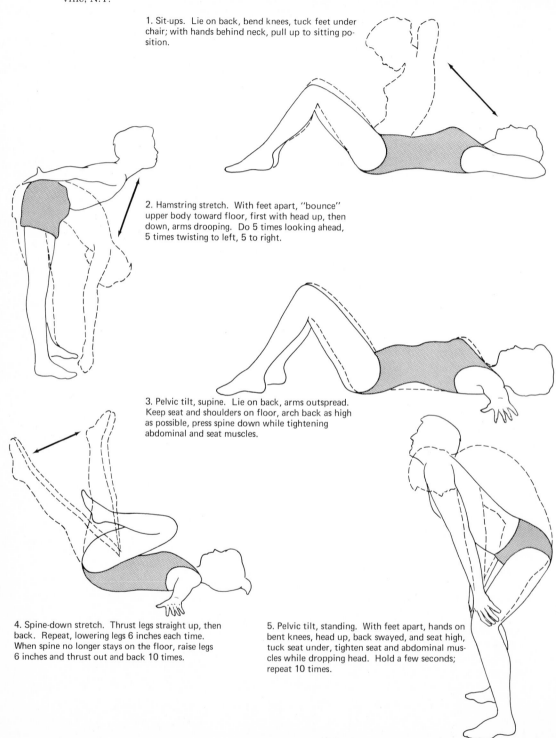

1. Sit-ups. Lie on back, bend knees, tuck feet under chair; with hands behind neck, pull up to sitting position.

2. Hamstring stretch. With feet apart, "bounce" upper body toward floor, first with head up, then down, arms drooping. Do 5 times looking ahead, 5 times twisting to left, 5 to right.

3. Pelvic tilt, supine. Lie on back, arms outspread. Keep seat and shoulders on floor, arch back as high as possible, press spine down while tightening abdominal and seat muscles.

4. Spine-down stretch. Thrust legs straight up, then back. Repeat, lowering legs 6 inches each time. When spine no longer stays on the floor, raise legs 6 inches and thrust out and back 10 times.

5. Pelvic tilt, standing. With feet apart, hands on bent knees, head up, back swayed, and seat high, tuck seat under, tighten seat and abdominal muscles while dropping head. Hold a few seconds; repeat 10 times.

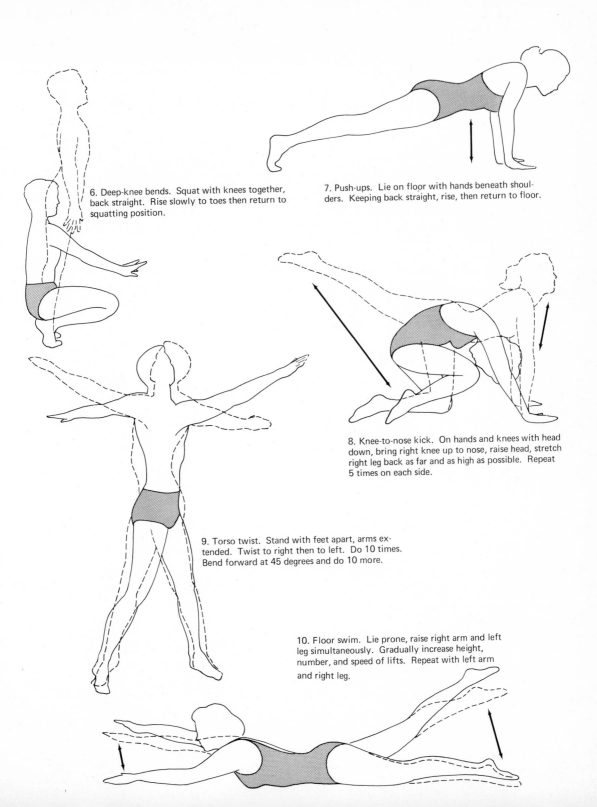

6. Deep-knee bends. Squat with knees together, back straight. Rise slowly to toes then return to squatting position.

7. Push-ups. Lie on floor with hands beneath shoulders. Keeping back straight, rise, then return to floor.

8. Knee-to-nose kick. On hands and knees with head down, bring right knee up to nose, raise head, stretch right leg back as far and as high as possible. Repeat 5 times on each side.

9. Torso twist. Stand with feet apart, arms extended. Twist to right then to left. Do 10 times. Bend forward at 45 degrees and do 10 more.

10. Floor swim. Lie prone, raise right arm and left leg simultaneously. Gradually increase height, number, and speed of lifts. Repeat with left arm and right leg.

Figure 13.2 Examples of posture.

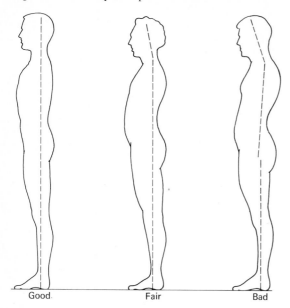

Good.   Fair   Bad

few who have the musculoskeletal attributes to hold an erect stance easily, but for others careful training in youth and regular exercise to maintain body tone are important.

For those whose bad posture is severe, careful evaluation of the individual's muscular and skeletal problems is desirable, and individually designed exercises should be prescribed. For others, exercises to strengthen the muscles of back and abdomen and to keep all joints limber are desirable, plus conscious thought to maintain erect carriage when standing and sitting.

BACK AND FEET

The feet, the legs, and the back carry the entire body. When fatigue, strains, poor posture, poor function, and ill-fitting and ill-supporting shoes interfere with normal weight bearing, then backaches, pains, and increased fatigue result.

The feet were originally designed for climbing and for walking on soft ground. When they are pounded on hard surfaces all day and confined within ill-fitting shoes, they give trouble which may be reflected throughout the back and may contribute to general fatigue and discomfort. A good shoe, without being loose, gives the foot plenty of room to spread. It gives support to the longitudinal and transverse arches of the feet. If these arches

are improperly constructed or are damaged, as in flatfoot, a competent medical consultant, rather than a shoe salesman, should advise on shoes.

Over the years, women's shoes have been serious offenders against health. Fashion has dictated the almost constant use of high heels and widths too narrow for proper support and function. In the mid-1960s, however, there appeared at least a temporary movement toward the sanity of lower heels and comfortable widths for everyday use.

Backaches may result from poor shoes or mechanical problems concerning the feet; they result also from beds which give poor support. Beds and mattresses should be large enough so that the sleeper can stretch out and move around; they should not sag. Many backaches and headaches result from sitting or standing still for long periods. Desk workers who get little exercise are particularly susceptible to such aches; when studying or otherwise immobilized in one position, it is helpful to get up and move around every half hour.

Other measures to protect the back against strain and pain include avoiding athletic and working activities for which you are not prepared, sitting down smoothly instead of roughly, and lifting heavy objects with the legs rather than the back muscles (see Figure 13.3)—in addition, of course, to good general exercise.

Figure 13.3 How to lift heavy objects properly.

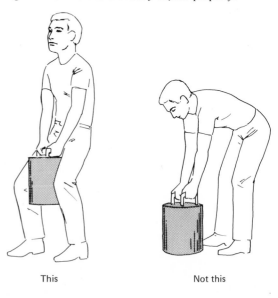

This   Not this

SLEEP AND REST

The need for sleep is obvious and yet mysterious. Unlike the positive benefits of exercise, the benefits of sleep are describable chiefly in terms of what happens after sleep deprevation. With prolonged lack of sleep, the capabilities for accurate seeing, hearing, and feeling diminish. After 100 to 120 hours of sleeplessness, hallucinations and paranoid thoughts increase rapidly and progressively.

A person who has shorter periods of sleeplessness or weeks of insufficient sleep at night can usually meet emergencies and perform routine tasks, including physical activity, satisfactorily; but for other tasks of moderate difficulty and for those which require creativity, both his performance and his perseverance diminish.

Sleep is probably regulated by a nerve center in the lower brainstem. During sleep the brain and the systems under its control show wavelike periods of activity, covering about 90 minutes in adults. At one extreme of the cycle the heart rate and blood pressure are slow and steady, and arousal is difficult. At the other extreme of the cycle there are irregular high levels of activity of the autonomic nervous system; when wakened during such periods, sleepers frequently report hallucinoid dreaming.

This suggests that sleep is an activity of the nervous system and is not just an inactivity of wakefulness. Obviously, therefore, sleep is a period of rest for the body but not for the brain. Sleep thus may entail dangers for patients with certain types of heart disease.[2]

The need for sleep varies just as other biological characteristics do. Observations on a group spending a long period in Greenland showed that the average need for sleep in 24 hours was 7.9 hours in either the continuous light of midsummer or the continuous dark and gloom of midwinter. Some notable persons function well with less sleep, but many of them have the excellent habit of "dropping off" for a few moments' or a few minutes' nap in the midst of a busy day.

The effect on health of chronic lack of sleep over many years is not known. Sleep and rest are essential in the treatment of many conditions,

[2]Editorial, *Journal of the American Medical Association*, Mar. 3, 1970, p. 1536.

such as rheumatoid arthritis, peptic ulcer, many neurotic symptoms and even psychoses, and heart disease. This does not mean, however, that lack of sleep causes the conditions.

The nonpsychic effects of sleeplessness and sleep are not impressive and cannot be used as arguments for or against a specific amount of sleep. Though the pulse, blood pressure, respiration, and metabolic rates decline in sleep, no changes in blood constituents or other body properties appear.

Insomnia, or involuntary wakefulness, is a common affliction. Only rarely is it due to some physical disorder; emotional tensions and anxieties cause most insomnia.

Students frequently have insomnia when they get insufficient exercise and study up to the moment they pop into bed. For these insomniacs, a period of recreation just before bed, preferably including some physical activity and a warm shower, is often helpful. Where emotional tensions are severe and do not respond to the simple measures of rearranging the details of life, help is necessary from a physician.

The use of sleeping pills has increased enormously in the United States since World War II. Used cautiously and preferably not every night, they are of help to some, but the dangers of habituation and overdosage are so great that most physicians hesitate to prescribe them freely. (See page 119.)

FATIGUE

Fatigue is familiar to all. Muscular fatigue, following vigorous physical exertion, is often pleasant, though if the exercise is pursued too far, the fatigue becomes pain. Changes in the blood and muscles, notably an increase in lactic acid, accompany muscular fatigue. The chronic fatigue of nervous tension and lack of sleep has no biochemical counterpart, and may be relieved by physical activity.

Both acute and chronic illness can bring a sense of fatigue which protects the victim by encouraging rest and sleep. Fatigue which does not respond readily to rest, or which recurs, demands a careful medical evaluation for tuberculosis, diabetes, a low-grade infection (such as infectious mononucleosis), or mechanical problems of the back and feet, as well as for the psychological factors which commonly cause fatigue.

The psychological factor most commonly responsible for chronic fatigue is boredom. Relief follows not more rest but more interests, activities, and enthusiasms. Forgetting oneself is the first step toward zestful living.

Drugs may modify fatigue. The use of coffee or other forms of caffeine to relieve minor and transient fatigue is common and harmless. The amphetamines ("pep pills") are sometimes prescribed by physicians, but their indiscriminate use may be habituating, and they reduce efficiency as often as they sustain it by abolishing sleepiness.

Industries, studying the work records of employees throughout the day, find that efficiency declines toward the latter part of the morning, improves after lunch, and then declines again more rapidly as the afternoon progresses. Accidents are most frequent during times of accumulating fatigue. These observations have led to the introduction of the "coffee break" so that a brief period of rest (and nourishment to increase blood-sugar level) can increase efficiency again.

RECREATION

Much of the previous discussion in this chapter has referred to the necessity of taking time away from one's daily work routines for the purpose of re-creation of the natural, energetic self. Sometimes recreation means physical activity; sometimes it means rest or a "coffee break"; at other times it means attention to intellectual and aesthetic needs.

During this century and particularly since World War II, recreation has become an increasingly important part of American life. Public authorities, private agencies, and business concerns have all played an important role in the growth of recreational activities and facilities.

The increase in the need for recreation stems partly from the changing nature of work. Man's labor used to consist primarily of physical exertion; now it consists largely of intellectual activities and skilled motions which consume little energy. In 1910, man supplied one unit of mechanical labor, while animals supplied four units and machinery seven. By 1945, for every unit of labor which man supplied, animals supplied one but machinery supplied over twenty. The trend has continued.

In 1957 for the first time in the United States persons engaged in service occupations outnumbered those engaged directly in production. The work week is shorter and some employees are working a 4-day week with 9 to 10 hours of work on each day, leaving 3 days of free time each week. Over 60 million workers have vacations with pay. Improved transportation allows more time for recreation and easier access to varying types of recreation.

In response to the need, cities, counties, states, and the federal government, plus some private industries and labor unions, have provided increasing numbers of indoor and outdoor recreation areas and facilities. One of the major problems in providing outdoor recreation is the constant shrinking of open and natural areas near cities. A valuable part of the recreational movement has been the increasing reservation of natural areas for posterity by purchase or gift. Even those who do not use these areas directly profit by a diminished sense of crowding.

QUESTIONS FOR DISCUSSION AND SELF-EXAMINATION

1   How have opinions and facts about healthy daily habits changed over the years?
2   How do the benefits of exercise to comfort differ from the benefits of exercise to health?
3   What is the difference between fresh air and healthy air?

4 Under what circumstances does oxygen deficit occur in human life, and what is its effect?

5 How does the body protect itself in extremes of temperature, and how may one assist in the protection?

6 Do the benefits of sunshine exceed its dangers? Document your answer.

7 What relationship does exercise have to the prevention, development, and care of heart disease?

8 Compare the effects of lack of sleep on physical function of the body and on emotional and mental function.

9 Compare the contributions of physical and psychological factors to fatigue.

10 How does interval training compare with other forms of physical training?

REFERENCES AND READING SUGGESTIONS

BOOKS

Isometric Exercises for Physical Fitness, Institute of Physical Medicine and Rehabilitation, New York.

Based on practical experience, this little book is a splendid guide to isometric exercises for physical fitness and rehabilitation.

Luce, Gay Gaer, and Julius Segal: *Sleep,* Coward-McCann, Inc., New York.

A prize-winning science writer and a psychologist have collaborated on this summary of current scientific knowledge about the mysterious state in which man spends about a third of his life.

Values in Sports, American Association for Health, Physical Education and Recreation, Washington

Report of conference on the role of athletics in developing personal value systems for boys and girls.

PAMPHLETS AND PERIODICALS

Rakstis, Ted J.: "New Help for Non-sleepers," *Today's Health,* September 1971, p. 16.

A consideration of insomnia—types, causes, methods of treatment, and research—which is sometimes said to be this country's most frequent medical complaint.

Segal, Julius, and Gay Gaer Luce: "To Sleep: Perchance to Dream," *Today's Health,* October 1969, p. 48.

A fascinating review of present scientific knowledge concerning sleep and dreams, of research in progress, and of important questions still unanswered.

14

EYES, EARS, NOSE, AND THROAT

Do you know the story of Helen Keller? Born in 1880; rendered deaf and blind by illness (probably encephalitis) at the age of 18 months; an uncontrolled, raging little beast until the age of 7; was taught to communicate with others by a hand language which transmitted letters and words by touch; brilliant graduate of Radcliffe, one of the foremost of woman's colleges; author; incessant worker for the blind and for the deaf throughout the world; friend of the great; noble human being who died in 1968. This woman, unable to see, to hear, or to speak, felt that hearing was the sense that she would most have preferred to have added to her faculties, for without it a human being is cut off from the fellowship of others. Both vision and hearing often are taken lightly by those who have them; like many aspects of health, their true value can be judged best by those who lack them.

THE CONSERVATION OF VISION

The eye is an extremely efficient instrument, functioning almost contiuously to provide clear vision for close work in school, office, or shop. In so doing it acts with surprising rapidity, performing upward of a thousand movements in 5 minutes of reading. It has been estimated that one-fourth of the daily energy expenditure of persons in sedentary occupations is utilized for the purpose of seeing.

Physiologically the eye is a mechanism much like a camera, which brings the rays of light to focus upon light-sensitive nerve endings in the retina. (See Figure 14-1.) These, in turn, transmit a

Figure 14.1 Vertical cross section of the eye—front to back.

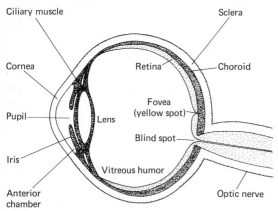

stimulus to the brain, where the visual image is perceived. In the lowest types of seeing animals the eye consists merely of a few pigmented cells, sensitive to light, at or near the surface of the body, and connected with some simple nerve structure. In the higher forms of life the eyes are more complex and are connected with the brain. In addition to their more highly developed eyes, insects and worms retain some simple, supernumerary eyes. Most spiders, for example, have eight such eyes, and some worms have four or more. (See Figure 14-2.)

The simplest type of eye can perceive only light, but as animals become biologically more complex the visual apparatus also becomes more complex and begins to perceive size, shape, distance, and color. Since accurate vision is an asset in the struggle for existence, the animals with the most efficient eyes tend to rise in the biological scale.

Hermann Helmholtz, the noted physicist who in 1850 invented the ophthalmoscope, which enables examination of the interior of the eyeball, is credited with saying that he would have returned to an instrument maker a piece of apparatus as imperfect as the human eye. Truly the eye is far from perfect, but the process of evolution has provided us with a visual instrument which adapts itself amazingly well to the changing demands made upon it.

Until times that are comparatively recent in biological terms, man lived outdoors and used his eyes chiefly for distance vision. Some changes of focus were necessary even then, but the demands made upon the visual apparatus were but a fraction of what they have been since man changed his mode of living. Several million years of reading the printed page may bring about a better adaptation of these outdoor eyes to the manner in which we now live.

THE CAUSES AND PREVENTION OF BLINDNESS

One of the greatest calamities that can befall a person is blindness. The occasional genius, however, such as Milton or Helen Keller, can rise far above this calamity, and many blind people are remarkably persistent and successful in making a life for themselves despite their handicap. Many develop an amazing acuity of hearing which enables them to sense the presence of objects and their relative distance on the basis of reflected sounds.

According to informed estimates, there are more than 10 million blind people in the world. Blindness is frequently thought of as "total absence of sight." Yet only about a third of the people recognized as blind are totally blind. Most of them can perceive light and motion, and many can count fingers at arm's length. Some see only a portion of an object because their visual field is limited. Some can spot a pin on the floor but fail to see a moving van on the road.

Legal and medical attempts to define blindness vary greatly. In France, people with one-twentieth of normal vision are entitled to carry a white cane and benefit from measures for the blind. In the United States "economic blindness" (inability to perform useful work for which sight is essential) is considered to be anything less than one-tenth of normal vision.

At the beginning of this century 28 percent of the blindness in this country was due to gonorrheal infections of the eyes of newborn infants, but this cause of blindness has been reduced to 0.5 percent. In the past 50 years, blindness in the United States due to infectious diseases has been reduced 75 percent. In spite of this, there has been an overall increase in blindness, primarily because people are living longer and therefore developing eye diseases that cause blindness.

More than half the blind, however, lose their

sight in infancy or in childhood. Fully two-thirds of the blindness which exists results from conditions which could be prevented or cured.

TRACHOMA

Also called *granular conjunctivitis*, trachoma is the world's greatest single cause of serious and progressive loss of sight. It is estimated that 500 million people, one-sixth of the population of the entire world, suffer from trachoma. In some areas essentially the entire population is infected. A survey in 1962 of American Indian high school children in southwestern states revealed that up to 40 percent showed evidence of having had trachoma.

Trachoma is caused by a virus and is spread by contaminated fingers, towels, clothing, etc. It is common in many tropical and subtropical countries and exists in countries of southern Europe and in parts of North and South America. The World Health Organization (WHO) European Conference on Trachoma stated that in countries where virtually whole populations are affected with trachoma, it is not uncommon to find that more than 1 percent of adults are totally blind, that more than 4 percent are economically blind, that more than 10 percent have serious impairment of vision, and that a much higher percentage have less severe visual defects.

Trachoma can be cured by modern drugs and can be prevented by soap, water, personal cleanliness, and sanitation. Many countries, with assistance from WHO and UNICEF, are staging mass campaigns for the control of this disease.

ONCHOCERCIASIS

A widespread disease in Central America and in large areas of Africa, onchocerciasis is caused by a tiny worm, filaria, carried to human beings by the lymph-sucking *Simulium* fly. The invasion of the eye by hordes of these worms results in blindness. Since the fly breeds in running water, the disease is limited to the neighborhood of streams and is therefore often called *river blindness. In infected areas there are villages in which every adult is blind, and children lead their elders about until they themselves become blind. This disease can be prevented by the use of insecticides—such as DDT —to wipe out the Simulium fly. In instances such* as this, insecticides are more of an aid than a hazard.

GERMAN MEASLES

German measles is a mild disease but one that may have serious consequences when contracted by a

Figure 14.2 Types of eyes.

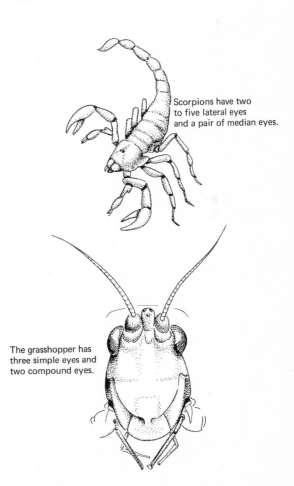

Scallops have two rows of simple eyes inside the shell.

Scorpions have two to five lateral eyes and a pair of median eyes.

The grasshopper has three simple eyes and two compound eyes.

mother during the first 3 months of pregnancy. When this occurs, up to 30 percent of the babies suffer from cataracts and other disabilities such as deafness or abnormalities of the heart. The only sure method to prevent this is for every girl or woman who has not had German measles to be vaccinated against it. (See page 267.)

HERPES SIMPLEX

An important cause of defective vision results from infections of the cornea by the herpes simplex virus—the virus which causes "cold sores." Fortunately a new drug, idoxuridine (IUD), effective against this virus is now available. It is reported that 75 to 80 percent of acute infections and 60 percent of chronic inflammations have responded to the drug.

CONJUNCTIVITIS OF THE NEWBORN

Until recent years an important cause of blindness in children was gonococcal infections of the eyes, acquired in the process of birth. Although this remains a serious danger in many parts of the world, it can be prevented if the doctor or midwife puts a preventive solution or ointment in the baby's eyes at birth.

HEREDITARY DEFECTS

Blindness may result from inherited predispositions. It is estimated that the danger of blindness resulting from hereditary conditions is 20 times higher among children of related parents than among those of ordinary marriages.

CATARACTS

Various changes which impair vision may occur in the eye during the later decades of life; most common of these is a cloudiness of the crystalline lens or its capsule, called *cataract*. Some degree of opacity, or cataract, is present in 34 percent of people between the ages of 40 and 50 and in about 90 percent of those over 70. This is a slowly progressive disorder.

Cataract occasionally is due to injury, to hereditary or congenital conditions, or to disease, but the most common type is the senile cataract, the cause of which is not understood. In the past a cataract was considered a hopeless sentence to blindness for the rest of one's life, but now useful vision can be restored in almost all patients by means of a simple but delicate operation.

GLAUCOMA

Glaucoma is a serious eye disease which accounts for 13 percent of recognized blindness in this country. It is responsible for much of the blindness after 40 years of age. Mechanically, glaucoma is due to an increased pressure within the eyeball. This much we know, but since the basic cause for the increased pressure is not understood we do not have the key to its prevention. However, if glaucoma is recognized early and proper treatment instituted, its progress frequently can be arrested. Glaucoma is an insidious disease which in early stages may produce no symptoms. If the increased pressure within the eye continues, the pressure has an effect on the optic nerve and causes marked damage, principally in the outer fields of vision at first, and finally affecting central vision. Headache, pain in the eye, seeing colored halos around lights, and loss of vision occur if the tension becomes high. Because of the usually insidious character of the condition, adequate periodic examination of the eyes is advisable, including for persons over 35 measurement of intraocular pressure. This is a simple procedure, using an instrument called a *tonometer*.

EYE INJURIES

Injuries constitute an important cause of blindness in this country. Some of these injuries can hardly be considered preventable, but the vast majority could be avoided with reasonable precaution. Individuals can learn to take necessary precautions. Industry can increase its efforts to safeguard the vision of employees. Children can be taught that they should not play with sharp instruments and that sharp objects must be handled carefully. They should be made aware that certain toys and games are hazardous. The National Society for the Prevention of Blindness, in a survey of eye accidents some years ago, showed a shocking amount of damage to the eyes of children by air rifles, especially in towns and cities.

Most industrial eye injuries occur in such occupations as machine operating, chipping, grinding and polishing, mining and quarrying, riveting, welding and cutting, glassmaking, sandblasting, and woodworking operations. In these and other occupations in which fragments of metal, wood, or stone may be thrown about, safety glasses, goggles, or masks should be worn. According to the National Society for the Prevention of Blindness, 45,000 Americans in a recent 10-year period avoided serious eye injuries by wearing safety glasses at work.

First aid in eye injuries Cleanliness is of the greatest importance in the care of eye injuries. A slight scratch on the surface of the eye may become so seriously infected that the eyesight is lost. Since the tissues of the eye are extremely delicate, expert medical attention should be secured whenever there is an injury to the eye.

The tears provide protection for the eyes not only by constantly washing the conjunctiva which covers the front of the eye but also because they contain proteins which inactivate bacteria and other infectious agents.

PARTICLES IN THE EYE
Dust, cinders, and other small particles of foreign material frequently lodge on the surface of the eyeball. The irritation thus produced results in a flood of tears which usually washes away the offending particle. Occasionally, however, such particles become lodged under a lid and for this or some other reason refuse to be dislodged. In such cases gently drawing the upper lid down over the lower one often dislodges the particle, and the accumulated tears wash it out. Rubbing of the eyes only irritates the tissues and embeds the particle. Using dirty fingers or a soiled handkerchief may result in infection. Furthermore, such methods can easily cause injury to the eyeball's surface. A physician's services should always be sought if the particle is not dislodged by tears or by the gentle measures described.

EYE INFECTIONS
Mild infections of the eye, called *conjunctivitis*, which may accompany colds, usually clear up with simple treatments. The more severe infections, on the other hand, require medical attention. These may be acute and self-limited or they may be due to serious disease, such as trachoma or gonorrheal ophthalmia, which, if not properly treated, will result in blindness. Almost all infections of the eye are communicable by means of hands, towels, etc., and care is necessary if infection is to be avoided.

Inflamed, granular conditions of the margins of the eyelids and the development of styes are frequently associated with eyestrain and with general ill health. For such conditions a complete physical examination and a careful refraction are more important than local treatments. Some such conditions, however, are due to allergic reactions to bacterial products, principally staphylococcus, and require treatment.

POISONS AFFECTING VISION
Among the poisons which may produce partial or complete loss of vision are tobacco, wood alcohol, and quinine.

Many persons use tobacco for years without any apparent effect on visual acuity, but others are definitely harmed by it. The eyes tire easily, visual acuity becomes progressively diminished, color vision is lost, and use of the eyes causes severe headache. Such symptoms occur most commonly in pipe smokers, particularly if both tobacco and alcohol are used in excess. If tobacco and alcohol are discontinued completely the symptoms usually disappear rapidly and vision returns to normal.

Quinine probably has caused more blindness than any other single drug. Ringing of the ears, headache, partial deafness, and dizziness are the common toxic symptoms produced by quinine. Less frequent but more serious is loss of vision, which may be partial and temporary or absolute for days, weeks, or life. A knowledge of the possibility of serious harm from the use of this drug should make people less willing to consume it, without medical advice, in various patent medicines for the treatment of colds, fever, and malaria. Concern is also being expressed about the increasing use of gin and tonic (quinine water) as a beverage.

EYEWASHES
Advertisements for eyewashes with fancy names suggest that these preparations should be used regularly if one desires bright, sparkling, healthy eyes. Physicians, on the other hand, never recommend such practices. Dust and dirt are constantly

settling on the eyeball, but nature removes them by maintaining a constant flow of tears which are gently carried over the eyeball by blinking of the lids. If there is unusual exposure to dust, smoke, or other irritating substances, a few drops of a saturated boric acid solution frequently are soothing.

COMMON VISUAL DEFECTS

The most common visual defects are nearsightedness, farsightedness, and astigmatism. These rarely lead to blindness but are responsible for an enormous amount of discomfort and inefficiency. Except for the farsightedness of advancing age, these condition are due to developmental abnormalities in the shape of the eyeball. Relatively little is really known concerning their actual cause.

In taking a picture with a good camera one first makes the necessary adjustments of focus, so that the objects which one wishes to photograph are clearly reproduced on the focusing ground glass. In a somewhat similar manner a picture of whatever is in front of the eye is thrown upon the retina. The retina is the innermost lining of the back of the eyeball and contains the nerve endings of vision. (See Figure 14.1.) If the rays of light from the object at which one is looking are brought to focus upon the center of this retina, where the vision is most acute, a clear visual picture is ob-

Figure 14.3 Focusing of light rays on retina.

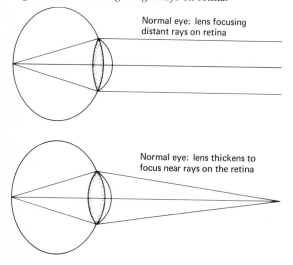

Normal eye: lens focusing distant rays on retina

Normal eye: lens thickens to focus near rays on the retina

COSMETICS WHICH MAY BE DANGEROUS TO EYES

Among the cosmetics offered for the enhancement of beauty are dyes for eyebrows, eyelids, and eyelashes. Some of these contain chemicals which are injurious to the delicate structures of the eye.

tained. If not, the image is blurred and indistinct. (See Figures 14.3 and 14.4.)

The mechanism of vision requires, first, that rays of light be reflected from an object to the eye. On a dark night we are unable to see objects about us because insufficient light rays are reflected from them, but we can see the moon, whose surface is reflecting light from the sun. After reaching the eye these rays of light must be bent, or refracted, so that they will come to focus upon the proper part of the retina. About 80 percent of this bending, or refraction, of light rays is done by the curved surface of the front of the eyeball and about 20 percent by the crystalline lens which is suspended within the eyeball. The thicker this lens, the greater will be the curvature of its surface and the more sharply will the rays of light which pass through it be focused. The thickness of the lens is controlled by a ring of tiny muscles, the ciliary muscles, which surround it within the eyeball. (See Figure 14.1.)

When one looks at a distant object, a near one in the same line of vision is indistinct. Also, if one focuses upon the nearer object, the distant one is not seen so well. This is because a clear image is obtained only of the object which is brought to focus upon the most sensitive portion of the retina. The other becomes indistinct as it goes out of focus. This shifting of focus is accomplished by a change in the thickness of the lens. In a perfect eye the rays of light from a distant object come to focus upon the retina when the eye is at rest, i.e., when the ciliary muscles are inactive and the lens is thin. This is called *emmetropia*.

FARSIGHTEDNESS (HYPEROPIA)

This is a universal condition at birth which usually disappears before there is much use of the eyes for near vision. In hyperopia, the rays of light with the eye at rest come to focus not on the retina but behind it. Blurring of vision results. The ciliary muscles correct this by contracting and making the lens thicker, thereby bringing the point of focus forward until it is on the retina. This results in clear vision, but it requires excessive work on the part of these muscles. For short periods of time this gives rise to no difficulties; but if it is continued, muscular fatigue is inevitable. This in turn causes headache, pain in the eyes, nervousness, and general fatigue. This type of visual defect is the one which causes the most severe symptoms of eyestrain. (See Figure 14.4.)

Important though farsightedness is as a cause of eyestrain, it is rarely discovered by the ordinary vision test, because during the test clear vision is secured by excessive use of the ciliary muscles. Hence, if a child brings a report from school that his vision test shows 20/20 in each eye, this should not be accepted as conclusive evidence that his vision is satisfactory. If symptoms of eyestrain are present, a further examination is indicated.

The use of drops for eye examinations   Much misunderstanding and misinformation exist concerning the use of "drops" for the examination of the eyes. The drops contain a drug, such as atropine or homatropine, which temporarily paralyzes the ciliary muscles. Unless this is done, the activity of these muscles in persons under about 40 years of age makes the accurate measurement of certain visual defects impossible. Everyone who needs glasses should have a thorough eye examination, and for a young person this implies the use of drops.

SQUINTS AND CROSS-EYE

Squint is the result of improper functioning of the external muscles of the eye so that both eyes do not focus on an object at the same time. The condition is often referred to as *strabismus*. This term is said to have originated from the fact that Strabo, a noted Alexandrian geographer, had a marked squint. The person with a squint has double vision and eventually comes to use only one eye.

Sometimes the degree of farsightedness in one eye of a child may be greater than in the other, or one eye may be farsighted and the other normal or relatively normal. When these conditions obtain and both eyes are used, one eye is under greater strain than the other. Since reasonably good vision can be obtained with the use of only one eye, in

time the overworked eye ceases to function, first when it gets tired and then continuously. The child does not know that he is using only one eye, and for a time no change is noticeable. Eventually, however, the muscles which turn the nonfunctioning eye toward the object of vision seem to realize that, since the eye is not being used, their work is unnecessary; consequently, they too stop working and the condition called *cross-eye* develops. At first this appears only when the child is tired, but eventually it becomes constant. After the unused eye has been fixed in one position for some

Figure 14.4   Correction of visual defects by lenses.

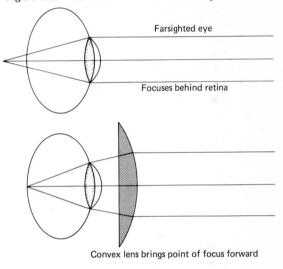

Farsighted eye

Focuses behind retina

Convex lens brings point of focus forward

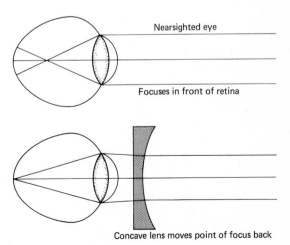

Nearsighted eye

Focuses in front of retina

Concave lens moves point of focus back

time, the muscles on the one side of the eyeball become shortened, and those on the other side stretched. This muscular change, however, is the end result and not the cause of cross-eye.

The prevention or treatment of cross-eye clearly must be based on a thorough eye examination with all muscles, overacting and underacting alike, put at rest. On the basis of such an examination, glasses can be prescribed which will tend to equalize the work of the two eyes and so prevent further progress of the condition. If the disuse of one eye has become an established habit, it may be necessary to cover the other eye temporarily in order to put this one back to work. To have the best chance of success, these procedures should be carried out in early childhood, just as soon as squinting is observed. Eye exercises may be of help; sometimes surgical intervention is required. The sooner attention is given to a child's squint, the better the condition can be handled.

PRESBYOPIA (THE SO-CALLED FARSIGHTEDNESS OF ADULTS)

The crystalline lens of a young child is very elastic and the ability to focus the vision upon near objects correspondingly great. With increasing age the lens loses its elasticity, and the power of accommodation is reduced. At 30 years of age the power of accommodation is only one-half as great as at 10 years of age, and at 45 only one-half as great as at 30. At the approximate age of 45 the near point for comfortable vision reaches the range of distance ordinarily used for reading. After this age most persons need glasses in order to read with comfort; and since the condition tends to be progressive, the glasses need to be changed every 1 to 3 years. For those already wearing glasses for myopia, this is the time to change to bifocals, the lower portions of which enable the eyes to focus on points near the eyes.

NEARSIGHTEDNESS (MYOPIA)

Nearsightedness occurs when the eyeball is longer than it should be. For this reason, with the eye at rest the point of focus of distant objects falls in front of the retina and indistinct vision results. The use of the ciliary muscles to make the lens thicker would move the point of focus farther forward and so make matters worse. Hence, the only way for a nearsighted person to obtain clear vision, without

glasses, is to bring the object closer to the eye. The glasses prescribed for myopia throw the point of focus backward toward the retina, thereby increasing the acuity of vision. (See Figure 14.4)

Although nearsightedness tends to run in families and is more common in some races than in others, its actual cause is unknown. It frequently appears in childhood and increases somewhat until about the age of 17 or 18. Some studies report that children who do a great deal of reading or other close work at this age are more likely to develop myopia than those who do not.

Nearsightedness occasionally becomes progressive and if not arrested may lead to serious impairment of vision. Some such cases are associated with malnutrition, focal infections, or general ill health. Thus the boy or girl with progressive nearsightedness should be placed under the care of a competent oculist and a general physician.

ASTIGMATISM

Astigmatism is a type of visual defect due to irregularity in the curvature of the portions of the eyeball through which the light rays enter, i.e., the cornea and the lens. Some eyes are relatively flat in one direction and excessively curved in the other, and the abnormal curvatures called astigmatism may be associated with either nearsightedness or farsightedness. Such visual defects frequently cause severe eyestrain. To obtain relief a careful eye examination and accurately prescribed and fitted glasses are essential.

COLOR BLINDNESS

When light strikes an object, some of the rays are absorbed and some are reflected. The reflected rays which reach the cornea give rise to the sensation of color. If an object reflects all the light rays, it is said to be white. If it absorbs all the light rays and reflects none, it is said to be black. Objects which we perceive as red, blue, etc., reflect the rays of light of the wavelengths which, when they stimulate the nerve endings, give rise to the sensations of these particular colors.

Color blindness is a condition in which the nerve endings are not sensitive to all the colors. This defect is hereditary. Approximately 1 man out of 12 and 1 woman out of 200 have some degree of color blindness. A male will be color-blind if he inherits the trait for this defect from either of his parents; the female will show the defect only if she inherits it from both parents. For this reason women who inherit this defect from only one parent may transmit it to their sons without themselves showing it.

Complete color blindness is very rare. Persons who have it see all objects without color, i.e., as the blacks, grays, and whites of an ordinary photograph. The most common form of color blindness is the inability to distinguish red from green. This is a distinct handicap in many activities. Traffic lights can usually be distinguished because of their brilliance. The color-blind driver also learns that the top light in the semaphore means "stop" and the bottom light means "go."

It is important for a person to know whether or not he is color-blind and, if so, to what extent. Today the Ishihara or similar plates are used. These charts show figures which are outlined by dots in the primary colors; the background of the figures consists of dots in confusing colors.

NIGHT VISION

The human eye is able to make certain adjustments to improve vision in dim light. First, and most obvious, it can tighten the muscles of the iris, thereby causing enlargement of the aperture and admitting more light. We see this as an increase in the size of the pupil. In bright light the iris expands and the pupil becomes smaller. The eye makes these adjustments reflexly.

Second, and even more important, the eye uses a different portion of the retina for night vision. The central posterior area, which is called the *fovea*, or yellow spot, and which provides the clearest vision in the daytime, is blind at night; the nerve endings in the area surrounding the fovea are more sensitive to dim light. For this reason one's vision is best at night if he does not look directly at the object he wishes to see.

Third, chemical changes occur in the cells of the retina which make them more sensitive to light. This change takes time and is spoken of as adapting the eyes to the dark. Adaptation is rapid at first but is not completed for half an hour. Pilots who are night fliers are carefully instructed in how to develop and utilize their night vision. Their life depends on this as much as on their planes and their ability to fly them.

Vitamin A deficiency causes night blindness, but there is no evidence that the addition of vitamin A to an adequate general diet improves night vision.

EYE SPECIALISTS

There are several groups of people who, with more or less justification, consider themselves eye specialists. It is important to be able to distinguish among them and to understand the service which each is qualified to render.

The *ophthalmologist,* or *oculist,* is a graduate physician who first had a basic education in general medicine and surgery and then specialized in diseases of the eye. He realizes that eyestrain or visual defects are frequently associated with and may be the first recognizable sign of disease, either in the eye itself or in some other part of the body; and he considers all such possibilities when making an eye examination. If, after a careful examination, glasses are deemed necessary, the oculist writes a prescription which is taken to an optician to be filled.

An *optician* is a craftsman, skilled in the grinding of lenses and the making and fitting of glasses according to prescriptions. If eyestrain is to be relieved, lenses must be accurately ground and glasses carefully fitted. It is essential also that frames and nosepieces be kept in proper adjustment. In some cases of astigmatism even a slight displacement of a lens from its proper position will cause discomfort.

An *optometrist* is a licensed, nonmedical practitioner, who measures refractive errors—that is, irregularities in the size or shape of the eyeball or surface of the cornea—and eye-muscle disturbances. In treatment, he uses glasses, prisms, and exercises. The educational requirements to become an optometrist are now 6 years of specialized college training at one of the twelve schools and colleges of optometry in the United States.

A word of sound advice for anyone who has or who thinks he has eyestrain is to investigate thoroughly before consulting those who advertise "Eyes examined free." Such establishments are business, not welfare, institutions. They give free eye examinations, but they make their profit by selling glasses. Hence, people who may need glasses should be careful about whom they consult. It is normally not necessary to worry about the glasses themselves, as in 1970 the U.S. Food and Drug Administration announced that to protect the public from eye injuries only impact-resistant lenses may be used in eyeglasses.

CARE OF THE EYES AND PREVENTION OF EYESTRAIN

Eyes will stand considerable abuse; but if one expects efficient service from them day after day and year after year, he must give them reasonable care. When used for close work, the eyes should be rested at frequent intervals by looking at a blank wall or at some distant object. During illness and convalescence they are susceptible to fatigue and so should be used sparingly. They need protection during infectious diseases, particularly measles.

Reading in bed frequently produces eyestrain because the book, magazine, or paper is not held in a proper position and lighting is inadequate and poorly placed. Likewise, reading with an unsteady light or on a moving train is fatiguing and likely to cause severe eyestrain. Adequate, steady, and properly located illumination is essential for comfort in the use of the eyes.

Goggles are useful to protect the eyes from dust and wind and are the most important single measure for the prevention of eye injuries in numerous occupations. Tinted lenses reduce the irritation from the glare of the sun in summer and the reflected light from the snow in winter.

Failure to correct myopia or presbyopia does not influence the progress of these conditions. Myopia tends to decrease after the growth period, while presbyopia tends to increase with advancing age. On the other hand, children with uncorrected visual defects are greatly handicapped. They tend to avoid playing with others and may be considered mentally retarded and queer. Early provision of proper glasses, therefore, is important, not only for the improvement of vision but also for social adjustment.

When symptoms of eyestrain or of defective vision occur, the eyes should be examined by a competent ophthalmologist or optometrist. However, not everyone with symptoms of eyestrain needs glasses. It is important also to realize that the condition of the eye and the general health are closely related. Defective vision may be due to a specific disease or may be aggravated by poor general health, and eyestrain may give rise to symptoms in remote parts of the body. Finally, when the eye is involved, the best service is none too good, for the possibility of preventing progressive loss of vision and eventual blindness may depend on the early recognition and proper treatment of glaucoma, trachoma, progressive myopia, or certain general diseases or toxic conditions.

EYE EXERCISES

Exercise of the eye muscles is a valuable adjunct in the treatment of certain types of muscular imbalance in the eyes, especially in cross-eyed children. Correction of refractive errors by lenses and in some cases muscle surgery are primary treatment measures, but if such measures are supplemented by proper eye exercises better results are usually obtained. Eye exercises, however, are not a substitute for other accepted means of treatment and should be employed only on the advise of a physician or an optometrist.

CONTACT LENSES

Lenses to be placed directly on the front of the eyeball were first produced in Germany 70 years ago, but only in very recent years have they gained any general acceptance. It is because of substantial improvements in these lenses that they are gaining favor. Originally contact lenses were made of glass and were large and heavy. Today they are made of plastic and are very lightweight and measure only $\frac{1}{3}$ to $\frac{1}{2}$ inch in diameter. They cover only the cornea of the eye, i.e., the pupil and the colored portion of the eye known as the "iris."

Certain types of visual defects can be corrected satisfactorily by contact lenses, while others cannot. In fact, contact lenses are helpful in some conditions in which it is impossible to obtain satisfactory vision with ordinary glasses. In certain occupations and activities contact lenses are preferable to ordinary glasses. Most contact and corneal lenses, however, are purchased for the sake of appearance. This may be a justifiable reason, just as people buy many other things in an attempt to improve personal appearance. On the other hand, extravagant advertising claims which depict glasses as unsightly and contact lenses as glamorous entice certain young people to enter into ill-advised contracts for their purchase.

Frequently, the charges are exorbitant and the lenses unsatisfactory or even dangerous. A survey by the American Academy of Ophthalmology of 50,000 contact lens users revealed that in 1 year 14 eyes were blinded or had to be removed; 157 were otherwise permanently damaged; and 7,607 were damaged but not permanently.

Contact lenses should be purchased only on the advice of a qualified eye specialist who does not profit from their sale. The fitting of contact lenses requires skillful, professional, and exacting service. Even with correct fitting, damage to the cornea sometimes occurs. Careful observation of the condition of the cornea must be maintained by a competent ophthalmologist or optometrist during the fitting procedure and at regular intervals thereafter. Contact lenses must not be kept in the eye for longer than the period recommended and never when there is irritation of any part of the eye.

Recently, "soft" contact lenses have been developed whose posterior portion conforms to the surface of the cornea. These promise to be a great improvement for people difficult to fit with ordinary contact lenses.

ILLUMINATION

Although poor lighting is an important factor in the development of fatigue and eyestrain, there is no satisfactory evidence that poor illumination is a cause of defective vision. Human eyes were developed, however, for use out of doors where the intensity of light, even on a cloudy day, is many times as great as in a well-lighted room indoors.

Direct sunlight in the middle of the day gives an illumination of approximately 10,000 foot-candles.[1]

The essentials of good lighting are that the light be adequate, uniform, and steady, and that glare and shadows be avoided. Under no circumstances should the source of light be in the line of vision. For reading and close work the whole room should be well lighted, with additional light centered on the work. A well-lighted room is bright and cheerful, a poorly lighted one gloomy and depressing. Good lighting improves the spirits, increases efficiency and productivity, and decreases accidents.

In rooms where no close work is done, 60- to 75-watt light bulbs are sufficient; classrooms, libraries, and desks should have at least 75- and possibly 100-watt light bulbs on top of the desk; and for finer work, such as drawing or sewing, 100- to 150-watt bulbs should be provided.

The colors of the walls and ceiling of a room have a distinct influence on the amount of light necessary to give adequate illumination. Light colors reflect the light; dark colors absorb it. The illumination at any point in a room is received in part directly from the source of illumination and in part from light reflected from the walls and ceiling. The type of shade or reflector over a light makes a great difference in the degree of illumination obtained from it. In fact, many of the most decorative shades render light practically useless for illumination. The degree of illumination available can be accurately measured by a light meter containing a photoelectric cell which indicates on a dial the intensity of light. In the planning of office buildings, schools, factories, and even homes an illuminating engineer should be consulted. And in the selection of a lamp to be used for reading or close work, the stamp of approval of the Illuminating Engineering Society (IES) gives assurance that the lamp is properly designed to give good illumination.

GLARE

Bright light which strikes the eye directly from an unshaded source or is reflected from objects such as glossy paper, polished furniture, clean white snow, or the hood of an automobile, causes con-

---

[1] A foot-candle is the amount of light at a distance of 1 foot from the flame of a candle of ordinary size, i.e., approximately 1 inch in diameter.

traction of the iris with resultant unequal stimulation of the retina. This is commonly described as "glare" and is responsible for a considerable amount of unnecessary eyestrain.

Sunglasses of various sizes, shapes, and hues have become synonymous with sports and vacations from Florida to Alaska and from seashores to mountaintops. As a result they are worn much more extensively than any real need for them would justify. Our eyes possess the capacity to adjust themselves to varying degrees of light intensity. It is a mistake therefore to make a habit of wearing sunglasses whenever one is in bright light. On the other hand, there are situations in which the light is so brilliant or accompanied by so much glare that the eyes are more comfortable if some of this light, particularly the ultraviolet light, is filtered out by special glasses. As a general rule, such glasses should not be worn indoors and should be put on out-of-doors only when the light is particularly bright. Many kinds of sunglasses are offered for sale, and many of them are reasonably satisfactory. However, some such glasses contain irregular curvatures or flaws that will contribute to eyestrain.

For persons whose eyes are particularly sensitive to light, a little tinting in the glasses they regularly wear provides comfort.

CONSERVATION OF HEARING

The deaf live day after day, year after year, in isolation imposed by silence. It is a small wonder that they may become depressed, seclusive, irritable, and dependent. It is estimated that 7 million Americans have subnormal hearing. Only about 10 percent of these are aware of and admit that they have hearing loss, and approximately 125,000 have little or no useful hearing and are classified as deaf.

Rates of impaired hearing per 1,000 persons in the United States are: 7.6, under the age of 25; 22.2, ages 25 to 44; 51.2, ages 45 to 64; 129.6, ages 65 to 74; and 277.4, ages 75 and over.

Although impairment of hearing increases with age, a survey in the Wisconsin public schools revealed that 5 to 8 percent of the schoolchildren in the state had hearing loss and that 3 percent were considered to be in need of medical care. Communicable diseases, tonsillitis, adenoiditis, excess earwax, injuries, and hereditary factors were responsible for many of these cases. Among very young children the problem of deafness is compounded by the fact that this handicap makes it extremely difficult for the child to learn to speak. Therefore, early diagnosis is particularly important among infants and preschool children, since speech training is most effective when begun before a child reaches school age.

CAUSES OF HEARING LOSS

There are two basic types of hearing loss: the conduction type, in which there is some interference with the passage of sound from the outside world to the inner ear; and the sensorineural type (or "nerve type"), in which hearing loss is due to some defect in the perception of sound in the inner ear, in the pathways to the brain, or in the brain itself. (See Figure 14.5.)

The *conduction type of hearing loss*, often called *conduction deafness*, may be caused by something in the external ear canal, such as impacted cerumen (earwax); by inflammation of the middle ear which results in swelling and accumulation of fluid; by scar formation in the middle ear as an aftereffect of infection; or by a bony disorder known as *otosclerosis*. Otosclerosis most commonly causes hearing loss by preventing movement of the stapes or "stirrup," the innermost of the three small bones of the middle ear by means of which vibrations caused by sound waves are transmitted to the nerve endings of hearing. This disease process, however, may invade the capsule of the cochlea and produce impaired hearing by involvement of the auditory nerve without immobilization of the stapes.

In recent years there have been marked advances in the treatment of all these middle-ear conditions. Plastic procedures on the damaged middle ear, known as *tympanoplasty*, are restoring useful hearing in many cases that could not be successfully treated a few years ago.

The majority of progressive hearing impairments in adults under 65 years of age are probably caused by the formation of spongy bone in the capsule of the inner ear—called *otosclerosis.* This condition prevents movement of the bones of the middle ear that transmit sound vibrations, and so results in deafness. This type of deafness can be treated successfully by modern surgery if little nerve damage has occurred. With the knowledge now available, permanent improvement should result in a high percentage of the patients treated if they have the type of deafness for which surgery is indicated.

Sensorineural hearing loss has numerous causes. Every person, if he lives long enough, will suffer some hearing loss as a result of degenerative changes in the auditory nerve. Such changes are often noticed at about 60 years of age by an inability to hear high tones, and then are progressive until between 70 and 80 years of age. Most elderly persons experience considerable hearing loss as a result of this change.

Exposure to loud or continuous noises, particularly of high pitch, is recognized today as a potential cause of loss of hearing. Industry has become increasingly alerted to this risk. Most industrial plants where the noise level is high now require preemployment screening tests for hearing, as well as the wearing of suitable protection by the employees.

It has recently been discovered that vibration below the audible range, such as that from explosions, earthquakes, aircraft, etc., can cause nausea, headache, and lassitude and even rupture of the eardrum.

One of the common causes of sensorineural loss of hearing in childhood is the virus of mumps. Injury may occur without the person's actually being ill. Scarlet fever and measles also may affect hearing. Ménière's disease, a condition in which dizziness, hearing loss, and head noises are usually present, is accompanied by sensorineural loss if the disorder is not controlled. Certain drugs such as quinine and some of the antibiotics—e.g., streptomycin, neomycin, and kanamycin—also may damage hearing. Even aspirin and other salicylate drugs used in large doses for the treatment of arthritis may impair the hearing of some persons. Cigarette smoking contributes to the progress of this type of hearing loss. Once sensorineural loss occurs there is no effective therapy, although a few persons recover some degree of hearing spontaneously. The principal hope lies in prevention.

Figure 14.5 Structure of the ear.

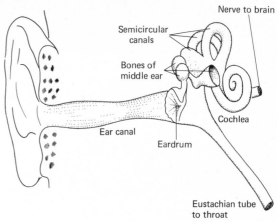

PRECAUTIONS IN SWIMMING AND DIVING

Swimming and diving, in the opinion of most otologists, are not dangerous to the ears of people with intact drumheads (commonly called *eardrums*), provided certain precautions are taken. However, diving feet first so that water forcibly enters the nose, improper exhaling with the head submerged, and vigorous blowing of the nose after emerging from the water may allow water to get into the sinuses or Eustachian tubes and may so irritate the nasal passages that an inflammation of the membranes lining these spaces results. Whenever a person has even a semblance of a cold, he should refrain from diving and should keep his head out of the water while swimming. Persons who have repeated ear infections or damaged drumheads or who have had certain types of mastoid operations should use special precautions to prevent water from reaching the middle ear. For such persons diving or swimming with the head partially submerged is unwise.

SERVICES AND AIDS TO HEARING

Life for a deaf person is difficult at best, but if the handicap is recognized early and faced intelligently, much can be done to minimize its seriousness. Proficiency in speech reading (lip reading) enables many deaf persons to lead a normal or a relatively normal life, but in order to attain proficiency the study of speech reading needs to be started early.

Improvements in electronic hearing aids are making it possible for many of the partially deaf to maintain contact with the world. A person considering the use of a hearing aid should consult an otologist who can advise the best type for the particular situation. The use of hearing aids should be started before the hearing is very seriously impaired. These instruments, properly selected and utilized, bring many pleasant and happy hours to the deafened.

Life for the partially deaf could be made much easier also if, in speaking to them, their friends would first attract their attention and then speak distinctly and slowly rather than loudly. Shouting is annoying, irritating, and difficult to understand. Speech and hearing clinics are offering helpful services to the deaf and hard-of-hearing in many communities.

CARE OF THE NOSE AND THROAT

Most of the acute infections to which man is heir are contracted through the nose and throat. Common colds, influenza, tonsillitis, pneumonia, scarlet fever, diphtheria, infantile paralysis, and so on, through a long list of diseases, find their way into the body through this portal. Measures which reduce the amount of infective material which gains access to the nose and mouth, such as washing the hands frequently and keeping them away from the face, the use of individual drinking glasses, and the avoidance of exposure to persons with these diseases, are all worthwhile.

The regular use of gargles, nasal douches, jellies, sprays, or drops, the so-called *control by nasal hygiene* without medical advice, is pernicious. Such preparations usually give temporary relief of nasal stuffiness, but they also interfere with the normal protective mechanism of the nasal mucous membranes and in time may cause sufficient irritation to give rise to a chronic catarrhal condition. When this occurs, the medication still gives temporary relief, and so the natural inclination is to use it more frequently.

There is a possibility also that over a period of time there may be enough absorption of these substances to be deleterious. Sniffers of cocaine or of snuff soon learn that absorption from the mucous membrane of the nose is prompt and efficient. In like manner, other substances are absorbed; and in some cases the effects may well be cumulative and toxic

OBSTRUCTION TO BREATHING

The most frequent cause of obstruction to breathing is the common cold. (See pages 274–279.) Uncomplicated colds rarely last more than a week, but the sinus infections which may complicate them are frequently protracted. The other common causes of chronic nasal obstruction are adenoids in children; and allergic conditions, nasal polyps, and abnormalities of the nasal septum. Lasting relief can be expected only by eliminating the cause of the obstruction. Self-medication merely aggravates the trouble.

ADENOIDS

The dull, pinched, stupid expression of the mouth-breathing child cries for relief. Susceptibility to colds and ear infections, impaired hearing, and a deformed upper jaw are among the other results of chronic mouth breathing by children. The most common cause of this is adenoids, an overgrowth of tonsil-like tissue located in the upper part of the pharynx behind the nose. (See Figure 14.6.) Fortunately the adenoids can be removed by surgery.

ABNORMALITIES OF THE NASAL SEPTUM

The septum is the partition between the two sides of the nose. (See Figure 14.6.) It is composed in part of cartilage and in part of bone. Theoretically the septum should be straight, but it rarely is. In fact, a perfectly straight septum is just as rare as an artistically perfect nose. Although many deformities of the septum are of little or no consequence, they occasionally are of sufficient seriousness to interfere with breathing, particularly if associated with other narrowing of the nasal passageway from trauma or developmental abnormalities. This not only is annoying but also predisposes to colds and sinus infection. In such cases an operative procedure may be indicated.

THE HUMAN BODY

a *If the vertebrae in the middle of the back are crushed, why may it be impossible to move the legs?*

b *If the thyroid gland becomes massively enlarged, why may swallowing and breathing be affected?*

c *Why is a nonpenetrating blow to the abdomen unlikely to injure the aorta —the large artery that carries blood from the heart through the chest and abdomen?*

The answers to these questions, and many others, are anatomical: you can derive them for yourself by examining the "Trans-Vision" plates in this insert. The anatomy of the body is intimately associated with its function, and every educated individual should know something of the interrelationships of the internal organs and structures of the body with their functions.

As you study these "Trans-Vision" plates, keep in mind the *purpose* of each of the organs pictured. If necessary, look up the name of the organ in the index of the text and read about it in the appropriate section; try to remember the names and the positions of the other organs to which it is attached or related. The organization of the body into *systems* is of great help in this. Although the "Trans-Vision" plates do not show the continuity of organ systems completely, you should readily be able to reconstruct this continuity.

The principal systems are these:

1 **The gastrointestinal system:** the mouth and throat; the esophagus; the stomach; the small intestine, into which the pancreas and liver pour their secretions, including the first part, or duodenum; and the large bowel, or colon, which is divided into the ascending, transverse, and descending colons and the rectum.

2 **The cardiovascular system:** the peripheral veins, which empty into the venae cavae that returns blood to the heart; the heart itself; the pulmonary arteries and veins, which lead to and from the lungs; and the aorta, which leads to the peripheral arteries that take blood to the tissues.

3 **The urinary tract:** the kidneys, ureters, and bladder.

4 **The nervous system:** the brain; the spinal cord, which runs from the brain down through the vertebrae; and the peripheral nerves, which run out from the spinal cord to the entire body.

a *If the vertebrae are crushed, the spinal cord may also be damaged and the nerve impulses may be unable to travel from the brain to the legs.*

b *If massively enlarged, the thyroid gland, which is just in front of the trachea and esophagus, may compress these structures, thus impeding their functions.*

c *That part of the aorta that supplies blood to the abdomen is protected by the muscles of the anterior abdominal wall as well as by the other organs and structures which lie in the abdominal cavity.*

(continued on back of insert)

PLATE I
Back view

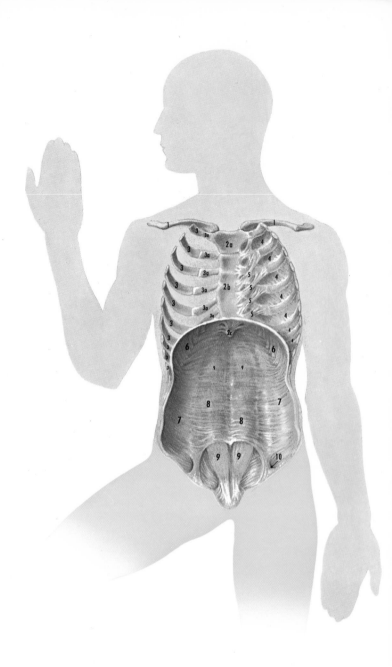

This plate shows the inside
surface of the front wall
of the chest cavity
and the abdominal cavity.

1. Clavicle
2a. Manubrium
2b. Body of the sternum
2c. Xiphoid process
3. Ribs
3a. Costal cartilage
4. Intercostal muscles
5. Transverse thoracic muscles
6. Diaphragm
7. Transverse abdominal
    muscles
8. Sheath of rectus abdominis
    muscles
9. Rectus abdominis muscles
10. Deep inguinal ring

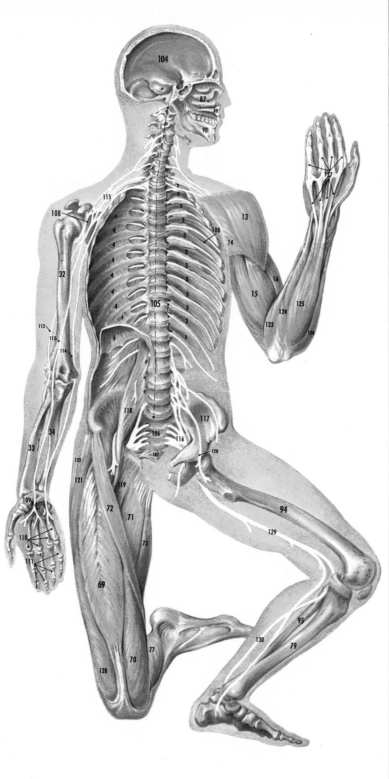

PLATE VI
Front view

104. Skull bones
87. Nasal conchae
89. Maxillary bone
90. Mandible
105. Vertebral column
106. Sacrum
107. Coccyx
108. Scapula
32. Humerus
33. Radius
34. Ulna
109. Carpal bones (wrist)
110. Metacarpal bones
111. Phalanges (finger bones)
112. Radial nerve
113. Median nerve
114. Ulnar nerve
4. Intercostal muscles
3. Ribs
115. Brachial plexus
116. Lumbo-sacral plexus
6. Diaphragm
117. Ilium (pelvic bone)
118. Psoas muscle
119. Pectineus muscle
71. Adductor longus muscle
72. Sartorius muscle
73. Gracilis muscle
77. Gastrocnemius muscle
69. Rectus femoris muscle
70. Vastus medialis muscle
120. Vastus lateralis muscle
121. Tensor fasciae latae
    muscle
122. Gluteus medius muscle
13. Deltoid muscle
14. Pectoralis major muscle
    (cut)
15. Biceps muscle (of arm)
16. Triceps muscle
123. Flexor carpi ulnaris m.
124. Extensor carpi ulnaris m.
125. Extensor digitorum
    communis m.
126. Extensor carpi radialis
    longus m.
127. Extensor tendons
    & sheaths
128. Femoral nerve
94. Femur
129. Peronaeus communis
    nerve
130. Tibial nerve
79. Tibia
95. Fibula

PLATE I shows the inside surface of the front wall of the chest and abdomen as it would be seen from within.

PLATE II shows the organs and structures of the chest and abdomen with the front chest and abdominal walls removed. It also shows the muscles of the arm and back of the neck.

PLATE III shows the organs of the chest and abdomen as seen from the back against the front wall of the body. It also shows the bones and arterial structure of the arm.

PLATE IV shows a cut section of the lungs, the heart, many blood vessels of the chest and abdomen, and the more posterior organs and structures of the abdomen, as well as the musculature of the leg.

PLATE V shows the contents of the chest and abdomen as seen when the structures of the back are removed. It also shows a cross section of the head and the bones and arterial structure of the leg.

PLATE VI shows the structures of the back, including the ribs, as seen with all the contents of the chest and abdomen removed. Some principal structures of the nervous system, the skeleton, the musculature of the arm and leg, and the interior portion of the skull are also shown.

Figure 14.6 (a) Section of the head showing tonsils and adenoids. (b) Section of the head showing internal nasal structure and relation of sinuses to the nasal cavity.

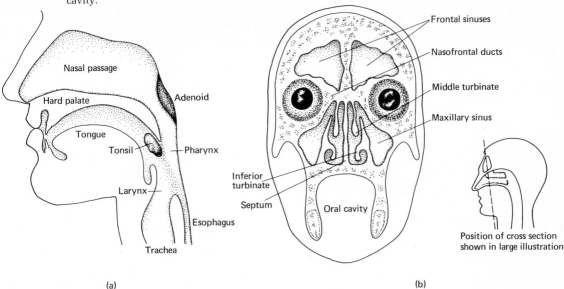

(a)

(b)

Position of cross section shown in large illustration

SINUS INFECTION

The term *sinus infection* or *sinusitis* is now used almost as loosely as *nasal catarrh* was in the past. Many persons who because of nasal stuffiness think they have sinus infection do not have it at all. On the other hand, sinus infection is of such frequency and seriousness that it merits careful diagnosis and treatment.

The nasal accessory sinuses (also called *paranasal sinuses*) are cavities in the bones of the skull, connected by small openings with the nasal cavity and lined with mucous membrane which is continuous with the mucous membrane of the nose. The sinuses bear the names of the bones they occupy (frontal, maxillary, sphenoid, ethmoid). They vary considerably in size and shape. It is probable that when an acute cold has existed for several days without much improvement, the inflammation has extended to the membranes lining the sinuses, especially the maxillary sinuses, which do not drain so easily as the upper group.

The spread of infection from the nasal passages to the sinuses may be increased by violent blowing of the nose—the nose should be blown gently with both nostrils open; by a hypersensitive allergic nasal mucous membrane; by diving; by swimming with the nose in the water; possibly by damp climates; and by the promiscuous use of sprays, oils, and antiseptics in the nose during acute colds. Also, the National Health Survey in 1966 reported 2 million more cases of sinus infection than would have occurred if the rate for nonsmokers had prevailed for the general population.

Acute sinus infections often clear up without treatment or with the application of such simple measures as heat, steam inhalations, rest, and improved nasal drainage. Occasionally, however, the infection is so severe or drainage so inadequate that pus accumulates in the sinus. This, also, may clear up promptly or may develop into a subacute or chronic condition. In acute sinus infection local symptoms of nasal discharge, pain, and headache, as well as general symptoms of fever, fatigue, general aching, and cough, are the rule. In chronic sinus disease, on the other hand, the local symptoms may be entirely absent. Occasionally infection from a sinus may be carried by the blood to other parts of the body, such as the joints, kidneys, heart, or brain. A condition potentially so serious calls for adequate medical supervision and treatment.

NASAL CATARRH

A generation ago "nasal catarrh" was a common complaint. Today it probably is just as prevalent but is known by other names such as *sinus trouble* or *postnasal drip.* This condition is due to chronic irritation of the mucous membrane, such as is produced by cigarette smoking or by the ill-advised use of "nose drops" or nasal inhalers. To be successful, treatment must be based on the elimination of the cause.

NASAL POLYPS

Chronic sinus infection usually is accompanied by a mucopurulent nasal discharge which produces an irritation of the nasal mucous membranes. This causes the membranes to swell and to obstruct breathing. If the membranes are hypersensitive, the development of grapelike growths called *polyps* may eventually result. In other words, polyps develop when sinus infection is superimposed upon an allergic nasal mucous membrane. The obstruction to breathing in such cases can be relieved by removing the polyps; but unless the allergic condition and the sinus infection are also corrected, the recurrence of the polyps may be expected.

HAY FEVER

The sneezing, sniffling, and nose blowing commonly called *hay fever* occur with greater or less frequency the year round. In fact, hay fever and related allergic conditions—such as asthma, hives, certain eczemas, headaches, and digestive disturbances—occur whenever a substance to which a person is sensitive gains access to the body in sufficient quantities.

The exact nature of the allergic process is uncertain. It is known, however, that heredity is one of the factors in its development; that a person may become sensitive to a wide variety of substances; that a healthy person can be rendered sensitive for a short period of time by injecting the blood of someone who is sensitive; that it is usually possible to identify the substances which cause trouble; and that a tolerance to offending substances may be built up by injecting them first in very minute and then in gradually increasing doses.

The symptoms considered typical of hay fever may be produced by pollens of plants, grasses, or trees; by the dander or hair of animals; by lint; by feathers; by foods; and by many other substances. The pollens, however, are the only substances of this sort which are definitely seasonal. In most areas of the country, pollens from the blossoms of trees cause the first seasonal hay fever in the spring of the year. These are followed by grass pollens in the early summer and by the pollens of ragweed and other weeds in the late summer and fall.

The pollens of grasses, trees, and many other plants are wind-borne and spell misery to hundreds of thousands of persons each year. Air currents may carry such pollen grains enormous distances and to great heights. A few have been found as high as 12,000 feet. From the upper air they frequently settle hundreds of miles away from their natural habitat and many months after the plants or trees from which they come have ceased pollinating. These pollens, however, may not give rise to hay fever, for symptoms occur only when the concentration of pollen in the air is high. During the pollinating season it is not uncommon to find 1,500 to 2,000 grains of a particular pollen to a cubic yard of air.

An accurate diagnosis of the pollen or pollens responsible for hay fever can be made by placing a minute amount of the pollen on a slight scratch of the skin. Swelling and redness indicate sensitivity to that particular pollen. If, in addition to this evidence of sensitivity, the plant is actually pollinating during the period when symptoms occur, one can be reasonably certain that this is at least one of the pollens causing trouble. It is unusual, however, for a person to be sensitive to one and only one pollen. Hence, in order that diagnosis may be complete, tests must be made with pollens from all the plants which are pollinating during the period of symptoms in the region in which the patient lives.

After the cause of hay fever has been determined, the simplest way to prevent it is to live, at least during the hay fever season, in a region in which the pollens to which one is sensitive do not exist. Another way to reduce exposure to pollen is to spend most of the day during the hay fever season in filtered air. This gives relief to many persons.

For the unfortunate hay fever victims who cannot move away during the hay fever season and whose homes and places of work are not air-conditioned, there is still considerable hope of obtaining relief, for it is usually possible so to increase a person's tolerance that he will be free from symptoms or at least reasonably comfortable even though exposed to high concentrations of pollen. Increased tolerance is accomplished by giving a series of injections of the pollens to which the patient is sensitive. In order to be effective this treatment must be based on an accurate diagnosis of the causes of the hay fever and the inclusion in the treatment material of all the pollens which are responsible for symptoms. Failure to do these two things has been the reason for many of the unsatisfactory results from this type of preventive treatment of hay fever in the past.

Temporary relief in hay fever and other allergic conditions can frequently be obtained by the use of a group of drugs called *antihistamines.*

TONSILS

The tonsils are masses of lymphoid tissue located between the pillars at either side of the opening between the mouth and the pharynx (throat). (See Figure 14.6.) They are part of the ring of lymphoid tissue of the throat region called *Waldeyer's ring,* which also includes the pharyngeal tonsils ("the adenoids"), which have been previously mentioned; the lingual tonsils, located toward the back of the tongue; and other small amounts of lymphoid tissue. Strictly speaking the masses of tissue commonly called the *tonsils* should be called the *palatine tonsils* or *faucial tonsils* because of their location. However, they usually are just called the *tonsils.*

Tonsils are so frequently removed that one is, inclined to wonder whether they can have any function at all. Actually there is no positive evidence of their purpose, although it is generally thought that they have some sort of protective function, ineffective though this seems to be in most cases. With repeated infections, changes may occur in the structure of the tonsils and adenoids which make them more or less constant sites of infection and a menace to general health.

In childhood, tonsils and adenoids are naturally large, but both decrease in size after adolescence. There are three definite conditions under which the removal of the tonsils and adenoids is advisable: (1) repeated attacks of acute tonsillitis or quinsy; (2) enlargement of tonsils and adenoids to the extent of causing obstruction to breathing, interference with the normal mobility of the soft palate, or obstruction of the Eustachian tube; (3) reasonable evidence that the tonsils are serving as a focus of infection. In this age of antibiotic drugs the need for tonsillectomy is reduced, but the indications just given for the procedure are still sound. The concept of focal infections is that infections at one point or focus in the body, such as the tonsils or the roots of teeth, are responsible for infections in other parts of the body or for certain general diseases, such as arthritis. To this concept medical opinion attaches less importance today than in the past. Tonsils, therefore, are less often removed on the suspicion that they are serving as focuses of infection.

Tonsillectomy is not a dangerous procedure if adequate precautions are taken to safeguard against accident. Undoubtedly many tonsils have been needlessly removed in the past, and more will be sacrificed in the future. On the other hand, the indications for the removal of tonsils and adenoids are being more accurately defined, and medical opinion on the subject of tonsillectomy is becoming more and more conservative.

QUESTIONS FOR DISCUSSION AND SELF-EXAMINATION

1 How do the major causes of blindness in the United States differ from the major causes of blindness in any other country? What is the implication to the several countries of these causes and their effects?

2 Compare and differentiate the effect on vision of cataracts, glaucoma, and trachoma and their treatments.

3 Describe the training and function of each of the following: ophthalmologist, oculist, optician, optometrist.

4 How do definitions of blindness differ and why?

5 What are the three conditions most needing correction by eyeglasses, and how do they differ in cause and effect?

6 In what ways can problems in the nose affect both ears and sinuses?

7 What parts of the ear are involved in the different types of deafness and by what mechanisms?

8 In what ways are treatment, diagnosis, rehabilitation, social problems, and adjustments in the blind and in the deaf similar? In what ways are they different?

9 How do the different causes of obstruction to breathing through the nose vary in significance?

10 What is the role of pollen in producing obstruction and other difficulties in the respiratory tract?

REFERENCES AND READING SUGGESTIONS

BOOKS

Davis, Hallowell, and Sol R. Silverman (eds.: *Hearing and Deafness: A Guide for Laymen*, rev. ed., Holt, Rinehart and Winston, Inc., New York.

An excellent book which not only discusses hearing and hearing loss, auditory tests, and similar topics, but also considers rehabilitation procedures and social and economic problems associated with hearing difficulties.

PAMPHLETS AND PERIODICALS

Allergy: A Story of Millions, Public Affairs Pamphlet, New York.

Prepared by the Committee on Public Education of the American Foundation for Allergic Diseases.

Bulletins of the National Association for the Prevention of Blindness, New York.

Cataract: Shadows that Need Not Be, National Society for Prevention of Blindness, New York.

A good explanation of the cataract problem and treatment procedures.

Conservation of Vision Pamphlets, American Medical Association, Chicago, Ill.

Publications of the American Hearing Society, Washington, and the American Medical Association, Chicago, Ill.

"World Health: Eyes," *Magazine of the World Health Organization*, 77 United Nations Plaza, New York, N.Y. 10017, June 1970.

An entire issue devoted to eyes, with splendid articles on safeguarding your eyesight; trachoma; cataract; the barrier of blindness; and detachment of the retina.

15

TEETH, SKIN, AND HAIR: THEIR HEALTH AND THEIR CONTRIBUTION TO HEALTH

The overemphasis on beauty that has become a daily part of our reading diet in newspapers and magazines does not lessen the actual physical and psychological importance of healthy teeth, skin, and hair. It is difficult to avoid being judged first by appearance, but more important, it is difficult to avoid being embarrassed by the loss of teeth, inflammation of the skin, or loss of hair that accompanies poor health. Fortunately, many of these disfiguring conditions are preventable.

SOUND TEETH

The relationship between the teeth and general health has been recognized for many years. Even horse traders inspected the teeth of their prospective purchases before making a selection. In recent times a great deal of attention has been given to the care and preservation of the teeth.

Teeth obtain support through contact with the skeleton. Each tooth has three parts. The crown projects above the gums and is covered with a layer of enamel. The root lies below the gum line; it has a bonelike covering called *cementum*. The crown and root come together at the neck. Underneath the hard outside coverings is a softer material called *dentin*. There is a small space inside the tooth, the pulp cavity, which contains blood vessels, lymph vessels, nerves, and the spongy material known as *pulp*. (See Figure 15.1.)

Every person has two natural sets of teeth. The first set of twenty is known as the *deciduous, primary, baby,* or *milk teeth*. The first deciduous

Figure 15.1   Cross section of normal tooth.

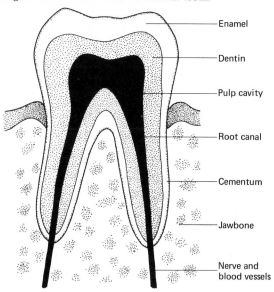

- Enamel
- Dentin
- Pulp cavity
- Root canal
- Cementum
- Jawbone
- Nerve and blood vessels

Figure 15.2   Sets of primary and permanent teeth.

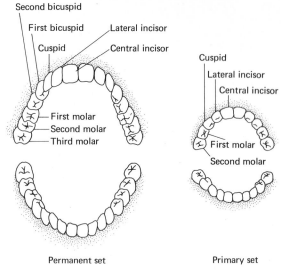

Second bicuspid
First bicuspid
Cuspid
Lateral incisor
Central incisor
First molar
Second molar
Third molar

Cuspid
Lateral incisor
Central incisor
First molar
Second molar

Permanent set

Primary set

teeth to appear are usually the lower central incisors. They generally erupt during the sixth and seventh months after birth. The last of the deciduous teeth to erupt are the upper second molars, which usually appear at the end of the second year. The time and order of the eruption of these teeth varies. When the deciduous teeth are completely erupted, there are ten teeth—two central incisors, two lateral incisors, two cuspids (also called *canines* or *eye teeth*), two first molars, and two second molars in the upper and in the lower jaw. (See Figure 15.2.)

The permanent set of teeth numbers thirty-two. The first permanent teeth to appear are usually the 6-year molars. They are the sixth teeth in order as we count back from the central incisors. They do not replace any of the "baby" teeth. They are sometimes mistaken for deciduous teeth and

thus may be neglected. Yet these four first molars are the largest and really the most important of our permanent teeth. When the permanent set of teeth is complete, there are two central incisors, two lateral incisors, two cuspids (canines), four bicuspids, and six molars in the upper and in the lower jaw. The second molars are called the 12-year molars; the third molars, the "wisdom teeth." They usually erupt between the ages of 17 and 21; but they may appear later, or they may not erupt at all. (See Figure 15.2.)

A survey by the U.S. Public Health Service estimated that 21.6 million persons in the United States and 29 percent of persons over 35 years of age are without any natural teeth; that only 36 percent of the population had visited a dentist during the past 12 months; and that 41 percent of the visits made were for fillings and 20 percent involved extractions.

DENTAL DECAY

Caries is the decay process which causes cavities. Caries is a very common disease; in fact, it is believed that over 95 percent of teen-agers show some evidence of dental caries. This is a localized disease process in which the enamel and later the

dentin are destroyed. Certain bacteria found in the mouth act on fermentable carbohydrates to form acids which can dissolve tooth structure. The action of these acids may begin in a crevice, irregularity, or break in the enamel, or even on the smooth surface. Surfaces in contact with other teeth and grooves in the back teeth are usually involved first. (See Figure 15.3.)

After the decay process has penetrated into the softer dentin, it proceeds more rapidly and enters the pulp cavity, where blood and lymph vessels and nerves are involved. There, an abscess may form, with accompanying swelling and pain.

The size, shape, and arrangement of teeth and their susceptibility to decay depends largely upon hereditary and nutritional factors during calcification and maturation. Crooked teeth are more susceptible to caries than straight ones. However, the causes of cavities are many: lack of sufficient fluoride, mechanical injury, composition of saliva, composition of the tooth—including fluoride content—and oral hygiene. Other major factors that increase the incidence of dental caries are oral microorganisms and carbohydrates on tooth surfaces.

DIET AND DENTAL CARIES

Skulls of Eskimos buried for hundreds of years and excavated by explorers in the Arctic, where the natural diet is high in fish and meat and low in carbohydrates, usually contain complete sets of teeth with little or no evidence of dental decay. On the other hand, skulls of Aztecs show abundant evidence of decay and root abscesses, as do skulls from the ancient Nile Valley, where cereal grains constituted a major portion of the diet, and skulls from the Hawaiian Islands, where natives lived chiefly on poi, from taro root, which consists largely of carbohydrates. Further support for the view that diet affects teeth is found in the increase of dental decay among Eskimos who have changed their native diet to American foods.

Proper diet is exceedingly important in providing sound, healthy teeth. Since the foundation of dental health is laid before birth, any deficiency in the diet of the pregnant woman should be corrected early in pregnancy. During the period of development and growth of the teeth a child needs a good diet if he is to have good dental health throughout his life.

Important though diet admittedly is, there does not seem to be any one dietary factor which is responsible for dental caries. Calcium and phosphorus, the two minerals found in bones and teeth, and vitamin D, which regulates the utiliza-

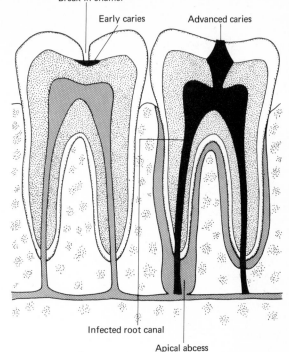

Figure 15.3 Cross section of tooth, showing decay.

Break in enamel

Early caries

Advanced caries

Infected root canal

Apical abcess

tion of these minerals by the body, are clearly essential while teeth are forming. Milk, certain vegetables, and fish foods are rich sources of both calcium and phosphorus. Vitamin D is likely to be deficient in natural foods during the winter months but is easily provided by vitamin D milk, cod-liver oil, or viosterol.

A well-balanced diet which is good for general health is satisfactory also for dental health. Sticky foods with a high carbohydrate content are cleared slowly from the oral cavity and should be restricted. From the standpoint of dental and general health, fresh fruits, vegetables, fruit juices and milk are much preferable to candies, cakes, and other sweets for desserts or snacks.

FLUORIDES AND DENTAL CARIES

During recent years investigations of dental caries have shown the great importance of adequate intake of fluoride salts in controlling this disease. (See Table 15.1.) Chemical analyses show that carious teeth contain less fluorine than noncarious teeth. Fluorine is a chemical that is always present

Table 15.1 Fluorides and dental caries: frequency of dental caries in school-children and natural fluoride content of drinking water in twenty-one cities.

City and state	No. of children examined	Percent of children caries-free	No. DMF* per child with caries experience	Fluoride parts per million
Galesburg, Ill.	273	27.8	2.36	1.9
Colorado Springs, Colo.	404	28.5	2.46	2.6
Elmhurst, Ill.	170	25.3	2.52	1.8
Maywood, Ill.	171	29.8	2.58	1.2
Aurora, Ill.	633	23.5	2.81	1.2
East Moline, Ill.	152	20.4	3.03	1.2
Joliet, Ill.	447	18.3	3.23	1.3
Kewanee, Ill.	123	17.9	3.43	0.9
Pueblo, Colo.	614	10.6	4.12	0.6
Elgin, Ill.	403	11.4	4.44	0.5
Marion, Ohio	263	5.7	5.56	0.4
Lima, Ohio	454	2.2	6.52	0.3
Evanston, Ill.	256	3.9	6.73	0.0
Middletown, Ohio	370	1.9	7.03	0.2
Quincy, Ill.	330	2.4	7.06	0.1
Oak Park, Ill.	329	4.3	7.22	0.0
Zanesville, Ohio	459	2.6	7.33	0.2
Portsmouth, Ohio	469	1.3	7.72	0.1
Waukegan, Ill.	423	3.1	8.10	0.0
Elkhart, Ind.	278	1.4	10.37	0.1
Michigan City, Ind.	236	0.0	10.37	0.1

*Decayed, missing, or filled teeth.
SOURCE: David Ast and Edward Schiesinger, "Fluoridation and Caries," *American Journal of Public Health*, March 1956.

in minute amounts in bones and teeth. An investigation conducted by the U.S. Public Health Service showed the fluoride content of drinking water in areas in which dental caries are rare to be about 1 part per million, but in areas in which dental caries are prevalent, the fluoride content was much less. (See Figure 15.4.) This suggested the possibility of reducing caries by the addition of fluorides to the drinking water of municipalities whose water contains less than this amount of fluoride.

The initial experiment with this type of preventive measure was made by the U.S. Public Health Service in Grand Rapids, Michigan. In 1945 sodium fluoride was added to the city's water supply to bring its content up to 1 part per million, the amount that occurs naturally in the water of many cities. The technique of this study was to determine at the beginning and the end of the experiment the amount of caries in schoolchildren of various ages in Grand Rapids as compared with

Muskegan, Michigan (the control area), where the water supply contained less than 0.2 parts per million of fluoride.

The results after 10 years were that the caries rate for permanent teeth of children born after fluoridation was put into effect was about 60 percent less in Grand Rapids than in Muskegan. In children 6 years of age (the peak of caries prevalence in deciduous teeth) the rate was reduced by 54 percent. The results also suggested some benefit to persons whose teeth had already formed or erupted when fluoridation was begun.

Studies made in Newburgh and Kingston, New York, cities with similar populations located on the Hudson River about 35 miles apart, showed similar results after 10 years of fluoride experience in Newburgh. For example, children between 6 and 9 years of age in Newburgh who had been drinking fluoridated water all their lives had a DMF (decayed, missing, or filled) rate for their permanent teeth that was 58 percent lower than in children of the same age in Kingston where the water is deficient in fluorides. No evidence of disfiguring mottled enamel was found among Newburgh children 7 to 14 years of age.

A later study showed that 92 percent of the children of Newburgh had not lost a single permanent tooth, while in Kingston 44 percent of the children of the same age had lost at least one permanent tooth; also that only 9 percent of the children who drank fluoridated water had teeth so "crooked" as to be physically handicapping, as compared with 22 percent of children who did not drink such water.

In view of these studies, one wonders why all municipalities with low fluoride content in their water do not adopt this measure for the reduction of dental caries. The reasons are many: some are political, some are financial, some have to do with inertia, and some have to do with organized opposition. The opponents of fluoridation question its safety, pointing out that fluorides are used as poisons for rats and other rodents. It is true that fluorides in sufficient quantities are poisonous, but so is chlorine, which is regularly added to water supplies to destroy disease-producing or-

ganisms; and so is iodine, which is added to table salt to prevent goiters.

In some communities in which the natural content of fluorides in the water exceeds 2 parts per million, a stained or flecked condition of the teeth, called *mottled enamel* or *dental fluorosis*, sometimes occurs. There is, however, no evidence or even suggestion that a fluoride content of drinking water of 1 part per million is in any way harmful or deleterious.

In communities where drinking water contains insufficient fluoride, parents should ask their dentists or family doctors for recommendations on adding fluorides to the diet of infants and children. This is easily done by adding fluoride drops to milk or orange juice, by using sodium fluoride tablets, or by using vitamin preparations which include some fluoride.

Studies have shown also that applying a fluoride solution directly to the teeth will help to reduce dental decay. The amount of reduction varies from child to child. The teeth must first be cleaned by a dentist or dental hygienist who then applies the fluoride solution and sets a schedule for further applications. Toothpastes which contain stannous fluoride have been shown to be of

Figure 15.4   Protection of teeth of schoolchildren by natural fluoride in drinking water.

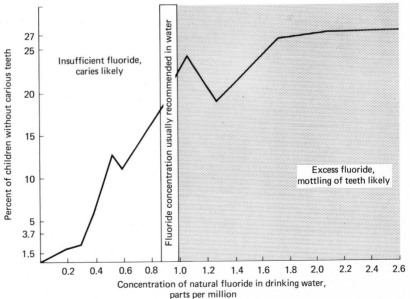

some value in the prevention of caries if used regularly.

CLEANLINESS

It is frequently said that "a clean tooth never decays." Whether this is true depends on the definition of cleanliness. If cleanliness implies freedom from bacteria, the statement probably is correct. But with bacteria constantly present in the mouth and in the food we eat, it is impossible to have the teeth bacteriologically clean. The action of acids produced by bacterial action upon carbohydrates on the teeth is greatest when there are gross accumulations of food substances. In fact, decay most frequently begins between the teeth or in pits or grooves where it is difficult to prevent accumulations of food. Hence, although cleanliness of the teeth is not the only important factor in the prevention of dental decay, it is highly significant.

Among the factors which play a part in determining the health of teeth is the presence of dental plaques or *tartar* (also known as *calculus*), the gelatinlike adherent films that form on the teeth and afford protection for the bacteria which produce the acids that dissolve the enamel. Still another factor is the length of time the acid is in contact with the teeth. When a dentist urges you to brush immediately after a meal or snack, "Immediately" is the key word. An hour later, even half an hour later, will do much less good.

One method of preventing decay that is being investigated is to paint the teeth, after thorough cleaning, with a liquid plastic that will harden quickly and will fill any pits, crevices or breaks in the enamel, thus preventing the bacteria and the sugars and starches that cause decay from getting into the structure of the teeth.

Dentists and other scientists believe that it will be possible to greatly reduce dental caries in the future by wider and more effective use of fluorides and by the application of other measures currently available or being developed.

ABSCESSES OF THE ROOT CANAL

The apical abscesses which develop around the roots of the teeth are the most dangerous type of mouth infection. Infective organisms usually reach these areas by traveling from deep cavities through the pulp of the tooth to the end of the root canal. At other times abscesses occasionally occur around the roots of apparently healthy teeth. (See Figure 15.3.)

An infection at the root of a tooth begins as a small inflammatory area in the periodontal membrane (around the tooth) and the bone in which the tooth is embedded. Unless an abscess forms and works its way to the surface, becoming a gumboil, these infections cannot drain except through the decayed tooth. Abscesses at the roots of certain teeth of the upper jaw may extend directly into the maxillary sinus and produce maxillary sinus infection. The development of these root abscesses is usually accompanied by pain; but they may develop, particularly at the roots of "dead" teeth, without any warning whatsoever. Drainage of an infected tooth can often be achieved by making an opening into the pulp cavity. In many cases a tooth can be saved by appropriate treatment.

Abscesses often form when the nerves in the tooth have died, but have not been removed. The dead organic material then provides a good medium for bacterial growth, and an abscess develops. One way to prevent such problems is to be aware of the danger signals for the death of a nerve. If a tooth is sensitive to hot or cold liquids, or if clenching the teeth is even mildly painful, one should immediately see a dentist. He can determine whether or not there is nerve damage.

GINGIVITIS AND PERIODONTITIS

Gingivitis is an inflammatory condition of the gums; *periodontitis* implies that the underlying structures are involved as well. The normal gums are pink or light red in color, thin and firm. If they become bright red or purplish, if they are soft, swollen, and spongy, or if they bleed easily, they need dental treatment. The cause of an unhealthy condition of the gums may be faulty diet, mechanical irritation, tobacco chewing or smoking, or bacterial infection.

Mechanical injury to the gums may result from faulty use of the toothbrush or from an accumulation of calculus on the teeth at the gum margin. Such mechanical injury produces an inflammation of the gums which is frequently followed by bacterial infection and periodontitis if the gingivitis is not treated and controlled.

It is important also that teeth be kept in proper repair so that they will be used regularly and uniformly. Missing teeth and poor fillings prevent the proper use of the teeth in chewing. They may allow the teeth to shift, giving an improper and painful bite. Brushing the gums and teeth will help remove the debris which accumulates around the gum margin and will thus aid in the prevention of periodontal diseases. Regular dental cleaning and scaling of the teeth by a dentist or dental hygienist is an important preventive measure.

Periodontitis, commonly called *pyorrhea*, is a severe infection of the gums that has become the major cause of lost teeth. The supporting bone breaks down, and serious infections may occur. The treatment of periodontitis depends on its type and severity, and can only be prescribed by the dentist after a careful study of the patient's condition. There are no available toothpastes, powders, or mouthwashes that in themselves will cure the condition. Bleeding of the gums while brushing the teeth, the separation of gums from the teeth, looseness or sometimes shifting of the teeth, and persistent "bad breath" are disturbances which should lead a person to early consultation with his dentist.

Recent studies show that gingivitis, periodontitis, and the loss of teeth are much more frequent in men and in women who smoke than in non-smokers (see page 98); and that for men from age 30 to age 59 and for women from age 20 to age 39 smoking doubles the risk of losing teeth.

One other cause of loss of teeth is the habitual grinding or clinching of the jaws. This action, which usually is unconscious or is done while asleep, causes the connection of the teeth with the jawbone to weaken and can result in the loss of teeth if not corrected. The use of a plastic mouth plate or simply autosuggestion frequently alleviates this problem.

CARE OF THE MOUTH AND TEETH

Cleanliness of the mouth and teeth is important from an aesthetic as well as from a hygienic point of view. It is difficult to keep the mouth clean in view of the irregularities in the shape of the teeth and the crevices between them. Nevertheless, by the regular use of the toothbrush and dental floss the teeth may be kept relatively free from deposits of food. The mouth should be cleansed in the morning, after each meal, and before going to bed in the evening.

THE TOOTHBRUSH

The toothbrush should have a flat brushing surface and firm bristles. It should be small enough to get at all surfaces. The number of tufts is not as important as the size and shape of the brush. Cold water should be used in brushing the teeth, for hot water softens the bristles. Afer use, the brush should be washed and hung up where it will become thoroughly dry before being used again. It is well to have several brushes which may be used alternately.

The teeth should be brushed on all surfaces which the brush can reach. Other surfaces should be cleaned with dental floss. A frequently taught method of toothbrushing is this: Place the bristles of the brush against the gums, just beyond the necks of the teeth, and pointing toward the roots of the teeth. Move the brush firmly so that the bristles sweep over the gums and the teeth. Brush the upper teeth downward and the lower teeth upward. Brush the chewing surfaces with a scrubbing stroke. Check with your dentist to assure yourself that your tooth brushing method is effective.

Electrically powered toothbrushes, in which the small brushing head oscillates, are suitable for general use. They are especially helpful for persons who have difficulty brushing their teeth because of physical handicaps. Powered toothbrushes are helpful also in brushing teeth of invalids or others who may need assistance. A dentist can give advice about powered brushes.

Within the past several years an instrument that delivers a jet of water under pressure for cleaning the teeth and massaging the gums has been marketed in this country. Concerning this the American Dental Association says: "The Water Pik Oral Irrigating Device is an effective aid to the toothbrush in a program of good oral hygiene. However, patients should consult their dentists regarding possible contraindications to its use and for guidance as to the appropriate degree of pressure to be used."

TOOTHPASTES AND POWDERS

Although brushing without a dentifrice is beneficial to dental health, a good dentifrice will aid in the cleaning. Clinical studies have shown that dentifrices containing stannous fluoride are of value in helping to prevent tooth decay if there is insufficient fluoride in the water.

Questions have been raised about the abrasiveness of certain dentifrices. However, according to the American Dental Association most of the widely marketed toothpastes do not have a level of abrasiveness that should be of concern to the average person.

MOUTHWASHES

The only real merit which can be ascribed to mouthwashes is that they give a pleasing sensation of cleanliness. They have no antiseptic properties

of any importance. If the mouth is healthy, they are unnecessary; and if not, they are valueless.

HALITOSIS

Disagreeable odor of the breath may come from decayed teeth, from collections of decomposing food between the teeth, from infections in the nose, sinuses, or tonsils, or from malodorous volatile substances eliminated from the bloodstream through the lungs. If decay or infection is present in or around the teeth, a dentist can take care of the problem. If decomposing food is frequently present, the situation can be corrected by brushing the teeth after each meal and by using dental floss at least once a day. Nose and throat infections can be cured by medical care, and the excretion of unpleasant odors from the lungs can be reduced if not eliminated by diets of low fat content. Mouthwashes may temporarily mask unpleasant odors, but they never really eliminate the odor or remove its cause.

DENTAL CARE

Regular visits to the dentist for all ages are important in dental care. Teeth should be cleaned at regular intervals of 6 months or as often as the dentist suggests. If cavities are properly filled when small, the progress of decay is arrested and the structure of the tooth is saved. To postpone or neglect necessary dental work is no economy. Dentistry is expensive and even the most skillful reconstructive work is not nearly so satisfactory as sound, natural teeth.

THE SKIN

The average person spends more time and more money on the care of the skin, the hair, and the nails for the sake of appearance than on medical and health services. However, the long-term appearance of the skin and hair is dependent more upon the general health of the body than upon the use of cosmetic preparations.

The skin, of which the hair and nails are inert appendages, performs several important functions:

1 The skin protects underlying organs and tissues against injury. Very few germs can

penetrate the unbroken skin. Blisters and calluses develop to help protect underlying tissues from injury. Tanning keeps out the irritating rays of the sun.

2 The skin plays an important role in the regulation of body temperature. The various metabolic and vital processes of the body produce heat which must be eliminated. If this heat were accumulated in the body, heat stroke or heat exhaustion would follow. Most of this heat is lost through the skin by radiation to the surrounding air or by the evaporation of

perspiration. When the body is hot and heat loss is essential, the blood vessels of the skin dilate, causing an increase in blood flow and a flushed or red appearance of the skin. The increased blood flow in turn causes an increase in heat loss and a stimulation of perspiration. Excessive heat loss or chilling causes constriction of the blood vessels, with blanching and discontinuance of perspiration.

3 The skin provides a sensory covering for the body. The nerve endings in the skin give rise to sensations of touch, pressure, pain, heat, and cold. These sensations enable us to respond voluntarily and involuntarily to noxious and threatening stimuli.

4 The skin serves as an accessory excretory organ. Most metabolic waste products are picked up by the blood and eliminated through the kidneys. The skin, however, contributes to this function. Under ordinary conditions with moderate activity, 2 to 3 quarts of perspiration, containing salt and some urea and uric acid, are eliminated each 24 hours.

The skin is a complicated and complex organ. For example, 1 square centimeter—about ⅙ of a square inch—contains 3 million cells, 100 sweat glands, 15 sebaceous (oil) glands, 10 hairs, 1 yard of blood vessels, 4 yards of nerves, 3,000 sensory cells at the ends of nerve fibers, 200 nerve endings sensitive to pain, 25 pressure apparatuses for the perception of tactile stimuli, 12 sensory apparatuses for heat, and 2 sensory apparatuses for cold. (See Figure 15.5.)

CARE OF THE SKIN

The most important factors in maintaining the health of the skin are the factors important for maintaining the health of the rest of the body—adequate rest, exercise, proper diet, and cleanliness. Attention to these general rules of hygiene will do more to produce a clear, attractive skin than the application of the many different types of so-called *skin foods* advertised so freely. In fact, lack of sleep, an unbalanced diet, and fail-

Figure 15.5 Microscopic section of skin, showing its structure.

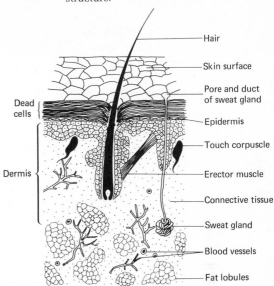

ure to wash the face frequently can undo all the care and effort put into a hairdo or the careful application of lipstick and powder.

The face should be washed at least once daily with warm water and a mild soap. For unusually oily skin, a cleansing with soap twice a day may be necessary. Cleaning the face with facial cream is scientifically unsound. The skin of the face is constantly exposed to dirt which adheres to the fatty secretion from the oil glands of the skin. If oils and creams are used as a substitute for soap and water, this accumulation of oily dirt is never completely removed and may be a cause of skin infections and other disorders. For unusually dry skin, an application of facial cream at night after the face has been thoroughly cleansed with soap and water may be beneficial. It is not harmful even for less dry skin but may be harmful for those who have a tendency to acne.

Chapping of the skin occurs most frequently in cold weather when the activity of the oil glands in the skin is reduced. Too frequent washing with soap removes oil from the skin and makes it more susceptible to chapping. Protection of the skin against wind and cold and the use of oil, cold cream, or glycerin reduce the likelihood of chapping. Thorough drying of the hands and face after washing makes chapping less likely.

SKIN DISORDERS

WRINKLES

With age changes in the skin occur. Oil glands become less active, elastic tissue fibers weaken, and underlying fat becomes thinner. As a result the skin becomes dry and wrinkled. There is no way to prevent this, and no "miracle cream," no matter how expensive, will safely and effectively remove wrinkles. However, their development may be retarded by avoiding excessive exposure to sunlight and by the regular use of good-quality softening creams or lotions. Cosmetic surgical procedures can temporarily lessen wrinkles.

BIRTHMARKS

"Birthmark" is a term applied to discoloration or pigmentation of the skin which is present at birth or appears shortly after birth. The superstition that birthmarks are due to some prenatal influence or fright of the mother is without foundation. Although birthmarks are rarely dangerous, they should not be irritated. Most red-colored or so-called *strawberry* birthmarks will disappear before school age and need no treatment. Such birthmarks, which are called *hemangiomas*, consist of blood vessels and occur in one out of every ten infants.

WARTS

Warts are caused by a specific virus which produces cauliflowerlike overgrowths of the horny layer of the skin. They may be spread from one part of the body to another by handling, and in susceptible people from person to person by both direct and indirect contact. At times they appear and disappear without apparent cause. Warts may occur on the soles of the feet and become so painful that removal is essential. The removal of a wart should be done by a physician, although small warts may yield to commercial removers.

ACNE

Acne, an inflammation around the oil glands of the skin (see Figure 15.6), is one of the common skin disorders of young adults and may be a source of great discomfort and humiliation. Acne develops as a result of an abnormal secretion of oil. Blackheads are frequent. Only a few lesions may occur, or they may be numerous. The most common locations are the face, chest, and back. Picking at these lesions contributes to infection, from which permanent scarring may result. Thorough cleansing of the skin several times a day with soap and warm water is important, followed, if inflammation is not severe, by drying with a rough towel. Eating oils and fats, pastry, and large amounts of carbohydrates and chocolate should be avoided. Milk and butterfat frequently contribute to the development of acne. Some physicians think that the chocolate, rather than the sugar, in candy and ice cream is responsible for acne in susceptible persons. It is possible to test yourself for this by discontinuing all chocolate for a month to see whether the acne improves.

The measures usually recommended for the prevention of acne are adequate sleep, a well-balanced diet, exercise and recreation, cleanliness of the skin and scalp, avoidance of creams and greases on the face and hair, and gentle removal of blackheads, using an "extractor" after soaking the face in warm, soapy water. Sunlight is beneficial to some complexions but bad for others.

When more than minor, acne should be treated by a physician. Persistent scarring can be alleviated in some persons by surgical abrasion of the superficial layers of the skin. Physicians experienced in the care of acne also can select medications which will substantially improve the condition; in certain cases, long-term treatment with antibiotics or hormones is useful. While acne may be very distressing during early adult years, the condition usually disappears in the early twenties.

FURUNCLES OR BOILS

Boils are infections usually caused by a staphylococcus that enters the skin along hair follicles. The common belief that boils are due to "bad blood" is erroneous. Diabetes mellitus, which causes an excessive amount of sugar in the blood, increases the susceptibility to boils, but this is hardly "bad blood." Persons with persistent boils should be checked for diabetes.

Boils are infectious and may be spread from one part of the body to another or from person to person by contact, clothing, towels, etc. Boils should be covered and should be cared for by a physician. If located on the upper lip or on the nose they are especially dangerous because of the possibility that the infection may spread to the brain.

ATHLETE'S FOOT AND RINGWORM

Athlete's foot is a widespread condition caused by a fungus (mold) which penetrates the superficial layers of the skin. It occurs most frequently in the damp, warm skin between the toes. Early signs are areas of moist whitish skin between the toes and cracking of the skin. Unless there is a secondary infection, damage caused by this fungus is rarely incapacitating.

The fungus or mold which causes athlete's foot is widespread. The infection is usually contracted from the floors of locker rooms, showers, bathrooms, and swimming pools, where people walk barefoot. Personal susceptibility, however, is a major factor in the development of disease. The fungus may be carried on the feet, particularly around the nails, for weeks, months, or even years before the disease becomes evident. Careful washing of the feet—including the areas between the toes—with soap, followed by thorough drying, helps avoid infection. Individual towels, washcloths, and bath slippers should be used.

A fungus known as *ringworm* may also become established on the skin or in the hair. Although usually acquired from another person, some types of this fungus may be acquired from animals, such as dogs or cats. On the skin, ringworm causes circular scaly patches which tend to heal in the center and extend peripherally. In the scalp the fungus may penetrate the shafts of the hairs, causing them to break off and leave small, round bald areas; or it may produce fine scaling in round areas on the scalp. Certain cases of ringworm are recognizable only under a Wood's light, a form of ultraviolet-light inspection. In its epidemic form this condition is found in schoolchildren. It is spread primarily by direct or indirect contact, e.g., by combs, brushes, caps, and hats that have been used by infected persons.

A fungus-killing antibiotic drug, taken by mouth, and applications to the skin of some new medicinal preparations are effective treatments for many superficial ringworm infections. Improper treatment may cause more trouble than the disease.

Figure 15.6   Oil-gland lesions.

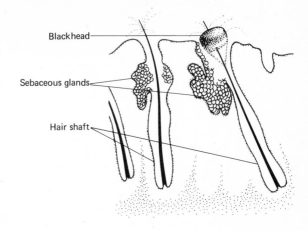

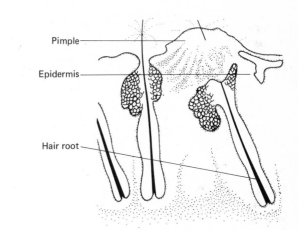

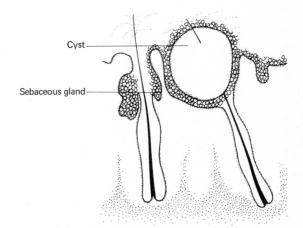

SCABIES

Scabies (the itch), which used to be one of the most common skin diseases, became very rare but has been making a recent reappearance. It is caused by the itch mite, which burrows under the skin and lays its eggs. Scabies is transmitted from one person to another by direct contact and indirectly by the use of bedding, gloves, or underclothing of an infected person.

SWIMMER'S ITCH

Persons wading or swimming in certain freshwater lakes or in certain bays of the ocean sometimes acquire a severe skin irritation named *schistosome dermatitis* and commonly known as *swimmer's itch*. This disease is caused by microscopic wormlike larvae which hatch in snail shells from eggs contained in the droppings of water birds. These larvae enter the pores of the skin, where they die but cause intense itching. The condition is acquired most frequently in warm, shallow water. Vigorous cleansing after being in infested water is helpful in preventing the disease.

PEDICULOSIS

Pediculosis is an infestation with lice. Three kinds of lice infest human beings: the head louse, the body louse, and the pubic louse (crab louse). Pediculosis can be controlled by recognition and the utilization of proper measures to remove and destroy the lice and their nits (eggs). One's physician and health department can give advice on the best measures to accomplish this.

IMPETIGO CONTAGIOSA

Impetigo is an infectious dermatitis which characteristically develops as small blisters, weeping sores, and crusts. It is most common on the face and hands. Impetigo is caused by either staphylococci or streptococci. It is transmitted from one person to another by direct or indirect contact. The person who has impetigo may spread the disease from one part of the body to another by scratching. Though impetigo is more commonly found among children, especially in warm weather, it may occur also in adults. For treatment the local application of specific antibiotic ointments is effective. In severe cases antibiotics are also given internally. The prevention and control of impetigo depend on the recognition, isolation, and prompt treatment of infected individuals.

HERPES

Herpes simplex (cold sores) and herpes zoster (shingles) are both caused by viruses, with the virus of herpes zoster identical to the virus of chickenpox. Cold sores usually occur on the lips; shingles usually appear in a circular line around the middle of the body. In both conditions, the skin lesions are first red, then tiny blisters, and finally crusts. Cold sores are usually of short duration and merely annoying, but shingles may be exceedingly painful, incapacitating, and long-lasting. In both conditions the virus apparently remains inactive in the cells of the body indefinitely unless or until something happens, such as a cold or exposure to the sun and wind, to stimulate the virus or to lower the resistance of the cells in which the virus is present.

URTICARIA OR HIVES

Urticaria, commonly known as *hives*, consists of small pink and whitish elevations of the skin which have the general appearance of insect bites. They are of various sizes, ranging from the size of the head of a large pin to a wheal of $1/2$ inch or more in diameter, and are accompanied by severe itching. They usually indicate an allergic reaction to a substance that is either brought into direct contact with the skin or absorbed by the respiratory or intestinal tract and carried throughout the body in the bloodstream.

Localized urticaria may result from insect bites if a person is sensitive to the formic acid introduced by the bite of the insect. It may also be due to some substance such as wool, dyes, or lacquers to which the person is sensitive. Elimination of such substances from the environment is the most effective preventive measure. Emotional stress and disturbances are important factors in chronic urticaria in some people. Antihistamine drugs are helpful in the treatment of many types of urticaria, particularly those due to specific sensitization rather than to emotional stress.

POISON IVY

Many plants, such as poison ivy, poison oak, and poison sumac (see Figure 15.7), give rise to a rash in susceptible persons. Individual susceptibility changes, so that a person who believes himself immune to ivy poisoning may later find that he is susceptible. The severity of the reaction varies from a few small, red itchy spots to swelling and blister formation over large areas of the body.

Poison ivy usually grows as a small shrub but it may take the form of a vine, growing just below the surface of the ground or on fences, telephone poles, or other structures that enable it to reach sunlight. The leaves are the key to the recognition of poison ivy. They grow in threes and, while their shape may vary, even on the same plant, their edges are deeply notched and their upper surfaces are glossy. The plant is native to North America and has a wide distribution. California and Nevada are the only states where it is rare. It is not found in dry areas, at high altitudes or in the shade of dense forests.

The irritating substance from these plants is an oil or a resin. This may reach the skin by direct contact or through clothing, shoes, tennis balls, garden tools, or dogs. The oil or resin may remain on such articles for long periods of time. Inflammation of the skin may appear in 6 to 12 hours, or it may develop 4 to 10 days after exposure. Apparently, man is the only animal affected.

Very minute amounts of the oil are sufficient to cause severe reactions in sensitive persons. The spread from one part of the body to another occurs early by means of hands, clothing, towels, etc., or later by absorption and spread through the lymphatic system. Such spreading may occur before as well as after inflammation develops. The more frequently a person has been affected by poison ivy the earlier the symptoms appear.

The disease runs a course of from several days to 1 or more weeks, depending on its severity. Treatment, at least of severe cases, should be under the direction of a physician. Cortisone derivatives in some cases are of great benefit. If a person has been in contact with these plants, washing the area immediately afterward with soap and water may remove the irritant oil and so prevent the development of the disease.

DRUG RASHES

Various drugs have long been known to cause skin rashes in some people. However, with the development and widespread use of various potent new

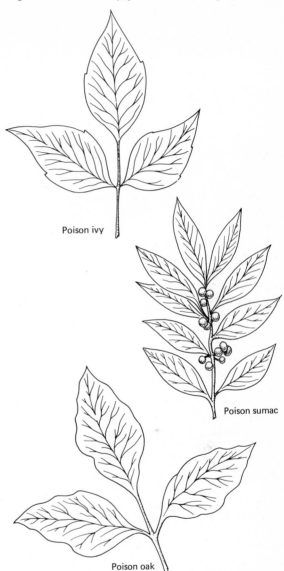

Figure 15.7   Poison ivy, poison sumac, and poison oak.

Poison ivy

Poison sumac

Poison oak

drugs for the treatment of heart disease, cancer, nervous conditions, etc., the frequency and severity of such reactions have been increasing significantly.

Such rashes may be localized or may cover the entire body and may be accompanied by sensitivity to light. Therefore, when persons who are taking medications develop skin rashes, they should consult their physicians without delay.

SKIN CANCER

Almost 200 years ago Sir Percival Pott, distinguished British surgeon and scholar, suspected that the cancers of the skin of the scrotum, common among chimney sweeps, were due to soot. We now know that soot contains carcinogens. Although Pott had no such information, he did prove his theory to be correct by demonstrating that these cancers did not occur when the chimney sweeps bathed frequently.

This was an epoch-making discovery—the first clue to the relationship of chemical agents and chronic irritation to cancer. Today it is common knowledge that excessive exposure to sunlight, ultraviolet light, coal tar, pitch, paraffin, certain lubricating oils, arsenicals, and other irritants may cause cancers of the skin. Fortunately, these cancers are on the surface of the body where they can be observed, and early diagnosis and prompt treatment usually result in cure.

Currently about 120,000 cases of skin cancer with 5,000 deaths occur annually in the United States. Skin cancer develops more frequently in persons with light or ruddy skins than in persons with dark skins. It is rare in Negroes.

Some cancers seem to develop from normal, healthy skin tissue, but most of them develop in areas where abnormal conditions have been present for a long time. These conditions are called *precancerous* because, while not cancerous themselves, they sometimes develop into cancer. (See Figure 15.8.)

Figure 15.8 How skin cancer develops: (a) The beginning growth of malignant cells in the skin; (b) a later stage; (c) a still later stage.

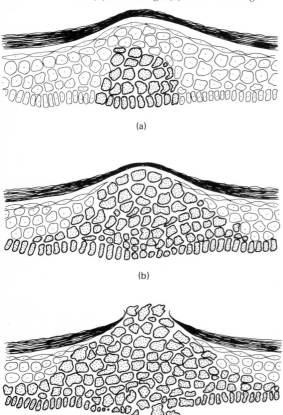

(a)

(b)

(c)

PRECANCEROUS SKIN CONDITIONS

Keratosis This is the most common of the precancerous skin conditions. It is a dry, scaly patch, or clump of patches, usually darker than the surrounding skin, which appears on exposed surfaces such as the face, neck, ears, and hands after years of exposure to the sun. When the top, scaly layer is removed, the base is seen to be made up of red, thickened "new skin." Especially if bleeding occurs, there is a possibility of early cancer. Keratoses vary greatly in different people and frequently cannot be distinguished from cancer without removal of a small bit of tissue for microscopic study by a pathologist—a procedure known as *biopsy*.

Leukoplakia This is a white, scaly thickening on the lip or membranes of the mouth, which may predispose to cancer. If this condition is present, it should be examined by a physician.

Moles Moles are an overgrowth of the deeper pigment layers of the skin. Most moles are harmless, but occasionally one develops into a rare but extremely serious form of skin cancer know as *malignant melanoma*. (See below.) The usual freckle, skin-colored mole, or reddish birthmark is not precancerous. These may, however, become dangerous when they are on the feet or so located that they are irritated by friction such as by a collar or belt. If moles are irritated or show a tendency to change in color or size, they should be examined by a doctor without delay.

MALIGNANT MELANOMA

The most dangerous, but fortunately rare, type of skin cancer is malignant melanoma. This type spreads early to other parts of the body. Malignant melanoma may arise independently or from a mole, as discussed above. One of the most definite signs of danger in a mole is the appearance of a dull, diffuse brownish zone spreading from it. If a mole is irritated and becomes larger or changes color, or if it bleeds, it should be seen at once by a physician. Moles on the feet are constantly being irritated but are easily overlooked.

BASAL-CELL CANCER (EPITHELIOMA)

This is the most common type of skin cancer. It rarely, if ever, spreads to distant parts of the body. In its simplest and most common form it appears as a small, firm, translucent gray nodule or bump on the skin, usually on the forehead, cheeks, nose, or other exposed areas. Since it is painless and rarely bleeds, this form is often unnoticed until it begins to grow more rapidly and its size calls attention to it. A fully developed basal-cell cancer is easily recognized. It has a central area of ulceration circled by a raised, gray, pearly edge. It is a painless, slow-growing ulcer which does not heal.

EPIDERMOID CANCER

Epidermoid (or squamous-cell) cancer is a less common form of skin cancer. This type may appear much like basal-cell cancer, but it spreads more rapidly. The epidermoid type of skin cancer usually starts in the form of a warty, crusty keratotic area or several such areas on the cheek, ear, neck, or back of the hand. The ulcerating form of epidermoid skin cancer is usually a shallow nonhealing ulcer which spreads on the surface of the skin—

sometimes over a wide area. On unexposed areas of the body, epidermoid skin cancer may arise in old scars of burns or infections, appearing as a nontender, raised, firm, pinkish, flesh-colored, small area on the normal skin.

EARLY DIAGNOSIS, PREVENTION, AND TREATMENT

In looking for the signs and symptoms of skin cancer, one should remember: Any increase in size, change in shape, deepening of color, bleeding or ulceration of a painless sore or mole which does not heal may be cancer unless proved otherwise.

The following rules of skin hygiene help guard against the development of skin cancer:

1 Ample use of soap and water by workers in industries utilizing materials suspected to be cancer-producing, to cleanse the skin of these irritating substances.
2 Protection of the skin from suspected cancer-producing substances. Workers should wear clean gloves and avoid long use of sooty, tarry, or greasy clothing.
3 Avoidance of overexposure to the sun. This rule applies particularly to light-complexioned people. All outdoor workers should wear protective clothing and use skin ointments to prevent the skin from becoming cracked or thickened.
4 Frequent examination, by a physician, of skin blemishes which may be subject to constant irritation or friction from clothing, and their early removal if any change in appearance occurs.

If skin cancer develops, it can be treated effectively by surgery, cautery, or x-radiation. The particular form of treatment depends on the type of cancer and the stage of the disease. The proper treatment can be selected only by a qualified physician.

COSMETICS

A clear skin and healthy hair are assets to personal attractiveness and so are desired by every person, young or old. That the appearance of the skin and hair is related to the general health of the body is too frequently forgotten. Cold cream or hair lotion, however, cannot be a substitute for the attractiveness that good health gives to the skin and hair, and cosmetics should be used only to complement the beauty with which nature has endowed the healthy person.

The commonly used types of cosmetics are face creams of various types, face powders, lipstick, and rouge. When first using a new type of cosmetic it is well to try it out on the wrist, where any undesirable reaction is less serious than on the face.

FACE CREAMS

The function of a face cream is to lubricate the skin and to prevent roughness and chapping. Ordinary plain facial or hand cream is probably the safest and most satisfactory type to use. The cost of the cream varies with the manufacturer. The formulas of the many special-purpose creams may be somewhat different, but the physiological effect on the skin is only that of lubrication.

The type of cream called *vanishing cream* is actually a kind of soap. When such creams are rubbed into the face, it is the equivalent of leaving soap on the face after washing. Because of this, vanishing creams tend to dry the skin. For women who have an oily skin, usually no irritating effect from the vanishing cream will be noted, and the face powder will stay on for a longer period of time. For the dry skin, however, vanishing cream will increase the dryness and may cause actual scaling and roughness of the skin.

FACE POWDERS

Face powders usually contain talcum, magnesium, French chalk, and starch or rice powder. Few face powders made by reputable manufacturers contain undesirable ingredients.

ROUGE AND LIPSTICK

Rouge and lipstick are usually harmless cosmetics and if used skillfully may contribute to attractiveness. The chief danger is in those which contain dyes to which some people may be allergic. Consumers Research has had a number of popular brands of lipstick and rouge analyzed, and the commonly advertised brands were found to be free from most undesirable substances. Even these, however, may not be safe for the occasional individual who is sensitive to a certain perfume or dye which may be harmless for the majority of people.

SUNTAN LOTIONS

Tanned skin carries an aura of leisure, of outdoor life, and of good health. Because of this, millions of Americans become sunbathing addicts. Others tan their skin by taking suntan pills or by using lotions containing a chemical called *dihydroxyacetone* (DHA). Natural tanning of the skin protects against the irritating effects of ultraviolet rays; chemical tanning of the skin does not do so.

Sunbathing and the air bath which accompanies it are pleasant and relaxing if not carried to excess or continued over too long a period of time. However, dry, wrinkled skin, as in premature aging, must be expected if one insists upon a deep suntan year after year.

Suntan lotions and creams contain chemicals which absorb certain wavelengths of ultraviolet rays. Among the most effective sun creams are those which contain para-aminobenzoic acid and its derivatives, the salicylates, and a digalloyl trioleate compound. These preparations do not increase the speed of natural tanning, but they do give protection against excessive sunburn before one has developed a tan. Creams and lotions which lubricate the skin are helpful in preventing the excessive drying effects of the sun.

DEPILATORIES

A depilatory is a substance that removes hair. For this purpose the common methods are shaving, scraping the skin with pumice stone or emery board, or using hair removers, of either the chemical or the wax variety. None of the above methods removes the hair permanently, since they have no effect on the root of the hair, which is the source of growth. The only safe method of permanently removing hair is by electrolysis. In this method an electric needle is inserted into each hair follicle, thus destroying the hair root. Unless electrolysis is done by an expert, it may cause scarring. Because each hair must be removed separately, this is an expensive method.

There is a common belief that shaving causes hair to grow out thicker and coarser than it was before. This idea, however, is false.

Chemical and wax hair removers are not entirely safe to use. In some individuals they cause irritation of the skin and may even result in skin infections. Manufacturers of some of these preparations falsely claim that they remove the hair permanently.

The simplest way to remove hair is with a razor. One can be sure that there is no danger of skin irritation or poisoning from a chemical and need have no fear that shaving will cause the hair to grow out coarser than it was before. Plucking the hair is also safe but obviously is very time-consuming. Hair should never be plucked from a mole, as this may cause irritation of the mole; the hair may, however, safely be cut short.

DEODORANTS AND ANTIPERSPIRANTS

For individuals who perspire excessively the prevention of body odor may be an important consideration in personal hygiene. Since body odor is caused by perspiration and the fatty acids formed from the sweat, prevention may be accomplished by frequent bathing, frequent changing of the clothes, and, in some instances, the use of a deodorant. Two types of deodorant are commonly advertised—those which deodorize the perspiration without restricting its flow, and those which both deodorize and stop the flow of perspiration. The first type, which depends for its action on such ingredients as boric acid, benzoic acid, zinc stearate, and antibiotics, may be obtained in either a dry or a paste form. It is usually harmless to use. The second type, which also diminishes the flow of perspiration, depends for its value on aluminum salts, tannic acid, or zinc sulfate. Though most people may use this type of deodorant without harm, in some preparations the solution may be so strong that it will cause a rash or other discomfort in sensitive individuals. This type of preparation should be used no oftener than is absolutely necessary. Deodorants should not be used immediately after shaving.

CARE OF THE HAIR

The same general principles of good hygiene which are used for the care of the skin also apply to keeping the hair healthy. Cleanliness is one of the most important aids in keeping the hair attractive. The hair, like the skin of the face and hands, is exposed to smoke and dirt. To keep the scalp and hair clean, the hair should be washed at least once every 2 weeks with a pure, mild soap. For many people a shampoo each week or oftener is necessary. Daily brushing of the hair will aid greatly in preventing the accumulation of dirt and in keeping the hair attractive; but in brushing, particularly with nylon brushes, care should be taken not to irritate the scalp.

Excessive dryness, excessive oiliness, excessive dandruff, or falling out of the hair are not normal and indicate that something is wrong. A physician should be consulted. Certain types of dandruff which cause a thick, oily scale to appear on the scalp are due to a germ infection and should be treated as such by a physician. The more common type of dandruff, causing dry scales to appear on the scalp, seems at times to be related to unhygienic habits of living, such as lack of sleep or excessive nervous strain, or sometimes to improper diet. Most of the so-called *dandruff*

cures which are advertised are of no more value in curing dandruff than are soap and water, though they may improve the appearance temporarily. Hair oils may be used by those with dry hair and scalp. The oil need not be expensive. Mineral oil or olive oil, with perfume if desired, is satisfactory.

Bald and balding American men and women are spending large amounts of money for futile hair-saving and dandruff-curing treatments. Baldness in most persons is hereditary. In others the cause in unknown.

The loss and replacement of hair are a natural process. In fact, everyone loses about 100 hairs a day. Yet, dermatologists report that in recent years the number of women who consult them about severe hair loss (alopecia) has increased greatly, some say as much as tenfold.

No single cause seems responsible for such balding. Heredity is a factor. Excessive oiliness, certain medicines, and a temporary decrease in the female sex hormones (estrogen) after pregnancy and after the menopause are others. Most important, however, seems to be the excessive pulling, stretching, and manipulation of the hair involved in some hair styles. Certain specialists advise women not to use brush-type rollers. For prevention and treatment of baldness, the American Medical Association's committee on cosmetics recommends regular, usually weekly, shampooing with a liquid soap which contains no detergents or other additives such as foaming agents, perfumes, or coloring; and a few minutes of daily brushing with a moderately soft natural-bristle brush. This type is recommended because many nylon brushes have square-cut bristles which may split and fray hairs.

Hair dyes have come to be extensively used.

Although most of them, even when used over a considerable period of time, cause no apparent ill effects, some contain substances to which an individual may be sensitive. The possibility of using a dye to which one is sensitive can be reduced by applying some of the dye as a patch test to the skin before using it on the hair. The bleaches that remove the color from the hair and enable a brunette to become a blonde at her pleasure are probably not harmful, although they may leave the hair dry and brittle.

QUESTIONS FOR DISCUSSION AND SELF-EXAMINATION

1 In what ways can bacteria damage structures in the mouth?
2 Why does the incidence of caries vary from community to community? Detail the mechanism(s) involved.
3 Why is fluoridation of public water supplies not medication?
4 Compare the effectiveness of the various personal and public ways of protecting against caries.
5 In what way is diet important to formation and maintenance of teeth?
6 What is the relationship between exposure to sunlight and skin health?
7 What is meant by *precancerous lesions*? How do they arise, what are they, and why are they important?
8 What dangers are attributable to cosmetics?
9 Describe the difference in danger to life in the various skin cancers.
10 When should loss of hair be an indication for consulting a physician? Document your answer.

REFERENCES AND READING SUGGESTIONS

BOOKS
Fluoride Drinking Waters, U.S. Public Health Service Report, Washington.

A 630-page collection of research reports on fluoridation.

Simons, R. D. G.: *The Color of the Skin in Human Relations*, Elsevier Publishing Company, Amsterdam, 1961.

In this paper-covered monograph, the author discusses the part that skin color plays in human life—the significance of such matters as the color bar, shade bar, hair bar, group solidarity, mixed races, caste systems, status symbols, and their resultant cultural and psychological implications. The monograph is thought-provoking and soul-searching without resorting to sermonizing.

PAMPHLETS AND PERIODICALS
The American Medical Association, Chicago, Ill., publishers.

Comprehensive and reliable pamphlets concerning the skin and hair.

Answers to Criticisms of Fluoridation, American Dental Association, Chicago, Ill.

Cleaning Your Teeth and Gums, American Dental Association, Chicago, 1972.

A pamphlet of latest information about how to care for your teeth and gums.

Kaplan, Ethel: "Be Glad You're Not Beautiful," *Today's Health,* August 1966, p. 22.

Beauty can be a problem. It may interfere with happiness, handicap a woman in her roles as wife and mother, and even pose the threat of emotional illness.

Kiester, Edwin: "Ugly Truths about Beauty Aids," *Today's Health,* June 1971, p. 16.

Ratcliff, J. D.: "How to Handle the Summer Sun," *Reader's Digest,* July 1971, p. 106.

Ross, Milton S.: "Acne—Tough Problems for Teenagers," *Family Health,* April 1971, p. 30.

Snyder, Jean: "How to Use Your Head when Your Hair Starts Falling Out," *Today's Health,* July 1971, p. 32.

A helpful consideration of this common and distressing condition.

16

COMMUNICABLE DISEASES

Paracelsus, Swiss-born physician of the sixteenth century, believed that it was possible to transplant diseases from the human body into the earth by means of magnets. Paracelsus had many followers who took his teachings seriously. A powder which used the magnetism principle in the next century was endorsed by King James, the Prince of Wales, the Duke of Buckingham, and many other noble Englishmen.

Today, folk remedies persist and some are written up in serious fashion. Those who find magical thinking comforting endorse these methods, whether they be copper bracelets, honey-and-vinegar, or huge doses of vitamin C.

On the other hand, today we also have specific knowledge of the causes and natures of many diseases, and specific knowledge of what medications and other treatments will affect these diseases and

how. The chapter that follows is devoted to a discussion of diseases caused by living organisms: bacteria, viruses, parasites, and other germs.

Many diseases which a generation ago struck fear into the hearts of people in every community are little more than names today. Yet there is a distinct hazard in the current widespread feeling of security and lack of concern about epidemic diseases. Sources of infection are still present; these diseases can spread into major epidemics if there are susceptible people and if control measures are relaxed.

One convenient way to classify diseases is: (1) communicable diseases, which sometimes are called *infectious* or *catching*, and (2) noncommunicable diseases. Communicable diseases may be transmitted from one person or animal to another in any number of ways.

When a communicable disease occurs in an isolated instance it is said to be *sporadic;* when a communicable disease occurs more or less continuously in a community or region, it is said to be *endemic.* If the disease attacks large numbers of people in a community or region, it is said to be *epidemic.* And if it spreads over a large region or over the world it is called *pandemic.*

Noncommunicable diseases such as arthritis, diabetes, hypertension, mental disorders, and coronary heart disease are not caused by microbial agents—bacteria or viruses or their products.

CAUSES OF COMMUNICABLE DISEASES

The communicable diseases are caused by microorganisms, commonly called *germs* or *pathogens.* Most of the microorganisms which cause diseases in man have adapted to living under the conditions that exist in the bodies of human beings or of animals. Consequently, they are able to survive only a relatively short time outside the body, unless they are cultivated in the laboratory under conditions which approximate those of the body. Under favorable conditions of heat, moisture content, and food supply similar to those found in the body, these organisms may multiply rapidly.

Some of these microorganisms are *animal parasites;* they may be single-celled, such as the malarial parasite, or multicellular, such as the worms which cause trichinosis, hookworm disease, etc. *Plant parasites,* which include certain fungi and molds, form another group of disease agents. Athlete's foot is caused by one of these plant parasites. *Bacteria* make up a third group of disease-producing organisms. Not all bacteria, however, cause disease. In fact, some bacteria— the saprophytes—which are present in the soil help to decompose dead organic matter, thereby enriching the soil. Other bacteria are always present on the skin and in the intestinal tract, but cause no harm unless the body's defenses are broken down by injury or disease.

Bacteria have various shapes as seen under the microscope. Some, called *bacilli,* are straight rods, e.g., the organisms causing diphtheria, typhoid fever, and tuberculosis. Others, called *cocci,* are round and form different kinds of groupings. For example, streptococci, which cause various types of infections, including scarlet fever, occur in chains; staphylococci, which cause boils and other infections, occur in clusters; and diplococci, which cause gonorrhea and other diseases, occur in pairs. Still other microorganisms are spiral-shaped, e.g., the *spirochete* of syphilis.

Viruses are still smaller microorganisms, frequently called *ultramicroscopic* because they cannot be seen with the ordinary microscope. They can, however, be studied with the electron microscope, which magnifies up to 1 million times. Using such microscopes, it has been found that viruses vary greatly in size and in shape.

The name *virus* means poison. Viruses seem to occupy an intermediate position between living things and inanimate materials. A virus may remain inactive for years, yet become active when it makes contact with a vulnerable cell. After entering a cell, the virus loses its identity and becomes active within the cell, almost like a chemical. It may then reproduce and destroy the cell that it has entered, liberating thousands or millions of virus particles to infect other cells. On the other hand, after entering a cell a virus may become latent and completely incorporated into the genetic material of the host cell. The host cell may later multiply and carry along the virus through successive cell generations.

A virus is essentially a parasite, able to reproduce itself only within a functioning cell. Viruses are responsible for more than half the infectious diseases of man and for hundreds of diseases of plants and animals. Certain viruses, called *bacteriophages,* are parasites of bacteria and are able to enter bacterial cells and destroy them.

Among the human diseases caused by viruses are smallpox, chickenpox, poliomyelitis, influenza, measles, German measles, hepatitis, mumps, and yellow fever. A number of tumors, some of them malignant, of plants and animals are caused by viruses, and it is possible that viruses may cause some human cancers.

Rickettsiae, intermediate in size between bacteria and viruses, constitute a fifth group. Rickettsiae, like viruses, can multiply only within living cells, but they are more complex organisms than viruses. They are carried by ticks, lice, and other insects and cause several important diseases, including Rocky Mountain spotted fever (tick typhus) and epidemic typhus (louse-borne typhus), a great scourge for generations of mankind living in poverty and filth.

INFECTIOUS AND CONTAGIOUS DISEASES

All communicable diseases are infectious: that is, they may spread and infect others. Of these diseases the ones that can be transmitted directly from person to person are also called *contagious*. For example, smallpox and diphtheria may properly be called *communicable, infectious,* and *contagious;* while malaria, typhus fever, and tetanus are *communicable* and *infectious* but, since they are not transmitted directly from person to person, are not *contagious.*

The entry and development or multiplication of a particular disease-producing organism in the body of man or animal is called *infection*, whereas the term used for the presence of a disease-producing organism in a nonliving article or substance or on a body surface is *contamination*. Thus one should speak of contaminated, not infected, milk or water.

With all communicable diseases there is an interval between the time an infectious organism enters the body of a susceptible person or animal and the time the symptoms or signs of the disease appear. This time interval, which may be a few hours or several years, according to the disease, is called the *incubation period.*

SOURCES OF INFECTION

Practically all communicable diseases are contracted from human or animal sources, which may be called *reservoirs of infection*. In fact, the most usual source of infection of man is some other person. This person may be one who is actually sick with the disease or one who has such a mild attack of the disease that it is not diagnosed, in which case he usually continues to expose others. The source of infection may also be someone who has recently convalesced from the disease or who, although himself immune and well, harbors the microorganisms of disease in his body and may scatter them about to infect others. This last type of source is commonly called a *carrier.*

Thousands of years before microorganisms were known there was some realization that persons who were in contact with patients ill with certain diseases were themselves likely to develop the diseases. Lepers have long been treated as outcasts. In the Middle Ages the Venetians, observing that epidemics, particularly of bubonic plague, followed the arrival of ships from certain foreign ports, passed a law requiring that ships with cases of "pestilance" aboard be held in the harbor 40 (*quaranta*) days. From this practice is derived the modern word *quarantine*. The reason a 40-day interval was selected is not known. It has been suggested that a period of 40 days was mentioned in the Bible in various connections, and that Hippocrates considered the fortieth day of a disease a critical day.

ROUTES OF ESCAPE AND TRANSMISSION

Disease-producing organisms are obviously of no danger to others as long as they are retained within the body of the patient or carrier. It is the microorganisms which get out of the body that cause infections in others. The routes by which these microorganisms escape from the body depend on the portions of the body infected. Most common of all routes are the nose and mouth, whose discharges, often in the form of an aerosol as from a cough or sneeze, are responsible for a large number of diseases and are most difficult to control. Among the more important of the diseases spread in this way are colds, influenza, pneumonia, tonsillitis, scarlet fever, diphtheria, measles, whooping cough, mumps, meningitis, tuberculosis, and German measles.

Disease agents which escape through discharges of the intestinal tract are, for the most part, those which enter the body with food and drink and localize primarily in the intestinal tract. Most important among these are typhoid fever, paratyphoid fever, dysentery, cholera, trichinosis, infectious hepatitis, and various intestinal parasites.

Among the intestinal parasistes, hookworm differs from the others in that its usual portal of entry is not through the mouth but through the skin between the toes. Hookworm eggs are discharged with excreta from the intestinal tract and hatched in warm soil into tiny larval worms. These larvae get into the skin of the feet of people who walk barefoot on contaminated soil. They enter the body through the pores of the soft skin between the toes and work their way into the bloodstream. They are carried by the blood to the lungs, where, being too large to pass through the tiny capillaries, they burrow through the thin membranes into the alveolar air sacs; thence, they pass up through the bronchial tubes and trachea to the mouth to be carried with the saliva to the stomach and the small intestine, where they set up the infection which is characteristic of the disease.

Other routes of escape for disease-producing organisms from the body are the urinary tract, the skin, and the mucous membranes which line the cavities of the body communicating with the exterior. The organisms which cause syphilis and gonorrhea most commonly escape from the mucuous membrane of the genital tract. Streptococcal infections, including scarlet fever, may be disseminated by discharges from the nose and mouth of infected persons, by the pus from infections which discharge to the surface of the skin or mucous membranes, or from infected middle ears or sinuses. Trachoma and the various types of conjunctivitis are disseminated by infectious discharges from the eye. From infected areas of the skin itself numerous diseases are contracted; most common among these are boils, impetigo, pediculosis, scabies, and ringworm, one type of which is called *athlete's foot*.

Mechanical puncture of the skin by insects or sharp instruments may result in the dissemination of disease-producing organisms. For example, mosquitoes ingest the virus of yellow fever and the parasites of malaria with the blood of infected persons and then by biting other persons inoculate them with these disease-producing organisms. Tetanus may result from skin puncture by a contaminated instrument such as a rusty nail, a rake blade, or a hypodermic needle used by addicts.

Disease agents may also be spread indirectly by insects or by articles or substances contaminated by disease-producing organisms, such as food, water, milk, soil, air, and certain other nonliving materials called *fomites*. The part played by fomites in spreading disease is not so great as it was formerly believed to be.

PRINCIPLES OF PREVENTION

The prevention of communicable diseases in general depends on three measures:

1 The blocking of the usual routes of transmission of infected material. This is the purpose of most of the measures of modern sanitation, such as water purification; sewage disposal; pasteurization of milk; use of individual paper drinking cups; sterilization of dishes, glassware, and other eating utensils; and washing of hands.

2 The prevention of the dissemination of infected material from the person who is the source of infection. This involves isolation, quarantine, and disinfection of bodily discharges and objects which may have been contaminated.

3 Immunization of susceptible individuals. Artificial immunization constitutes an important preventive measure against certain diseases. (See Chapter 17.)

QUARANTINE AND ISOLATION

By definition of the American Public Health Association, quarantine means "the limitation of freedom of movement of persons or animals who have been exposed to communicable diseases for a period of time equal to the longest usual incubation period of the disease to which they have been exposed." A similar public health measure called *isolation* provides for "separating of persons suffering from a communicable disease, or carriers of the infective organism, from other persons in such places and under such conditions as will prevent the direct or indirect conveyance of the infectious agents to susceptible persons."

In practice both isolation and quarantine are frequently modified by the application of scientific knowledge concerning the diseases in question. For example, malaria and yellow fever are controlled by preventing people from being bitten by infected mosquitoes; a case of smallpox is of little or no danger in a thoroughly vaccinated community; bubonic plague is controlled by eliminating rats; typhus fever is combated by measures against body lice or rat fleas, and Rocky Mountain spotted fever by measures against ticks. Intelligent isolation of patients with these diseases must take such basic facts into consideration.

DISINFECTION

Strictly defined, *disinfection* is the destruction of all organisms and their products which are capable of producing disease, while *sterilization* is the destruction of all microorganisms, saprophytic as well as disease-producing. *Antiseptics* prevent the multiplication of microorganisms but may not destroy them. *Deodorants* destroy and neutralize unpleasant odors, but many of them have no dis-

infecting powers. *Fumigation* is the use of fumes or gases to destroy microorganisms, vermin, or insects.

Disinfection may be accomplished by physical or chemical means. Physical methods of disinfection are chiefly dry heat, steam, boiling, drying, and ultraviolet light. Chemical disinfectants for the most part are applied in liquid form but may be gaseous.

Disinfectants destroy bacteria through physical or chemical changes of the cell substance of the organisms; consequently *time* and *temperature* are important in all disinfection. Usually the stronger the solution the more quickly the disinfectant will act, but *none acts instantly*.

RESISTANCE TO DISEASE

We frequently speak of increasing resistance to disease by exercise, fresh air, good food, and rest. All these measures are important for the maintenance of health, but they do not afford specific protection against communicable diseases. An athlete in the best of health may be just as susceptible to measles, smallpox, or scarlet fever as is his friend who leads a sedentary life. On the other hand, malnutrition, fatigue, and general ill health increase general susceptibility to such communicable diseases as colds or pneumonia, against which the body develops little if any specific immunity.

The white blood cells (see Figure 16.1), which usually number about 8,000 per cubic millimeter of blood, constitute a major line of defense against most bacterial infections. When an infection such as a streptococcic sore throat, pneumococcal pneumonia, or a wound occurs, the white blood cells immediately concentrate at the site of infection and are produced—primarily in the bone marrow —in greatly increased numbers. At the site of infection there is a death struggle between the infecting organisms and the white blood cells, the white blood cells ingesting and destroying the infecting organisms and the infecting organisms killing many white blood cells. The pus which accompanies infections consists largely of dead white cells.

In virus infections, such as influenza, measles, and poliomyelitis, there is no increase and fre-

quently a decrease in white blood cells. The only role, therefore, that white blood cells play in virus infections is their contribution to the development of antibodies.

Specific resistance to communicable diseases depends on the possession by the body of specific protective substances, called *antibodies*, which destroy infectious organisms or counteract their poisonous products. (See Figure 16.2.) The body may procure these protective substances either by manufacturing them itself or by being given them from some other person or some animal which has produced them.

Figure 16.1 White blood cells ingesting bacteria (streptococci).

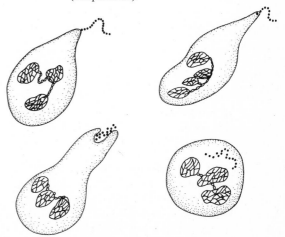

Figure 16.2 Antibodies in action.

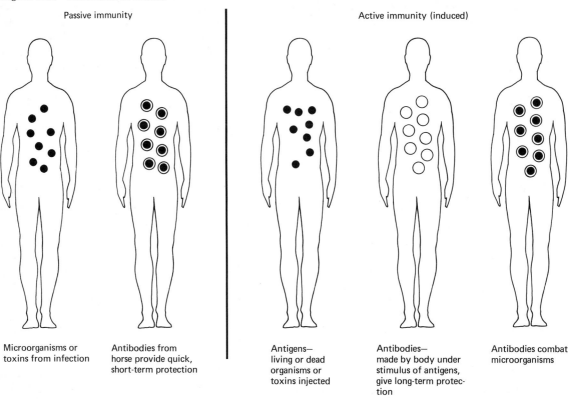

Passive immunity — Active immunity (induced)

Microorganisms or toxins from infection

Antibodies from horse provide quick, short-term protection

Antigens— living or dead organisms or toxins injected

Antibodies— made by body under stimulus of antigens, give long-term protection

Antibodies combat microorganisms

The human or animal body produces specific antibodies when stimulated to do so by the presence of disease-producing microorganisms or their poisonous products. (*Specific* in this context means "acting only against the organisms or toxins against which they were produced.") Antibodies may be produced as a result of an actual infection with the microorganisms of a disease. Antibodies may be developed also when a person has repeated small contacts with the disease agent, even if there is no clinical evidence of infection. The production of antibodies can be stimulated by introducing into the body dead or greatly weakened microorganisms or minute amounts of their poisonous products. This is called *artificial immunization.*

The resistance obtained in the ways just described is spoken of as *active immunity* because the body produces its own protective substances. Such immunity is relatively slow in developing but tends to last a considerable period of time. In some

instances this may be a few months, in others a few years, in still others a lifetime. Substances which stimulate the body to produce antibodies are called *antigens*. Antigens may be living or dead organisms, or the toxins produced by organisms. Strictly speaking, the term *vaccine* should be used only for antigens which consist of living or dead organisms. Thus, it is correct to speak of *smallpox vaccine* and *typhoid vaccine* because these antigens consist of organisms. On the other hand, when modified bacterial toxins are used as antigens to produce immunity, they are called *toxoids* rather than vaccines, e.g., *diphtheria toxoid* or *tetanus toxoid.*

The other type of specific resistance or immunity is *passive immunity* in which antibodies are received from some other person or animal and are not produced by the body itself. Whereas in active immunity the body can be compared with a factory because it makes its own antibodies, in passive immunity the body can be compared with a storage warehouse which receives the antibodies made by another person or animal and takes no active part in the process. An unborn child may receive antibodies through the placenta of the mother. Such protection lasts only for several months after birth. Passive immunity may be obtained by injecting into the body some of the protective substances which have been produced by a person who has had the disease or by a horse into which the microorganisms or their poisonous products have been injected. In either instance the protective substances are found in the blood. If taken from some other person, the liquid part of the blood, with or without the corpuscles, may be injected directly; or the constituent of blood which contains the antibodies, called *gamma globulin*, may be extracted, concentrated, preserved, and used as needed. If the protective substances are obtained from horses, they are removed from the blood and concentrated, and their strength is standardized before injection. The resistance or immunity thus obtained is present immediately after the injection but lasts a relatively short time.

The difference in the duration of active and of passive immunity results from the fact that in active immunity the body has learned to produce its own antibodies and keeps producing them or reproduces them as needed over a considerable period of time, in some instances even throughout life. In passive immunity, on the other hand, the antibodies injected into the body are foreign substances and are gradually eliminated or destroyed.

The degree of protection in passive immunity depends on the quantity of protective substances injected. Passive immunity is utilized when there is need for immediate protection, as when one is actually ill with a disease or when infants, who are particularly susceptible, have been exposed to a disease against which such protective substances are available. An example of passive immunization is the use of diphtheria antitoxin. Chapter 17 discusses certain immunizations which have proved of value in disease prevention.

INTERFERON

In recent years a protein, called *interferon* has been identified and shown to be of great importance in combating virus infections. It is produced by body cells in response to stimulation by a virus. It in-

creases resistance, however, not only to this virus but to other viruses as well. In fact, it has been called the body's all-purpose virus fighter. Some studies suggest that in experimental animals it destroys cancer cells which contain a virus without injuring normal cells. Present research aims to produce interferon in quantities that can be tried in the treatment of various virus diseases. There are also experimental methods to stimulate an individual's production of his own interferon.

IMMUNITY IS RELATIVE

Immunity is relative and depends both on the amount of antibodies which one possesses and on the amount and virulence of the infection to which one is exposed. One may be immune to a small dose of a mild infection but susceptible to a similar dose of a highly virulent infection or to a larger dose of the same infection. During epidemics of virulent smallpox, persons who had been vaccinated some years before have contracted the disease and some have died, even though the immunity which they possessed would have protected them against mild infections.

ALLERGY AND IMMUNITY

In the development of immunity the body produces antibodies against disease organisms or their products. Similarly, the body develops antibodies against other antigens, such as proteins and chemicals. This process is spoken of as *sensitization*. In one who is thus sensitized, the reaction between antibodies and antigens may produce illness— sometimes sudden, serious, and even fatal illness. Such reactions may be caused by horse serum, antibiotics, or drugs and occasionally by the sting of insects. They occur most frequently in persons who have received previous administrations of the substance. It is not certain just what the mechanism is that produces such allergies, but the reactions are sufficiently serious and occur frequently enough to cause physicians to urge that penicillin and other antibiotics be administered only when specifically and urgently needed. Otherwise, because of their ill-considered use, people may become sensitized to antibiotics and therefore not be able to use them at a later time when the need may be critical. Approximately 300 deaths from reactions to penicillin are reported to occur annually in this country.

DRUGS IN THE CONTROL OF COMMUNICABLE DISEASES

Invaluable also in the control of certain communicable diseases are various drugs, some of which are chemicals, some antibiotics. Probably the oldest example of such drugs is quinine, which for centuries was used both for the treatment and for the prevention of malaria. In recent years this "classic drug" has been largely replaced by synthetic chemicals; first by atabrine and more recently by chloroquine. The development of Salvarsan, an arsenic-containing chemical, for the treatment of syphilis represented one of the great forward steps in medicine. However, this "magic bullet," as it was sometimes called, has been replaced by penicillin and other antibiotics which are more effective and simpler to use.

Pencillin was the first to be developed of a group of drugs known as *antibiotics*. These drugs, which are produced by molds or similar living organisms, destroy a large number of microorganisms, thereby making possible the effective treatment of the infections or diseases which they cause. In some instances, such as the use of penicillin to ward off heart damage in rheumatic fever, they are proving valuable also for prevention. The antibiotics are truly "miracle drugs."

DRUG-RESISTANCE INFECTION

In recent years, certain strains of microorganisms, first staphlococci and more recently bacteria known as *gram-negative bacteria,* have developed resistance to penicillin and other antibiotics. As a result such antibiotics are no longer effective in the treatment of patients infected with these organisms.

In many hospitals, antibiotic-resistant bacteria are giving rise to serious infections, particularly following operations. The indiscriminate use of antibiotics for the treatment of minor infections encourages the development of resistant strains of infectious microorganisms. These drugs therefore should be used only when definitely needed, and then only in adequate dosage and under the direction of a physician.

The occurrence of antibiotic-resistant organisms has become so widespread as to constitute a serious public health problem. Fortunately, several semisynthetic—that is, partly chemically produced—penicillins are now available which destroy staphylococci that are resistant to ordinary penicillin.

COMMUNICABLE DISEASES

In other chapters of this book various communicable diseases are considered: diseases for which there are known immunizations in Chapter 17; mononucleosis in Chapter 2; the respiratory diseases in Chapter 18; the diseases acquired from food and drink in Chapter 12; and veneral diseases in Chapter 20. In addition several important communicable diseases are considered in this chapter.

INFECTIOUS HEPATITIS

Hepatitis means inflammation of the liver. Infectious hepatitis has become one of this country's major communicable diseases. Although little was heard about it until recent years, it is not a new disease. In epidemic form it occurred in the armies of Napoleon; it was prevalent among the soldiers during the Civil War in this country. In World War I and World War II it was an important problem because of the long period of time needed for convalescence from an attack of the disease. In

fact, during World War II more than 300,000 United States soldiers were hospitalized because of infectious hepatitis, and on the Italian front at times both American and German troops were rendered essentially ineffective because of it. This disease has been known by other names such as *camp jaundice, field jaundice, infectious jaundice, yellow jaundice,* and *catarrhal jaundice.*

Infectious hepatitis is caused by a virus and is most common among children and young adults. After an incubation period which is usually 25 days but may vary from 15 to 50 days, the disease develops suddenly with varying symptoms such as fever, headache, dark urine, abdominal discomfort, and mild nausea or diarrhea or both. Usually, after a few days the yellow coloring of the skin and of the whites of the eyes, known as *jaundice*, appears. Not all patients, however, show jaundice. This stage of the disease, which lasts a variable length of time, is followed by a period of prolonged convalescence frequently lasting several weeks or months. Many unrecognized cases of infectious hepatitis can be diagnosed by laboratory studies. Severe cases may develop chronic liver disease, and occasionally death may result.

The virus can be found in the stools and in the blood of infected persons. It is spread primarily by personal contact, most frequently through the intestional-oral route. Outbreaks, however, have been traced to milk, water, and various foods, including clams and oysters harvested illegally from beds unapproved by the U.S. Public Health Service because of contamination with human sewage.

In the fall of 1969 Holy Cross College after playing only two football games canceled the rest of its schedule because practically the entire squad became ill with hepatitis, contracted from polluted water from a drinking fountain on the practice field.

Personal cleanliness and community sanitation, such as proper sewage disposal, provision of safe water supplies, and food sanitation, are useful methods for controlling the disease. Gamma globulin is effective for passive immunization prior to or during the first 2 weeks after exposure. Prospects for the early development of an effective vaccine appear encouraging.

SERUM HEPATITIS

Serum hepatitis is another inflammatory disease of the liver caused by a virus similar, but not identical, to the virus of infectious hepatitis. Although both types of hepatitis confer an immunity which is usually lifelong, this immunity is only against the particular type that the person has had. Serum hepatitis is usually more severe than infectious hepatitis, fatality rate—6 to 12 percent for serum hepatitis as compared with 2 to 5 percent for infectious hepatitis. Serum hepatitis is transmitted by blood transfusions, by the injection of blood products, and by needles and syringes which have not been adequately sterilized. Drug addicts frequently become infected in this manner. Physicians and nurses have been infected merely by pricking a finger with a hypodermic or intravenous needle.

HEMOLYTIC STREPTOCOCCAL INFECTIONS

Hemolytic streptococci produce a number of acute and severe infections in man. The most common of these is streptococcal sore throat, commonly called *strep throat*. If a streptococcal infection causes a generalized rash, the disease is called *scarlet fever*. There are more cases of streptococcal disease reported to the U.S. Communicable Disease Center than of any other kind of infection: about half a million annually, and the number is increasing.

The streptococcus organisms enter the body through the nose or mouth and set up an infection in the throat. If the particular organism is not a good producer of toxin, or if the person has immunity to the toxin produced, there is no rash. The complications of sinus, ear, and mastoid infections are due to the extension of infection from the pharynx. The nephritis which occasionally occurs is due to the toxin. Similar hemolytic streptococci cause rheumatic fever; erysipelas, an infectious skin disease with a rash; and puerperal fever, a febrile infectious disease that may follow childbirth. (See page 331.)

The streptococci are contained in the nose, throat and ear discharges of patients, of those with mild cases—which are frequently unrecognized—and of carriers. Transmission of the infection from person to person is principally by contact with patients or carriers, or by means of droplets of moisture expelled from their noses or mouths. However, the organisms may be transmitted also by milk or other materials contaminated with streptococci.

Fortunately, the sulfonamide drugs, penicillin, and certain other antibiotics have greatly reduced the seriousness of streptococcal infections.

CHICKEN POX

Hardly anyone escapes this relatively mild viral disease. Chicken pox has a sudden onset with slight fever, mild general symptoms, and a rash characterized by tiny blisters on a red base, followed by crusts or scabs. After the patient's recovery the virus of chicken pox apparently remains quiescent in the body, but occasionally it may produce the localized infections known as *herpes zoster* or *shingles*, for which there is no immunization or specific treatment.

LEPROSY

Although not an important health problem in the United States, leprosy merits special mention as one of the most dread diseases of mankind and one of the first diseases to be recognized as communicable. From earliest biblical times lepers were considered unclean; they were driven from their homes and communities and forced to exist and to die by themselves. The fear and loathing of this disease were due largely to the disfigurement which it produces: thickened, wrinkled, nodular skin; open sores; and frequently, missing fingers and toes. Involvement of nerves, with numbness and loss of sensation, is frequently the first identifiable symptom of the disease.

The cause of leprosy, a bacillus similar in appearance to the tuberculosis bacillus, was discovered in 1873 by Dr. G. A. Hansen, a Norwegian scientist. Leprosy is therefore sometimes called *Hansen's disease*. The mode of transmission is not known, but prolonged intimate exposure seems necessary for infection. The long incubation period, usually 3 to 5 years, makes the identification of sources of infection exceedingly difficult.

Leprosy today, with an estimated 12 to 15 million cases throughout the world, exists primarily in tropical or semitropical areas, particularly in Africa, southeast Asia, the eastern Mediterranean, Brazil, and parts of the Caribbean. In the United States there are a few cases in Hawaii and occasional cases in Texas and Louisiana.

There is no specific vaccination against leprosy, but the tuberculosis vaccine BCG (page 284) has been found to provide considerable protection.

In the treatment of leprosy several relatively new drugs are quite effective. Among these is the sedative drug thalidomid, which, however, causes children to be born deformed if the drug is taken by the mother during pregnancy. (See page 328.) In the treatment of leprosy patients, this drug is reported to be 90 percent effective. Unfortunately, not more than 25 percent of known leprosy patients are receiving adequate treatment. Social prejudice against lepers makes many victims unwilling to reveal the early symptoms of their disease.

ANIMAL DISEASES TRANSMISSIBLE TO MAN

When we speak of animals, we usually think of those which range in size from mice to elephants. By definition, however, animals include all living things endowed with sensation and independent motion. The animals related to diseases of man are not only the larger animals, but also an extensive group of animals known as *arthropods*. The arthropods include all small animals with articulated bodies and limbs, such as insects, spiders, ticks, and mites.

Larger animals are associated with disease of man primarily because man is susceptible to certain communicable diseases and parasites of these animals. The arthropods are important primarily because they serve as a means of transmission of disease-producing organisms from man to man or from animal to man. More than 100 animal diseases are known to be transmissible to man. Of these the more important are brucellosis, bovine tuberculosis, trichinosis, rabies, tapeworm, plague, tularemia, anthrax, psittacosis, leptospirosis, equine encephalitis, and several types of fungus infections. (See Table 16.1.)

BRUCELLOSIS

Foremost in importance among the animal-borne diseases in this country is brucellosis, known also as *undulant fever, Malta fever, Bang's disease*, and *contagious abortion of cattle*. In human beings brucellosis can be a prolonged debilitating disease with recurrent periods of fever. Man becomes infected from cattle, swine, or goats; rarely, if ever, from human beings. In 1946 it was estimated that 5 percent of the cattle of breeding age in the United States were infected with brucellosis. Fortunately, this infection rate has been reduced to less than 1 percent as a result of the federal-state cooperative brucellosis eradication programs. Infection in human beings may occur from the use of contaminated raw milk or milk products or from contact with infected animal tissues or their secretions. At present brucellosis of man is almost wholly a rural occupational disease of butchers, veterinarians, and others working with infected animals or handling infected carcasses and tissues.

Until recently, there was no effective treatment for brucellosis. Fortunately, however, some

Table 16.1 Major zoonoses* in the Americas

Diseases	Animals involved	Mode of human infection	Geographical distribution
Virus diseases:			
Encephalitis, arthropod-borne	Horse, mule, birds	Mosquito bite	Widespread
Psittacosis	Parrot, parakeet, pigeon, turkey hen, duck	Inhalation, contact	Brazil, Canada, United States
Rabies	Dog, cat, wolf, fox, bat, skunk	Animal bite	Widespread
Jungle yellow fever	Monkey, other vertebrates	Mosquito bite	Jungle areas
Richettsial diseases:			
Q fever	Rat, cow, sheep, horse, dog, goat	Inhalation, tick bite	Widespread
Spotted fever (Rocky Mountain, Brazilian, Colombian)	Wild rodents, other animals	Tick bite	Brazil, Canada, Colombia, Mexico, Panama, United States
Typhus fever (murine)	Rat	Flea bite	Widespread
Protozoal disease:			
Chagas' disease (trypanosomiasis)	Cat, dog, rodents	Insect bite (*Reduviidae*, *Triatoma*), skin abrasions, mucous membrane	Throughout Central and South America
Bacterial diseases:			
Anthrax	Cow, horse, sheep, goat, swine, wild animals	Contaminated wool, hair, hides, air, food, water	Widespread
Brucellosis	Cow, swine, goat, sheep, horse, dog	Occupational exposure, milk, meat, or other contaminated food	Widespread
Leptospirosis	Rat, dog, cow, swine, rodents	Contact of skin or mucous membrane with contaminated water or dust	Widespread
Plague	Rodents	Flea bite	Areas in Argentina, Peru, United States, Brazil, Venezuela, Ecuador, Bolivia
Salmonellosis	Cow, swine, hen, sheep, rat, dog, cat, turtle	Contaminated food	Widespread
Tuberculosis, bovine	Cattle, goat, swine, cat	Contact, milk and dairy products	Widespread
Tularemia	Wild animals, birds	Tick bite, skin contact, water	Canada, United States
Helminth diseases:			
Hydatidosis	Dog, ruminants, swine, fox, rodents	Contact, contaminated food, water	Throughout South America
Schistosomiasis	Ruminants, swine, dog, cat	Skin contact with water contaminated with intermediate host snails	Brazil, Caribbean Islands, Surinam, and Venezuela
Trichinosis	Swine, rodents, wild carnivores	Contaminated meat	Argentina, Canada, Chile, Honduras, Mexico, United States

*Animal diseases that can be transmitted to man.

antibiotic drugs, notably the tetracyclines, cure a large proportion of the patients with this disease.

Prevention depends on the eradication of the infection among domestic animals (vaccination is helpful in accomplishing this), on the pasteurization of all milk before drinking or before processing into milk products, and on the use of rubber gloves and antiseptic measures in handling diseased or potentially diseased animals or their products. By observing these simple precautions and by giving continued support to the program for eradication of brucellosis in animals, hundreds of people each year can avoid this infection which saps vitality and produces prolonged invalidism and disability.

BOVINE TUBERCULOSIS

A generation ago children crippled from tuberculosis of the bones and carrying scars from tuberculosis of the lymph nodes were common sights. Children contracted these infections by drinking raw milk from cattle infected with tuberculosis. Today in this country both conditions are exceedingly rare.

When the attack on bovine tuberculosis began about 50 years ago, 10 to 50 percent of the cattle in many sections of the country were infected. To eradicate tuberculosis, cattle were tuberculin-tested and the reactors were slaughtered.

The eradication of tuberculosis among the dairy herds was the chief reason for the disappearance of this infection in children. Another public health measure, however, which contributed to this is the pasteurization of milk. Pasteurization kills tubercle bacilli, so that pasteurized milk can be used with safety even when there is no assurance that the milk comes from dairy herds that are free from tuberculosis. In some countries bovine tuberculosis is more prevalent among the cattle population than in the United States. Therefore travelers abroad as well as at home should use only milk and milk products which have been properly pasteurized.

TRICHINOSIS

Although all carnivorous animals may be infected, trichinosis is a disease primarily of swine and of rats. Man usually becomes infected by eating inadequately cooked pork or pork products from infected hogs. Since it is neither practical nor accurate by present methods to examine meat for trichinae, fresh pork products should always be thoroughly cooked. Government-inspected meat which has a cooked appearance must, by law, have been sufficiently heated to destroy any trichinae.

The prevalence of this disease in the United States, where 5 to 10 percent of the people have been infected, led to a national conference on trichinosis, which made the following recommendations for the control and ultimate eradication of trichinosis in man:

1 The adoption of state laws or regulations requiring that all garbage and waste products of butchered animals fed to hogs be adequately cooked

2 Enforcement of the section of the Interstate Quarantine Regulations that prohibits the shipping of uncooked garbage across state lines for the purpose of feeding swine

3 The prohibition by federal law of the moving of live hogs or raw pork out of any state that does not have and enforce garbage-cooking regulations

4 The education of the farmer to exclude all raw pork scraps and offal from his own household garbage that is to be fed to swine

5 The dissemination of information on incineration and alternative methods for garbage disposal

6 The prohibition by state law of the sale of garbage-fed hogs for slaughter at plants not having federal inspection or its equivalent

7 Continuation of the program of informing housewives and other food handlers of the necessity for cooking all pork and pork products thoroughly

RABIES

All warm-blooded animals may be affected by rabies, or hydrophobia, a disease that is almost always fatal once symptoms appear. For many years rabies was considered primarily a disease of dogs and, to a lesser degree, of cats, wolves, and other animals. Recently reported cases among dogs have decreased while the number among squirrels, foxes, and skunks has increased substantially. In 1965, 1 human case and 4,574 cases of wildlife rabies—primarily in skunks and foxes—were reported in the United States. Rabies has been diagnosed also in insectivorous bats from eighteen states in widely separated parts of the country.

The cause of rabies is a virus that infects the brain. The infection is accompanied first by excitement, then by paralysis and death. The virus is present in the saliva of infected animals and is transmitted primarily by the bites of these animals. In a few cases infection has resulted when the saliva of an infected dog or cat has gotten into a scratch or tiny break of the skin. Airborne spread of rabies from bats to man in caves where bats are roosting has been demonstrated but rarely occurs.

Dogs with rabies are commonly called *mad dogs.* In the excitement stage they may run great distances and snap at everything they meet. In the paralytic stage, which may occur without the period of excitement, the animals drool and appear "drunk." The name *hydrophobia,* meaning "fear of water," is given to this disease because when paralysis of the muscles of swallowing occurs, the animals cannot drink and therefore avoid water.

After the rabies virus gets into the body, it travels along the nerves to the brain. For this reason the length of the incubation period depends on the location of the bite, bites on the face having a much shorter incubation period than bites on the hands or the legs. In general, rabies has a long incubation period, varying from 10 days up to 10 weeks or occasionally even up to 6 months.

This long incubation period makes it possible to treat persons with a vaccine even after they have been bitten by rabid dogs and in many instances to build up a good resistance or immunity before the disease develops. The vaccine, which consists of killed virus, is given hypodermically in a series of injections. It is essential that the injections begin at the earliest possible moment.

This type of preventive treatment was developed by Louis Pasteur in 1885 and is commonly known as the *Pasteur treatment.* Before this, human rabies was widespread and uniformly fatal. Pasteur's work with this disease was truly dramatic and epoch-making.[1] Recently, a safer vaccine, manufactured by growing the rabies virus on duck embryos, has replaced the Pasteur vaccine.

Eradication of rabies in dogs depends on (1) registration or licensing of all dogs, (2) elimination of all stray dogs, (3) proper restraint and confinement of dogs, (4) rabies immunization of all dogs. Vaccination does not give lasting immunity; therefore it should be repeated at intervals as recommended by the veterinarian. Programs for rabies vaccination of all dogs have been shown to be extremely effective in the prevention of rabies epidemics in many communities in this country.

Every dog which has bitten a person, particularly in areas where rabies has occurred, should be kept under careful observation for 10 days. This procedure also applies to other animals which bite human beings if their capture and confinement are possible. If the dog was capable of transmitting rabies at the time of the bite, it will show symptoms of the disease within the 10-day observation period. Every person who is bitten by a dog known to be rabid or suspected of being rabid should receive preventive treatment, as recommended by a physician, without delay.

TAPEWORMS

Tapeworm infestations are contracted by eating beef, pork, or fish containing the larvae of these parasites which have not been destroyed by adequate cooking or freezing. Beef or pork tapeworm infections are detected when animals are slaughtered in meat-packing plants which have government meat-inspection service. Under the supervision of government veterinarians, infected carcasses are properly disposed of to prevent human infection. Prevention may also be accomplished by destroying the parasite through adequate cooking or freezing.

PLAGUE

Plague, caused by a microorganism called *Bacillus pestis,* is a disease primarily of rats and other rodents and only secondarily of man. The infection is primarily spread from rat to rat and from rat to man by the bite of the rat flea. In man the disease may take either the bubonic or the pneumonic form. Bubonic plague is transmitted only by the bite of a flea which has fed on an infected rodent or human being. In the pneumonic form of the disease, the germs are present in the sputum and are communicable directly from person to person, in the same way as other respiratory infections.

In the bubonic form in man the lymph nodes, usually in the groin, which drain the area of the

[1]See Paul de Kruif, *Microbe Hunters,* Harcourt, Brace & World, Inc., New York, 1954; paperback, Pocket Books, Inc., New York, 1959.

flea bite become swollen and filled with pus. Such nodes are known as *buboes,* from which the disease derives its name. When the plague germs are carried to the lungs and cause a pneumonia, the condition is called *pneumonic plague.* Bubonic plague has a fatality rate of 25 to 50 percent or more when untreated. The fatality rate for the pneumonic form is nearly 100 percent.

For a period of more than a thousand years Europe was swept by epidemic waves of plague. The most serious of these epidemics, called the *Black Death,* occurred in the fourteenth century, with a death toll estimated to have been in excess of 25 million people, one-fourth of the total population. The last great European epidemic of plague occurred in London in 1664–1665, when approximately one-third of the population of that city died within a few months. After this epidemic, plague rapidly decreased and almost disappeared. However, it reappeared in Hong Kong in 1894 and was rapidly carried by rats on trading ships to all corners of the globe. In 1950, 42,000 cases were reported throughout the world; and in 1970, 1,500 cases and 148 deaths. Plague is still endemic in parts of Burma, India, Java, Ceylon, and Madagascar.

In this country plague has become entrenched among the ground squirrels of the West Coast and is gradually spreading eastward. Wild rodents form a natural reservoir of plague. In the United States among human beings, 5 cases and 1 death were reported in 1969, 13 cases and 1 death in 1970, and 2 cases, 1 in New Mexico and 1 in Oregon, with no deaths in 1971.

A vaccine of value has been developed against plague, but the control of the disease depends primarily on the control of rats. Ships which come from plague-infested ports are routinely fumigated to destroy all rats and rat fleas. In countries where, because of poverty, rat control is impossible, plague will doubtless continue to spread. In the United States, in spite of the reservoir of infection among wild rodents, it is improbable that plague will ever reach epidemic proportions.

TULAREMIA

Tularemia is a highly fatal, infectious disease of wild rabbits. To a lesser extent it is found among other wild animals, such as field mice, squirrels, opossums, skunks, and coyotes; and occasionally it is accidentally transmitted to man. At times tularemia becomes so widespread as almost to wipe out the rabbit population. Bloodsucking insects, such as wood ticks and deerflies, transmit the infection from animal to animal. Infection of man usually results from handling infected rabbits. It may occur, however, from the bite of infected ticks or biting flies, especially among persons associated with sheep raising and shearing.

Tularemia is reported to be increasing in various parts of the country, although it can easily be prevented. Since probably 90 percent or more of human tularemia infections come from rabbits, hunters should not bring home or even pick up rabbits which appear weak, sick, or sluggish, or which have been found dead. Rubber or plastic gloves should be worn by everyone who handles, skins, or dresses rabbits. Wild game should be cooked until no "red juice" remains around the bones. These are simple but effective precautions against a serious disease. Domestic rabbits raised in captivity have not been reported to have acquired the disease or to have transmitted it to man.

ANTHRAX

Anthrax is a serious disease primarily of cattle, horses, sheep, goats, and swine, and only secondarily of man. The anthrax bacillus was the first disease-producing microorganism ever seen under a microscope. Vaccination against anthrax was developed by Pasteur in 1881, when this disease threatened to wipe out the sheep and cattle in France. This was the first disease against which animals were successfully vaccinated.

Today human anthrax is rare in this country, although it still occurs as an occupational disease associated with handling of hides and wool. Anthrax of animals does occur although not so frequently as in the past, and treatment of the disease is more effective.

PSITTACOSIS

Psittacosis, also known as *parrot fever* or *ornithosis,* is a disease of birds and fowl which may be transmitted directly to man. People contract this disease by inhalation of the virus from infected birds or their cages, primarily from dried excretions on the feathers or the floor of the cage. Parrots, parakeets, love birds, and turkeys are the most common sources of infection for human beings.

although canaries and pigeons also may be sources of infection. More than 70 varieties of birds have been found to be infected with and capable of spreading the virus.

Prevention of spread from parrots, parakeets, and love birds to human beings depends on awareness of the danger of making pets of birds of the parrot family, particularly when they have been recently imported or may have had recent contact with other birds in stores and pet shops. A new medicated bird food containing antibiotics may be helpful in eliminating the virus from the bird's system. Several wholesalers of pet birds in this country feed all birds this medicated food prior to sale to prevent transmission of the disease.

Psittacosis may occur also in turkeys, and a number of epidemics in poultry-processing plant workers have occurred as a result of processing infected turkeys. Others affected have included farmers and turkey handlers on farms where the turkeys were being raised. Poultry-plant workers contract this disease by inhaling the virus from the air and from aerosols created in the processing. Prevention of this type of outbreak in human beings depends on recognition of the disease in the turkeys and on effective treatment or disposal of the birds.

CRYPTOCOCCOSIS

This relatively rare but serious disease is caused by a fungus and disseminated by the droppings of pigeons. The New York City Health Department reports about 20 cases and 4 deaths each year.

EQUINE ENCEPHALITIS

Equine encephalitis, is a virus disease which produces an inflammation of the brain in horses, pigeons, pheasants, prairie chickens, domestic fowl, man, and probably other species of animal and bird life. *Encephalitis*, which means inflammation of the brain, is occasionally transmitted to man by one of several varieties of mosquitoes and possibly in other ways. The name *equine encephalitis* was applied to it in 1937 when over 70,000 horses in the United States (most of which died) were diagnosed as having this disease, which was frequently called *blind staggers*. In man this disease is sometimes spoken as *sleeping sickness*. Fatality rates are about 60 percent in man and about 90 percent in horses. Recent researchers suggest that birds are the principal reservoir of infection and that the disease is secondarily transmitted to horses, as to man, by mosquitoes. In 1966, 2,123 cases in animals were reported in the United States.

INSECTS AND DISEASE

A considerable number of diseases of man and the lower animals are transmitted by insects, some mechanically, others biologically.

Mechanical transmission implies that the insect carries the infective microorganisms from one place to another but is not an essential link in the transmission of infection. Infective material may be carried on the body of the insect or on its proboscis, or it may be taken into the insect's intestinal tract and regurgitated or discharged with the excreta. Common examples of diseases that are mechanically transmitted by insects are typhoid fever, bubonic plague, and tularemia.

Typhoid fever is transmitted by the housefly. The habits of flies are such that they are very likely to carry infective material from excreta to foods to which they have access.

Bubonic plague is transmitted by the fleas of rats or other rodents. The fleas take the *Bacillus*

pestis into their stomachs with the blood of infected animals, then regurgitate the organisms into wounds caused by biting other animals or human beings.

Tularemia is transmitted by the rabbit tick, wood tick, horsefly, deerfly, etc. These insects pick up the *Bacterium tularense* with the blood of infected animals and inoculate other animals or human beings in much the same manner that the *Bacillus pestis* is transmitted by fleas.

Biological transmission means that the microorganism undergoes some stage of its development within the body of the insect; i.e., the disease is not transmitted naturally from one person or one animal to another except by passage through the insect, which acts as its intermediate host. The more important among the diseases transmitted biologically by insects are malaria, yellow fever, typhus fever, and Rocky Mountain spotted fever.

MALARIA

At least three-fourths of mankind live in malarial zones. In 1950, about 300 million people were attacked by malaria and 3.5 million died. As a result of antimalarial campaigns, these figures have been cut by more than 50 percent, but the disease still presents a huge international health problem.

In World War II, during the Battle of Sicily, more American and British soldiers were put out of action by malaria than by the weapons of the enemy. In the battle areas of the South Pacific during the early years of the war the malaria rate reached 750 cases per 1,000 men per year. One of the great triumphs of modern medicine and sanitation was the control of malaria among the United States armed forces during World War II. Hundreds of thousands of our men lived and fought in areas of the world so badly infested with malaria that never before had white men been able to survive in them. The native populations had developed considerable tolerance from long exposure. The enemy made a serious miscalculation in believing that this could not be changed.

Today a similar determined attack on malaria is assuring vastly better health to millions of people throughout the world. In the United States fewer than 100 cases were reported in 1966 as compared with 62,763 cases in 1945. However in 1967, 2,885 cases; in 1968, 2,610 cases; and in 1970, 3,051 cases were reported, almost all of them soldiers returned from Vietnam. In southern Europe 4 million new cases a year were reported before DDT spraying; now there are fewer than 10,000 a year. In the Soviet Union there were some 4,300,000 cases of malaria immediately after World War II. In 1965 fewer than 10,000 new cases were reported. In the Americas three-fourths of the population are now protected, and complete protection is expected within a few years. Substantial progress is thus being made toward the goal of the World Health Organization to eliminate malaria from the world. (See Figure 16.3.)

In the eradication of malaria and other insectborne diseases, DDT is exceedingly effective. However, its toxicity to birds, animals, and possibly fish raises the question whether its use should be permitted. (See page 36.) Some countries of northern Europe have outlawed its manufacture and sale. However, in countries in which serious diseases that can be controlled by DDT are present, the decision is difficult: Do the benefits from the use of DDT outweigh the harm to the environment which results from its use? Serious concern about this is stimulating searches for insecticides which will be effective but will not be harmful to other forms of life.

Malaria is caused by a tiny parasite which lives inside the red blood cells and is transmitted by the female anopheles mosquito. Approximately 12 days after an anopheles mosquito has its meal of blood containing malarial parasites, the development of the parasite in the body of the mosquito is complete and the mosquito has become infective. The name *malaria*, which means "bad air," was given to this disease centuries ago by the Romans, who noticed that the disease was prevalent in the swamps and lowlands and rare in the mountains.

The typical symptom of malaria is a severe chill followed by a high fever which lasts for several hours; hence the name *chills and fever* or *ague*. These attacks occur with great regularity at intervals usually of 24, 48, or 72 hours, depending on the type of parasite. Although few attacks of malaria in otherwise healthy people are fatal, a person with malaria is half sick all the time.

Prevention of malaria depends on the following measures:

1 Elimination of the breeding places of mosquitoes by drainage of swamps.
2 Destruction of mosquito larvae with oil, insecticides, or fish.
3 Safeguarding patients from mosquitoes until their blood is free from parasites, to prevent further spread.
4 Blood examinations of persons living in malarial districts to determine which ones are infected so that they may be treated and will cease to be reservoirs of infection.
5 Screening of porches and houses and in general taking particular precautions against being bitten by mosquitoes.
6 The use of safe insecticides to destroy mosquitoes in or around human habitations.
7 Administration of small doses of antimalarial drugs, such as quinine, atabrine, or chloroquine, during periods of probable exposure. A recent report states that chlo-

Figure 16.3 Cases of malaria in the United States, 1933 to 1970. Source: U.S. Public Health Service.

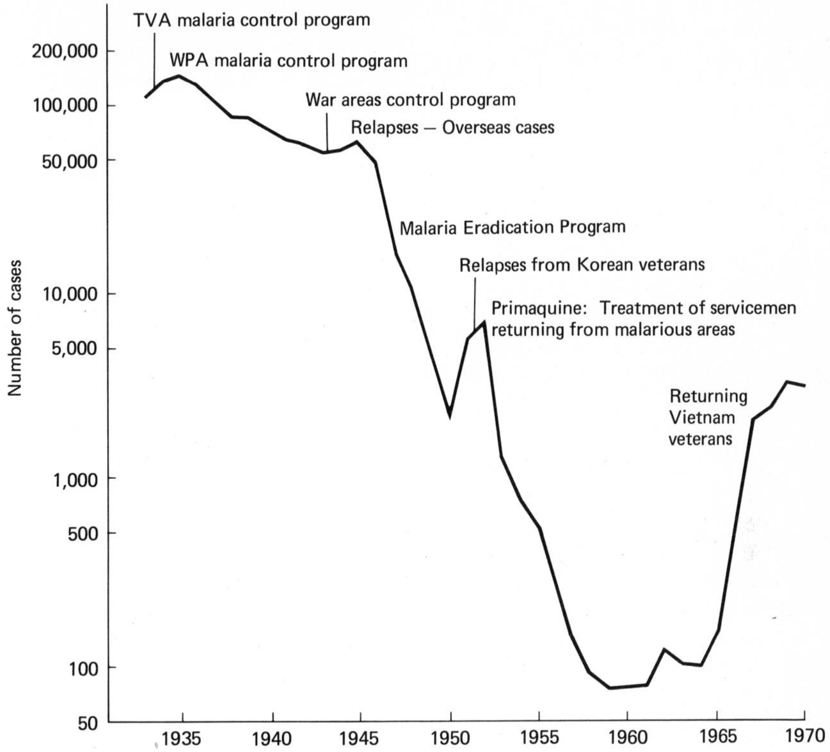

*The reported number differs from the more complete count from the case surveillance system.

roquine is proving so highly effective and so nontoxic that in certain South American countries it is being mixed with table salt for use by the general population. Preliminary results suggest that this may be a simple, inexpensive, and effective way to prevent and eventually eradicate malaria. Still better, however, may be a new drug, a single injection of which seems to have protected a group of volunteers for almost a year.

In spite of these precautions, malaria has become a serious problem among United States armed forces in Vietnam because of the presence of a severe form of malaria that is resistant to the usual antimalaria drugs. Fortunately, several new drugs have been developed which, used in com-

bination, give promise of being effective against this type of malaria.

YELLOW FEVER

Yellow fever is a serious disease caused by a virus and transmitted by the female *Aëdes aegypti* mosquito. In 1793 yellow fever caused panic among the citizens of Philadelphia, taking a death toll of one-tenth of the population of that city in the space of a few months. Periodically thereafter it made sections of the Gulf Coast almost uninhabitable. It drove the white man out of the Canal Zone during the building of the Panama Canal. Then the United States Army Yellow Fever Commission, headed by Dr. Walter Reed, proved that it is spread by the Aëdes mosquito. Yellow fever was eliminated in the Canal Zone, and construction proceeded. Thereafter, one by one, its strongholds were attacked. The story of the studies on yellow fever and the application of the knowledge gained thereby is a brilliant page in the history of our nation. In fact, in 1969 only 118 cases were reported to the World Health Organization by the countries of the world.

The virus of yellow fever is present in the patient's blood only during the first 3 or 4 days of the disease, and it takes 12 to 14 days after ingestion of the virus by the mosquito before the insect is able to transmit the disease. This period is known as the *extrinsic incubation period*. Its length varies with the temperature. A mosquito, once infected, remains so all her life. The disease is not spread from one person to another by contact or by fomites.

Yellow fever is usually a fatal disease, but those who recover have a high-grade immunity. An effective vaccination has been developed against this disease; but prevention of yellow fever, at least in developed communities, depends primarily on the extermination of the Aëdes mosquito. This task, compared with the extermination of the Anopheles mosquito, is relatively simple because the Aëdes mosquito breeds almost exclusively in artificial containers of water located in the vicinity of human habitations. A second effective preventive measure is careful screening of patients from mosquitoes, particularly during the first week of the disease.

A type of yellow fever, known as *jungle yellow fever*, was recognized in South America in 1933. It is transmitted from monkey to monkey and from monkey to man by forest mosquitoes which are tree-living insects. Jungle yellow fever is sometimes called *woodcutter's disease* because the adult mosquitoes live in trees and attack woodcutters when the trees are felled. In recent years this disease has extended into the Central American countries. Of the 118 cases of yellow fever reported world wide in 1969, 46 were in South America.

TYPHUS FEVER

Typhus fever is an acute infection accompanied by high fever and a rash. There are three forms of this disease: epidemic typhus (louse-borne, or classical typhus); endemic typhus (flea-borne, or murine typhus); and scrub typhus (mite-borne typhus, or Tsutsugamushi disease). All these diseases are caused by rickettsial organisms named in honor of Dr. Howard Taylor Ricketts, an American physician who died in 1910 while engaged in research on these microorganisms.[2]

Epidemic typhus (louse-borne typhus) has always accompanied wars, causing an enormous amount of illness and death among both military and civilian populations. It was an important contributory factor in Napoleon's defeat in the Russian campaign of 1812–1813. During World War I it killed hundreds of thousands of people in eastern Europe. By World War II much had been learned about typhus; but even so, it occurred in epidemic proportion among refugee groups and in many camps for war prisoners and displaced persons. Typhus fever disappears spontaneously with the observance of personal cleanliness. Specifically, its prevention depends primarily on the avoidance of lice. To aid in this, some extraordinarily effective insect repellents and insecticides, most notable DDT, were developed and utilized in World War II.

Between the World War I and World War II, a vaccine against typhus was perfected in this country and was given to all American military personnel sent into typhus areas. The result of these measures was that practically no typhus occurred among American troops, even though it was present in the civilian populations and among the unvaccinated troops of other armies in the same areas.

Endemic typhus (flea-borne typhus), which has been reported in several states along the Gulf of Mexico and along the South Atlantic coast, is much milder than epidemic typhus. Its reservoir is primarily the domestic rat, from which it is occasionally transmitted to man by the rat flea. Control measures are directed principally to the destruction of rats, or at least to keeping them out of human habitations. Inoculation with recently developed vaccine may be useful in special circumstances. Since 1944 there has been a marked decline in endemic typhus, with fewer cases in urban than in rural areas. Many factors such as new housing, better care of garbage, ratproofing of buildings, the extensive use of insecticide dusting programs, and the newer rodenticides have aided

---

[2]See Hans Zinsser, *Rats, Lice and History*, Little, Brown and Company, Boston, 1935, for a fascinating story of the effect of typhus on the history of the world.

in the control of this disease. In 1969, 28 cases were reported in Texas with fleas from cats implicated as vectors in several cases.

Scrub typhus (mite-borne typhus) was a serious problem among United States troops in certain areas of southeastern Asia during World War II. The mites get onto people from jungle grass or underbrush. If at all possible, areas in which the disease occurs should be avoided. Clearing of brush and grass from camp sites and the wearing of protective clothing are control measures. No effective vaccine has been developed.

ROCKY MOUNTAIN SPOTTED FEVER

Rickettsial organisms are responsible also for Rocky Mountain spotted fever (also called *tick-borne typhus*). This infectious disease is widely distributed throughout the United States but is most prevalent in the Rocky Mountain, Middle Atlantic, and Southern seaboard states.

This disease has been especially studied in the Bitter Root Valley of Montana, where the occurrence of the malignant form is limited to the western slope of the valley. During the past few years, an "Eastern" type of Rocky Mountain spotted fever has been described. Both types are transmitted by ticks—the Western type by the wood tick, the Eastern type by the dog tick. In the southwestern United States the "Lone Star" tick has served as a vector. In this disease ticks serve both as reservoirs of the infection and as vectors which transmit it. In recent years there has been a great increase in reported cases, particularly in the East, with Virginia the major endemic area. Tick-infected areas should be avoided when possible. Preventive measures consist in frequent examination of the clothing and body for ticks and, if they are found, their careful removal without crushing.

In removing ticks from animals or human beings, the person should protect his hands. Vaccines containing killed Rickettsiae reduce the chance of infection and lower fatality rates of those who develop the disease.

RICKETTSIALPOX

Another rickettsial disease, called *rickettsialpox*, was recognized in New York City in 1946[3] when an epidemic occurred in a housing development. The disease is accompanied by chills, fever, and a rash; the fatality rate is negligible. The reservoir of the infection is the house mouse, and it is transmitted to man by a rodent mite. Thus prevention of the disease depends on the elimination of mice and mouse harborages. The disease is not spread from one person to another.

OTHER INSECT-BORNE DISEASES

Several diseases transmitted by insects from animals to man have been discussed earlier, namely, plague, tularemia, and encephalitis. Others of interest include dengue ("breakbone fever"), transmitted by the bite of various mosquitoes (the *Aëdes aegypti* and others); trypanosomiasis (African sleeping sickness), transmitted by the tsetse fly; trench fever, an important cause of loss of manpower hours in World War I, transmitted by the body louse; relapsing fever, transmitted by lice and by ticks (In 1968 10 out of 20 Boy Scouts contracted this disease after sleeping in old, rodent-infested cabins near Spokane, Washington); Colorado tick fever, transmitted by ticks; and onchocerciasis (river blindness), transmitted by the simulium fly. (See page 203.)

[3]Berton Rouché, "The Alerting of Mr. Pomerantz," in *Eleven Blue Men*, Little, Brown and Company, Boston, 1954, pp. 48–66.

QUESTIONS FOR DISCUSSION AND SELF-EXAMINATION

1 Compare the various microorganisms which can infect human beings. How do they differ in structure, way of life, transmission, and effects?

2 When are drugs useful in the treatment of communicable diseases, when are they ineffective, and when are they dangerous?

3 Does the word *infectious* mean the same thing in the terms *infectious mononucleosis* and *infectious hepatitis*? Defend your answer. (See also Chapters 2 and 12.)

4 Explain the relation between "reservoirs of infection" and "carriers." Be specific.

5   What diseases have occurred most frequently in major epidemics?

6   What communicable diseases have occurred widely and frequently but not in epidemics?

7   What are the two major types of immunity to infection and how are they induced?

8   What is the importance of animals and of insects in human disease? Are the two always involved together in a human disease if one is involved? Document your answer.

9   Describe the differences and similarities of isolation and quarantine. Of what use are they in the control of infectious disease, and how has their usefulness changed?

10 What do you consider the three most important measures in controlling the spread of communicable disease? Defend your answer.

REFERENCES AND READING SUGGESTIONS

BOOKS

Anderson, Gaylord W., Margaret Arnstein, and Mary R. Lester: *Communicable Disease Control*, 4th ed., The Macmillan Company, New York, 1962.

A vast amount of information on communicable diseases and measures to control them; not only is personal protection against communicable diseases discussed, but emphasis is placed on protection of the community.

de Kruif, Paul: *Microbe Hunters*, Harcourt, Brace & World, Inc., New York, 1954. (Also in paperback, Pocket Books, Inc., New York, 1959.)

Written over 30 years ago, this series of biographies has served as a fascinating introduction to the history of achievements in health for untold numbers of readers. The book has been reprinted many times.

Beneson, Aleron S. (ed): *Control of Communicable Diseases in Man*, 11th ed., American Public Health Association, Washington, 1970.

The official 5-year report by the American Public Health Association of current knowledge concerning the nature, occurrence, cause, reservoir of infection, mode of transmission, incubation period, period of communicability, susceptibility resistance, immunization, and methods of control of the communicable diseases of man.

Vallery-Radot, René: *The Life of Pasteur*, paperback, Dover Publications, Inc., New York, 1960.

The standard biography by Pasteur's son-in-law, reprinted from the translation by Mrs. R. L. Devonshire (1901). The introduction by Sir William Osler is excellent.

Williams, Greer: *The Plague Killers*, Charles Scribner's Sons, New York, 1968.

A fascinating story of one of mankind's greatest achievements, the control of many diseases which for centuries undermined personal health and national vitality. Prominent among these are malaria, yellow fever, typhus fever, and hookworms—diseases which have been virtually eliminated in many countries but which are still serious handicaps to social, economic, and political progress in most of the developing countries of the world.

PAMPHLETS AND PERIODICALS

Edelson, Edward: "The Battle against the Virus," *Family Health*, April 1971, p. 18.

A dramatized report of some of the research that is in progress concerning *interferon*, a substance produced by body cells which helps protect against certain virus infections.

Roueché, Berton: "Annals of Medicine: The Simpsons and the Hepatitides," *New Yorker*, p. 72, Aug. 21, 1971.

A fascinating story of an epidemiological investigation (medical detective work) to determine the source of an epidemic of 76 cases of infectious hepatitis, centered in a community of 2,025 population in northeastern Michigan.

Rhodes, Lynwood Mark: "Why Cholera Is the Disease Nations Try to Hide," *Today's Health*, June 1971, p. 51.

A summary of current outbreaks of cholera, the methods by which it is spread, its treatment, and its social and economic consequences.

17

IMMUNIZATIONS OF VALUE[1]

The most dramatic and far-reaching achievement of medical science has been the development of vaccines and other immunizations which provide protection against diseases that for centuries were a constant menace to health and to life and frequently took an awesome toll in localized epidemics or in worldwide pandemics. (Figure 17.1.)

Immunization is extremely valuable not only to the individual whose health, and perhaps life, is protected by it but also to the community in which he lives. To spread in a community, a contagious disease needs a number of people in frequent contact with each other who are susceptible to the disease. When immunization or a previous attack of the disease or a natural immunity has resulted in 80 percent or more of the people in a community being immune to the disease, epidemics cannot occur. If a random case of the disease develops in such a community, it will spread to only one or two other people, or not at all, for the chances of many susceptible individuals having sufficient contact with the disease to contract it are very, very small.

The most important immunizations now available and in use are listed in Table 17.1 and discussed in this chapter.

SMALLPOX

A person living today cannot possibly realize what smallpox meant before the days of vaccination. Smallpox was as inevitable then as chicken pox is today. In fact, it was then considered primarily a children's disease, for one rarely reached adult life without having had it. It has been estimated

[1]Statements concerning immunizations are based upon the recommendations of the U.S. Public Health Service Advisory Committee on Immunization Practices, Department of Health, Education, and Welfare.

Figure 17.1   Immunizations in a rural area. (Photograph from United Nations.)

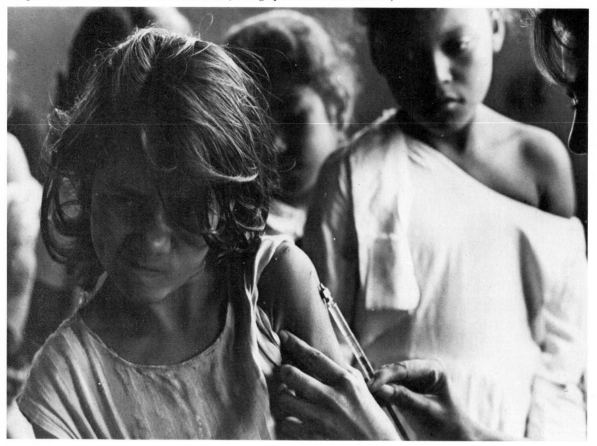

that 60 million people in Europe died of smallpox during the eighteenth century. Smallpox was prevalent in India, China, and Egypt for thousands of years, but it did not appear in Europe until about the fifteenth century. Charles IX and Louis XIV in France carried scars of the disease, and Louis XV died of it. George Washington contracted smallpox in the West Indies. Queen Mary, wife of William III, died in London of smallpox in 1694 at the age of 33.

Smallpox was brought into Mexico by the Spaniards soon after the discovery of America. Within a short period 3.5 million persons were said to have died of the disease in Mexico alone. Rapidly the disease spread to the North American Indians, and it has been estimated that half of them died of it in a short time.

Smallpox is caused by a virus which is present in discharges from the nose and throat and in the pus and crusts. It is spread primarily through the air and is highly contagious. It is a severe febrile disease accompanied by a rash that is first red spots, then raised red areas. These are followed by vesicles (small blisters) which fill with pus, then dry and become crusted, and eventually drop off.

Smallpox varies enormously in severity. In prevaccination days it was always severe, being fatal to between 20 to 30 percent of its victims. But just prior to the beginning of the twentieth century a very mild form of smallpox appeared in Florida and spread rapidly over the whole of the United States. Since then this mild, nonfatal type of the disease has predominated to such an extent that people have become careless about maintaining

Table 17.1 Immunizations of public health importance in the United States

Disease	Immunizing material	Immunity produced Type	Dependable duration	Recommended For whom	When
Smallpox	Cowpox virus	Active	5–10 years	All normal persons in areas in which smallpox exits	1st: 3 to 9 months of age 2d: entrance to school Later: every 5 or 6 years and during epidemics
Diphtheria	1. Toxoid	Active	5–10 years	All normal children and susceptible adults especially exposed, such as nurses and physicians	1st: 3 to 6 months of age 2d: entrance to school and at 5-year intervals to age 15
	1. Antitoxin	Passive	2–3 months	Exposed infants and young children	If not immunized and closely exposed to disease
Typhoid and para-typhoid fever	Dead germs	Active	2–3 years	Susceptibles	On exposure to disease or before traveling in foreign countries
Whooping cough	Dead germs	Active	Several years	Infants, children	4 months of age
Measles	1. Attenuated virus	Active	Prolonged	Infants	9 months of age
	2. Immune blood serum, gamma globulin, or placental extract	Passive	Few weeks	Exposed infants	On exposure to disease
Mumps	Attenuated virus	Active	Probably life	Children	1 year or older
Tetanus	1. Toxoid	Active	Probably 5–10 years	Children Adults	In infancy When likely to be exposed
	2. Antitoxin	Passive	Few weeks	Exposed children Exposed adults	After injuries likely to be contaminated, if toxoid has not been administered
Rabies	Attenuated virus	Active	Undetermined	Anyone exposed	On exposure to saliva of suspected animal
Combined immunization	Diphtheria and tetanus toxoid and whooping cough vaccine	Active	5–10 years	Infants	3 months of age Repeat at school age without whooping cough vaccine
Poliomyelitis	Dead or attenuated virus	Active	Not yet known	All persons under 40 years of age	In infancy or later
Rubella	Attenuated virus	Active	Not yet known	All children	1 to 6 years of age

*Combined immunization may also contain poliomyelitis vaccine.

immunity to it. This is unfortunate, for whenever a sufficient proportion of the population becomes susceptible an epidemic of smallpox is possible. Whether an epidemic is mild or severe depends on which type of infection happens to be introduced.

In the winter of 1924–1925 such a calamity occurred. People had become negligent about vaccination, and when the malignant type of smallpox was brought into this country several serious epidemics occurred. In Minneapolis alone during December and January of that year there were approximately 1,000 cases of smallpox, with 300 deaths. During that winter seventeen cities of 100,000 population or more reported deaths from smallpox; and some of these, notably Detroit, Toledo, and Camden, had very high rates. In localized outbreaks of smallpox in 1962 and 1963 in England and Sweden, the fatality rate in unvaccinated persons was 40 percent.

These facts and other similar considerations have made some public health authorities skeptical of the wisdom of the withdrawal by the U. S. Public Health Service, in 1971, of support for required smallpox vaccination. Travellers entering the United States are now required to have current smallpox vaccination *only* if they have come from a country where smallpox is known to be endemic. Furthermore, the Public Health Service recommended that states, communities, and institutions drop any requirements for smallpox vaccination. Their reasoning is that smallpox is now uncommon in the world, having been eliminated from large areas. Furthermore, the complications of vaccination, even though extremely rare, have recently been causing more illness and even death than smallpox itself in the United States. It was believed that if a case of smallpox were diagnosed in the United States, danger of an epidemic could be eliminated by vaccinating all contacts and the entire local community. Other authorities, however, remembering the Minnesota epidemic and other such episodes, expressed concern that once a nonimmune population has developed, perhaps in 20 or 30 years, serious epidemics of smallpox could occur again in the United States.

The occurrence of smallpox is in no way influenced by climate, soil, age, or occupation. It affects alike the rich and the poor, the clean and the dirty. It spreads wherever the contagion finds

susceptible people. The one and only method of controlling it is to raise individual resistance by means of vaccination.

Vaccination as we know it today was developed after 20 years of experimentation by Edward Jenner in England in 1796. Before this, many persons were immunized by inoculation with material taken from a sore on a patient with a mild case of smallpox and rubbed into a slight abrasion of the skin of the person to be protected. This practice had been in vogue for centuries in India and China. Mild cases of smallpox and lifelong immunity usually developed in persons thus inoculated. It is said that an English physician was granted a life annuity of 10,000 pounds for performing this service for Catherine the Great of Russia.

During a serious epidemic of smallpox in Boston shortly before the American Revolution two hospitals were set aside for such inoculations. Treatment consisted of "inoculation, festering, diet and medicines, drying up and convalescence." Patients were kept in the hospital for 3 or 4 weeks and then were isolated at home for 2 or 3 weeks.

Smallpox was so prevalent in the Continental Army during the first two years of the Revolutionary War that the number of available troops was greatly reduced and the fear of the disease discouraged recruiting. On January 6, 1777, General Washington said that smallpox was "the greatest enemy of the Continental Army" and ordered the inoculation of all troops and new recruits. Smallpox inoculation involved a risk of death of 3 per 1,000 as compared to 160 per 1,000 for naturally acquired smallpox. After inoculation the army was essentially free of smallpox, and its effectiveness was so greatly improved that this procedure is reported to have been "an important factor in saving the army from disintegration and in securing the successful outcome of the Revolutionary war." Smallpox vaccination, after its development by Jenner, was ordered for the U.S. Army on May 26, 1812, the eve of the outbreak of the War of 1812.

Dr. Edward Jenner, a practicing physician in rural England, investigated the folklore belief of peasants that persons who contracted a mild disease of cattle called *cowpox* did not get smallpox. His studies convinced him that this was true, and in 1796 he published a report to this effect. His proof was that persons who were inoculated with cowpox and then after recovery were exposed to smallpox or were inoculated with the discharge from a sore of a smallpox patient did not develop the disease. There was skepticism at first concerning this, but his results were confirmed by others and his method of vaccination came to be used wherever smallpox occurred.

Smallpox vaccination, although still confused in the minds of some with inoculation of smallpox material, is an entirely different procedure. Vaccine is obtained not from patients with smallpox but from healthy calves which have been inoculated with cowpox, or from laboratory cultures of cowpox virus on chick-embryo culture medium. In the preparation of this vaccine the most careful surgical technique is used, after which the vaccine is tested for purity and then accurately standardized.

The technique of vaccination is to introduce a very small amount of vaccine into the skin, usually of the arm. In a few days the skin becomes red and swollen and one typical cowpox lesion develops. This should be protected from dirt, kept dry, and not touched. Shields should not be worn. Usually no bandage is necessary.

Complications of vaccination occasionally oc-cur but the risk is infinitesimal in comparison with the protection conferred by vaccination.

Immunity developed as a result of vaccination is variable in degree and duration, and decreases with time. It usually provides a high level of protection for at least 3 years and a waning immunity for 10 years or longer. The first vaccination has been recommended during the third year of life: that is, between the second and third birthdays. The chances of reactions at this age are less than during the first year. However, vaccination should be performed at any time that there is a risk of exposure to smallpox, as in foreign travel. Revaccination has been recommended when the child enters school and subsequently every 5 years. Revaccination is recommended also whenever there is an outbreak of the disease in the community and whenever a trip abroad is planned that includes areas in which smallpox exists. It must be remembered that smallpox has not yet been placed in the "museum of medical curiosities" and that possibilities of infection still exist. However, only 31,000 cases of smallpox were reported for 1970 throughout the world, and the World Health Organization believes that this dread disease can soon be eliminated.

DIPHTHERIA

Over the past 5 years, the annual median number of diphtheria cases reported in the United States was 187. In 1940, 30 years earlier, there were 30,018 cases and 3,065 deaths. Yet the possibility that outbreaks of diphtheria may still occur is illustrated by nine reported cases and three deaths in Miami in October and November 1969. Within the next month 70,000 children were vaccinated to put an end to the possibility of an epidemic. Many cases of diphtheria in the United States in recent years have occurred in adults whose immunity has declined since their childhood immunization.

Diphtheria is caused by a bacillus which sets up an infection in the throat and gives off a toxin (poison) which is absorbed into the bloodstream and carried throughout the body. This may affect the nervous system, causing paralysis, and the heart muscle, causing heart failure. For a patient to recover from the diphtheria, this toxin must be neutralized by antitoxin which the body produces or which is injected for treatment.

Diphtheria organisms are disseminated in the nose and throat discharges of patients and carriers. They are transmitted principally through direct contact with the infected droplets. Diphtheria bacilli may be spread also by articles soiled with discharges from diphtheria patients and carriers. Before the days of pasteurization various epidemics were traced to milk.

The most important measure for the prevention of diphtheria is the active immunization of children. This is accomplished by the injection of modified diphtheria toxin, called *toxoid*. This is safe and effective. To infants and young children triple antigens (tetanus and diphtheria toxoids combined with whooping cough vaccine) are frequently administered. For adults a mixture of tetanus toxoid and diphtheria toxoid is commonly used in order to maintain immunity to both diseases.

Diphtheria antitoxin, which is prepared from the blood serum of a horse previously injected with diphtheria toxin, contains protective substances which neutralize the diphtheria toxin, and so is useful for treatment or for temporary protection. Before the use of antitoxin, which was developed about the beginning of the present century, approximately one person out of every three who got diphtheria died. With antitoxin available there would be practically no deaths if the antitoxin were administered at the very onset of the disease and in sufficient dosage.

The Schick test, a dependable test of immunity against diphtheria, involves the injection into the skin of the forearm of a very small, definitely measured amount of diphtheria toxin. If redness results, the reaction is considered positive and indicates that the person is susceptible to diph-

theria. No redness in 2 days indicates immunity. With infants and young children this test is rarely used, because so many of them are susceptible that it is better to immunize them all than to attempt to pick out the few who might be naturally immune. Among older children and adults, however, the proportion of immune individuals is greater, and hence, the test gives information of distinct value.

If reasonable use were made of available scientific knowledge, diphtheria would soon become as unknown in the United States as cholera and yellow fever. There is a test which determines who is susceptible; there is an immunizing agent which gives prolonged immunity; there is an effective antitoxin for treatment of the susceptible people who develop the disease. Nothing more could be desired. But it remains for the public to maintain universal immunity by cooperation with their physicians and public health authorities.

TETANUS

Tetanus is the scientific name for the disease called *lockjaw*. The cause is a bacillus which in the absence of oxygen produces a toxin that causes violent muscular spasms. The jaw muscles are among the ones first affected; hence, the name *lockjaw*. Tetanus bacteria, in the form of spores, stay alive in dirt, but they do not produce toxin as long as they are exposed to air. In deep wounds, where they are shut off from air, they grow and produce toxin. Tetanus has occurred as a result of superficial scratches, however, and the bacteria have caused the disease by growing in ulcerated areas on the legs of people with vascular disease. The fatality rate for this disease averages about 35 percent.

The normal habitat of tetanus germs is the intestinal tract of horses and other herbivorous animals. Hence, the tetanus organisms are most likely to be found in the excreta of these animals. Barnyards, highways, fields, and gardens in which manure is used as a fertilizer are practically certain to abound with the spores of this organism.

The widespread belief that tetanus is likely to develop in wounds contracted by stepping on a rusty nail has a valid basis. A nail can make a

deep, penetrating wound which may seal itself and thus provide a good environment for the growth of tetanus organisms; there is also a good chance that a rusty nail which has been lying on the ground or on the barn floor may be carrying the tetanus bacillus. The danger from the rusty nail about which mothers for so long have warned their barefoot youngsters is neither in the nail nor in the rust. The danger lies in the probability that the nail is heavily contaminated with tetanus organisms.

On a cattle range or where manure is used as fertilizer, the soil is practically certain to be heavily contaminated; the machinery and tools a farmer uses are also heavily contaminated; thus, the farmer is constantly exposed to the danger of tetanus. Long-lasting protection through the use of tetanus toxoid is therefore especially important for him. Stockyard workers and sheepherders are among other occupational groups constantly exposed to this organism. And in this age of automobiles, urban dwellers frequently go to rural areas where they may come in contact with the tetanus organism. Furthermore, in recent years, a considerable proportion of tetanus cases occurred in nonrural areas following abrasions of the skin. They occur also among narcotic addicts who become infected by the use of nonsterile needles.

Active, prolonged immunity against tetanus is obtained by the injection of tetanus toxoid. It is now recommended that tetanus toxoid be given to all children in infancy. This is important since children often suffer minor injuries playing in potentially contaminated soil or street dirt. Such injections will provide prolonged protection, but "booster doses" should be given about the time of entrance to school and every 10 years thereafter. Tetanus toxoid is usually given along with diphtheria toxoid and whooping cough vaccine in the "triple antigen," or with the new "four-in-one" antigen, which also contains poliomyelitis vaccine.

When a person who has been immunized by toxoid injections is injured and contamination of the wound by tetanus organisms is considered a possibility, a "booster shot" of toxoid should be given.

Tetanus antitoxin, which, like diphtheria antitoxin, is prepared from horses, gives a passive protection against tetanus toxin. This is useful for the prevention of the disease in persons who receive deep wounds in areas where tetanus organisms are likely to be present and who have not been immunized with tetanus toxoid.

WHOOPING COUGH

Whooping cough, or pertussis is most serious for infants. In fact, in 1970 whooping cough caused 20 deaths in this country, most of which were of children under the age of 4. Pneumonia is the complication which causes most of the deaths.

The disease is caused by an organism present in secretions from the nose and throat and usually is spread directly from one person to another. The early symptoms are those of a common cold. The cough gradually increases in severity and then comes in series of explosive coughs followed by the characteristic "whoop." Whooping cough is a disease for which the seriously sick child needs constant nursing attendance.

An active immunization is now available in pertussis vaccine. In routine immunizations of infants the vaccine can be given along with the immunizing agents against diphtheria and tetanus. Hyperimmune gamma globulin and pertussis immune serum are available to give passive immunization either for treatment or for the protection of young children who have been exposed to the disease.

POLIOMYELITIS

Poliomyelitis, or *infantile paralysis,* as it has been known for many years, is a disease of great antiquity. An ancient Egyptian carving shows the wasted leg muscles of a polio victim. Poliomyelitis is an apt name for the disease in which inflammation of the gray matter of the central nervous system occurs (*polio* in Greek means gray, *myelos* means marrow, and *itis* means inflammation).

Poliomyelitis is an acute communicable disease caused by a virus and usually characterized be a fever, headache, stiffness of the neck and back, and general discomfort. The early signs and symptoms are vague or may be absent. Thus many cases of poliomyelitis are overlooked. The virus affects the cells of the spinal cord, causing weakness and paralysis. The paralysis may be temporary or, if enough of the motor nerve cells to the muscles involved are destroyed, it may be permanent. When nerve cells in the spinal cord which control movements below the neck are damaged, the disease is often spoken of as *spinal polio.* In *bulbar polio,* cranial nerves and nerve centers in the base of the brain, the most vital of which control breathing, circulation, and swallowing, may be affected. The fatality rate varies from 5 to 60 percent in the bulbar type, and from 2 to 10 percent for all cases during an epidemic.

The disease agent which causes poliomyelitis

is a virus, of which there are three types. An attack makes an individual permanently immune against the type of virus involved. It provides, however, little if any protection against infection by one of the other types of virus. After the onset of poliomyelitis the virus is found in the secretions of the nose and throat. Later it appears in the fecal discharges, where it continues for a period of several weeks.

Intimate association and droplet spread from infected persons account for most of the transmission. In the dissemination of this disease, mild, unrecognized cases are of greatest importance. There is no evidence that milk, water, other foods, sewage, or insects play significant roles in the transmission of the disease agent. A person most often comes down with the disease 10 to 12 days after exposure and is most infectious to others during the latter part of this period and the first few days of the acute illness.

Before the development of immunization procedures, studies of the blood serum of the adult population in different parts of the country showed that 50 to 80 percent of persons contained antibodies against the virus of poliomyelitis. These figures indicate that most persons at some time or other have been infected with poliomyelitis virus and that paralysis is infrequent.

A safe and effective vaccine against poliomyelitis became available in 1954. This vaccine, which was developed by Dr. Jonas Salk, contains all three strains or types of poliomyelitis virus killed by treatment with formaline, and is called the *inactivated poliovirus vaccine* (IPV). This vaccine is exceedingly effective in preventing paralytic poliomyelitis. However, its use has been largely replaced by a vaccine that is given by mouth, developed by Dr. Albert Sabin. This consists of live attenuated virus and is called the *oral poliovirus vaccine* (OPV). This vaccine is available either against each of three individual types of poliomyelitis virus separately or as a combined vaccine against all three types of virus. This combined trivalent vaccine is now used almost exclusively because of the ease of its administration. An initial vaccination with three doses of this vaccine will produce immunity to the three types of poliovirus in well over 90 percent of persons.

The three-dose immunization series should be started at 6 to 12 weeks of age, commonly with the first dose of diphtheria-tetanus-pertussis vaccine. On entering school, all children who have had the three-dose primary series of oral vaccine should be given a single dose of the same vaccine. Children or adults who did not receive the vaccine as infants should be given the primary series of three doses. There is no need for routine booster doses beyond the time of entering school. However, a single dose of the trivalent vaccine can be given to persons who are likely to be exposed to poliomyelitis because of travel or occupation.

Very rarely paralysis has occurred in persons who have received the oral vaccine or among their close contacts. However, only one case of "vaccine-associated" paralysis in recipients and two in close contacts have been reported for each 9 million doses of vaccine given.

These vaccines, which represent one of the great triumphs of medical science, are associated, and properly so, with the names of Dr. Salk and Dr. Sabin. However, much of the work which made these and other vaccines possible was done by a brilliant, unassuming man practically unknown to the public, working in an unpretentious laboratory in Boston in the 1930s, 1940s, and 1950s: Dr. John F. Enders. His peers respected him, and the experts gave him the Nobel Prize for his work with viruses. It was he who made most of the progress in getting viruses to grow in tissue cultures. His early methods were laborious, difficult, and by today's standards undeveloped. But they established the principles which made it possible to safeguard the health and the lives of millions.

Since these vaccines have been in use, paralytic poliomyelitis has almost disappeared in this country. However, low immunization rates still prevail in certain disadvantaged urban and rural groups, particularly among infants and young children born since the mass immunization campaigns conducted between 1958 and 1962. Most of the cases of paralytic poliomyelitis in recent years occurred in these groups. To ensure continued freedom from this disease, it is necessary to continue regular immunization of all children from early infancy. The increasing numbers of unprotected children in this country are causing great concern among public health authorities.

MEASLES

Measles, although frequently considered trivial, is a serious disease in infancy. Before the advent of modern drugs to combat complicating pneumonia, the fatality rate in infants sometimes reached 30 percent or more. About 97 percent of measles cases in this country occur below the age of 15 years. In 1960 there were 380 deaths and in 1968, 24 deaths from measles in the United States. Among the serious complications of measles are encephalitis, middle-ear infections, pneumonia, and bronchitis.

Two historic examples of the virulence which measles can attain when introduced into nonimmune populations are the epidemics in the Faroe and Fiji Islands. In the Faroe Islands no measles had occurred for 65 years; but when it was reintroduced in 1846, it killed a quarter of the population. In the Fiji Islands, measles had been unknown until it was introduced by some trading vessels and killed 40,000 persons in a population of 150,000. It is reported that measles is today one of the serious health problems in rural Africa.

The cause of measles is a virus spread by discharges from the nose and throat. The incubation period is 14 days. Early symptoms resemble those of an ordinary cold. It is in this stage that measles is most highly contagious. Later stages are characterized by a general rash, by spots in the mouth, and by fever.

A vaccine for active immunization against measles was licensed by the U.S. Public Health Service for general use in 1963. This vaccine, which consists of attenuated measles virus, occasionally causes a mild febrile reaction, but it provides a high level of protection against a disease that has been practically universal and can be very serious in infants. Administration of this vaccine at 12 months of age is recommended.

Experience with more than 35 million vaccinations in the United States indicates that live measles virus vaccines are among the safest immunizing agents available. Officials of the U.S. Public Health Service state that if all children were vaccinated before school age, measles could be completely eradicated in the United States.

Measles vaccination will usually prevent the disease if it is administered before or on the day of exposure to someone with the disease. Protection is not conferred when vaccine is given after the day of exposure.

Passive immunization is available for the protection of unimmunized children known to have been exposed to measles. Gamma globulin or placental extract may be used. Depending on the amount of gamma globulin used and the time when it is given, the disease may be either prevented or modified in its severity. The protection from such injections is temporary but usually long enough to safeguard a child during a current epidemic. The child will soon be susceptible again, unless he has had a mild form of the disease. Each year, however, that an attack of measles can be postponed means a material reduction in the danger to the child.

Vaccination programs have brought a 95 percent reduction in the incidence of measles. However, the percentage of children immunized against measles has been declining over the past several years and cases of measles have been increasing: 47,351 cases and 120 deaths in 1970 as compared with 22,231 cases and 24 deaths in 1968, an increase of 100 percent in cases and 400 percent in deaths in 2 years. This trend is a matter for real concern.

RUBELLA

Rubella, also called *German measles* or *3-day measles*, is a mild virus disease, frequently accompanied by a rash that may resemble either measles or scarlet fever. A child may have such a mild case that parents do not realize that he is sick. However, during pregnancy the disease may cause serious problems in the unborn baby. These were first noted in 1941 when an Australian ophthalmologist called attention to the occurrence of cataracts in the offspring of mothers who had had German measles in the early months of pregnancy. Other studies followed these original observations and showed that congenital defects not only of the eye but of other organs, such as ear, heart, and teeth, had occurred. Thus a disease to which little attention had been paid assumed great importance.

The most extensive epidemic of rubella in recent years occurred in 1964–1965, when 8,000 fetal deaths and more than 1,800,000 cases, including 247,000 women in the first 3 months of pregnancy, were reported in the United States. This epidemic caused an estimated 20,000 children to be born with serious birth defects.

Just how often congenital anomalies occur as a result of this disease is not known. It has been estimated that up to 50 percent of children born after the mother has had German measles during the first 3 months (the first trimester) of pregnancy have abnormalities of one kind or another and that in smaller numbers abnormalities may occur if the mother contracts the disease between the third and sixth month of pregnancy. It is most important, therefore, that young women be immune to this disease. An attack gives lifelong immunity; but if an attack occurs during pregnancy, the results may be tragic.

Fortunately, a safe and effective attenuated live virus vaccine against rubella has become available. Public health authorities recommend that children 1 to 14 years of age be vaccinated. They believe that if 60 to 70 million children were given a single injection of this vaccine, the disease would be wiped out.

If, in spite of attempts to avoid exposure to German measles during early pregnancy, such exposure does occur, the physician may recommend use of passive immunization in the form of immune serum globulin (gamma globulin). However, its effectiveness is uncertain.

MUMPS

Mumps, one of the common communicable diseases, is caused by a virus and occurs most frequently in childhood. Its onset is sudden, accompanied by fever and by swelling and tenderness of one or more of the salivary glands, most frequently the parotid glands at the angles of the jaw. The ovaries and testicles may be involved, particularly in persons past puberty. For this reason mumps, unlike most infectious diseases, is less serious in children than in adults. Meningitis, encephalitis, and nerve deafness are serious but infrequent complications.

The peak season for mumps is late winter and early spring. Most cases occur in children between the ages of 5 and 15, but the most serious cases are likely to occur in adult and adolescent males.

The incubation period of mumps is 12 to 26 days, commonly 18 days. The virus is present in the saliva of infected persons and is spread by droplets of moisture in the air, by direct contact, or indirectly through articles freshly soiled by the saliva of infected persons.

Mumps vaccine, made from an inactivated virus, has recently become available. This provides substantial protection in about 95 percent of persons. Only one dose given by injection is required. How long immunity will last is unknown, but observations over a 3-year period show continuing protection. Immunity following an attack of mumps is usually lifelong.

This vaccine may be given to children at any age after 12 months. It is of particular value for children approaching puberty, for adolescents and for adults, particularly males, who have not had mumps. It is not known whether mumps vaccine will provide protection after exposure to the disease, but there is no contraindication to its use at this time.

A combined vaccine for measles, mumps, and German measles is proving just as effective in early trials as the three vaccines given separately.

TYPHOID FEVER

Typhoid fever, discussed more fully in Chapter 12, has been almost wiped out in many parts of the world by sanitation of water, milk, and food supplies. In the armed services and certain other groups, however, sanitary measures are supplemented by the use of typhoid vaccine, which consists of dead typhoid organisms.

The efficacy of typhoid vaccination in increasing resistance to this disease is beyond question. Studies indicate that it provides 70 to 90 percent protection. However, the hazard of typhoid fever has been so greatly reduced that few people in civil life consider it necessary to keep up individual resistance by means of vaccination. This is a reasonable course to follow when the sanitary status of the available water, food, and milk is known. On the other hand, travelers, particularly in foreign countries where sanitary conditions are primitive, will find in typhoid vaccination cheap insurance against a serious disease. Such vaccination, however, does not mean that an individual may drink contaminated water or eat contaminated food with impunity, both because typhoid vaccination does not give complete protection and because of the danger of other intestinal infections.

OTHER IMMUNIZATIONS

Numerous other vaccines and serums are available. Cold vaccines, influenza vaccine, and BCG vaccine against tuberculosis are considered elsewhere (Chapter 18.) Certain other immunizing materials such as botulinus antitoxin and vaccines against plague, typhus, cholera, yellow fever, and Rocky Mountain spotted fever are of definite value but are used only in specific situations.

IMMUNIZATION PROCEDURES FOR INTERNATIONAL TRAVEL

Today more than ever before Americans are traveling abroad and literally journeying to all areas of the earth. Whether the trip is for business or for pleasure, it is possible for the tourist to become infected with communicable diseases. If this occurs, the infected person may endanger not only his own health but the health of persons in countries where he is traveling; and upon his return home, he may endanger the health of his own community.

Certain sanitary regulations for international travel have been established, to a large extent as a result of agreements made between governments. Unless such rules are observed, travelers may experience delays and even serious interferences with travel plans.

Since there are changes from time to time in immunization requirements, they should be checked well in advance of a trip. The Division of Foreign Quarantine of the U.S. Public Health Service has prepared a booklet[2] for the information of persons planning international travel. Information can be procured also from state and local health departments, from branches of the U.S. Public Health Service, or from shipping and airline offices. It should be borne in mind that the International Certificate of Vaccination form is the only one accepted for foreign travel.

[2]The booklet *Immunization Information for International Travel* may be purchased from the Superintendent of Documents, U.S. Government Printing Office, at a nominal cost.

MISCONCEPTIONS CONCERNING IMMUNIZATIONS

In spite of the demonstrated safety and value of vaccines, there is still much misinformation and misunderstanding concerning them. Some of this is based on lack of understanding or honest doubt, but people should realize that there is definite, organized propaganda against immunization procedures. Some of the enemies of immunization are merely misinformed, misguided individuals. Others are interested in securing adherents to a particular form of treatment or disease prevention. Some practitioners of the so-called *healing cults* have been known to seek vaccination for themselves while advising their patients to avoid it.

The question most frequently raised concerning artificial immunization is whether it may be deleterious to inject foreign substances such as dead or weakened organisms or their products into the body. This is a natural and perfectly proper question, particularly when several immunizations are suggested. The answer is obvious, however, if one considers that when a person contracts these diseases and recovers, recovery is almost always complete, even though enormous quantities of the infectious organisms have permeated the body. In vaccinations the quantities introduced into the body are definitely known and are far below the amounts which can cause damage. Such injections may not produce so great or so prolonged an immunity as usually follows an attack of the disease; but neither do they carry the hazards of prolonged illness, serious complications, and even death that accompany natural infection.

QUESTIONS FOR DISCUSSION AND SELF-EXAMINATION

1 How do cowpox and smallpox differ? How is vaccination related to these two diseases?

2 What are the relative places of active immunity and passive immunity in public programs of disease control? (See also Chapter 16.)

3 Why is active immunization against tetanus preferable to passive immunization? Give details.

4 Which programs of immunization may have saved the most lives? Document your answer.

5 Describe the diseases which can be eliminated in the United States by more vigorous immunization programs but which are now represented by at least a few cases each year?

6 What factors prevent immunization from being completely effective in eliminating contagious disease?

7 Which disease has had two major vaccines developed to combat it? How do they differ?

8 Describe the variation in the effects of measles in different populations. What accounts for this variation?

9 Which diseases are known to cause defects in some unborn babies when suffered by the mother? What are the defects which occur?

10 What are "booster doses," and what are their importance and function?

REFERENCES AND READING SUGGESTIONS

BOOKS

Benenson, Abram S. (ed): *Control of Communicable Diseases in Man*, 11th ed., American Public Health Association, Washington, D.C., 1970.

Carter, Richard: *Break-through: The Saga of Jonas Salk*, Trident Press, a division of Simon & Schuster, Inc., New York, 1966.

A dramatic and accurate story of the life, vicissitudes, and final success of Jonas Salk in developing a vaccine against poliomyelitis—one of the great medical breakthroughs of our time.

Panum, Peter L.: *Observations Made during the Epidemic of Measles in the Faroe Islands in the Year 1846*, Bibl. Lager, Copenhagen, 1847 (translation published by American Public Health Association, New York, 1940).

This famous study of measles is a classic in the field of communicable diseases. Students interested in the historical background of such diseases will find the reading of this account, prepared when Panum was 26 years of age, a stimulating experience.

Peacock, D. B., and E. R. Gold: *Introduction to Immunology*, The Williams & Wilkins Company, Baltimore, 1965.

A not-too-technical discussion of the principles of immunology and their application to the prevention of disease.

PAMPHLETS AND PERIODICALS

Pediatrics Panel: "Give the Shots Earlier and Skip Smallpox," *Medical World News,* Nov. 5, 1971.

A summary of the recommendations of the Committee on Infectious Diseases of the American Academy of Pediatrics.

Editorial: "Smallpox Vaccination," *Journal of the American Medical Association,* Chicago, Ill., Nov. 8, 1971, p. 876.

An excellent review of the development of smallpox vaccination, its effectiveness in controlling this disease, and why the U.S. Public Health Service is now recommending that routine smallpox vaccination of all children in this country be discontinued.

Immunization Information for International Travel, U.S. Public Health Service, Communicable Disease Center, Atlanta, Ga.

This information, which is constantly being updated, is available also from local offices of the U.S. Public Health Service, from state and local health departments, and from travel agencies.

18

RESPIRATORY DISEASES

Dick S. had had five colds in the previous 6 months, and went to his college health service for help. He received a thorough examination, including consultation with a specialist in nose and throat disease who could find no abnormalities. In most people's lives the frequency of colds varies from time to time; any sort of medication, from vitamin C to injections of plain sterile water may appear to reduce the frequency of colds. In Dick's case, there was no disease which was undermining his health, the diet which he reported eating was adequate, and there was no local factor in his nose, throat, or sinuses which rendered him susceptible to colds. The physician did discover that his colds often lingered unusually long, with pain over the sinuses upon pressure, which suggested that he had sinusitis as a complication to some of his colds. Dick also told him that he blew his nose vigorously, and the physician pointed out that he might be causing his own sinusitis by forcing nasal secretions, including bacteria, into the sinuses from the nose. Fortunately, Dick was able to accept this advice and did not waste his money on unnecessary popular preventatives or treatments.

The most common portal of entry into the body of disease-producing microorganisms, noxious fumes, gases, and other deleterious substances is the respiratory system. Some of these agents produce generalized infections; others give rise to diseases that affect primarily the respiratory organs: the nose, pharynx (throat), larynx, trachea, bronchi, and lungs.

COLDS

The common cold has been simply but well described as an infectious "runny nose." Other conditions, such as allergies, chilling, or emotional disturbances, may produce a runny nose, but these are not colds. The common cold is caused by viruses which are present in nasal discharges and can be spread to others by sneezing, by blowing the nose, or by direct or indirect contact.

The common cold is never fatal, and rarely serious. Yet it is the leading cause of illness in this country and, according to estimates by the U.S. Public Health Service, is responsible for the loss of 150 million work-days annually. In a 9-year study of a large number of families in Cleveland, Ohio, it was found that respiratory diseases accounted for two-thirds of all the illnesses in these families and that colds are the most frequent type of respiratory illness.

COLD VIRUSES

Many researchers have shown that viruses present in the nose and throat secretions of patients with colds, when introduced into the nasal cavity of others, will produce colds in approximately 50 percent of volunteers.

The usual symptoms of virus colds are stuffiness of the nose, sneezing, watery nasal discharge, dryness and soreness of the throat, and occasionally mild headaches. Mild general aching and discomfort may occur, but there is little or no elevation of temperature. The usual duration is 4 to 5 days. Secondary infections with other germs (bacteria) that attack the nose and throat or lungs may follow. Colds with similar symptoms may be caused by different viruses and the same virus may produce different symptoms in different people or under different conditions.

A number of other viruses, some of which are called *adenoviruses*, also cause acute upper respiratory infections. Fever, sore throat, headache, general aching, and conjunctivitis are the common symptoms of infection with adenoviruses. Outbreaks are most common among military recruits but may also occur in civilian institutions or summer camps. A vaccine has been developed which is effective in protecting against several strains of adenoviruses. However, these viruses are responsible for not more than 5 to 10 percent of acute upper-respiratory-tract infections in the civilian population and are clearly different from the viruses of the common cold.

CHILLING

Although chilling has little if any effect upon the development of virus colds, it is common experience that exposure to drafts and chilling of part of or the whole body may result in sneezing and nasal stuffiness and discharge. Just why these symptoms occur is not entirely clear, but the probability is that they are due primarily to changes in the blood flow to the skin and mucous membranes. These reactions are not likely to occur in people who regularly take active physical exercise and have accustomed themselves to rapid changes in temperature.

CLIMATE

Climate is believed by many to be an important factor in the development of colds. This belief is due largely to the fact that colds are many times as prevalent during the winter months as during the summer. Yet seasonal incidence occurs in the balmy South, in Rio de Janeiro, in Honolulu, and in California, just as it does in Minnesota and New York. Furthermore, the change of seasons does not explain the several quite distinct waves of colds which occur during the winter.

PHYSICAL FACTORS

Anything that produces irritation or injury to the membranes of the nose and throat will cause sneezing, nasal discharge, and the other symptoms characteristic of colds. Usually these symptoms are of short duration unless the injury to the mucous membrane opens the way to bacterial infection.

Many things may irritate the mucous membranes of the nose and thus contribute to the development of colds. When the autumn wind fills the atmosphere with dust, colds increase. Tobacco smoke irritates the membranes of the throat and nose of most people. As a result some smokers have a chronic low-grade irritation. The gases in storage battery shops, garages, and chemical industries may produce congestion of the nose; and dry overheated air, such as occurs in most American homes and buildings during the winter months, may predispose to colds.

ALLERGIES

The symptoms which allergies produce in the nose are essentially the symptoms of an acute head cold: sneezing, nasal discharge, stuffiness, and obstruction to breathing.

People who suffer with allergic nasal symptoms periodically or continuously throughout the year may think that their symptoms are due to repeated colds or to chronic sinus infection, and studies indicate that a high percentage of "cold-susceptible persons" have allergies or come from allergic families. Sinus infection may develop as a result of a nasal allergy. Allergy is of sufficient importance to be considered as a possibility in every case of chronic or recurrent colds or chronic sinus infection.

OTHER FACTORS

Other nonspecific factors seem to be related to susceptibility to colds in many people. Most important among these are malnutrition, fatigue, overeating, lack of exercise, constipation, nervousness, and malformed nasal passages.

EPIDEMIOLOGY OF COLDS

Colds occur in every section of the world; all ages are susceptible, but children have many more colds than adults, with the highest rate in infants under 4 years of age. After age 4 the rate declines to a low point in the age group 15 to 24, rises from 25 to 34,

and then again declines until it reaches a minimum in the age group of 55 years and over. In childhood boys have more colds than girls, but after the age of puberty women have more colds than men. Complications are most frequent and most serious in infants. The family studies in Cleveland indicated that almost three-fourths of common colds are acquired in the home. The very young schoolchild frequently introduces colds into the household.

Various studies show that the virus is present in the nasal discharge of patients during the first 3 or 4 days of an attack of a cold, and that it remains infective for about 5 hours after leaving the body. During these few days, therefore, it may be spread by sneezing and coughing. Likewise, drinking glasses, cups, forks, doorknobs, and handrails may transmit cold viruses, as well as other microorganisms, from one person to another.

Approximately 100 viruses have been identified which are capable of producing what we call *colds*; about 20 of these seem to be responsible for a large proportion of colds.

COMPLICATIONS AND ALLIED CONDITIONS

The importance of colds lies not so much in the colds themselves as in their complications. Of these, the most common are sinusitis, otitis media (middle-ear infections), and infections of the lower part of the respiratory tract, such as laryngitis, tracheitis, bronchitis, and pneumonia. Influenza, tonsillitis, pharyngitis, and other acute respiratory-tract infections produce symptoms similar to colds but are distinct disease entities.

PREVENTION OF COLDS

NATURAL RESISTANCE

It is common knowledge that certain persons are much more susceptible to colds than others. Hereditary immunity or susceptibility has been suggested as the explanation for these differences. Studies by Johns Hopkins investigators, however, indicate that susceptibility is not a fixed quality. By studying the occurence of colds among a large group of individuals over several years, they concluded that in most persons individual susceptibility varies over a period of several years.

Though the general factors responsible for natural resistance to colds are rather vague, nature

has provided certain definite local defenses against the introduction of infections into the upper respiratory tract. (See Figure 18.1.) Most important among these are:

1 The tiny hairs, or vibrissae, at the entrance to the nasal passages. These filter out coarse particles of foreign material inhaled with the air.
2 The mucous secretion of the membranes lining the nose. Tiny glands located throughout these membranes are constantly producing a moist, slightly sticky

Figure 18.1 Natural defenses against colds.

Mucus-covered membranes
of nose warm air, catch
dust and germs; cilia
carry germs to pharynx

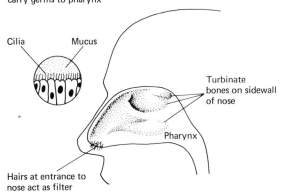

Cilia   Mucus

Turbinate
bones on sidewall
of nose

Pharynx

Hairs at entrance to
nose act as filter

secretion which covers their surfaces. This mucous film is in constant movement toward the pharynx (throat) and is renewed approximately every 10 minutes. It serves to warm and moisten the air as it is inhaled, thereby conditioning the air for contact with delicate tissues of the lower respiratory tract. Thin sheets of air passing over these surfaces deposit at least three-fourths of their bacterial content on the mucous membranes. Some of these are destroyed by the mucus itself; others are attacked by white blood cells contained in it; and still others are carried away by the flow of mucus to the pharynx, from which they are either expectorated or swallowed. The mucus also protects the delicate membranes of the nose from mechanical injury by particles of dust or smoke which are contained in the air.

3 The cilia, which cover most of the membranes of the respiratory tract. These cilia, which are in constant motion, pick up particles of foreign material and carry them to the pharynx, from which they are discharged or swallowed. Cigarette smoke and medicated oils first slow and eventually stop the action of these cilia.

These are the more obvious local defense measures that nature has provided to protect peo-

ple against colds and other infections introduced through the upper part of the respiratory tract. It is important in efforts to prevent colds that one not destroy or interfere with these natural defenses.

AVOIDANCE OF INFECTION

Under the conditions of modern life it is obviously impossible to avoid exposure to colds. The best we can hope for is to reduce the degree of exposure, thereby reducing the probability of infection. This can be accomplished by keeping one's distance from people who have colds; by prohibiting persons who have colds from any association with infants; by thorough washing of the hands before meals and after contact with objects likely to contain infective material; by keeping the hands away from the nose and mouth; by routine sterilization of dishes and silverware; and by the use of individual drinking glasses even within the family.

AIR DISINFECTION AND DUST SUPPRESSION

Since respiratory infections seem to be transmitted primarily through the air, it is logical to assume that they could be substantially reduced if we could rid the air of disease-producing organisms.

Dust-suppression measures to reduce contamination of the air we breathe are feasible and recommended. For the disinfection of air, ultraviolet radiation and germicidal vapors are effective under experimental conditions, notably in hospitals. They have not, however, reduced respiratory infections when utilized in schools, factories, or military barracks. For community control, therefore, practical measures in this area must await future developments.

VENTILATION

The ventilation of sleeping quarters should be regulated in accordance with outside atmospheric conditions, keeping in mind that drafts are undesirable and that sleep is most restful in an atmosphere which is cool rather than warm or cold.

DIETARY MEASURES

Many dietary measures are recommended for the prevention of colds, but none is based on scientific evidence or established fact. For the maintenance of health a complete, adequate, and balanced diet is necessary, however.

The administration of well-selected vitamin mixtures among University of Minnesota students led to the conclusion that large doses of vitamins A, B_1, B_2, C, D, and nicotinic acid have no demonstrable effect on the number or the severity of infections of the upper part of the respiratory tract when administered to young adults presumably on a reasonably adequate diet.

VITAMIN C FOR COLDS

Vitamin C (page 166) has been promoted for many years by the citrus fruit industry for the prevention and treatment of colds, but critical studies fail to substantiate these claims.

Since 1970, however, tremendous interest in this subject has been stimulated by a small book entitled *Vitamin C and the Common Cold*,[1] written by Linus Pauling, a most distinguished chemist. In the book the author states that for the past several years he and his wife have been taking large doses of vitamin C daily and "noticed an improved feeling of well-being and especially a striking decrease in the number of colds we caught and their severity." As pointed out above, however, most people have fewer colds as they grow older. Pauling states that he is convinced that the daily massive doses of vitamin C which he recommends are harmless; but scientists are not certain of this. For example, acidification of the urine by vitamin C could promote the formation of kidney stones.

Professor Pauling also says, "I do not know how effective this regimen really is. Professor Robinson and I are carrying out a rather small study. I hope that other investigators in the field of public health will carry out some large scale studies."

This obviously should be done, but until the results of such studies become available, there seems no scientific support for the statement that large doses of vitamin C over a period of time are harmless or will prevent or cure colds.

VACCINES FOR COLDS

Cold vaccines, consisting of heat-killed cultures of microorganisms ordinarily found in the nose and throat during colds, have been available and

[1]See Vitamin C for Colds, editorial, *American Journal of Public Health*, p. 649, April 1971.

used for a considerable number of years. In order to determine their effectiveness, several of these vaccines were included in the studies of colds which were conducted some years ago at the University of Minnesota.

At the beginning of this research program students who volunteered to take the treatments were assigned alternately and without selection to control groups and to experimental groups. The students in the control groups were treated in exactly the same manner as those in the experimental groups, but they received blanks instead of vaccine. All students thought that they were receiving vaccine and so had the same attitude toward the study. The students in all groups were instructed to report to the health service whenever a cold developed and to keep a record of each cold of more than 24 hours' duration. The physicians who saw the students at the health service when they contracted colds had no information about the group to which they belonged.

The students who received by injection the oldest and most widely used cold vaccine reported that during the previous year they had averaged 4.7 colds per person, but that during the year that they were taking the vaccine they averaged only 2.1 colds per person. This is a reduction of 55 percent, apparently an excellent result. In fact, it is just as great a reduction as had been reported in studies which concluded that these vaccines are of value.

Unfortunately for the hopeful side of this picture, the control group, who received injections of sterile water, reported that they had had an average of 4.9 colds during the previous year and 1.9 colds during the year of the study, a reduction of 61 percent. In other words, the group which got nothing of any possible value for the prevention of colds reported just as good results as did the group which got the vaccine.

Such results reported by a control group are exceedingly significant because they show how easily and how unjustifiably enthusiastic one may become concerning any procedures or preparations, no matter how worthless, for prevention of colds or, for that matter, for the prevention or treatment of other diseases, when skillful advertising or well-meaning but uncritical friends recommend them. Furthermore, how completely one can be misled or mistaken in judging the value of preparations for the prevention of colds is illustrated by telephone calls and letters received from physicians the winter following this study, stating that people who had been university students the year before and had participated in the cold-prevention studies had come to them asking for the same kind of vaccine that they had received at the university. What could be more convincing, except for the fact that the records showed that many of these were in the control group and that the injections they received contained only sterile water.

Now that viruses have been implicated as a cause of colds, the possibility of developing vaccines has been suggested. However, it will be difficult or impossible to develop an effective vaccine against a disease which may be caused by a large number of different viruses and which itself confers little if any immunity.

NASAL SPRAYS, MOUTHWASHES, GARGLES, AND ANTISEPTICS

Nasal sprays, mouthwashes, gargles, and antiseptics may destroy germs in test tubes if given sufficient time, but none of them acts instantaneously, nor are they effective in the weak solutions which can be tolerated by the membranes of the nose and throat. Furthermore, only a very small proportion of these membranes can possibly be reached by such preparations.

TREATMENT OF COLDS

It is frequently said that if you treat a cold, you can cure it in 7 days; and if you do nothing about it, you will be well in a week. And a favorite prescription is a couple of dozen soft linen handkerchiefs and several days in bed. Such skepticism about the value of treatment of the common cold is amply justified. Yet, most people have their favorite remedies in which they have great confidence and which they are glad to recommend to others.

BED REST

Following the advice "Go to bed when you have a cold and stay there until you are well" protects others from exposure, may increase general resistance, and keeps the body warm.

HOT BATHS

Hot baths for the treatment of colds may consist of hot water, hot air, or steam. The effect of these baths is to dilate the blood vessels of the skin and mucous membranes and to increase blood flow through them. As a result, the nasal passages may be widened and nasal congestion and stuffiness reduced. However, the cold is not cured.

Similar effects may be obtained with massage or other forms of physiotherapy or with hot or cold compresses, mustard plasters, and certain medicated ointments. If such treatments are followed by rest in bed with sufficient covers to prevent cooling, the effect is prolonged.

EXERCISE

Exercise is frequently utilized by athletes for the treatment of colds. They describe it as "sweating out" a cold. What they may experience is relief of nasal stuffiness, and discharge, as a result of the exercise. This occurs, as with hot baths, because of the increased flow of blood to the muscles and the skin. Such relief is only temporary, but occasionally for unknown reasons it does seem to prevent further progress of the cold. Usually, however, the symptoms recur when the body cools.

LIQUIDS

Large quantities of liquids in the form of water, lemonade, orange juice, or other drinks have long been considered a valuable aid in the treatment of colds. Actually, however, the practice of forcing fluids for colds is based on assumption rather than on evidence of its value.

MEDICATIONS

The treatment of colds is palliative, that is, aimed at the suppression of symptoms and the support of the natural processes which combat infections rather than at destroying germs.

Medication may help suppress the symptoms of colds. Aspirin, taken as two 0.3-gram (5-grain) tablets every 3 hours as needed, relieves aching and headache. However, people with peptic ulcers and some other types of upper intestinal disorders should not take aspirin. Some older but effective cold medications, such as a codeine-papaverine mixture, are sold only on a physician's prescription and may be difficult to obtain. These have now been largely replaced by capsules or tablets which contain an antihistamine and a decongestant. The antihistamines, at least by themselves, are of dubious effectiveness, but the decongestants, chemical derivatives of epinephrine (adrenalin), shrink the swollen mucous membranes of the nose and diminish their excessive secretions. Many of the commercially available "cold tablets" sold in drugstores contain such decongestants. Physicians may prescribe nose drops, cough medicine, and other agents for special circumstances.

Penicillin, the other antibiotics, and the sulfonamides ("sulfa drugs") are completely ineffective against viruses, including those which cause colds. However, these agents may be effective against the bacteria which cause the complications of colds. They should be taken only when recommended by a physician and in the dosage prescribed. Taken before complications occur, they may cause antibiotic-resistant organisms to invade the body.

THE COMMERCIAL ASPECTS OF COLDS

The sale of preparations for the prevention and treatment of colds has become a multimillion dollar business promoted by intensive public advertising. Mention should be made of results obtained from testing two nationally advertised medications for the treatment of colds. One of these is an internal medication which was purchased on the open market, removed from the original containers, and administered unlabeled to a series of students in this study. The directions given with this medication were those recommended by the manufacturer. The results were not significantly better than those obtained with sugar tablets, 44 percent as compared with 35 percent reporting benefit. Furthermore, 14 percent of the students who took this medicine reported unpleasant symptoms after its use.

The other commercial preparation studied was the most extensively advertised and widely sold nose drops for the prevention and treatment of colds. A supply of the drops was purchased at a local drugstore, transferred to unlabeled bottles, and dispensed to students with the directions recommended by the manufacturer. Thirty-one percent of the students who used this medication reported benefit from it, thereby putting it in the same class as sugar tablets so far as the effective treatment of colds is concerned. Yet, the public spends millions of dollars for this preparation each year.

The brand tested is just one of many advertised preparations to be dropped or sprayed into the nose for the prevention or cure of colds. People think that they are benefited by such preparations because they give temporary relief of congestion and stuffiness. Little do they realize that medicated oily preparations in the nose, whether applied by spraying or dropping, interfere with the action of the cilia and may even destroy respiratory epithelium. For this reason, as well as because of the irritation which many of these preparations produce, most nose and throat specialists advise against using drops, sprays, or other medications in the nose, except when they are definitely indicated for some specific condition.

INFLUENZA

Influenza and *grippe* are terms used to designate acute infections of the respiratory tract in which constitutional symptoms are more pronounced than in the common cold. Although coryza (symptoms of the common cold) frequently accompanies influenza and grippe, these conditions are characterized more particularly by headache, sudden onset, backache, fever, chills, prostration, sore throat, and cough. The fatality rate from influenza is low, most patients recovering in 3 to 4 days, but cough and weakness may persist for some time.

The precise distinction between grippe and influenza is not clear. The symptoms and physical findings are similar. In general, however, the term *grippe* is used to designate the relatively mild infections which occur with greater or lesser frequency almost every winter, while the term *influenza* is used for the more severe infections which occasionally occur in epidemic form.

At intervals of 10 to 12 years, pandemics of

influenza have occurred. The most serious of these on record occurred in 1918–1919 when a new strain of influenza appeared, spread rapidly, and caused the greatest disease holocaust of modern history. Within a year and a half, this pandemic is estimated to have infected 700 million persons throughout the world, of whom 20 million died; more than half of the latter were Americans. In the American army during World War I, 24,000 troops died from influenza, as compared to 34,000 killed in battle.[2] We now know that this disease was due to a virus that was a mutant only slightly different from the virus which for hundreds of years has caused the relatively mild influenza or grippe familiar to us all.

In 1957 another pandemic occurred. First noted in Asia, the influenza spread rapidly to Europe and South America, and then in the fall and winter swept the United States from coast to coast. Because of its origin, it was called *Asian influenza*. This pandemic affected many millions of persons over a period of several months, but the duration of illness was usually only 3 or 4 days and deaths were rare. (See Figure 18.2.)

Influenza is an acute infectious disease, caused by a filtrable virus. A vaccine developed against this virus has been widely used during and since World War II with results which indicate that it

reduces the occurrence of influenza among vaccinated persons to about one-third the rate among the unvaccinated. Unfortunately, the general usefulness of this vaccine is limited by the appearance of new strains of the virus against which the vaccine is not effective.

Such a new strain was responsible for the Asian influenza pandemic of 1957. Fortunately the World Health Organization gave advance warning of the spread of this disease in other parts of the world and the probability of an epidemic in this country. Acting promptly on this information, the U.S. Public Health Service arranged for the preparation of a vaccine against this particular strain of influenza. The vaccine was produced with unprecedented speed and administered to millions of persons. Results indicate that it was about 50 percent effective in preventing the disease.

In 1968–1969 a mutant of the Asian influenza virus appeared in Hong Kong and spread to many parts of the world. This epidemic, which was known as the *Hong Kong flu*, was reported in 44 states of this country and caused a great deal of illness and absenteeism from school and work but resulted in relatively few deaths. The prompt identification of this virus made possible the preparation of a vaccine against it within several months.

Another major epidemic of influenza is anticipated for the late 1970s. It is hoped that a more effective vaccine will be available by that time.

[2]For a comprehensive survey of this epidemic see *American Journal of Public Health*, vol. 58, no. 12, p. 2192, December 1968.

Figure 18.2 Deaths from influenza in the United States, 1900 to 1965. Source: Public Health Service.

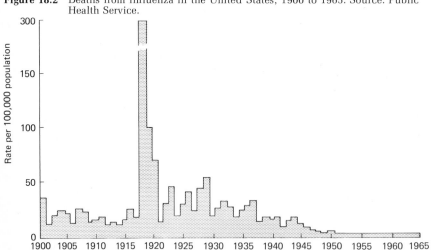

The influenza vaccines currently available contain the Asian strain as well as the previous strains of influenza virus. Their use is recommended for infants, for elderly and debilitated persons, and for people who are very likely to be exposed to infection. Reports indicate that they are 60 to 70 percent effective in providing protection. They do not, however, protect against mutant strains which from time to time appear and may spread with great rapidity.

The virus of influenza is highly infective and is transmitted from person to person by means of discharges from the nose and mouth. Measures to reduce contact with infected persons should be observed, although they are not very effective.

The great danger from influenza is not the disease itself but the pneumonia and other complications which so frequently follow it. These may develop in spite of all precautions, but they occur most frequently among persons who remain up and about while ill. Consequently, the most valuable advice which can be given to patients with influenza is, "Go to bed when you have any fever and remain there until thoroughly recovered." Other measures are helpful but should be prescribed by a physician in accordance with the needs of the individual patient.

Influenza in relation to the college student is discussed in Chapter 2, Health Problems in the College Years.

PNEUMONIA

Pneumonia is an inflammatory infection of the lungs which causes one or more portions of one or both lungs to be filled solidly with blood serum, red blood cells, white blood cells, and bacteria. The cause of pneumonia is a microorganism—most commonly in young people a tiny organism called *Mycoplasma pneumoniae*. Other causes of pneumonia include viruses and several bacteria: the pneumococcus, the streptococcus, occasionally the tubercle bacillus, the staphylococcus, and other organisms.

In infancy and old age pneumonia is largely a terminal process; i.e., it is the actual method by which death comes to a large number of people previously weakened by infectious disease, by injury, or by the lowered vitality characteristic of extreme youth or extreme age.

Pneumococcal pneumonias, caused by the pneumococcus, of which more than 75 different types are known, frequently infect one or two entire lobes of the lung at a time and so are called *lobar pneumonias*. They are considered primary pneumonias, although patients often report having had a cold before the onset of the pneumonia. It seems that, even with virulent pneumococci present in the nose and throat, some temporary lowering of body resistance from fatigue, alcohol, chilling, malnutrition, or a cold is frequently necessary for pneumonia to develop.

Pneumococci are disseminated with the nose and throat discharges of patients and of carriers. During seasons of pneumonia prevalence there are many more healthy persons carrying pneumococci in their noses and throats than there are actual cases of the disease.

Immunization of the general population against pneumococci is not practical. On the other hand, penicillin, other antibiotics, and—to a lesser extent—the sulfonamid drugs save the lives of most of the victims of this disease, many of whom could not possibly have survived in former years when 20 to 40 percent of pneumonia patients died.

Streptococcal pneumonias are usually secondary to some other disease, such as measles, whooping cough, or influenza, and produce small areas of inflammation scattered throughout the lungs. These areas of infection begin around small branches of the bronchi (bronchial tubes), and the condition is frequently spoken of as *bronchopneumonia*. The reduction of deaths from such pneumonias depends primarily on prevention, and on early and adequate care of the primary disease.

Children with measles or whooping cough should be carefully protected from all contact with persons who have colds and from conditions which tend to lower their resistance. In the treatment of streptococcal pneumonia, penicillin, other antibiotic drugs, and the sulfonamides give excellent results in most cases.

Virus pneumonia, a type of pneumonia caused

by several different viruses, is uncommon. It is probably spread directly by nasal and throat discharges. One type (psittacosis) spreads from parrots, parakeets, and other birds. Not much is known about the duration of immunity after an attack. Complications are uncommon. Death is rare in most types of virus pneumonia. There is no specific treatment.

Primary atypical pneumonia (also called *mycoplasmal pneumonia*) first recognized by physicians about the time of World War II, is the name attached to many mild pneumonias not associated with the pneumococci or with other bacteria. Late in the 1950s it was demonstrated that a tiny organism, later classified as *Mycoplasma pneumoniae*, was the cause of primary atypical pneumonia. The tetracycline antibiotics cure most cases.

For the prevention of pneumonia one can suggest only the avoidance of anything which tends to reduce vitality. Care should be given to acute respiratory infections, such as colds, influenza, bronchitis, and sore throats. Persons with fevers from such infections should be under a physician's care.

TUBERCULOSIS

Tuberculosis, long called the *captain of the men of death,* is a chronic infectious disease that usually affects the lungs but may involve every organ of the body. For many years tuberculosis was the leading cause of death in this country, and its current drop to approximately one-twentieth of the rate at the beginning of this century is therefore most impressive. This change came in response to improved standards of living, a definite plan of attack on the disease, an extensive educational campaign for its prevention, new drugs for treatment, and other factors.

In 1970, 5,560 people in the United States died of tuberculosis if the death rate of 1900 had prevailed in 1970, about 370,000 people would have died. This miraculous improvement might suggest that tuberculosis has become an unimportant disease. Unfortunately, this is not true, for the number of new cases is declining only slowly. It is estimated that 25 million persons in this country carry tuberculosis bacilli in their bodies and that 150,000 have the active disease. In 1970, 37,000 new cases were reported, of which 22,000 were in an advanced stage.

Tuberculosis is usually associated with poverty, malnutrition, overcrowding, and low standards of personal and community hygiene. It causes an estimated 3 million deaths annually throughout the world and is the major health problem in many countries.

In this country a number of significant changes have occurred in the incidence of tuberculosis. It is no longer a disease which takes its toll primarily among young adults. Today about half the deaths from tuberculosis are of persons over 50 years of age, and death rates are highest among older persons of poor socioeconomic status. The tuberculosis death rate among patients in mental institutions is about 25 times the rate among the general population.

Years ago milk was a serious mode of transmission of the bovine strain of this bacillus to children, but with the widespread adoption of pasteurization of milk and the effective program for eradication of tuberculosis among cattle, bovine infection of man has become rare in this country.

There has been much less progress in the control of human tuberculosis than in the control of the disease among animals. Yet all the scientific information necessary for eventual eradication of this disease is available. All that need be done is to apply it.

It is known, for example, that a person who has active tuberculosis with an abnormal chest x-ray has taken into his body, usually through inhalation, living tubercle bacilli which were discharged, usually by means of coughing, from the body of someone else. Hence, if we can discover the people who are disseminating tubercle bacilli and can isolate or treat them so that they will no longer be infectious, the chain of continuing infection will be broken.

That raises the question of how the disseminators of infection can be identified. One way is by the use of the tuberculin test.

TUBERCULIN TESTS

After the invasion of the body by the organisms which cause tuberculosis, the body tissues, including the skin, become sensitized to the proteins of the tubercle bacillus. This sensitization occurs even if there is not enough disease to be dectected in the chest x-ray. As a result, when these proteins later are introduced into the tissues there is a characteristic reaction. In the commonly used method of administering this test, a minute amount of tuberculin is injected into the skin of the forearm.[3]

If the area of injection becomes swollen after 2 to 3 days, the reaction is "positive" and indicates that tuberculosis organisms are present in the body. A positive test result does not indicate where the tuberculous infection is located or whether it is active or quiescent. X-ray and other examinations are necessary to determine these facts. When a tuberculin test once becomes positive, it usually remains positive throughout life.

A tuberculin test is considered "negative" if no skin reaction develops within 3 days. This indicates that no living tuberculosis organisms are present in the body.

Most colleges and universities now include tuberculin tests or chest x-rays of students as a part of their routine entrance physical examinations. This procedure is discovering each year in the colleges of this country some students who might have been active sources of infection to others. An example of what can happen if students with active tuberculosis live in close association with other students is the following report.

In early February several years ago, a young man reported to his college health service for examination. He was found to have extensive pulmonary tuberculosis involving both lungs, Tubercle bacilli were abundantly present in the sputum. He stated that he would go to his home physician immediately to arrange for treatment. Instead of doing so, he continued in the university until the school year ended in June, and he later died of tuberculosis. These facts did not come to light until 8 months later, when another young man who reported for examination because of recent symptoms was found to have active pulmonary tuberculosis. There had never been any clinical tuberculosis in his family, but the year before he had been the roommate of the first student.

The tuberculin test is a valuable procedure for determining whether someone has been infected with tuberculosis. If the original test indicates that the person has not been infected, the test should be repeated periodically, preferably each year if the person seems well, and whenever he exhibits any symptoms which suggest the possibility of tuberculosis infection. If a tuberculin test gives a positive result, it does not need to be repeated because in all probability it will continue to be positive. An x-ray examination of the chest should be made at least once a year, however, to see whether there is evidence that the infection has become active. Evidences of beginning activity of a tuberculosis infection of the lungs may be seen in an x-ray film $2\frac{1}{2}$ years, on the average, before symptoms appear. By the time recognizable symptoms bring the patient to the physician, 75 percent of cases are moderately or far advanced. Since the results of treatment of tuberculosis depend to a great extent on the stage at which treatment is begun, these months of delay may be of vital importance in determining the outcome of the disease.

TREATMENT AND CONTROL

Rest and good food, together with the use of antituberculosis drugs, make it possible for certain patients to be satisfactorily treated at home. Patients with more advanced disease, and particularly those who are infectious to others, need hospital care. A few of these cases can be rendered noninfectious and their recovery hastened by surgery.

A second line of approach to the control of tuberculosis is to search for the source of infection whenever an infected person is discovered. Disseminators of infection can be identified not only by the use of the tuberculin test but also by x-ray examination of the chest. Routine x-rays are particularly valuable in special groups such as hospital and clinic patients, military recruits, and impoverished older people. X-ray examinations of men for military service in World War II led to the discovery of more than 100,000 cases of active tuberculosis.

Everyone who develops tuberculosis has been

[3]According to the technique used for its application, tuberculin tests are called the *Mantoux*, the *von Pirquet*, the *Heaf*, and the *Tine* tests.

exposed to some person or some animal with the disease. When a child becomes infected, the source of infection is most likely within the family—possibly a parent, or a grandparent with "chronic bronchitis," an older brother or sister, or some regular visitor to the family.

VACCINATION AGAINST TUBERCULOSIS

Approximately 40 years ago scientists at the Pasteur Institute in Paris produced a vaccine against tuberculosis. This vaccine, called BCG (bacillus Calmette-Guérin), consists of a strain of tuberculosis organisms which were originally taken from cattle but have been grown in the laboratory so long that they are no longer able to produce disease. They do, however, produce a mild and harmless local skin infection which results in increased resistance to tuberculosis. The U.S. Public Health Service recommends that BCG vaccine be used in groups such as doctors and nurses working with tubercular patients, or in communities where exposure to the disease is unusually high and where other means of control are inadequate.

People who have received BCG vaccine develop positive tuberculin reactions. The value of the tuberculin test in identifying infected persons is therefore destroyed by this vaccination. Results with this vaccine indicate that it is approximately 80 percent effective for about 10 years. Its greatest value is in countries where tuberculosis is so widespread that children are almost certain to be exposed to infection.

BCG vaccination, although of great value in the control of tuberculosis, should be regarded as only one of many procedures to be used in tuberculosis control, and not as a substitute for hygienic measures or public health practices designed to prevent or minimize tuberculosis infection and disease.

PERSISTENT COUGH

Cough is a reaction to irritation within the respiratory tract. Coughs which accompany acute respiratory infections disappear as the infection subsides. Persistent cough, however, is a symptom of a serious underlying condition, such as emphysema, chronic bronchitis, tuberculosis, or lung cancer, which may require prompt remedial measures.

The findings of American and British investigators indicate that the most important factor in producing persistent cough is cigarette smoking. Nasal catarrh, i.e., sinusitis and postnasal drip, plays an important contributory role in persistent cough. This, too, is often attributable to cigarette smoking.

CHRONIC BRONCHITIS AND EMPHYSEMA

Chronic bronchitis and emphysema, frequently grouped as chronic obstructive pulmonary disease, are causing an increasing number of deaths in this country: 1,204 deaths in 1950 and 24,165 in 1968—a more rapid rise than has occurred for any other cause of death. Even more ominous is the rising toll of sickness and disability from these diseases. Patients with coronary heart disease or lung cancer usually either recover or die in a relatively short time. Patients with chronic bronchitis and emphysema are partially or completely disabled for many years.

Chronic bronchitis is a persistent or recurrent inflammation of the bronchial tubes. As a result of irritation, the cells in the lining of the bronchi produce an excessive amount of mucus, and a chronic cough develops because of the effort to expel the irritating material and the mucus. (See Figure 18.3.)

Emphysema, frequently associated with chronic bronchitis, is a disease in which the lungs lose their elasticity and cannot expand and contract normally to draw in and force out air. As the disease progresses, the walls of the air sacs become greatly overstretched and the air sacs are gradually destroyed (Figure 18.4). The result is a slowly progressive, crippling disease which seriously reduces the ability of the lungs to exchange oxygen and carbon dioxide. Pressure in the blood vessels of the lungs increases, which makes it necessary for the heart to work harder to maintain a flow of blood through the lungs. If the patient does not die from lack of oxygen, he is likely to die from heart failure.

Persistent cough, with or without expectoration, is the most common early symptom both of chronic bronchitis and of emphysema. This is frequently ignored or dismissed as "merely a cigarette cough." The most frequent reasons for seeking medical care given by bronchitis and emphysema patients are fatigue and shortness of breath. The symptoms may develop gradually, sometimes without significant cough. Unfortunately, by the time such patients see a physician more than half the lung tissue may have been destroyed. Lung tissue which has been destroyed is not regenerated. These patients, therefore, have to live the rest of their lives as lung cripples.

The causes of chronic bronchitis and emphysema are multiple and include chronic irritation, repeated or chronic infections, bronchial asthma, and injury from coughing. However, the rapid increase in these chronic pulmonary diseases is doubtless due to the presence of new irritating inhalants not common before this century. General air pollution is one of these irritants, but cigarette smoking is of vastly greater importance.

In the American Cancer Society's study of a million men and women, the death rate for bronchitis and emphysema for men aged 45 to 64 was 6.6 times as high for those who smoked cigarettes as for nonsmokers; in the age group 65 to 84 the corresponding rate was 11.4 times as high. For

Figure 18.3 Bronchioles, alveoli, and blood vessels. Source: E. Cuyler Hammond, "The Effects of Smoking," *Scientific American,* July 1962.

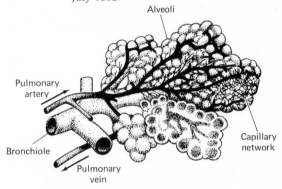

women the rate was 4.9 times as high for all smokers as for nonsmokers and 7.4 times as high for the "heavier smokers." For pipe and cigar smokers the emphysema rate was 1.4 times as high for nonsmokers.

Microscopic examination of the lungs of smokers and nonsmokers who died from causes other than lung cancer or emphysema shows that lung damage increases with the amount and the duration of smoking.

There is no cure for emphysema, but improvement usually follows cessation of smoking and a program of rehabilitation to improve pulmonary function. Emphysema has become the most rapidly increasing disabling disease in this country.

LUNG CANCER

For discussions of this major cause of deaths, see Chapter 5, page 70, and Chapter 7, page 95.

Figure 18.4 Effect of cigarette smoking on the microscopic appearance of alveolar walls. Source: Auerbach et al., "Changes in Bronchial Epithelium in Relation to Sex, Age, Residence, Smoking, and Pneumonia," *New England Journal of Medicine,* vol. 267, July 19, 1963.

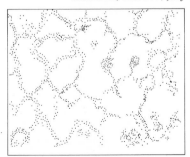

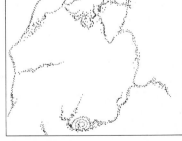

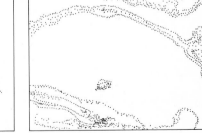

Normal   Moderate rupture (Emphysema)   Extensive rupture (Emphysema)

ASTHMA

Asthma is another chronic obstructive respiratory disease, characterized by recurrent attacks of difficulty in breathing, usually with wheezing, coughing, and a feeling of suffocation. It is due to spasmodic constriction or narrowing of the bronchial tubes, with secretion of thick mucus. Attacks may last from a few minutes to several days. During an attack the victim is unable to expel the air he takes in, which means that he is unable to supply enough oxygen to his lung capillaries. This may be severe and frightening.

Most attacks of asthma are on an allergic basis, the person being hypersensitive or allergic to substances in the air he breathes or, less frequently, in the food he eats. The substances that cause allergic asthma are similar to those that cause hay fever: pollens; emanations from animals such as dogs, cats, or horses; feathers; wool; house dust; and so forth. Allergic asthma most frequently develops between the ages of 20 and 40, while asthma due to infection may occur at any age but is most frequent in older persons. Chronic emphysema sometimes develops as a complication of prolonged asthma.

Certain drugs, particularly epinephrine or adrenaline, administered or prescribed by a physician, are effective in relieving acute attacks. Prevention depends upon identifying the substance to which one is allergic and then avoiding it. Periodic injections ("allergy shots") to desensitize the victim to the substance to which he is allergic may be of substantial help in some cases.

INSECTS AND ALLERGIES

It has long been known that allergic disorders of the respiratory system can be associated with insect particles, debris, and emanations present in the air; and that serious and occasionally fatal allergic reactions to insect stings may occur.

The insect population to which the human race is exposed is of staggering proportions. Swarms of grasshoppers, locusts, and butterflies may partially block out the sky and cover hundreds of acres of land. During the moulting season mayflies literally cover beaches and buildings. Along the shores of Lake Huron and Lake Erie, street-cleaning equipment at times is required to clear the streets of mayflies and caddis flies. Heavier and stronger insects remain near the ground, while smaller and weaker species densely populate the air up to 1,000 feet.

The reproduction rate of insects is phenomenal. The queen bee produces 2,000 eggs daily for 2 months of the year. Some termites produce 40,000 eggs in a day; the parasitic wasp may produce several thousand progeny from a dozen eggs. With such fantastic rates of reproduction, and with their dispersal from the tropics to the frozen north, on the ground and in the air, there is little opportunity, despite the use of insecticides and pesticides, to avoid contact with some form or other of insects.

Some insects are benefactors of man; others are annoying, pestiferous, and a constant threat to his comfort and well-being. The honeybee is commercially produced and used extensively to increase cross-pollination of crops. Silk is obtained from the cocoon of the silkworm. The resin secreted by the scale insect *Tachardia lacca* of India is converted into shellac. The ladybug feeds on insects and their eggs, while the dragonfly feeds voraciously on flies, gnats, and mosquitoes. On the other hand, man is constantly battling such crop destroyers and pests as weevils, potato bugs, Dutch elm beetles, and cutworms.

The insects most frequently involved in the production of allergies are the hexapoda, or six-legged insects, of which there are over a million varieties, including moths, butterflies, flies, mosquitoes, bees, wasps, hornets, yellow jackets, and beetles.

There is reason to believe that allergy to insects—next to pollen, mold, and fungus spores—is the most important cause of respiratory allergy in temperate and tropical regions. Asthma and other allergic disorders have been proved by careful studies to be due to such insect allergens. Desensitization with inhalant insect allergens has proved effective in controlling symptoms.

Immunological studies on whole-body extracts

of wasps, hornets, bees, and yellow jackets indicate that several antigenic protein fractions are shared in common, while other fractions are specific for each insect. This suggests that full protection against this group of stinging insects might be possible from a single extract.

A survey of 2,606 persons sensitive to insect stings revealed progressively severe reactions in about 65 percent of persons not desensitized. Following desensitization, reactions to subsequent stings are reduced in about 90 percent of treated persons. Protection may be maintained for years or may be lost in less than a year. Desensitization is recommended for persons who have had any degree of general systemic reaction following an insect sting.

QUESTIONS FOR DISCUSSION AND SELF-EXAMINATION

1 Through what route do most infectious diseases enter the body?
2 What do the following factors have to do with the common cold: (a) age, (b) geography, (c) chilling, (d) occupation, (e) viruses, (f) climate, (g) exposure to people with colds? Document your answers.
3 Distinguish between general resistance and specific local defenses against colds. Be specific.
4 What is the relation among allergy in the nose, the common cold, and sinusitis?
5 When are antibiotics useful in the treatment of colds? When are other medications useful?
6 What respiratory viruses are known to mutate

(change) every 10 years or more? What is the practical implication of this mutation? Be specific.
7 How has the prevalence, distribution, and mortality of tuberculosis changed in this century? What factors have influenced these changes?
8 How does a tuberculin skin test differ from chest x-rays in the detection of tuberculosis? What is the importance and significance of each?
9 What is the difference between chronic bronchitis and emphysema, and what is their relationship?
10 What causes of emphysema are known?

REFERENCES AND READING SUGGESTIONS

BOOKS

Andrews, Sir Christopher: *The Common Cold*, W. W. Norton & Company, Inc , New York, 1965.

An eminent British virologist who has devoted intensive study to the common cold reports on the present status of medical knowledge concerning this universal malady.

Diamond, Edwin: *The Beleaguered Lung*, The World Book Science Annual, Field Enterprises Educational Corp., Chicago, Ill., 1965.

Assaulted by a host of invaders and irritants, a remarkable organ withstands use and abuse—but only for so long. A splendid explanation of how and why our lungs work and of the common diseases which affect them. Excellent illustrations.

Dubos, René J., and Jean Dubos: *The White Plague*, Little, Brown and Company, Boston, 1952.

A story of man's fight against tuberculosis. It tells of many distinguished men and women who suffered from the disease and discusses its social aspects.

PAMPHLETS AND PERIODICALS

Chronic Bronchitis and Emphysema, U.S. Public Health Service, Washington.

A brief pamphlet summarizing the present knowledge about these serious and increasingly prevalent diseases.

Murray, Don: "Our Fastest-growing Health Menace," *Reader's Digest*, January 1967, p. 111.

Chronic bronchitis and emphysema—both

related to cigarette smoking—are taking a tragic toll in life and health and are increasing in number of cases more rapidly than any other disease. Here is what we must do if the trend is to be reversed.

Myers, J. A., Ruth E. Boynton, and H. S. Diehl: "Tuberculosis among University Students: A Thirty-five Year Experience," *Annals of Internal Medicine*, vol. 46, p. 201, 1957.

Ratcliff, J. D.: "I Am Joe's Lung," *Reader's Digest*, March 1969.

An excellent article on how the lung functions and the mechanism by which emphysema interferes with its functioning.

19

HORMONES

The widespread use of birth-control pills is only one indication that hormones have become much more familiar to the chemist, doctor, and patient alike than they once were. A less widespread use of hormones is in the control of diabetes, a disease for which no controlling drug was formerly available.

Hormones are manufactured by the body in great quantity and great variety. They have a huge variety of functions that have only begun to be investigated. These complex substances play a critical role in the healthy functioning of the body.

Manufactured by the endocrine glands from materials in the bloodstream, hormones are complicated chemicals which circulate in the blood and affect the growth, development, and functioning of the body. All life processes take place in body cells; it is here that the hormones make their contribution to life. Together with impulses from the nervous system, the hormones control the cellular and organic functions of the body, keeping them running smoothly and restoring them to their usual levels if they have been disturbed. The control is so automatic that we are usually unaware of hormones as a force in life until some deficiency or overproduction occurs.

The action of hormones is chemical. Hormones derive their name from a Greek word meaning "to stimulate or to excite," and they chemically influence the growth, development, and functioning of both body and mind. These chemicals are produced in the *endocrine glands*, the technical term for the small organs found in various parts of the body which manufacture the hormones from materials taken from the bloodstream. Unlike other secreting glands, such as the salivary glands, which secrete their output into the intestinal tract or onto other surfaces connecting with the environment (skin, eye, respiratory tract), the endocrine glands, or glands of internal secretion, secrete their

Figure 19.1 The glands of internal secretion.

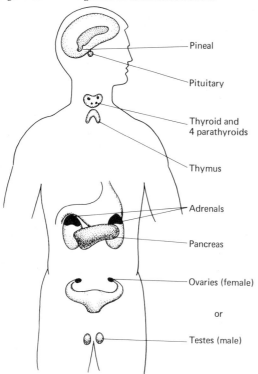

Pineal

Pituitary

Thyroid and 4 parathyroids

Thymus

Adrenals

Pancreas

Ovaries (female)

or

Testes (male)

duction has been demonstrated in very energetic persons or in those whose sexual inclinations are deviant. The changes of mood to which many people are subject are rarely associated with endocrine abnormalities.

The amazing influences of hormones on the body thus are influences not on temperament but on normal function. Even though our knowledge concerning their activities is far from complete, great progress is being made. Modern research techniques have obtained more and more hormones in pure form; thus they have been or are being analyzed and their effects on organs and individual cells determined. Some of these hormones have also been synthesized. As a result, knowledge of endocrine function and disorders and the treatment of endocrine abnormalities has advanced rapidly in the past generation.

Many of the hormones from the endocrine glands are absolutely essential for human existence; removal of the pituitary, thyroid, parathyroid, adrenals, or pancreas results in death sooner or later unless appropriate corrective treatment is instituted. The sex glands are essential not only to perpetuate the existence of the human race but also for the general development and well-being of the individual. Some hormones act in coordination with others; some hormones antagonize each other. Increased or decreased secretion of one hormone often produces changes in the secretion of other hormones.

Hormones were discovered and characterized through investigation of bodily malfunctions and diseases. It was discovered that some, like the thyroid hormones, act generally on many cells, while others act primarily on just a few, or even on just one kind of cell, like aldosterone, a salt-controlling hormone from the adrenal glands which acts only on certain cells in the kidneys.

The coordination of hormones and their actions takes place for the most part in the brain, particularly in the part of it known as the *hypothalamus*, and in the pituitary gland, which is closely associated with the hypothalamus.

products directly into the bloodstream, through which they are circulated to all the tissues of the body. (The word *gland* is also applied to the lymph nodes, as in the term *swollen glands,* referring to enlarged lymph nodes in the neck, but the lymph nodes are not glands which secrete.) (Figure 19.1.)

The chemical hormones circulating in the bloodstream influence virtually every cell in the body. Time was—and not so long ago—when it was popular to ascribe much of human behavior to the endocrine glands; Napoleon was described as the "pituitary type" and Charles Dickens as "the product of an exceptionally vigorous thyroid." The facts have not corroborated such speculation. Hormones account for very little of the *variation* of human temperament. No unusual hormone pro-

HYPOTHALAMUS AND PITUITARY

The central part of the brain—the *limbic system*—has the most to do with the physical expression of emotions. From above, it receives impulses and gives impulses to the part that controls motion,

sensation, and thought: the cerebral cortex. At the base of the limbic system is the *hypothalamus*, whose function is primarily the regulation of the central and controlling gland of the hormonal system: the *pituitary*. The hypothalamus thus earns the title "conductor of the endocrine orchestra."

The pituitary secretes the hormones which control the gonads and much of sexual life. The pituitary also produces a hormone which stimulates and regulates the thyroid gland. The pituitary's growth hormone, subject to genetic limits, not only determines the final height of a man or woman, but also influences carbohydrate metabolism.

The adrenal glands and their secretion of cortisone and related hormones are also under the direction of the pituitary and its hormone ACTH (adrenal cortico-tropic hormone). From the posterior portion of the pituitary comes an antidiuretic hormone which acts on cells in the kidney to prevent excessive secretion of urine. Indeed, of all hormones, only insulin, parathyroid hormone, and epinephrine are not under pituitary control or influence.

ADRENAL GLANDS

Perhaps the most important glands under pituitary control are the *adrenal glands*. They are divided into two portions and lie just above each kidney. The adrenal glands are essential in the body's resistance to stress, both physical and psychological, and the adrenal hormone known as *epinephrine*, or *adrenalin*, is under the influence of the sympathetic nervous system rather than the pituitary. Epinephrine, like the other hormones of the adrenal glands, helps a person to respond to emergencies by increasing his heart rate and blood pressure and by mobilizing sugar stores, making them available to the body for quick energy. Epinephrine is secreted by the central part of the adrenal gland, the medulla. (See Figure 19.2.)

The other adrenal hormones, such as cortisone, which *are* under the influence of the pituitary, come from another part of the adrenal, the cortex. A large number of synthetic hormones, referred to by physicians as *steroids* or *corticosteroids*, have been developed from cortisone, a glucocorticoid, and when a patient is given "cortisone" it is likely that he has actually been given a chemical relative of cortisone. Although these hormones have serious side effects, they are useful in the treatment of a large number of illnesses, particularly when only a short period of treatment is required. These hormones, for example, are often used to control cases of poison ivy and infectious mononucleosis and to treat some cases of leukemia. They are also used to treat such diseases as rheumatoid arthritis, gout, asthma, ulcerative colitis, and eczema.

There are actually seven major types of hormones similar to cortisone, collectively called *steroids*: each type may include several specific chemicals. These seven types include two different types of female hormones (also secreted by the ovaries and by the placenta during pregnancy), two types of androgenic or masculine hormones, two types of glucorticoids, which facilitate the metabolism of carbohydrates and which also suppress inflammation in the body, and the mineralocorticoid, aldosterone, which controls the way the kidney conserves sodium, possium, chloride, and water.

Some medical authorities believe that it is very important to keep the hypothalamus-pituitary-adrenal axis stimulated by vigorous physical exercise regularly throughout life, even into old age. They have presented evidence that this enables one to resist stresses, particularly psychological ones, more effectively than would otherwise be possible. They attribute the increased incidence of heart attacks and sudden deaths in sedentary people to functional atrophy of this system.

Figure 19.2   The adrenal glands.

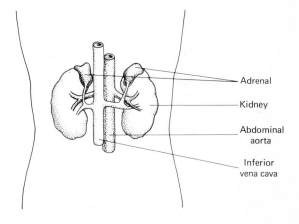

Adrenal

Kidney

Abdominal aorta

Inferior vena cava

THE SEX HORMONES

The hormones which control reproductive and sexual life come not only from the gonads, the ovaries and testicles, but also from the pituitary gland and, to a minor degree, from the adrenal glands. These hormones have five main functions:

1 They induce the attraction to the opposite sex which finds its ultimate physical satisfaction in sexual intercourse.
2 Beginning at puberty, increased secretion of testosterone in boys and of estrogen in girls leads to the development of secondary sex characteristics: the enlargement of the genitalia, the development of the breasts and other womanly curves in girls, the development of the muscles and lowering of the voice pitch in boys, and the adult patterns of body hair.
3 Under the stimulus of the gonadotropic hormones from the pituitary, the ovaries and testicles produce ova (eggs) and sperm, respectively.
4 The sex hormones are important in the building of proteins and in the maintenance of sturdy bones.
5 Besides making possible the development of the ovum and sperm and creating the conditions necessary for their union, they also prepare the lining of the uterus for implantation of the ovum and then are essential for the maintenance of the placenta through pregnancy. (Further information about sexual and reproductive anatomy and physiology appears in Chapter 20.)

Sex hormones are produced until the end of life. In women, the menopause or change of life occurs in the forties or early fifties; at this time there is a great reduction and change in the ratio of the various hormones secreted. In some, but far from all, women, unpleasant sensations such as "hot flashes" and emotional lability occur; such symptoms usually respond well to treatment with estrogens (female sex hormones) to replace the natural deficiency which occurs from this time on.

HORMONES, CELLULAR BIOCHEMISTRY, AND INTERMEDIARY METABOLISM
Within a living cell a vast number of chemical activities take place, all of them necessary to the survival of that cell or of the entire body. Some of these activities have to do with the structure of the cell or its storage function (such as protein and fat metabolism). Other chemical activities are connected with the methods of duplication of the cell or of its components and with the cell's manufacture of complicated chemicals such as enzymes.

Most of these processes take place in the central nucleus of the cell and in the tiny ribosomes in the cytoplasm outside the nucleus. Involved are the complex chemical structures, DNA and the various forms of RNA, which in essence contain the very secrets of life. But other chemical compounds in the cell are relatively simple, many of them derived primarily from sugars and other carbohydrates. The oxidation, or burning, of sugars and other simple chemical compounds provides the necessary energy for the functioning of the cells and indeed of the whole body. Without energy the rest of the chemical processes of the cell would come to a halt, the heart could not contract, food could not be digested, and the many other functions of the body, voluntary and involuntary, would cease.

This intermediary metabolism of the cell can take place only in the proper environment. The hormones of the body contribute much to creating this environment. Some hormones have specific effects on one or more of the chemical reactions in the cell. The maintainance of the optimal level of many ions and other chemical compounds in the body also falls under hormonal influence. Even the passage of water and chemical compounds through the wall of the cell may be influenced by hormones.

The hormonal changes in men are far less predictable, but there tends to be a decline in the amount of testosterone secreted in later life. These changes in hormonal secretion usually do not affect sexual desire or performance in either sex.

An interesting medical difference between men and women is the frequency of coronary artery disease in men below the age of 45 and its rarity in women before the menopause. This has suggested that estrogens may protect against coronary disease, and indeed clinical investigators have found some protection from second coronary attacks in men given doses of estrogens on a regular basis. Unfortunately too many unpleasant side effects occur when estrogens are given to men to make this a practical and acceptable treatment.

DIABETES

One of the most common hormone deficiency diseases, which illustrates the importance of hormones to health and the serious consequences of hormone deficiency, is *diabetes*. Diabetes is caused by a lack of insulin, a protein which makes it possible for the body to store and burn carbohydrates in ways not yet completely understood. (Insulin also appears to increase absorption from the intestinal tract.) In normal persons, insulin is secreted by the pancreas, a gland located just below and behind the stomach. It is secreted mostly during and after eating, and particularly after the absorption of carbohydrates into the bloodstream. But in diabetics the pancreas does not secrete sufficient insulin, so that their bodies are unable to metabolize sugar properly. This can lead to a serious, even fatal, condition.

Excessive urine and excessive thirst are the most characteristic symptoms of diabetes, the way in which the disease most often makes itself apparent. The name of the disease, in fact, is derived from a Greek word meaning to pour through, as the urine in fact does in the kidneys of a diabetic person.

In this chapter we will be concerned with the more common form of the disease, *diabetes mellitus*, sometimes referred to as *sugar diabetes*. (a less common form is *diabetes insipidus*, caused by a disorder of the pituitary gland.) Modern medical knowledge has separated diabetes mellitus into two types: juvenile or youth-onset diabetes and maturity-onset diabetes. The latter is milder, and afflicts mainly overweight people in middle age or later, especially those who are both older and fatter. Juvenile diabetes, which typically appears in childhood or early adulthood, is more severe, comes on more suddenly, and is usually more difficult to regulate. Juvenile diabetes almost always requires regular injections of insulin for its control, while mild cases of maturity-onset diabetes can sometimes be controlled by weight loss and diet.

Particularly in older people, the disease may develop gradually, and the symptoms that accompany it may not be noticed. In addition to increased frequency of urination, thirst, and perhaps increased appetite, the person may feel tired, have itching and sometimes even loss of sensation in the feet, or experience diarrhea at night. Doctors can often detect that a person has incipient diabetes through tests which show that the future victim has an unstable way of handling sugar: he is subject to rapid fluctuations in the amount of sugar in the blood, and frequently develops low blood sugar (hypoglycemia) 2 to 4 hours after a high-carbohydrate meal.

The onset of diabetes may be dramatic or slow, but the effects can be disastrous and tragic, particularly in patients who are not careful about following the diet and medication prescribed. Complications sometimes develop even in those who are most conscientious about following prescribed treatment, however. Diabetes affects not only blood sugar, but also the arteries all over the body. This artery damage can, in turn, affect the retina, the "seeing" part of the eye, where light waves are converted into nerve impulses: vision dims, and blindness may occur. There may also be damage to the arteries which supply the heart and the legs, causing heart attacks, impotence in men, and difficulty in walking. Infections are more likely to occur, especially in the kidney, and kidney failure due to the infection and to the arterial damage may result. These complications need to be kept in mind by the diabetic patient at all times, to remind him of the importance of following treatment recommendations.

THE TREATMENT OF DIABETES

Although diabetes was known in ancient times, only recently has an effective treatment been developed. The earliest medical document extant, the Ebers papyrus, dating from approximately 1500 B.C., mentions diabetes, but not until the late nineteenth century was it known that a secretion of the pancreas was involved in this disease. There were then many unsuccessful attempts to isolate the active antidiabetic principle from the pancreas in sufficiently pure condition for treatment of patients. In 1921, Dr. Banting and Dr. Best in Toronto isolated an extract of dog pancreas, which had been previously prepared by ligation of the pancreatic ducts leading into the intestinal tract, thus destroying all the pancreas except the islets of Langerhans, the specific groups of cells within the pancreas which secrete insulin. From this they succeeded in obtaining an extract which reduced the amount of sugar in the blood and urine of dogs which had been made diabetic by the complete removal of the pancreas. Then, with the aid of the biochemist Collip, they were able to prepare the hormone in a form which could be injected under the skin of human diabetics. This final success was heralded the world over. Within a few years, thousands of previously doomed sufferers were daily employing this lifesaving remedy, which was given the name *insulin* from the Latin word *insula,* meaning "island." In 1971 there was still alive an elderly social worker who had been near death when insulin first became available, but had lived another 50 years because of Banting and Best's discovery.

Before the discovery of insulin, practically all children who developed diabetes died within a few years, sometimes within days or weeks, in spite of the most expert care. Even middle-aged diabetics usually died prematurely, and older diabetics were subject to serious risks from infections as well as from diabetes itself. Today, average diabetics who take conscientious care of their disease under careful medical supervision can often live as long as their nondiabetic contemporaries.

Insulin injected every morning, and occasion-

ally more often, remains the lifesaving treatment for all severe and most moderate cases of diabetes. Equally important, however, is diet. Weight reduction and avoidance of sugars and starches will control many mild cases of diabetes and is essential in the treatment of moderate and severe cases. For some patients, particularly those with maturity-onset diabetes, new, insulin-potentializing drugs such as tolbutamide and chlorpropamide have been used to help control the disease. In 1970, however, a report appeared which indicated that these drugs may fail to control the complications of diabetes and may even increase the risk of death from heart disease. Although the report was promptly challenged by some diabetes specialists, it will be many years before the final status of these drugs is established.

In 1969 the first pancreas transplants were performed. This operation appeared to control diabetes very well. However, it seems unlikely that this will ever become a widely used method of treatment.

The most serious form of diabetes is the uncontrolled state known as *diabetic acidosis.* In diabetic acidosis, the body accumulates acid products which result from the incomplete or faulty burning of fats—a secondary manifestation of active uncontrolled diabetes. The patient has deep, rapid breathing, incredible thirst, vomiting, then uncontrollable drowsiness, and finally coma leading to death. This inexorable progression can usually be reversed by treatment with large amounts of insulin, fluids, and medications. Even today, this serious stage may be reached if the victim has ignored early symptoms. One of the most gratifying results of therapy that a physician is privileged to experience is the dramatic return of such a patient from the edge of death.

Despite these greatly improved methods of treatment, diabetes remains a serious disease. As late as 1970, diabetes caused 37,820 deaths in the United States, was the seventh leading cause of death in the entire population, and was the sixth leading cause of death among those between 65 and 74.

As noted above, the disabling and fatal complications of diabetes (blindness, kidney failure, heart attacks, loss of blood supply to the legs) cause death in diabetic patients more frequently than does the diabetes itself. These complications, as well as the dangers from the disease itself, make it imperative that there be early diagnosis and continued, effective treatment and control of the disease. Unexplained increase in thirst, increased amounts of urine, weight loss, or any of the other symptoms described above demand immediate investigation for possible diabetes mellitus. This investigation should include either a blood-sugar test, given 1 or 2 hours after a meal; or a glucose-tolerance test, in which a standard dose of pure sugar (glucose) is given the patient to swallow, and the level of sugar in the blood is determined at regular intervals for 3 to 6 hours thereafter. Anyone who has a close relative suffering from diabetes should have a blood-sugar test performed at least once a year. Early detection and early control are the only ways to prevent serious complications.

WHO GETS DIABETES?

Diabetes can appear in a family for the first time without warning, but it is more often passed from generation to generation by a recessive gene, which will not cause diabetes in the person who inherits it unless paired with another, matching, recessive gene from the other parent. Therefore, the chances of the children of a diabetic patient becoming diabetic themselves depend on whether the other parent has a recessive gene to transmit. The children of two diabetic parents will all have diabetes, and two normal parents can transmit diabetes to their children if both carry recessive genes. In practice, the risks to children work out this way:

Diabetes in relatives	Usual risk to child
One parent has close blood relative with diabetes	20 percent or less
One parent has diabetes	Variable: 0 to 50 percent
Close blood relative of both parents have diabetes	30 to 40 percent
One parent and a close blood relative of the other parent have diabetes	50 to 80 percent
Both parents have diabetes	100 percent

In interpreting these risks, remember that they do not indicate the time of life when diabetes will occur; the disease may not appear until old age.

HYPOGLYCEMIA

The "opposite" of diabetes mellitus is *hypoglycemia* (low blood sugar), in which the pancreas secretes an excess of insulin instead of too little. All of us probably have mild degrees of hyperinsulism and low blood sugar from time to time, especially during periods of great stress, when a high-carbohydrate meal can lead to a precipitous drop in the blood-sugar level. With the lowering of blood sugar, the individual feels faint and tired, usually sweats profusely, and feels hungry. He may have trouble concentrating. (In severe cases, such as the very rare cases caused by a tumor in the pancreas or the accidental injection of too much insulin, unconsciousness, convulsions, and even death can occur.) Any food will quickly relieve the symptoms of the mild cases of hypoglycemia. If such episodes occur regularly, they can be prevented by decreasing the amount of sugar and starch eaten and taking instead protein and fat. Protein and fat are absorbed more slowly than carbohydrates, and they stimulate the secretion of insulin into the blood-stream much less than do carbohydrates.

Fatigue, moodiness, and other symptoms of hypoglycemia at the end of the morning are often experienced by those who have busy schedules and eat a high-carbohydrate breakfast of, for example, juice, coffee with sugar, and pancakes. The late morning slump could be prevented by having an egg or bacon and a glass of milk for breakfast instead of the pancakes.

Unfortunately, lay people and even some physicians have exaggerated both the extent of hypoglycemia and the methods needed to control it. These people attribute many types of symptoms and illnesses to hypoglycemia, sometimes even when the blood-sugar levels in the patients involved are within the average range (which can extend down to 70 milligrams of glucose per 100 cubic centimeters of blood, or even lower). They than prescribe or adopt unnecessarily complicated diets and other therapy. An examination by a physician should be obtained by such persons.

OVERACTIVE AND UNDERACTIVE THYROIDS

The *thyroid* is a small gland in the lower part of the neck, usually weighing about an ounce and producing only a tiny fraction of an ounce of thyroid hormone daily. Largely under stimulus from the pituitary gland, itself under the control of the hypothalamus, the thyroid gland supplies its hormone, thyroxin, through the bloodstream to every cell in the body to keep the cells working chemically at an optimal rate.

Excessive thyroid hormone makes the cells work too fast chemically. Excessive hormone may be produced either by a thyroid gland which is generally enlarged and overproductive or by a small nodule in the thyroid which has gone out of control. What the individual feels and notices is a preference for cold weather over warm, excessive nervousness and restlessness, weight loss despite usually good appetite, palpitation, and excess sweating. Treatment of thyroid overactivity (variously called *hyperthyroidism, toxic goiter,* and *Graves' disease*) can be accomplished by certain drugs which prevent the production of thyroid hormone, by giving radioactive iodine, which damages the hormone-producing cells, or by removing a large part of the thyroid gland, after suitable treatment with medication.

In *hypothyroidism,* on the other hand, the thyroid is underactive and the patient is sluggish, sleepy, intolerant to cold, and perhaps overweight; the skin is dry and coarse, and the voice may become hoarse. Severe cases of this condition are called *myxedema.* Unfortunately, many people jump to the conclusion that their thyroid glands are underactive if they do not have the energy that they would like to have or if they tire easily. Hypothyroidism is an infrequent cause of fatigue. Likewise, most cases of obesity are caused not by hypothyroidism but by overeating. Careful laboratory tests are needed to determine whether thyroid underactivity is the cause of any given symptoms. Taking thyroid tablets unnecessarily may be harmful because it may cause a serious disease to remain undiscovered or masked; rarely, the patient may develop signs of thyroid overactivity while taking unnecessary thyroid medication, which may suppress his own thyroid production.

Both hyperthyroidism and hypothyroidism can be severe diseases, even leading to death if not treated effectively.

To produce thyroid hormone, the thyroid gland must have iodine. Deficiency of iodine in the diet over a long period of time leads to an inefficient overgrowth of the gland in a vain attempt to compensate. The result is a *goiter,* visible as a swelling in the lower part of the neck. Such goiters may become tremendous, even cutting off breathing through pressure on the trachea ("windpipe"). They are usually treated by surgical removal.

Fortunately, the number of cases of goiter is steadily declining in the world. In the past goiter was common in inland areas where there was a deficiency or lack of iodine. Such an area exists in the United States near the Great Lakes. In such goitrogenous areas, children may be born with severely deficient thyroid function, as a result of which their growth, both physical and mental, is severely stunted. These children are called *cretins* and their disease *cretinism.* This is one of the most tragic forms of mental retardation because it is preventable, and because it is also treatable if recognized early. Today both goiters and cretinism have been largely eliminated in the developed countries through the addition of iodine to the diet in the form of iodized salt. Though little appreciated outside afflicted areas, this is one of the great public health triumphs of modern times.

OTHER DISEASES CAUSED BY HORMONAL IMBALANCE

Many diseases, most of them rare and not of general interest, can result from hormonal imbalance. Below are brief descriptions of the most common ones.

Addison's disease, from which President John F. Kennedy suffered, is the result of a deficiency of hormones from the adrenal gland. Weakness, low blood pressure, darkening of the skin, and nausea and diarrhea are the common symptoms. Because it usually comes on gradually with vague symptoms, it is often difficult to diagnose. Since the discovery of cortisone and related drugs, however, it has been relatively easy to treat. Untreated, it is often fatal.

Hyperparathyroidism, an overactivity of the parathyroid glands (which are located next to the thyroid gland in the neck), causes the body to increase the amount of calcium in the blood to abnormal levels. Calcium is then withdrawn from the bones, giving rise to vague bone aches and pains, and is excreted in the urine, where it may be precipitated to form kidney stones. Weakness, heart irregularities, increased urination, and nausea and vomiting may result. Once diagnosed, it is easy to cure by removal of one or more of the parathyroid glands.

Gigantism, or growth to an unnatural height, results from excessive production of the growth hormone by the pituitary gland. Those who develop the disease before growth stops may continue growing to over 7 feet. If the disease first occurs after growth has stopped, only the jaw, nose, fingers, and toes enlarge, and the disease is called *acromegaly*. Because the growth hormone is antagonistic to insulin, a mild form of diabetes mellitus often occurs in gigantism and acromegaly. The diseases can be controlled or cured by x-ray therapy of the pituitary.

SOME PRACTICAL ASPECTS OF HORMONES

For the most part, the endocrine glands supply their hormones independently of the actions of the body or the mind. It seems that the control they provide for body functions is so essential that their production has to remain automatic.

However, the possibility of preventing three hormonal problems deserves attention: (1) the protection of the insulin supply and prevention of diabetes by avoiding overweight and excess consumption of carbohydrates; (2) the protection of the thyroid by adequate iodine intake—use of iodized salt in deficient areas; (3) protection of adrenal function by the stimulus of regular exercise.

In addition, it is sometimes useful to modify the hormone pattern for the benefit of the patient. For example, in some cases of retention of salt and water by the body, it is possible and desirable to block hormonal influences on the kidney and make the kidney get rid of the excess. The most familiar example, however, is the class of oral contraceptives collectively known as *the pill*; these are chemical compounds closely related to the female hormone progesterone which have the property of suppressing ovulation.

Finally, hormones are useful in the treatment of many diseases. Sometimes the treatment is merely the replacement of a deficiency in the body: thyroid hormone in myxedema or cretinism, or adrenal hormones in Addison's disease. But at other times, notably in the use of cortisone and its relatives in treating the many diseases mentioned above, the changes in the body's functioning produced by a hormone improve a disease condition.

QUESTIONS FOR DISCUSSION AND SELF-EXAMINATION

1 By what mechanisms do hormones affect the body?
2 Which of the endocrine glands are essential to life? In each case, what would be the threat to life?
3 What are the similarities and differences in the arrival of puberty in male and female?
4 What is the relation between iodine in the diet and thyroid disease?
5 What is the relationship between the brain and the hormonal system?
6 How do the adrenal glands contribute to the body's response to stress?
7 Compare the importance and significance of

the sexual effects of the sex hormones with their nonsexual effects.

8   What is the relationship of insulin to diabetes?

9   What are the symptoms of insufficient insulin and excessive insulin?

10   How does thyroid function affect one's tolerance of heat and cold?

REFERENCES AND READING SUGGESTIONS

BOOKS

Maisel, Albert Q.: *The Hormone Quest*, Random House, Inc., New York, 1966.

  An exciting and accurate story of the use of hormones to improve human health.

Weller, Charles, and Brian Boylan: *The New Way to Live with Diabetes: A Complete Guide*, Doubleday & Company, Inc., Garden City, N.Y., 1966.

  A useful handbook for patients and their families.

PAMPHLETS AND PERIODICALS

Cooley, Donald G.: "Hormones: Your Body's Chemical Rousers," *Today's Health*, part 1, vol. 40, p. 28, November 1962; part 2, vol. 40, p. 28, December 1962.

"Fight or Flight Trait Is Blocked in Humans: Harmful Effects of Epinephrine," *Science News*, Mar. 12, 1966, p. 169.

Maisel, Albert Q.: "The 'Useless' Gland That Guards Your Health," *Reader's Digest*, November 1966, p. 229.

  A good summary of recent research relative to the thymus gland.

"Stress Causes Rise in Hormone Output," *Science News*, May 14, 1966, p. 371.

Yolles, Stanley F.: "The Mystery Gland—The Pineal," *Today's Health*, March 1966, p. 76.

  A few years ago the pineal was considered a mystery gland with little or no function. This is a summary of research which has changed these ideas.

20

SEX AND SEXUALITY

What does it mean to be male? Female? Masculine? Feminine? The tradition of the nineteenth century was that the man was the breadwinner, the defender of the family against the outside world, the strong, the brave, and the absolute ruler of the home. The woman was gentle, meek, fragile, and the mistress of the details of housekeeping. There were certain sexual roles which went along with these social roles. Modesty to excess, silence and even ignorance about sexual matters (some Victorian girls were not taught the "facts of life" until the night before their marriage), strict abstinence from premarital sex, and passivity in sexual relations after marriage were the characteristics of the female role. Men were not so limited, but were expected to respect the "good women." "The other kind" of women were available, however, and though it was not spoken of, before marriage a gentleman might have sexual relations with such women. Even after marriage, a husband's extramarital affairs were neither so disastrous nor so surprising as a wife's infidelity, which was inexcusable.

Obviously the roles for both sexes have greatly changed. The belief still persists, it is true, that men have more initiative to make romantic and sexual approaches to women than vice versa, that men should be more vigorous, stronger in character as well as in muscle, and more strictly rational than women. But it is less and less frequently expected that there will be predictable differences between the sexes in personality traits and in behavior.

As sexual roles in our society have become less defined, many people have begun to question whether, aside from the most obvious physical differences, there are any differences at all which are actually innate in the sexes. Are there real emotional differences between the sexes, or are the apparent differences the result of conditioning from birth by the expectations of parents and society? If the differences are real, what is their physiological basis? Are there sexual limitations determining what men and women are capable of?

In the past few years, in addition to the growth of a strong Women's Liberation movement, an increasingly vocal Gay Liberation movement has been posing many questions to society. What is the cause of homosexuality? Is it a natural biological instinct in everyone that most people have repressed, or is it an emotional illness, an abnormal sexual role? Is a heterosexual relationship any more legitimate or "normal" than a homosexual relationship? Can a homosexual relationship be loving, satisfying, and stable? Is the concept of "sexual perversion" even valid any more? Does the law have any right to discriminate against homosexuals and other people whom society considers "deviant" in their sexual behavior? What are the legal implications of the possibility of sex changes through hormones and surgery?

As we attempt to look beneath the traditions and prejudices of society to find the essence of sexuality—what the basis of sex really is, what part sex plays in the emotional fulfillment of the total human being, and how a person's sex affects the rest of his life—we will often come up with more questions than answers. Today, many people turn more to the work of biologists, anthropologists, psychologists, and sex researchers than to the answers about sex that religion and conventional morality once provided. Yet there would still be the need for personal moral standards even if it were determined that certain modes of physical and psychological behavior are valid for the entire human race.

Paradoxically, with increasing freedom from fear, guilt, convention, ignorance, and repression in sex, our society is experiencing more confusion of sex roles, more commercial exploitation of sex, and a lack of love, meaning, and real pleasure in sexual relationships. Our increasingly sexual orientation in all aspects of culture is perhaps symptomatic of a search for the love, beauty, and emotional satisfaction that have been lost in the sexual lives of many people. No book can provide all or even most of the answers for the problems faced in

human relationships. This chapter will attempt only to pose some questions and to provide information about sex and sexuality.

Sexual differences start with the anatomical and other biological differences; it is these differences that are most commonly connoted by the word sex. Sexuality is composed of the emotional and psychological phenomena that accompany sexual anatomy and sexual functions. The recognition of sexuality as much more than the anatomical and physiological aspects of sex has been an important step in the development of modern attitudes toward sex and sexuality. To foster these attitudes the Sex Information and Education Council of the United States (SIECUS) was formed; its purpose is:

To establish man's sexuality as a health entity; to identify the special characteristics that distinguish it from, yet relate to, human reproduction; to dignify it by openness of approach, study, and scientific research designed to lead towards its understanding and its freedom from exploitation; to give leadership to professionals and to society, to the end that human beings may be aided towards responsible use of the sexual faculty and towards assimilation of sex into their individual life patterns as a creative and recreative force.

Though our knowledge about sexuality, particularly its psychological aspects, is incomplete, understanding of the basic facts about sex and sexuality can contribute greatly to making sex a satisfying and creative force in life. While psychological health is the most important ingredient in any relationship between two people, sexual misinformation and maladaptation can greatly hamper the chances for a sexually successful relationship. Parents, teachers, religious counselors, physicians, and others from whom young people seek advice should not be prevented by embarrassment or reserve from discussing sex intelligently, objectively, unemotionally, and helpfully.

A sexual relationship with the right person, at the right time, and under the right circumstances, is a magnificently satisfying experience. A prime object of knowledge about the biology of sex and about the psychological and social concomitants of sexual relations is to make possible a satisfying, creative, and complete relationship.

THE MALE ROLE IN SEX

The parts of the body which play a part in male sexual activity and reproduction are the penis, the scrotum, and the testicles, on the surface of the body; the vas deferens or spermatic cord, which runs from the testicles into the body and joins the urethra; and the prostate gland and seminal vesicles, which are located entirely within the body. Figure 20.1 shows the male genital system.

The penis becomes hard and erect when the spongy interior fills with blood during sexual excitement. Physical or psychological stimuli cause a sexual reflex: the veins which drain blood out of the penis constrict and cause the musculature at the base of the penis to clamp down on these veins. The result is that the main artery of the penis fills with blood so that the penis becomes firm and hard; this is called an *erection*. Other tissues which have similar properties are found in the clitoris of a woman and in the nipples.

The penises of different males vary in length. This variability has no relation either to the capacity to engage in sexual intercourse or to the ability to satisfy one's partner sexually. The head of the penis, and particularly the small raised band of tissue known as the *corona*, has very sensitive nerve endings which provide most of the pleasurable sensations of sexual activity.

At birth, the penis has a fold of skin—the foreskin—which comes down from the shaft of the penis over the head of the penis. The foreskin is frequently removed by circumcision shortly after birth, although this minor operation may be performed at any time of life. Circumcision facilitates cleanliness. It greatly reduces the risk of cancer of the penis in men, a rare disease; more important, the risk of cancer of the cervix of the uterus is much less in wives of circumcised men than it is in wives of uncircumcised men.

Widespread folklore claims that a circumcised man can give more sexual pleasure to his partner than an uncircumcised man can, largely because of supposedly increased ability to control the timing of his ejaculation. There is no proof of this claim, however. Except for a few men who have foreskins that are much too tight and must be circumcised, the foreskin is retracted behind the head of the penis during an erection and intercourse, so that actually the foreskin does not affect intercourse.

The testicles lie within the scrotum, the bag of skin which is located just behind the penis. In the testicles the male sex cells, called the *sperm* or *spermatazoa*, are formed, and many millions are released in each ejaculation. Beginning at the time of puberty, the testicles secrete the principal male sex hormone, testosterone, into the bloodstream. There are two different kinds of sexually important cells within the testicles, one to produce testosterone and the other to produce the sperm.

The cells which produce sperm line several miles of tiny tubes called the *seminiferous tubules*. They connect to a larger, tightly coiled tube at the top of the testicle called the *epididymis*, which stores sperm. From the epididymis the vas deferens or spermatic cord takes the sperm upward, within the body, to join the urethra, from which they are expelled in the sexual climax or ejaculation. As they pass by the seminal vesicles and prostate gland, the sperm are joined by and mixed with the oily, milk-colored fluid known as semen. The ejaculate or semen which spurts from the end of the penis at the sexual climax, therefore, is composed of sperm from the testicles and secretions from the

Figure 20.1   The male reproductive system.

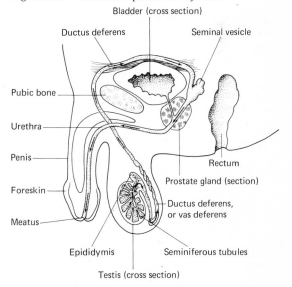

Bladder (cross section)

Ductus deferens

Seminal vesicle

Pubic bone

Urethra

Penis

Foreskin

Meatus

Rectum

Prostate gland (section)

Ductus deferens, or vas deferens

Epididymis

Seminiferous tubules

Testis (cross section)

seminal vesicles and prostate which lie near the bladder (as well as a tiny amount of secretion from glands along the urethra itself).

The prostate is the more important of these two organs, because it is the frequent location of disease in later life. Infections of the prostate can occur at any time in adult life. Cancer of the prostate is the third highest cause of cancer deaths among men. It is usually a slow-growing cancer and if diagnosed early it usually can be treated successfully. The prostate can also enlarge and cause obstruction of the flow of urine by compressing the urethra. Virtually all men have some noncancerous enlargement of the prostate by the time they are in their sixties, but in only a minority is the enlargement sufficient to cause obstruction. Before the flow of urine is completely shut off, the victim usually notices that he must urinate more frequently than usual and that that he has difficulty in starting to urinate.

Normal sexual activity, including the ability to father children, depends upon these structures being intact, and upon normal psychological and nervous-system functioning as well. The ability to have an erection and engage in intercourse is called *potency*. It is different from the ability to father children, which is called *fertility*, and which depends upon the ability to produce the many millions of healthy, vigorous sperm which are ejaculated in each sexual act. It is possible for a man to be fertile and yet unable to have sexual intercourse except on rare and isolated occasions. On the other hand, a man may be unable to produce enough healthy sperm to impregnate his wife and yet have enough testosterone released into his bloodstream by his testicles to lead an active sex life. For example, on rare occasions mumps can cause permanent damage to both testicles of an adult man; the damage is only to the cells of the seminiferous tubules, which produce sperm, and not to the Leydig cells, which produce testosterone. When both testicles have been thus damaged, the man is sterile (infertile) and yet potent.

THE FEMALE ROLE IN SEX

A woman's external genitalia, or sexual parts, are the two pairs of *labia* (lips), which lie on either side of the shallow depression known as the *vulva*, and the *clitoris*. The internal genitalia are the *vagina*, the *uterus* (womb), the *fallopian tubes*, and the *ovaries*.

Ordinarily the labia are all that can be seen of the external genitalia. With sexual excitement and separation of the legs, they part to show the vulva. At the forward part of the vulva lies the clitoris, a small knob of tissue which is composed of erectile tissue like the penis, though it is much smaller in size than the penis. With sexual excitement, it becomes engorged with blood: like the penis, it has important nerve endings which convey pleasurable sexual feeling when stimulated. The entrance to the vagina lies at the posterior end of the vulva (see Figure 20.2) with the entrance to the urethra just in front of it. With sexual excitement, the labia enlarge and part to allow easier approach to the vagina; glands on the inner aspects of the labia as well as in the vagina secrete mucus which lubricates the area during sexual intercourse. The external genitalia, then, are formed and act so as to promote the entrance of the penis into the vagina.

The vagina acts both as an organ to receive the penis during sexual intercourse and as the birth canal for delivery of the baby from the uterus to the outside world at birth. In a woman who has not yet had sexual intercourse the vagina is usually partially or completely blocked by the hymen, or maidenhead. The structure of the hymen can vary considerably. It may be so thick, firm, and strong that surgical removal is necessary in order for sexual intercourse to take place satisfactorily (unless the couple are willing to wait an extended period and to stretch it gradually). On the other hand, it may be so small and insubstantial that the first penetration of the penis into the vagina pushes it out of the way without pain or bleeding. Usually, its size and strength lie between these two extremes. Stretching it by inserting one or more fingers slowly and gently into the entrance to the vagina makes it possible in most such cases to have intercourse with a minimum of pain and bleeding. Stretched or not stretched, the hymen is usually not so much "broken" as it is torn or pushed out of

Figure 20.2 The female reproductive system, anterior-posterior section.

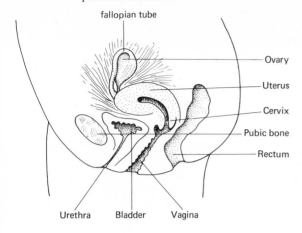

the way during the first few episodes of sexual intercourse.

The vagina, which slants toward the back rather than running vertically into the woman's body, has a muscular wall which enables it to contract firmly around the penis. At its upper end is the entrance to the uterus: the cervix, or neck, of the uterus. Both the vagina and the cervix of the uterus play an active role in sexual intercourse. The vagina actively responds by muscular contraction to the motion of the penis. At orgasm, the sexual climax, not only are there more vigorous vaginal contractions but also there are contractions of the cervix which promote the passage of sperm into the cavity of the uterus.

The function of the uterus is entirely to prepare for pregnancy and to make pregnancy possible. The lining of the uterus, called the *endometrium*, goes through cyclical changes culminating in the monthly bleeding called *menstruation*. (Note that the term *menstrual cycle* means the entire time from the beginning of one menstrual period, or bleeding, to the beginning of the next, usually a term of approximately 28 days.) Starting with puberty, hormones from the pituitary gland near the brain cause the ovaries to secrete two other hormones: estrogen and progesterone. Estrogen, secreted in the first half of the menstrual cycle, causes a gradual buildup of endometrium so that a fertilized ovum (egg cell) can readily become attached and start to grow. Then, during the second half of the menstrual cycle, progesterone is se-

creted into the bloodstream by the ovaries (specifically by the little group of cells called the *corpus luteum* or *follicle* which has just released an ovum). When progesterone stops being secreted because no pregnancy has occurred, the endometrium breaks down; the blood and surplus cells from the endometrium are shed for 3 to 5 days through the vagina. (See Figure 20.3.)

Menstruation can and should be a minor problem to most women, a bother only because of the need to wear a menstrual pad or tampon to absorb the menstrual flow. In some parts of the world, such as certain Polynesian islands, where no tradition of menstrual discomfort exists, it is rare for women to have cramps or pain during menstruation. On the other hand, girls who are brought up to expect incapacity during menstruation will often have excruciating cramps. To be sure, there are occasionally physical causes of excessive menstrual cramps. When severe cramps occur, they need medical evaluation and therapy. Women whose general health and resistance are good are less apt to have painful periods than women who are in ill health. Likewise, women who get regular, vigorous exercise are less apt to have menstrual cramps than inactive women. Women athletes can continue to exercise and compete in athletic contests during their menstrual periods. For the normal healthy woman, a long walk during menstruation is more beneficial than several hours in bed. Other normal activities can proceed without interference. Many couples find sexual intercourse unesthetic during menstruation, but there is no danger to health from intercourse at this time.

Figure 20.3 Internal female reproductive organs, cross section.

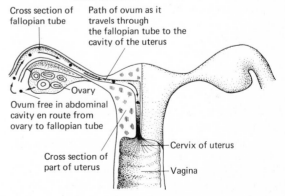

Mothers who have healthy attitudes towards their own menstrual cycles and teach these attitudes to their daughters contribute in an important way to their daughters' adult health.

Twenty-eight days is the average length of the complete menstrual cycle in American women. In 2,316 women who reported 30,655 menstrual cycles (from the beginning of one menstrual flow to the beginning of the next), 95 percent of the cycles fell between 15 and 45 days, with the average 28.1 days. Variation in cycle length is most common in women under 25 and women over 40 years of age.

When an ovum is fertilized and settles on the endometrium (technically, it becomes *implanted*), the corpus luteum in the ovary starts to produce even more progesterone, which in turn enables the pregnancy to develop and progress until the birth of the baby.

The endometrium, which makes all this possible, is thin. The muscular wall of the uterus is much thicker. The function of this muscle is to gradually expand during pregnancy and then, at the conclusion of a pregnancy, to contract periodically (in labor contractions) and finally to push the baby through the vagina to the outside world.

The remaining parts of the female genital system are the ovaries and the fallopian tubes. The fallopian tubes are attached to the upper portion of the uterus, one on each side, and extend a short distance into the abdominal cavity, where their shaggy ends help to capture an ovum when it is released from one of the ovaries. When an ovum is fertilized by a sperm cell, the event usually occurs in the fallopian tube. Only after fertilization does the fertilized ovum gradually drift into the main cavity of the uterus and settle on the endometrium.

The ovaries, one on each side of the uterus, are small oval structures which produce the hormones estrogen and progesterone and contain ova that are released once each menstrual cycle. Most of the several thousand ova in an ovary are already formed when a girl is born. These ova are held in small groups of cells called *follicles*. Under the influence of hormones from the pituitary gland, a follicle enlarges and pushes its ovum out of the ovary to be picked up by the shaggy end of the fallopian tube. The corpus luteum, or "yellow body," develops in the place in the ovary from which the ovum is expelled. If pregnancy occurs the corpus luteum continues to secrete progesterone until birth, after which it disintegrates and leaves only a tiny scar.

PUBERTY

Puberty is the time when boys and girls mature and become adults in sexual function. Characteristic changes in body configuration and body hair occur, as well as changes in function.

Just as menstruation is the event which defines puberty for girls, the ability to have ejaculations of semen defines puberty in boys. Erections of the penis can and do occur much earlier in life, even in infancy, but the ability to ejaculate semen does not exist until puberty. These ejaculations may result from stimulation of the penis or they may be spontaneous in the form of nocturnal emissions (commonly called *wet dreams*). These nocturnal emissions are normal and should be regarded as such by boys and by their parents. In healthy boys they may occur nightly over periods of time or not more often than once a month. Their regularity or irregularity has no significance. No effort to control them is necessary or desirable, for they do no harm to general health, strength, or any function of the body. Just as girls should be taught the facts about and proper attitudes toward menstruation, boys should be taught the facts about and proper attitudes toward ejaculation and nocturnal emission.

Puberty now occurs at a much earlier age than it did 50 or more years ago. At that time, the average age when girls started to menstruate was 16; now it is under 12. Puberty, the result of increased hormone production, usually occurs sometime after the age of 10 in girls and 12 in boys. Wide variation in timing is possible, and in some families puberty is delayed beyond the age of 15, or sometimes even later. Such delay does not produce any defect in adult sexual function.

The pituitary gland, lying at the base of the brain and under the control of the hypothalamus (see page 290), inaugurates the process of puberty by sending out increased amounts of hormones as the time for puberty arrives. These pituitary hormones act on the gonads—the ovaries and testicles—which in turn produce sex hormones themselves. The ovaries produce estrogen, causing the breasts to swell, the hips to become curved, body hair to form, the genitals to increase to adult size, interest in the opposite sex and in sexual activity to awaken, and ovulation and menstruation to occur. The changes in body form and hair are called the *secondary sex characteristics,* in contrast to the primary characteristics, the genitals themselves.

The pituitary in boys secretes the same hormones. These hormones act on the testicles, stimulating them to produce testosterone, which causes the development of the secondary sex characteristics of men: enlargement of muscles, lowering of the voice, growth of the genital organs, the ability to produce semen and have ejaculations, and awakening of sexual interest.

At the same time that these secondary sex characteristics are appearing, and indeed just before, boys and girls grow very rapidly—have a "growth spurt." Often within the course of 2 years they reach their full adult height. Several hormones contribute both to the growth and to the timing of the cessation of growth.

PHYSIOLOGY OF NORMAL SEXUAL FUNCTION

Although most sexual dysfunction is psychological in origin, a normal anatomy and physiology contribute to normal, satisfying sexual relations. Hormones make possible both the psychological interest and the physical responsiveness to attractive members of the opposite sex or to sexually exciting circumstances. The nervous system converts the psychological interest into actual physical response. Coordinated and stimulated by the endocrine hormones and by the nervous system, the sexual organs are readied for sexual intercourse.

The penis, the clitoris, and the entrance to the vagina contain special nerve endings which not only give pleasant sensations when stimulated but also create reflexes which promote or maintain sexual function. Stimuli go to the spinal cord and to certain nerve bodies called *ganglia,* and in return other stimuli return to the genital organs, causing the penis to swell and become erect, the clitoris to become erect and the labia to swell, and the small glands which line the vagina and the labia to secrete the mucus which lubricates sexual intercourse. Other reflexes cause muscular contraction of the vagina and dilation of small blood vessels in the body, particularly the pelvis. As sexual intercourse progresses, further reflexes result in the responses of orgasm and ejaculation. In both men and women, normal orgasm includes a general muscular tensing, flushing caused by dilation of small blood vessels, and a pleasurable heightening of general sensation, as well as the pleasant and satisfying peak sensation in the genitals. In men, ejaculation accompanies orgasm, with rhythmic contractions of the walls of the vas deferens and the urethra helping the muscular body of the prostate to force the semen out of the penis in pulses. In women, orgasm is accompanied by rhythmic contractions of the vagina and the cervix of the uterus.

Masters and Johnson[1] have observed scientifically the three stages of sexual intercourse which are known by many human beings through personal experience. These consist of arousal, during which the genitals are readied for intercourse; a plateau, during which the genitals remain aroused during sexual stimulation; and orgasm. Orgasm is normally followed by a period of profound relaxation. In either men or women, the whole process or any part of it may last a long time or may be over very quickly. For example, in the practice of *coitus reservatus* (which was used by a utopian New York settlement of the nineteenth century known as the *Perfectionists*) a man learns to keep sexual stimulation below the point at which orgasm and ejaculation take place. This enables him to continue sexual intercourse for an extended period, during which his partner may have several orgasms. On the other hand, when a couple have not had intercourse for a period of days or weeks and both are very excited, the whole cycle of

[1]William H. Masters and Virginia E. Johnson: *Human Sexual Response,* Little, Brown and Company, Boston, Mass., 1966.

arousal, plateau, and orgasm can take place for both in a very short time.

The sexual reflexes and their results have been presented as though they depend chiefly or exclusively on stimulation of the genitals themselves. However, stimuli which are primarily or exclusively psychological can bring about the same changes and processes. Reading erotic passages or seeing erotic scenes can be the stimulus, or the stimulus may be physical contact which does not involve the genitals, such as kissing. Occasionally these stimuli can bring a person to full orgasm.

PSYCHOLOGY OF NORMAL SEXUAL FUNCTION

Knowing the facts about the sexual structure and function of the human body contributes to healthy attitudes toward people's roles as sexual partners. But just as dangerous as ignorance of sex is the tendency to regard it as purely a physical phenomenon. We have strong psychological reactions to sex, whether or not we are aware of them; it is impossible to separate the two and may be unhealthy to try.

Sexual activity with a partner normally involves feelings of warmth, tenderness, and affection. When these feelings are absent or denied, both partners are deprived of gratification which is as important as the physical pleasure. To attempt to deny the emotional component of sex in one relationship may create conflicts which will interfere with full relationships with others on other occasions.

The famous psychologist and lay analyst Rollo May has noted that increasing numbers of patients are seeking help for lack of sexual satisfaction. These are adults who are "experienced" sexually. Frequently, there is little about sex that they do not know. They have studied "marriage manuals" and sexual techniques; often they have actually put a wide variety of techniques into practice. They are thoroughly sophisticated in terms of knowledge and experience. Yet they feel sexually unrewarded, lonely, and empty. Sex has let them down. Because they have not related well with others (except, perhaps, physically), their sexual lives have lacked emotional meaning. In many cases, even the joy of the physical relationship was not shared; they experienced sex as a solitary, lonely sensation, rather than as a union.

One might reply, "But isn't it true that many people get pleasure from uncommitted sex?" The honest answer is, "Of course, but not all people. And those who do get pleasure fail to experience the deep satisfaction of a relationship with strong emotional attachment. Even those who have no commitment to premarital chastity may dislike uncommitted sex." More problematic is the question of whether uncommitted sex is ever as satisfying as committed sex. Uncommitted sex, frequently promiscuous, is not emotionally meaningful. It would seem that those who consistently engage in uncommitted sex are not capable (at least, not at that particular stage of their lives) of forming a lasting, loving relationship.

The psychology of sex is not limited to the presence or absence of emotional commitment between partners. Men and women satisfy many other needs in their sexual relations: dependency, for example. All human beings need some emotional support and reassurance from others. Husbands and wives are normally dependent on each other to some extent: their sexual relations provide a natural way to express this dependency.

Sometimes, some desire to receive or inflict pain (as in masochism or sadism) may accompany sexual excitement and gratification. When such needs are balanced between the partners, and are not too strong, they need not disrupt the marriage or its sexual expression. It is unlikely, however, that strong urges of this sort would fail to make most partnerships discordant, even though in theory the needs of both partners were being met.

Almost all the sexual dysfunctions of marriage are psychological in origin. The most common and most obvious examples are impotence of men (inability or failure to achieve an erection of the penis) and frigidity of women (inability to enjoy sexual relations and to respond physically to sexual stimuli). Only rarely do hormonal deficiencies or other diseases produce these abnormalities in young people. Rather, they result from psychological problems. When a man has a poor image of himself as a man or a woman a poor image of herself as a woman, then sexual function may falter. Too, when a relationship loses warmth and affection, sexual difficulties often arise.

ATTAINING ADULT ATTITUDES AND BEHAVIOR

The development of a healthy psychological adulthood begins at birth. From his own genetic composition, from the familial and other environmental influences on him, and from what he chooses from his environment, a person's adult attitudes and other behavior develop. This is as true of sex as of other aspects of life.

At birth, when parents discover the gender of their new baby, they begin to project on him their own expectation of his roles in life. Although the child can adapt to either sexual role up to about the age of 2 or 3 (as proved by cases in which congenital defects have confused the actual sex of the child, but the defects have then been corrected surgically), the expectations have importance from the beginning. They profoundly affect how the child will act as boy or girl and, eventually, as a man or woman. Even though they may not have thought about the subject, the parents may expect that the young child will—or will not—have interest in the anatomic differences between boys and girls, and that he will—or will not—show this interest by getting undressed with other children, for example. Parents' attitudes can transmit themselves to children without specific instructions or other spoken words. A smile, a smirk, or a frown at an appropriate point can transmit an attitude as well as spoken words.

Genital activity, as well as the more general manifestations of sexuality, may begin early in life. Baby boys have erections, and though ejaculation of semen does not occur until puberty, stimulation of the baby's penis may bring on a type of sexual climax with profound relaxation following. Small children commonly show curiosity about each other's anatomy, and sexual play between children or by a child alone is not unusual or, under ordinary circumstances, harmful.

Parents can help or harm the healthy development of normal adult sexuality. Extreme permissiveness which sets no limits on behavior makes it difficult for children to develop internal psychological controls on their own impulses. To live in an adult world which does demand some conformity to standards is difficult for the grown child who had no rules as he was growing. Though he may or may not feel comfortable with his own, often overwhelming, whims and impulses, these whims and impulses will seldom mesh with the habits of others, even of others who are equally undisciplined.

At the other extreme, parents who become frightened or angry at a child's innocent sexual explorations will probably induce harmful feelings of guilt about sex in the child. If parents frequently punish sexual activity (such as touching the genital organs) and disapprove of interest in the opposite sex and other aspects of human sexuality, development of normal sexual attitudes and interests will be very difficult for the child, and he may grow into a lonely adult unable to accept his own sexuality or to have satisfying sexual relations with others.

Put in positive terms, childhood is the time to learn reasonable attitudes toward the facts of human sexuality. This is the time to learn the difference between shame and embarrassment, and the appropriateness of privacy. By instruction but even more by reaction, expression, and mood, parents teach children that interest in sex is acceptable and desirable, but that there are limits beyond which public physical expression of the interest cannot be tolerated. Examination of his own genitals in moderation and in private is acceptable, but in public is to be discouraged. Sexual play with other children is a premature expression of a natural interest rather than serious misbehavior to be punished severely. Parents can gently remove children from such play and quickly divert them into other interesting and absorbing play, thus avoiding guilt and undue shame over an innocent event.

The attitudes of the parents toward themselves and each other are of great importance in the development of the child's attitude towards sexuality. Parents who feel comfortable in their own roles and who show love and respect for each other provide a model for their children. Parents unable to feel or show love and respect for each other are likely to instill in their children a presumption that their own relations with the other sex will be cold and even hostile.

Many of the foundations of personality, including sexuality, are set by the age of 7. (Some experts believe that one's gender identity is irreversibly fixed by the age of 2 or 3.) Three of the groups in Western civilization who have been most interested in the development of the child—the

Jesuits, the communists, and the psychoanalysts (each from quite a different point of view)—have agreed on the importance of these first years in forming personality and attitudes. Although development of personality, including attitudes toward sex, continues through the school years and afterwards, and although far more dramatic changes in sexual *behavior* itself occur in puberty and just after puberty, the direction and basis of many of the later changes are already set.

The years from 5 or 6 to puberty are often called the *latency period*, although this term does not reflect the active interest in the changes of puberty which are not far off. Puberty brings an acute awareness of new sexual impulses, and the adolescent begins to learn how people must cope with and eventually satisfy these impulses. What goes on in the mind is more important, in most respects, than whether or not an adolescent actually engages in masturbation or sexual intercourse. Whether or not the arrival of overt sexual urges causes conscious anxiety, embarrassment, dismay, or other emotional discomfort, the establishment of an adult sexual identity always takes time and effort, and there is always some hidden uncertainty at first about how adequately one can fill the appropriate sexual role. Adult sexual identity is made up of comfort, pride, and pleasure in being a man or a woman, and these things do not come instantaneously.

MASTURBATION

A form of sexual activity which often starts at or near puberty is masturbation. Masturbation is self-stimulation of one's own genital organs for sexual gratification, normally resulting in a sexual climax. It is almost universal in boys and common in girls.

Although masturbation causes no harm to body or mind, most people come to recognize that it is an incompletely satisfying form of sexual behavior which can provide no more than release of sexual tension. Psychiatrists and psychologists agree that "excessive" masturbation is a symptom but not a cause of emotional disturbance, often accompanying a wide variety of psychological tension states ranging from simple anxiety to schizophrenia. Excessive masturbation cannot be defined in terms of frequency or absolute numbers: rather, masturbation becomes excessive when it is a preoccupation. When performing and thinking about masturbation occupies a major amount of time or emotional effort, it has become disproportionate to the rest of life.

SEX IN MARRIAGE

Most people recognize soon after puberty that their deepest emotional needs will be satisfied only by a complete relationship—physical, psychological, and spiritual—with someone of the opposite sex whom they love. Most human societies have institutionalized this relationship in something called *marriage*.

Even within marriage, sexual behavior varies greatly, without harm to health or happiness. In this most private part of life, why should anyone try to be average?

In a well-adjusted marriage, each partner considers the needs of the other in determining the frequency and the techniques of intercourse. In the first weeks or months of a union, sexual relations are usually frequent, in many cases once or more a day. As the other obligations and interests of life reassert themselves, the frequency usually diminishes somewhat, but many couples will find times when again their sexual interest in each other can be given full expression. The range of variation between human beings is wide, and adherence to an average or to a high rate of frequency of intercourse has little to do with happiness or a feeling of sexual fulfillment.

In both sexes, the decline of sexual performance in middle and later life is usually slow. Except in the latest stages of life, the decline affects merely the frequency with which sexual intercourse can be performed satisfactorily. The menopause seldom marks a significant decline in sexual interest among women, and there is serious doubt that there is such a thing as male menopause. In some women, sexual interest actually increases during or after the menopause.

A curious bit of folklore does seem to interfere with sexual activity in the middle years in some men. Sexual intercourse is falsely thought to represent a loss of general strength, and the busy, active man who is incorrectly informed chooses to reserve this strength for his business or profession or for the golf course. The facts are that although sexual intercourse takes muscular exertion and may produce transient fatigue, it has no effect on general health or strength aside from the promotion of mental health which may result.

The majority of men remain potent past retirement age provided their general health is good.

Forty percent of healthy married couples in their eighties are able to have intercourse, according to some studies.

Just as frequency of intercourse varies in normal healthy people, so does technique of sexual relations. The many marriage manuals now available give complete details about sexual technique. These manuals are of use in reassuring people that their natural impulses can be properly carried out and in helping inhibited people to respond normally to their impulses. However, when such manuals are used as a substitute for spontaneity, affection, mutual consideration, and tenderness in sexual relations, they can be a handicap to a satisfying sexual relationship rather than an aid.

OTHER SEXUAL BEHAVIOR

Heterosexual relations do not account for all human sexual experience. Not all humans are exclusively or even primarily attracted to a member of the opposite sex. Homosexuality is the most common example of a different sexual orientation. The term *homosexuality*, literally referring to sexual desire for, or sexual activity with, members of one's own sex, is often carelessly used to describe everything from a mild attraction to someone of the same sex to a sexual life devoted exclusively to relationships with others of the same sex. A large fraction of men (about 30 percent, according to Kinsey's figures of the 1940s) have had one or more homosexual experiences, and presumably another fraction have had fantasies of homosexual activity. The important thing to recognize about homosexual thoughts or one or two isolated homosexual experiences is that they do not commit a person to a homosexual life. Especially in childhood and adolescence, isolated homosexual experiences are more common than is generally realized.

Many so-called *homosexuals* are in fact bisexuals, who feel sexual attraction to people of both sexes. In contrast, confirmed homosexuals have little or no interest in the opposite sex. Homosexuals are no more dangerous to others than are heterosexuals, and are generally no more attracted than heterosexuals to fetishism, sadism, masochism, or sexual activities involving more than one partner.

The causes of homosexuality are obscure. So far, no genetic or hormonal differences have been discovered in homosexuals. For many years, scientists have disagreed about whether some homosexual behavior is a part of "human nature." Neither side has proved its point conclusively.

Many psychiatrists believe that "growing up straight" depends principally on having parents who are comfortable in their own roles as heterosexual adults. Conversely, the absence in the home of a successfully adjusted older person of the same sex, or the presence of unsatisfactorily adjusted adults of either sex, may predispose a person to homosexual activity. However, contradictory conclusions were reached in a study by the psychologist Evelyn Hooker of Los Angeles, in which 30 male homosexuals and 30 male heterosexuals were given an extensive battery of psychological tests which omitted only references to sexual activity and preference. Neither group had felt the need to consult psychiatrists, and both were functioning well in the nonsexual areas of their lives. A group of skilled and experienced psychotherapists who examined the tests without knowing the sexual history of the subjects were unable to find any psychological differences between the two groups.

Another study dealing with the relationships between female homosexuals discovered that only a minority of these arrangements provided for one partner to be exclusively active and the other exclusively passive (an observation also true for male homosexuals). Virtually all had been aware of sexual attraction to persons of the same sex before actual sexual experience, and this experience usually occurred after the age of 16, often after the age of 20.

Treatment for homosexuals who desire to change is available. Some therapists have had success with group therapy; behavioral therapy has also had some success. Many homosexuals, however, do not wish to change their sexual orientation; for them, therapy is directed toward achieving social adjustment and self-acceptance.

HEALTHY ADULT SEXUALITY

Sexuality is an important part of healthful living. Being a man or being a woman is an aspect of life that cannot be ignored without serious emotional consequences. Attaining complete comfort in one's sexual role takes time, and perhaps very few people are absolutely successful. However, fortunately for the human race and for the individuals who compose it, the great majority make their way, either slowly or quickly, and with varying degrees of anxiety and hesitation, through the steps which lead to a satisfying adult sexual role.

QUESTIONS FOR DISCUSSION AND SELF-EXAMINATION

1 How have changing roles of men and women affected marital relations?
2 Distinguish between the terms *sex* and *sexuality*.
3 What is the relationship between sperm and semen?
4 How is potency related to fertility? Does lack of one cause lack of the other? Explain the mechanisms involved.
5 What differences in meaning are there in these terms: *menstruation, menstrual period, menstrual cycle*? Explain the physiological events that determine each.
6 What is the role of endometrium in menstruation, sexual relations, and pregnancy? (See also Chapter 22.)
7 Which endocrine glands are involved with the advent of puberty and in what ways?
8 What accounts for the failure of attention to "good" sexual technique to result in sexual satisfaction?
9 What variations in the length of sexual intercourse can occur?
10 What are the primary influences on the development of adult sexual attitudes, and what factors can stimulate development of attitudes variant from the usual?

REFERENCES AND READING SUGGESTIONS

BOOKS

Brecher, Ruth, and Edward Brecher: *An Analysis of Human Sexual Response*, Little, Brown and Company, Boston, and Signet Books (paperback), New American Library, Inc., New York, 1966.

A splendid analysis of the recent study of Masters and Johnson, with comments on sexual patterns in the Southwest Pacific, frigidity, marriage counseling of the sexually maladjusted, and the sex problems of the aging.

Burt, John J., and Linda A. Brower: *Education for Sexuality: Concepts and Programs for Teaching*, W. B. Saunders Company, Philadelphia, 1970.

Careful, simple in approach. A good manual for teachers.

Crawley, Lawrence Q., et al.: *Reproduction, Sex*

and Preparation for Marriage, Prentice-Hall, Inc., Englewood Cliffs, N.J., 1964.

A frank, honest, readable, reliable, and well-illustrated discussion of sex and reproduction problems for young adults.

Dalrymple, Willard: *Sex Is for Real—Human Sexuality and Sexual Responsiblility,* McGraw-Hill Book Company, New York, 1969.

In the preface to this book Dr. George Packer Berry, former dean of the Harvard Medical School, says, "Dr. Dalrymple's book is a brilliant essay about human sexuality. He makes his points most effectively by his many examples. . . . His long and close relationship with students and his sympathetic appreciation of their feelings, problems, and behavior have made him an eagerly sought-out counselor and friend of generations of them. You will enjoy reading this book—and you will profit from doing so."

Hastings, Donald W.: *A Doctor Speaks on Sexual Expression in Marriage,* Little, Brown and Company, Boston, 1966.

A useful manual for young couples, dealing solely with the sexual side of marriage and incorporating recent scientific findings and reflecting modern attitudes. The author is professor of psychiatry at the University of Minnesota Medical School.

Hettlinger, Richard F.: *Living with Sex: The Student's Dilemma,* Seabury Press, New York, 1966.

A thoughtful, unprejudiced discussion of facts and issues.

Kirkendall, Lester A.: *Premarital Intercourse and Interpersonal Relationships,* The Julian Press, New York, 1961; paperback, Matrix House, New York, 1966.

A sound report and discussion in an area of vital importance and considerable confusion. The author has presented a documentation of facts and has raised thought-provoking questions which should challenge every parent and educa-tor and, most important of all, young people themselves.

Lieberman, Bernhardt (ed.): *Human Sexual Behaviour: A Book of Readings,* John Wiley & Sons, Inc., New York, 1971.

A good selection running from Freud through Masters and Johnson to Bartell on group sex.

Masters, William H., and Virginia E. Johnson. See footnote, p. 305; also *Human Sexual Inadequacy,* Little, Brown and Company, Boston, Mass., 1970.

These two books report the results of many years of scientific study of the physiology and psychology of the sexual function.

PAMPHLETS AND PERIODICALS

Hacker, Andrew: "The Pill and Morality," *The New York Times Magazine,* Nov. 21, 1965.

A professor of government at Cornell University considers the possible effects of the birth-control pill on campus morality and on the "sexual revolution."

Lader, Lawrence: "Three Men Who Made a Revolution," *The New York Times Magazine,* Apr. 10, 1966, p. 8.

A fascinating story of the development and acceptance of the birth-control pill and of ongoing research into other, still simple methods of preventing conception.

McBrown, P.: "Human Sexuality Explored," *Science News,* Apr. 30, 1966, p. 323.

Silberman, Arlene: "What Should I Tell My Son?" *Reader's Digest,* May 1966, p. 103.

Smart, M. S.: "What You Should Know about Homosexuality," *Parents' Magazine,* May 1966, p. 31.

————: *Have Your Next Baby when You Want To,* Planned Parenthood of America, New York, 1967.

A pamphlet rated excellent, brief, and to the point.

21

SOCIAL AND EMOTIONAL ASPECTS OF SEX

In the late 1960s, a boy in a Texas high school contracted syphilis from an unknown source. Within a few months, sixty-five other students at the same school had developed syphilis. About three-quarters of the cases were contracted by heterosexual intercourse, the other quarter by homosexual relations. Such epidemics of venereal disease are another aspect of sex, less attractive than the aspects discussed in the preceding chapter.

In this chapter we will discuss the "social problems" of sex, including venereal disease, illegitimacy, and abortion; the various kinds of relationships between the sexes, including dating, courtship and marriage; and the whole matter of decision making in sex. Since sex usually is part of a larger relationship between two human beings, it involves complex emotional and psychological attitudes.

VENEREAL DISEASE

One of the most unpleasant social consequences of sex is venereal disease. The word *venereal* is derived from "Venus," the name of the Roman goddess of love, and refers to anything having to do with sexual intercourse. Veneral diseases are the diseases which are transmitted by sexual intercourse.

There is a common idea that "nice people" don't get venereal disease, that it can be contracted only from prostitutes or other promiscuous "types." This is false. Venereal disease is found on all levels of society, and among people with varying habits. Obviously, the larger the number of sexual partners a person has, the more likely it is that he or she will contract venereal disease. But symptoms of venereal disease can be minor or even absent, particularly in women, and anyone who has had sexual relations with another person may be infected. Many people have venereal disease in an unrecognized, symptomless form which is nevertheless infectious. Seldom can one be sure whether a person has a venereal disease without a medical report.

GONORRHEA

The most common venereal disease is gonorrhea (also called *clap* or *gleet*). Its major symptom is usually a profuse discharge of pus from the urethra (the tube which discharges urine from the bladder) or from the vagina. Frequently there is pain on urination. The bacteria, called *gonococci*, which cause this disease need a warm, moist surface on which to grow and multiply. The urethra, the vagina, and the rectum furnish ideal homes. There the tiny bacteria multiply rapidly, causing inflammation, irritation, and damage to the local tissues. From these locations they can invade the neighboring tissues, penetrate into the bloodstream, and spread to other parts of the body.

In a man, the infection may spread along the path which the sperm travel, in the vas deferens (spermatic cord); an infection often involves the prostate gland, and sometimes the epididymis, next to the testicle. Sterility can result from the damage done by the infection and inflammation. In women, the infection can spread from the vagina through the uterus to the fallopian tubes and even to the general abdominal cavity. As in men, sterility may result. In both men and women, the bacteria of gonorrhea sometimes spread by way of the bloodstream from the sexual organs to the joints, causing an acute, severe arthritis, and on rare occasions to the heart, with potentially fatal results.

All these gonorrheal infections are painful and potentially serious. Before the antibiotic era, it often took weeks or months for them to subside. Today, most acute gonorrhea can be readily treated and promptly cured with penicillin or other antibiotics, provided that the patient seeks help early in the course of the disease. Particularly on the West Coast, many strains of the bacteria are resistant to penicillin, and valuable time may be lost while the doctor finds another antibiotic which will be effective.

The first symptoms of gonorrhea are the discharge of pus from the penis or from the vagina, and a burning pain on urination. The symptoms are usually milder in women than in men: a slight vaginal discharge occurring a few days after intercourse should never be ignored, because it can be the only sign of gonorrhea. The onset of gonorrhea usually occurs 3 to 8 days after sexual relations. Fever is unusual unless and until the infection spreads to other areas.

The pus of gonorrhea contains many bacteria and is very infectious. Furthermore, the bacteria can be passed from person to person during the incubation period before pus has appeared. But since the bacteria cannot live for long when exposed to air, it is almost impossible to contract gonorrhea from a toilet seat or any other object.

Doctors suspect the presence of gonorrhea when the symptoms described above are present. They prove the diagnosis by demonstrating and identifying the bacteria on a stained microscope slide or by culturing the bacteria (getting them to grow on a jelly like bacteriological medium).

In the United States in the late 1960s and early 1970s gonorrhea has increased and become epidemic. (See Figure 21.1.) Public health authorities estimated that close to 2 million Americans contracted gonorrhea in 1969. Stated the American Social Health Association: "Gonorrhea is clearly out of control and to date no systematic national program has been developed to attack the epidemic."

SYPHILIS

More dangerous than gonorrhea, but less common, is syphilis, once widely epidemic throughout the western world. Until very recently, syphilis was a common cause of insanity, heart disease (often with sudden death), and damage to other vital organs. Undetected and untreated, it can still be dangerous; over a thousand Americans were still dying each year from syphilis during the late 1960s (2,193 in 1966), but only 470 died from it in 1970.

Syphilis is more insidious in its onset than gonorrhea. The incubation period between sexual intercourse with an infected partner and the appearance of symptoms is 10 days to 10 weeks. The first visible manifestation of syphilis is a painless ulcer, known as a *chancre*, a small round area in which the skin or mucous membrane is irritated or destroyed. This ulcer will not be noticed if it is

Figure 21.1 Syphilis and gonorrhea in the United States, 1950 to 1972. Source: U.S. Public Health Service; *Journal of the American Medical Association,* July 3, 1972.

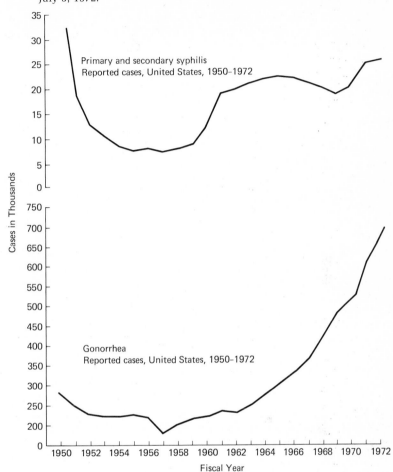

hidden inside the vagina or urethra. It occurs at a point of contact with the syphilitic germs, and so is most common on or in the genitals themselves; but it can occur in the rectum or mouth, or on any part of the skin, if the contact with infection has occurred there.

The second visible sign of syphilis comes within a few weeks of the appearance of the chancre, and consists of a widespread rash. Since the original chancre may not have been noticed, the rash may be the first sign seen by the victim. In some cases, the rash itself is absent or so faint as to be ignored.

Both the chancre and the small spots of the rash contain the syphilitic germs, the spirochetes.

If another person comes into intimate contact with any of these areas he may receive the spirochetes into his own body, where they will penetrate and cause a new case of syphilis.

Except for occasional fever and mild general discomfort, the acute stages of syphilis (the chancre and rash) are not incapacitating or dangerous to the victim. The danger comes years later. During the initial stages, the spirochetes spread widely through the body; then the disease enters a latent stage detectable only by blood tests. Ten or more years later, damage to the heart, brain, or other organs makes itself apparent. Chronic inflammation causes distortion of the aorta and the aortic valve of the heart, finally resulting in heart failure, possibly in sudden death. Syphilis may also cause chronic inflammation of the brain, resulting in loss of mental function and often symptoms of insanity, such as paranoid thoughts, delusions, or depression. Tumorous growths filled with spirochetes as well as with inflammatory cells may displace and destroy the liver, bone, or other parts of the body.

Fortunately, all these complications are unusual today in the United States. When the early signs of syphilis are noticed by their victim and diagnosed by a physician, prompt treatment leads to prompt cure. Blood tests done before marriage, during routine physical examinations, or on admission to a hospital disclose other cases which can then be effectively treated before permanent damage is done.

Doctors diagnose syphilis either by identifying the spirochetes in the chancre or rash or by blood tests. The prototype of these tests is the *Wasserman test*, a name often used by lay people to describe any blood test used to detect syphilis. Actually, there is a whole family of such tests, known collectively as *serological tests for syphilis* (STS).

Modern treatment of syphilis is effective. After decades of difficult and dangerous treatment with arsenic, penicillin began to be used in the 1940s; it has a cure rate near 100 percent. While previous treatment took weeks, months, or even years, penicillin cures patients within days. Most people who are allergic to penicillin can receive satisfactory treatment with other antibiotic drugs. If syphilis has already damaged the heart, brain, or other organs, the damage will probably not be undone, but relentless advance of the disease is often stopped by treatment.

OTHER VENEREAL DISEASES

Other types of venereal disease are rare. Soft chancre is a disease which occurs mainly in those with very poor personal cleanliness; lymphogranuloma venereum is even rarer; verruca accuminata, an uncomfortable type of wart, is particularly common around the anuses of male homosexuals.

Other diseases, usually not classified with the venereal diseases proper, are nevertheless spread by sexual contact. Pubic nits, *pediculosis pubis*, are often spread during such intimate contact. An inflammation of the male urethra known as *nonspecific urethritis* also appears after sexual intercourse. At least some of the cases are caused by a tiny organism, a mycoplasma, which is between a bacterium and a virus in size. Nonspecific urethritis, like gonorrhea, causes a discharge from the penis and burning on urination, but the symptoms usually start about 10 days after intercourse and are milder than those of gonorrhea. Unlike gonorrhea, it does not cause sterility or spread to other parts of the body, and it produces no symptoms in women.

SPREAD AND CONTROL OF VENEREAL DISEASE

Although the incidence of syphilis has increased little in recent years, gonorrhea has increased sharply. Venereal disease is the result of individual acts of sexual intercourse and afflicts individuals, but it is a major community problem as well. As long as any sexual contact takes place between partners other than those completely faithful to each other, venereal disease once existing in a community has a tendency to spread. The number of cases of venereal disease present in a community is referred to by public health authorities as a *reservoir*. If the reservoir of venereal disease in a community is low, the chances that an individual in the community will contract venereal disease are slight, even if he is promiscuous. If the reservoir is large, any casual or extramarital sex is much more likely to result in venereal disease. Therefore, elimination of venereal disease is beneficial to the community as a whole as well as to any individual exposed or infected.

The great increase in the amount of venereal disease in the United States is due to three factors. First, sexual intercourse outside marriage has increased in frequency, particularly among teenagers. Second, the condom, which prevents the transmission of venereal disease, has become a less popular method of contraception. Third, male homosexual intercourse has increased in frequency, and promiscuity is more common in the homosexual subculture than in other parts of society. Homosexual intercourse, particularly anal, is a very effective way to transmit a venereal disease from one infected person to another.

The twin weapons of public health against venereal disease are health education and case finding. Health education does not hope to eliminate extramarital sex, but it does try to discourage promiscuity, to encourage the use of condoms in casual sex, and to encourage the prompt treatment of disease. Education can be effective. When Los Angeles introduced venereal disease education, syphilis cases dropped 58 percent, while in nearby Long Beach and Pasadena (without venereal disease education) syphilis increased by 500 percent during the same period. The elimination of venereal disease remains a reasonable, if difficult, public health goal.

Case finding is the immediate weapon against the spread of venereal disease. *Case finding* means that public health workers interview all sexual contacts of someone who has venereal disease, and persuade them to have examinations for venereal disease and, if they are infected, to obtain prompt medical treatment. In all states, physicians treating a patient with a venereal disease are required by law to report the facts to the local public health authority. Police, other legal authorities, and parents never learn of the illness or the events which led to it, nor is punishment meted out to anyone involved. However, the other person or persons with whom the patient has had sexual relations can be investigated and treated.

Were this cycle of tracing, investigation, and treatment always complete and prompt, the United States could eliminate venereal disease within a year or two. But patients and even doctors are not always cooperative. In some areas, studies have shown four or more cases of venereal disease unreported for every case reported. Investigations may be slow. If a "contact" suspect is not investigated for a week or more after the first case is reported, and if the contact also has venereal disease, then other people may have been infected in the intervening time and the reservoir of venereal disease in the community may have expanded. Furthermore, some communities and some states have not appropriated enough funds to interview contacts and arrange for their investigation and treatment.

In some areas, on the other hand, intensive rapid investigation of all cases and their contacts has resulted in a marked lowering of the incidence of venereal disease. A team of public health workers interviews everyone with whom an infected person has had sexual relations, and conduct the interviews within a day or two after the first case has been diagnosed. Such prompt investigation has, in a few instances, discovered twenty or thirty cases of venereal disease in a community within a short time.

ILLEGITIMACY

Illegitimate pregnancy occurs in many different types of relationships: a couple in love and planning marriage, but careless about birth control, a couple with a stable relationship but without commitment to permanency, a couple with a frankly expedient exploitation of each other for sexual satisfaction, a couple overcome with physical passion but without an emotional relationship, a couple overcome with alcohol, a rape. As a result of the many variables involved, each illegitimate pregnancy is different. Not only may varying degrees of shame and distress be involved, but illegitimacy usually means various combinations of economic burden and disruption of personal plans.

The problems of illegitimate pregnancy do not consist just of discovering the fact of pregnancy and then making a decision on the course to be followed. Before that, there is the waiting to know: Am I (is she) pregnant or not? Is that the reason I am (she is) "late"? When will a urine test for pregnancy be positive? It is usually positive about 2 weeks after the first menstrual period is missed, but is that true for me (for her)? If the test is negative, can I (she, we) rely on its accuracy? Will the next menstrual period come on time? Or will the test have to be repeated, and when? These days or weeks of waiting are not pleasant.

Then, when the diagnosis is established as pregnancy and not nervousness or apprehension, there are more emotionally difficult moments. Is the father of the child concerned and involved? Is he present, or is he miles away? Do both partners agree on the course to be followed? If marriage is already planned, is the date to be moved or established? Are one or both sets of parents to be told, and if so, when? (Most parents, even conservative parents, are more understanding and helpful than their children expect.)

Illegitimate pregnancies, often leading to dangerous illegal abortions, unhappy marriages, and unwanted children, constitute a major social problem. Some authorities estimate that in many parts of the country one out of six unmarried girls under the age of 20 will become pregnant (or has become pregnant already). In a Canadian study, lack of a stable home environment was a frequent common factor in the lives of girls who became pregnant out of wedlock. Only half of the girls' mothers were at home full time, and the proportion was much higher for the mothers of the younger pregnant girls. Promiscuity was not a major factor; the majority of girls had had intercourse with only one partner. But only 50 percent of the girls themselves considered their sex education adequate (and probably many others had had inadequate sex education by objective standards).

For the individual girl, or couple, confronting an illegitimate pregnancy, three choices exist. One choice is for the girl to have the baby, without marriage, and raise it herself or place it for adop-tion. In some segments of society, girls are willing and even interested in these courses, but the practical difficulties are great for a family without a father, and the emotional difficulties are great for the mother who places her child for adoption.

Another choice is marriage. But almost all authorities agree that it is unwise for a couple whose relationship is not both loving and stable to be precipitated into marriage by an unwanted pregnancy. These marriages have at least two strikes against them: the unwanted child and the uncommitted relationship. They often fail, and they give little emotional support to the new child.

And then there is abortion. With its own risks to the mother's life and health, with the emotional and moral problems it presents to many, and with the difficulty of obtaining one in many states, abortion is not invariably an ideal answer to ille-gitimate pregnancy.

ABORTION

The status of abortion has been a burning issue secretly for generations and in the open recently. In most states only the most serious threat to the mother's life and health was legal justification for abortion until many states reformed their abortion laws in the late 1960s and early 1970s. Colo-rado, followed by other states, allowed legal abor-tion for pregnancy resulting from rape or from incest and for pregnancy which has a significant risk of resulting in a deformed child. Hawaii was the first state to allow abortion upon agreement of a woman and her physician, provided that the woman had been a resident of the state for at least 3 months; New York quickly followed with a simi-lar law that had no residency requirement. In 1968 the American Public Health Association advocated the repeal of all laws limiting medical abortions. (See also page 397.)

Literally, *abortion* is the termination of preg-nancy, by any cause, during the first third of the pregnancy's normal duration. Natural abortions may result from a deformed fetus or from an abnor-mality in the uterus or placenta (through which the fetus obtaines its nourishment). Abortions induced by artificial means sometimes are divided legally into *therapeutic* abortions, performed according to the traditional medical justifications; and *illegal* abortions, usually conducted by nonmedical per-sonnel, contrary to local law. With the rapid change in abortion laws, however, this distinction makes little sense today, except perhaps in states where the traditional laws are still in effect.

Chemical means have been used from time immemorial to terminate pregnancies, but up to the present time there has been no chemical safe to take by mouth (or by injection) which is guaranteed to terminate a pregnancy. Consequently, most in-duced abortions are performed by various direct actions on the pregnant uterus. The most tradi-tional method has been curettage—the introduc-tion of a long metal rod with a cuplike contour to its end which allows the operator literally to scrape the inside of the uterus, dislodging any pregnancy while doing so.

A recent, effective method of producing an abortion is to dilate the entrance to the uterus and then to apply suction to the contents. Another method is the introduction of chemical pastes into the uterus; and still another, used in some ad-vanced pregnancies, is the introduction of strong salt solutions into the amnionic sac (bag of waters) in which the fetus is suspended.

Complications can occur following abortions, even under ideal conditions. When the surroundings are not entirely sterile (free of harmful bacteria), the chance of introducing infection into the uterus is great. This infection can be purely local, or it may spread to the Fallopian tubes (causing sterility later) and even to the bloodstream, causing blood poisoning and threatening life. Another complication of abortion, particularly when performed outside hospitals but occasionally in the most competent professional hands, is hemorrhage. Hemorrhage can cause death through blood loss or secondary kidney failure. Finally, the instrument can rupture the uterus. Even in a hospital, the risks to life of abortion are much greater than the risk of the most effective contraceptive method, the birth-control pill.

The abortion debate continues both publicly and in the minds of women, married or unmarried, with unwanted pregnancies. Three issues enter into this debate. First, does a fetus possess life? And if it does, isn't an abortion murder? Roman Catholic belief states that life starts when the ovum is fertilized; many Protestant and Jewish theologians say that it begins when the ovum is implanted in the wall of the uterus (an important distinction when debating whether it is justified to use a method, such as high doses of estrogen hormones, to prevent a fertilized ovum from implanting). Others argue that life as we know it does not begin until birth and the beginning of consciousness.

Second, does a woman have the exclusive right to determine what happens within her uterus, or does that right belong partly or wholly to others: her sexual partner, society, or God? Finally, how much should society's need to restrict population be taken into consideration? Abortion helped Japan, which was severely overpopulated, reduce its population growth sharply. Organizations such as Zero Population Growth hold that abortion on request is highly desirable public policy. The problems of the population explosion and its implications for human health and the survival of the human race are dealt with in both Chapter 3, Human Ecology, and Chapter 22, Having a Family and Being a Parent.

The current trend makes it probable that in the near future legal, medically performed abortions will be readily available for women with unwanted pregnancies, either in their own states or elsewhere within the United States, with the agreement of a physician. Society, moreover, will have to ensure that uninformed women with little money will have the same free choice and opportunity that are available to, say, a college girl with a similarly unwanted pregnancy. But even when law and opportunity make abortion available, the woman herself, with whatever advice she seeks and accepts, will have to make the final decision about whether to seek an abortion, based on the factors we have just discussed as well as on the practical issues in her own life.

THE SEXES: DATING TO MARRIAGE

Many "lower" animals develop sexual interest only when the female is in heat; at other times they often behave toward each other as though sexual differences do not exist (the great apes and some monkeys would not be classified as "lower" in this sense). Humans usually have sexual interest in members of the opposite sex throughout their lives from puberty until old age. Even though few encounters between a man and a woman proceed as though a physical relationship were likely or even possible, nevertheless men and women usually behave toward each other with recognition of their sexual differences. In particular, the custom known as *dating* usually involves some sort of

physical relationship between the partners, perhaps not to the point of sexual intercourse, but with physical contacts which are different, and deliberately so, from contacts that occur with other people.

DATING

Dating is an American invention which started in the 1920s. Previously, social relationships between the unmarried in most circles were carried on under strict supervision. The church, the front parlor, the formal dance with a dance card, group activities, and other chaperoned occasions provided almost the only contact with the other sex for most young people. The girl's father expected to be asked for permission to call upon his daughter as well as for permission to marry her. In other parts of the world, such strictness still persists, and in some cultures marriages are still arranged by parents, with the couple barely meeting or sometimes not even seeing each other at all until marriage.

Dating provides autonomy for the unmarried. Young people are able to choose their own activities and to an increasing extent their own social practices. Dating is one of the factors responsible for the development of an independent youth culture.

Over the years dating has become less and less directly connected to future marriage. Dating is an end in itself, a satisfying aspect of social life. Physical relationships to some extent often occur, but they are not part of the definition of dating. In fact, however, with the increasing informality of relationships between the sexes, it is often difficult to define exactly what constitutes a "date."

Dating has other functions besides providing the company of a member of the opposite sex. It may provide status both for the individual and for his group. A man desires to be seen with an attractive and popular girl, and a girl to be seen with a handsome and well-known man. College fraternities and sororities and other groups often prefer that their members have dates that will bring prestige to the group.

Dating also allows the person to develop and "try out" his own personality, to test himself in a social situation. In dating, the young person begins to develop the qualities he will need in marriage—the qualities needed by father or mother, breadwinner, budgeter, homemaker, confidant, and so forth. Last comes the function most often commented on, though often not the most conscious function: dating as preparation for selecting a wife or a husband. The young person learns what qualities are desirable and congenial in a companion, and develops skills for handling relationships with someone of the opposite sex to whom he is emotionally close. There is usually an introspective analytic aspect to a close relationship, in which the couple openly discuss their personal feelings, desires, strengths, and weaknesses and apply their findings to their present and future relationship.

A series of steps often lead from dating to marriage: for example, group activities, casual dating, regular dating, going steady, having an "understanding," formal engagement, and finally marriage itself. These steps exist more as points on a continuous spectrum than as separate and formal steps through which people move in orderly fashion. Many a couple decides to go steady virtually as soon as they start to date, while others jump almost instantaneously from regular dating to formal engagement. Others marry almost as soon as they recognize a strong commitment to each other.

Is a young person entirely free to date and become close to anyone else of the opposite sex, then? Of course not. Depending on the family and community he belongs to, pressures, spoken or unspoken, are placed upon him to seek or avoid certain types of partners. He may or may not be free to date someone of a different race, religion, or ethnic background. His parents may make him uncomfortable if he dates someone of a different social or economic status. A person must decide whether to accept or reject these restrictions, knowing that rejecting them may mean cutting himself and his future husband or wife off from his family.

In many parts of the country in the early 1970s, however, dating as a social institution was declining or had even disappeared. The social climate which followed the conclusion of the "youth revolution" of the years 1964 to 1970 favored greater informality of life-styles and of relations between the sexes. Instead of planned events, especially with the man issuing an invitation to the woman for a specific event at some point in the future, young people preferred spontaneous activities, often in a group. Attraction to members of the opposite sex was as strong as ever, but "pairing off" would occur within the framework of group events or of spontaneous activities chosen by the couple as part of their continuing relationship. The effect that this development will have on marriage and on the choice of lasting partnerships remains to be seen.

CHOOSING A MATE

"Choosing a mate" is actually an oversimplified description of the process leading up to marriage. Many people think that choosing a mate is a process distinct from dating, although in fact, getting married is only a further step in an already existing relationship, a step by which the couple choose to declare their relationship permanent and have it recognized by law and society.

Despite criticism and scoffing, the idea of romantic love still serves as the basis for most decisions to marry in the United States today. Love is hard to define; it partakes of physical attraction, of tenderness or empathy, and of sharing. In its extreme, it includes a devotion blind to faults. Within a relationship, it implies faithfulness, commitment, and loyalty.

At one time romantic love and sexual love were regarded as distinct and sometimes even mutually exclusive. This was partly the case because of the nature of marriage at the time: sex was something that the wife owed her husband both legally and morally, whether or not there was any love between them. Today such a separation of sex and love would seem ridiculous to many people (although in fact, in many casual sexual relationships, there may be little or no love). The ideal of romantic love expects its culmination in the sexual relationship, the physical relationship contributing to and strengthening all other aspects of the relationship.

Romantic love, however, is not the only basis for a successful and happy marriage, although it is doubtless the primary thing that brings people together. Any couple must consider many other factors as well in predicting the success of their marriage. Although it is difficult to predict such success, various studies have been made and the incidence of divorce, which is certainly a good indication of an unhappy marriage, has been carefully measured. Through this method it is possible to determine that certain factors tend to increase the chances for marital success, while others decrease the chance of success, although of course much depends on the degree of love and commitment felt by a couple for each other. Some couples with many factors against them nevertheless are determined to make a marriage work, and do so successfully.

In general, men and women having much in common are more likely to have happy marriages than those with little in common, in terms of personal background and intellectual and cultural interests. Couples who share interests in music, theater, the arts, good books, and other forms of entertainment and self-expression are likely to be happier together than those whose interests conflict or who share no interests. Mixed marriages are more likely to result in divorce than marriages which are not mixed in race or religion. This is not to say that such marriages should not take place; they may have firm foundations and may contribute a great deal toward bringing ethnic and religious groups in the United States closer together.

A previously happy family life also contributes a great deal to the stability of the marriage. If the prospective bride and bridegroom's parents were happily married and have remained that way, their own chances for marital success are statistically good. If they see their own childhoods as happy, this is a favorable sign. Conversely, someone from an unhappy family or personal background may not have the capacity for a happy marital and family life himself.

A suitable prolonged period of acquaintance before marriage is a favorable factor in marital happiness. This represents not only the fact that the relationship *has* been tested before marriage, but also that the partners *were willing* to test it. They showed personality strength by postponing gratification in order to establish the best possible relationship and make sure that their relationship would remain strong under various circumstances.

Common expectations of marriage may be very important to its success; any couple considering marriage should discuss at length their hopes, plans, and expectations about finances, child planning, child discipline, vacations, residence, sexual relations, and possible careers for both husband and wife. How are they going to make their joint decisions in these important areas? Can they make joint decisions successfully? What are the values on which they intend to base these decisions? How will they meet adversity together when it comes in the form of financial troubles, family illnesses and deaths, job troubles, quarrels, or personal ill health?

There is remarkably little evidence about what kinds of personalities are compatible and increase the chances for happiness in marriage. Some argue that personalities that are similar should marry; others that dissimilar personalities make for a happier marriage.

Even though a couple should seriously consider in an "objective" way the chances that their marriage will be successful, ultimately the "irrational" factors involved are just as important. A well-known story tells of a bachelor who reported to a friend that he had met an eligible girl who met all the criteria he had for the ideal wife. The friend congratulated him and asked when they were to be married. "Never" was the surprising reply. "But why not?" "I don't like her."

Definitions of marriage are changing. Traditionally, marriage was defined as a relationship established by a wedding ceremony; but today, even theologically speaking, the emphasis is on the relationship. Many couples consider themselves to be married even though they have never had a wedding. Conversely, dissolving a marriage is easier today than it once was, both legally and otherwise, particularly for marriages that have not been established by a ceremony. But the emotional and psychological importance of the marriage relationship continues; both satisfaction and joy, on one hand, and suffering and psychological trauma, on the other hand, occur in informal as well as formal marriages.

MARRIAGE AND ITS SUCCESS

Marriage as a warm, loving, lasting relationship marked by devotion, commitment, and fidelity remains the ideal of a great majority of Americans, despite the increasing occurrence of extramarital sexual relations. Benjamin Franklin, though noted in his day for his attentions to many women, wrote in praise of marriage: "It is the Man and Woman united that makes the complete being."

The happy marriage does not happen automatically. Even the factors which predict that a marriage has a better than average chance for success are no substitute for the efforts the couple must make to promote happiness once they are married. A married couple can attempt to avoid discussing subjects known to be irritants, whether politics, a football team, or religion, and they can attempt to find common ground on which to discuss an important topic. They can give open praise and credit to each other for jobs well done and for talents usefully employed for the benefit of the marriage. When a husband or wife cooks well, keeps attractive, does something special for the children, receives an honor, makes an unusual professional or other accomplishment, or receives a raise in pay, he or she deserves credit for it, and the marriage will be stronger for a compliment enthusiastically given.

A partner can often learn to like the things that his spouse likes, whether opera or pumpkin pie. Agreement on philosophical topics may be more difficult. The importance of education, of a given method of child rearing, or of a financial campaign for the local hospital may command quite different loyalties from the two. Arguments may arise about small topics, such as where to spend an evening, on which there are honest differences of opinion. When arguments do arise—and they are not a sign of an unsuccessful marriage—a couple can conduct themselves so that the disagreement is limited to the subject at hand. The human tendency to generalize and accuse the spouse of multiple failings instead of one, or of malignant plotting instead of simple mistakes, or of worthlessness instead of human limitation, is a destructive tendency to be avoided. Statements made in the heat of argument will often be remembered even if they were not meant. At the end of an argument, willingness to admit error and to apologize for excesses can save the marriage.

Money often is a major point of disagreement in marriage. When students marry, there are often very real economic problems. Furthermore, differences in training about debt, about payment of bills, and about the priorities which different material things should receive are very common. Many of these differences can be avoided or resolved by careful and lengthy discussion. But it is surprising how deeply ingrained attitudes towards money are. It is not easy to become conservative in spending when one is used to being liberal, and vice versa.

Fortunately sex itself is less frequently a cause of marital unhappiness than it once was, but it is still common enough to be a leading cause of divorce. A marriage which does not give its physical component an important priority is unlikely to be strong and successful. The importance of sex in marriage has been stressed not only by law but by religious leaders. Muhammed emphasized the joys of sexual activity; the Old Testament contains the Song of Solomon, a poem in praise of sexual love; and Saint Paul, even though personally celibate, vehemently urged the appropriateness of sex in marriage: "The wife has no rights over her own body; it is the husband who has them. In the same way, the husband has no rights over his body; the wife has them. Do not refuse each other except by mutual consent, and then only for an agreed time, to leave yourselves free for prayer" (1 Corinthians, Chapter 7).

Sexual satisfaction in marriage is not difficult to attain, given the loving desire most couples have to satisfy each other. The manuals which describe the numerous ingenious variations of activities and positions possible are not nearly as important as a mature approach to sex and to each other, and open communication about what is most pleasurable. Sexual responsiveness is natural to both men and women.

But a couple must not expect too much of themselves or of each other. While major sexual incompatibility is now much less common than it was two or three generations ago, they should not expect the same ecstatic experience in each sexual encounter. Even though the woman is able to achieve orgasm on a fairly regular basis early in their sexual relationship, neither her climax nor his will always be identical in physical sensation and psychological meaning. Sexual experience varies from time to time; though it can and should be, and usually is, a major source of satisfaction, it is no more perfect than the human beings who engage in it.

There are directly important physical facts which influence sexual experience. The length of time taken in stimulation of each other's bodies (the foreplay), the methods used in such stimulation, the positions used in intercourse, and the length of time taken in intercourse are the most important of these physical matters. There are long textbook descriptions of these, but if a couple lack spontaneity and imagination, the textbook descriptions will be of limited help. Cookbook sex is not very satisfying.

There are other aspects of a couple's sexual relationship that need discussion, both before marriage and from time to time afterwards. Do they want a double bed or twin beds? Do they have reservations about appearing naked to each other? What are their feelings about what nightclothes should be worn or not worn—and when or whether they should be taken off? How much sleep does each need, and how important is it that sleep be uninterrupted? Do they have preconceptions on the frequency or timing of sexual relations either at the beginning of marriage or later on? How much fresh air do they want in their bedroom, and what temperatures do they tolerate well?

Not infrequently, although a couple have set the psychological and physical stages for their sexual relations with care and appropriate zeal, some disability will interfere with their early sexual satisfaction. Men may ejaculate very quickly (premature ejaculation), so that their wives are unable to come to orgasm, or they may be impotent (unable to have an erection). Women may fail to have normal vaginal secretions, may have limited sexual feeling, or may not have a full sexual orgasm for weeks or months after marriage. Any of these disabilities are disturbing to those who suffer them, for they may be misinterpreted as a sign of inadequacy, a failure to be a "real" man or woman. Usually, with understanding and sympathy from the partner, and with the passage of time, these problems are solved by the normal psychological and physical adjustments that occur. Discussion with and examination by a physician may be reassuring and helpful, particularly when the disabilities are prolonged. Consultations with a psychiatrist or psychologist will be effective in working out the psychological mechanisms which usually cause this type of disability.

DECISION MAKING ABOUT SEX

Although there are many people today who still hold to the traditional morality, it is obvious that this morality no longer commands universal loyalty. The religious beliefs which once served as a common denominator are becoming less important to many. Absolute standards persist in the minds of individuals and in some groups of people, but there is an increasing belief in society as a whole that each individual has the right and the responsibility to develop his own code of behavior. For those who lack a set of rules established by religious belief, maxims such as "Premarital intercourse is wrong" will be of little use. Instead, the formulation of personal ethics must depend on an assessment of other values in life.

Modern values place an emphasis on relationships, and physical contact, whether it includes sexual intercourse or not, is judged on the basis of whether it is appropriate to the emotional relationship between the two people. In considering the nature and extent of relationships, individuals and couples have to consider what they feel to be their responsibility to each other and to themselves. What are the qualities a person wishes to have himself and what are the qualities he wishes his relationship to have? How is a sense of the dignity of the human being best promoted in a relationship, and how do sexual practices increase or diminish it? How does a person see himself, and is his respect for himself increased or decreased by a given kind of behavior? What does he see as his ideal relationship with someone of the opposite sex? Will it have continuity? Fidelity? Will creating such a relationship be easier or harder if he has had previous physical relationships of one degree

or another? Will it be easier or harder for his partner?

What does the person believe to be the crucial landmarks in the journey to a lasting and complete relationship with someone he loves? What place does their open commitment to that relationship have? What place does their marriage ceremony have?

Clearly, the responses of different people to each of these questions will vary. But they are important to many people. It is not too difficult for most people in today's world to be comfortable with their own inhibitions, too. The development of a personal code of behavior is important both to the individual's happiness and emotional good health and to the health of society.

QUESTIONS FOR DISCUSSION AND SELF-EXAMINATION

1 Compare the symptoms, causes, and effects of syphilis and gonorrhea.

2 How does the incidence of venereal disease today compare with that of 1960? What accounts for any changes, and what methods are available to decrease the incidence of venereal disease?

3 What are the advantages and disadvantages of the different choices available to the girl illegitimately pregnant?

4 What are the advantages and disadvantages to individuals and society of abortion for unwanted pregnancy?

5 In what way(s) are abortions unsafe?

6 Compare the various motivations toward marriage and their importance.

7 Compare the importance of common interests with the importance of successful ways of solving disagreements, as factors in marital success and satisfaction.

8 How does sexual compatibility relate to other factors in marital success?

9 What are the most frequent types of sexual dysfunction in early married life, and what approaches are likely to result in their control or elimination?

10 In your opinion, what are the three most important goals for an individual's sexual life and how can they best be obtained?

REFERENCES AND READING SUGGESTIONS

BOOKS

Chesser, Eustace: *Unmarried Love*, David McKay Company, Inc., New York, 1965.

A British psychiatrist discusses a sexual code for single people, with emphasis on honesty rather than chastity.

Duval, Evelyn M.: *Why Wait till Marriage?* Association Press, New York, 1965.

A realistic consideration of the questions of premarital chastity and postmarital fidelity.

Mudd, Emily H., Howard E. Mitchell, and Sara B.

Taubin: *Success in Family Living*, Association Press, New York, 1965.

Based on research into the family life of 100 normal families, the book analyzes the factors that contribute to successful functioning of the family, including sexual behavior.

PAMPHLETS AND PERIODICALS

Barron, Jennie L.: "Too Much Sex on the Campus," *Reader's Digest*, May 1964, p. 59.

A lawyer-judge discusses this question from the points of view of society, the individual, and the college.

Masters, William H., and Virginia E. Johnson: "Sex and Sexuality: The Crucial Difference," *Reader's Digest*, February 1967, p. 123.

A discerning consideration of the differences between the physical aspects of sex and the pervasive role of sexuality in the development of personality and mature, satisfactory relationships between men and women.

Naismith, Grace: "The Plain Truth about VD," *Reader's Digest*, p. 65, September, 1972: and "How to Stop the VD Epidemic," *Reader's Digest*, p. 165, October 1972.

Two articles about the current epidemic of veneral diseases as it affects individuals and the community and what can be done to stop it.

22

REPRODUCTION: HAVING A FAMILY AND BEING A PARENT

Becoming parents is an emotional and economic crisis for most people. Photographs sometimes show the adoration of a parent for a child, or the trust of a child as he looks into his parent's face. Fiction sometimes captures the complicated moments which result from years of common experience, shared feelings, and tensions hidden or not so hidden involving three or more related people. But what does parenthood really involve? What preparation is possible? What are the choices, deliberate or not, which determine a pregnancy, and the attitudes, habits, and activities which determine the quality of parenthood? The answers are generally stated as scientific facts, but the facts are interwoven with the most powerful and moving emotions that human beings know.

Particularly in this contraceptive age, sex can be separated from reproduction, but reproduction cannot be separated from sex. Chapters 20 and 21 presented the physical, emotional, and social realities of sex; in this chapter, the personal and social implications of parenthood are discussed.

PREGNANCY

Nature has ensured that man, like other animals, will continue to exist as a species until his environment is destroyed or excessively altered. Parenthood is an easily attained goal for most people. Most human beings have a strong sexual drive during the fertile years of their lives. The great majority of women conceive within a few months of beginning sexual relations, if no contraceptives are used.

The physiology of sex sets the favorable stage

Figure 22.1 Ovum, sperm, and fertilization.

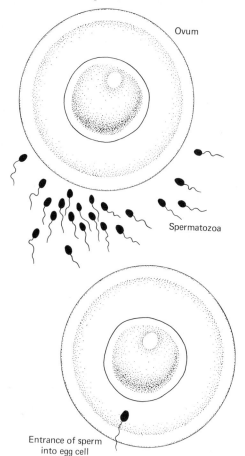

Ovum

Spermatozoa

Entrance of sperm
into egg cell

for fertilization and pregnancy when intercourse takes place near the time of ovulation. Of the millions of sperm ejaculated at or near the entrance to the uterus, many will make their way through the uterus, into the fallopian tubes, and to the vicinity of the ovum which has left the ovary and started down the fallopian tube toward the uterus. (See pages 301–303 for the anatomy and terminology.) That one single sperm penetrates a single ovum to fertilize it and produce an embryo is true, but the process is much more complicated than that. Enzymes in the wall of the ovum are necessary for penetration. Furthermore, a blocking chemical in the seminal fluid surrounding sperms usually destroys these enzymes. Only during a woman's fertile period are additional substances produced within the uterus to neutralize the blocking chemi-

cal and allow the sperm to penetrate and fertilize the ovum. Recent research on methods of contraception has attempted to find a way to stop this neutralization so that the blocking chemical can continue to prevent fertilization even during the fertile period.

The fertilized ovum drifts into the uterus, where it actually burrows into the wall. This process, called *implantation*, stimulates the formation of the placenta, which is composed largely of blood vessels and blood-filled spaces or lakes. In the placenta, the blood of the baby and the blood of the mother are separated by a very thin membrane. Across this membrane, the baby obtains its nutrition and oxygen from the mother. The umbilical cord links the placenta to the baby. The placenta is tiny at first, but grows as the embryo develops; after the baby is born, the placenta is delivered through the vagina as the afterbirth.

By the time the fertilized ovum burrows into the uterine wall, it has already increased from one cell, to two cells, four cells, and further stages; when it is about 6 days old and consists of about sixty cells, it implants. Only after 6 weeks of development will it look like a mammal, and only after 9 weeks will it look like a miniature human infant. Yet from the moment of conception its chromosomes (containing genes made up of DNA) are controlling its development and predetermining that its eventual form will be that of a human being instead of that of a monkey, a dog, a reptile, or a bird. Certain cells or groups of cells will develop into skin and nervous system, others into the parts of the intestinal tract, others into the parts of the circulatory system, and so forth. (See Figure 22.2.)

The critical differentiation of the different body organs and essential structures occurs during the first 3 months of pregnancy. During these 3 months, damage to the fetus is more likely than later in the pregnancy. German measles, other viral infections, chemicals (for example, thalidomide), x-rays, or poor nutrition may cause the baby to develop congenital defects, such as blindness, deafness, congenital heart diseases, or mental retardation.

Though the major structures of the body take their form during the first 3 months, most of the increase in size comes during the *last* 3 months of pregnancy. At the end of the first 6 months the average weight of a fetus is only 2 pounds, and only

Figure 22.2 Development of embryo and fetus.

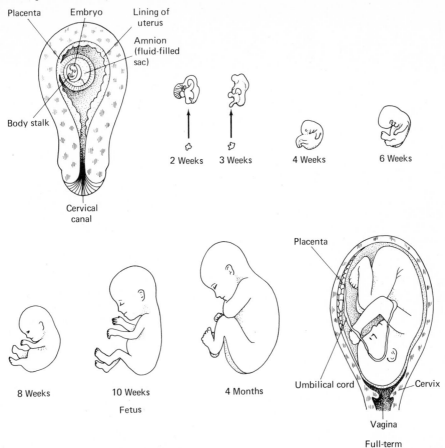

one in ten infants will survive if born prematurely at this stage of development, no matter how expert the medical care. At the end of a normal 9-month pregnancy, the average weight is 7 pounds 6 ounces, and 99 out of 100 full-term infants born in the United States survive.

Occasionally, not one embryo but two (or rarely, more) form at the same time. About a third of these dual pregnancies result from the splitting of one fertilized ovum, which then develops into identical twins. Since they come from the same fertilized ovum, identical twins share the same chromosomes and genes and their physical characteristics are extremely similar. The differences, usually minor, which develop between them are due to the differences in the physical and psychological environments to which they are subjected.

Unlike identical twins, fraternal twins result from the fertilization of two different ova; they have different placentas. The resulting twins can be as different as any other pair of siblings, and can be of opposite sexes.

Twins of either sort are almost always smaller than the average newborn infant; they are born within a few hours of each other at the most, usually within a few minutes. In the United States, twins occur about once in every 90 births, triplets once in every 9,300 births, and quadruplets once in every 490,000 births. A fertility-inducing drug introduced in the 1960s, clomiphene, stimulates the release of several ova at the same time, sometimes leading to multiple simultaneous pregnancies, up to and including quintuplets. These will not be identical siblings.

SYMPTOMS AND CARE DURING PREGNANCY

The first symptom of pregnancy is failure to menstruate. When a woman between 15 and 45 years of age who has had intercourse without contraception close to the time of ovulation is a week or more overdue for her monthly period, the most likely cause is pregnancy. Illness, emotional tension, and even strict dieting, however, can cause delay or temporary cessation of menstruation. A few women continue to pass small amounts of blood at the time of their expected menstruation for several months of pregnancy.

Shortly after the first menstrual period is missed, but occasionally before that time, morning queasiness and mild nausea may be experienced, progressing to vomiting in perhaps 50 percent of pregnant women. The breasts become full and enlarged, and the lower abdomen is slightly protuberant even though the size of the uterus is not yet significantly increased.

In most cases, a positive diagnosis of pregnancy can be established with great confidence about 2 weeks after pregnancy has prevented a menstrual period. A pregnant woman's urine contains unusual amounts of progesterone, the hormone secreted in large amounts in pregnancy.

As pregnancy advances, its manifestations change. Any nausea and vomiting (morning sickness) present early in the pregnancy usually subside within a month or two. Later in the pregnancy, the breasts secrete a sticky yellowish fluid. Appetite varies, but usually is increased in the last half of pregnancy. The expectant mother gains weight. This weight gain must be carefully monitored, so that the amount gained is consistent with the size of the baby. Because of the baby's increasing weight against the kidneys, the need to urinate is frequent; and constipation may occur as well.

Somewhere between the sixteenth and twenty-second weeks of pregnancy, most mothers begin to feel their babies move. Motion, often very vigorous, continues intermittently until delivery. At about the same time, a physician can detect the baby's heartbeat by listening to the mother's lower abdomen with a stethoscope.

The length of pregnancy is variable, with an average duration of 280 days. At the end of this time, because of influences not entirely understood, the process known as *labor* starts. The baby has already descended within the uterus, with its head usually downward and resting against the lower walls of the uterus just above the cervix. The cervis of the uterus enlarges. Labor contractions start, slow contractions of the uterus which force the baby down toward the birth canal and enlarge the uterus still further. In some pregnancies, particularly first pregnancies, temporary or false labor may occur one or more times before the final event. In a few pregnancies, particularly when the mother has already had several children, only a few labor contractions are necessary to deliver the baby through the birth canal.

Millions of women, since the human race evolved, have delivered babies successfully without the assistance of trained physicians or midwives. What modern obstetrical assistance to the delivery of the baby has accomplished is the near-abolition of deaths from hemorrhage, infection, and other complications, plus the promotion of a prompt and healthy return to normal pre-conception anatomy and physiology. If labor is prompt and effective, the obstetrician may have to do very little; he may make a small, readily repaired cut at the lower end of the birth canal (an episiotomy) to make the final emergence of the baby easy and to prevent tearing of tissue.

When labor is prolonged, difficult, complicated, or ineffective, or when the baby does not come out head first, the obstetrician's role becomes increasingly important. In the unusual circumstance in which delivery through the birth canal is impossible, the obstetrician performs a Cesarean section, so named because tradition says that Julius Caesar was born in this manner. An incision is made in the lower abdomen and into the uterus itself. The baby and the placenta are removed, and the incision is repaired.

Health care during the entire pregnancy is important, as well as general good health and good care at the time of delivery. In 1930, of every 10,000 mothers giving birth, 67 died; in the 1960s this number dropped to 4. Diet and nutrition, with emphasis on adequate protein, minerals, and vitamins and on restriction of weight gain and of salt in the diet, and regular checkups by the personal physician are the most important parts of prenatal medical care.

Major changes in everyday life during pregnancy are no longer thought desirable. However, cigarette smoking by the mother during pregnancy reduces the size of the newborn child and slightly reduces the chances of having a live baby, especially a live baby boy. Clothing should be comfortable, and support for the enlarging breasts and abdomen may be desired. Most women need more sleep early in pregnancy but have difficulty getting uninterrupted sleep late in pregnancy because of their inability to find a comfortable position. Sexual relations need not be interrupted until late in the pregnancy, unless bleeding or "spotting" from the vagina occurs after intercourse, in which case the physician should be consulted promptly. Physical activity, including such vigorous pursuits as swimming, tennis, or horseback riding, need not be abandoned, or at least not until late in the pregnancy.

In general, the improvement in general health during pregnancy, the diminishing number of restrictions placed on the pregnant woman, and the vanishing risk to life from pregnancy have meant that the psychological pleasure and fulfillment of pregnancy can be enjoyed by most women. These factors have helped to convert the female role in sex from that of an apprehension-ridden, acquiescing object to that of a joyful partner in the complicated physical and psychological process which is human sexuality.

HAZARDS OF PREGNANCY

Figure 22.3 shows the causes and rates of maternal deaths; note that deaths from *all* causes have decreased in recent years. Some of these hazards were once the cause of many deaths. Most notable of these was "puerperal fever," which was essentially an infection of the uterus often due to unsterile methods used during delivery. In 1843, Oliver Wendell Holmes, a physician and the father of the Supreme Court justice of the same name, declared in a paper entitled "The Contagiousness of Puerperal Fever" that physicians, nurses, and mid-

Figure 22.3   Maternal mortality by cause, United States, 1950 and 1965. Source: U.S. Public Health Service.

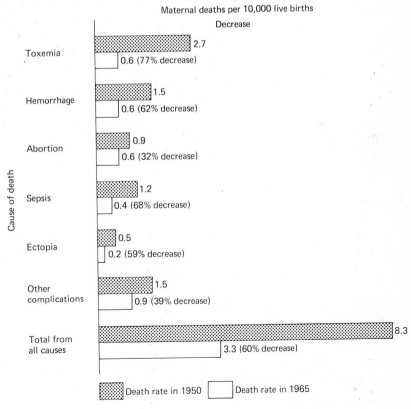

Maternal deaths per 10,000 live births

Cause of death	Death rate in 1950	Death rate in 1965 (Decrease)
Toxemia	2.7	0.6 (77% decrease)
Hemorrhage	1.5	0.6 (62% decrease)
Abortion	0.9	0.6 (32% decrease)
Sepsis	1.2	0.4 (68% decrease)
Ectopia	0.5	0.2 (59% decrease)
Other complications	1.5	0.9 (39% decrease)
Total from all causes	8.3	3.3 (60% decrease)

wives were responsible for most of the infections which occur during childbirth. That was a bold and shocking statement, since it came before Pasteur's discovery of the relationship of microorganisms to disease and before Lister's introduction of asepsis and antisepsis. But the simple practices which were adopted on Holmes' recommendation, such as careful washing of the physician's hands before delivery, the use of surgical gloves, the cleansing of the entrance to the birth canal, and the use of sterile surgical sponges, the incidence of puerperal fever fell dramatically. Modern antibiotics have succeeded in eliminating it almost entirely.

Another common hazard which has been largely eliminated is toxemia of pregnancy, an illness characterized by high blood pressure and convulsions. With modern dietary and drug treatment and early detection, this hazard has become much less serious.

A rare form of cancer which is usually fatal if untreated may follow pregnancy: choriocarcinoma of the uterus. In this country it occurs following 1 in 25,000 pregnancies. Two modern drugs, methotrexate and actinomycin D, now cure most of the cases, making it the most curable type of cancer next to skin cancer.

CONTRACEPTION AND FAMILY PLANNING

The changing attitudes towards female sexuality have been closely associated with the development of modern methods of contraception (birth control) and widespread knowledge and approval of contraception. The fear of pregnancy has been a traditional· block to sexual fulfillment in many women. The abolition of this fear by modern contraceptive methods has been closely associated with the awakening of female demands for equality with men. With the chance of pregnancy nearly eliminated, women can make the same decisions about sex as men do. Contraception gives men and women the opportunity to make sex a joyful, spontaneous manifestation of their continuing relationship.

Although contraception is never 100 percent effective in preventing pregnancy, modern methods approach complete effectiveness, and have had major effects on attitudes, social policy, and perhaps behavior. At least five major results may be cited.

1 Individual families can and do restrict the number and spacing of their children, with important psychological and economic advantages and without resorting to sexual abstinence.

2 National birth rates have fallen, diminishing the population explosion and the increase in pollution, as discussed in detail in Chapter 3, Human Ecology. The potential for maintaining earth as a place habitable by mankind now exists.

3 Demands on hospitals, schools, and manufactured goods for children have diminished, and relative changes in other parts of the economy have occurred and will continue to occur.

4 The sex lives of many people have been made vastly more satisfying by the removal of the fear of unwanted pregnancy.

5 Contraception may have contributed and may be contributing to a more liberal attitude toward sexual activity before and outside marriage, although it is more likely that the increased openness about sex in our society has contributed more to the acceptance of contraception than vice versa.

The term *contraception* refers to methods of avoiding pregnancy without avoiding sexual intercourse. Techniques of contraception have been known for centuries, perhaps millennia, but effectiveness and esthetic acceptability are recent improvements. Contraceptive techniques can be divided into three groups: first, those which use no mechanical or chemical devices but which attempt to avoid pregnancy by utilizing special techniques of intercourse (mainly, withdrawal) or timing of intercourse (rhythm system); second, those which mechanically attempt to prevent sperm from reaching an ovum or prevent a fertilized ovum from implanting in the uterus; and finally, substances given by injection or by mouth to prevent ovulation or to prevent implantation of a fertilized ovum.

Experts describe the "ideal contraceptive" as one that would be effective, safe, inexpensive, reversible, easy to use, and acceptable to a diversity of people and cultural groups. These experts also doubt that a single contraceptive will ever be found to meet all these conditions.

Many methods have been used to limit the number of children in a family or in a community. Infanticide, or killing of newborn babies by various means, is looked upon with abhorrence in Western society today, but it has been used in many parts of the world to control family size. (Abortion is discussed in Chapter 3.) Sexual abstinence is the only method of birth control presently approved by the Roman Catholic Church for married couples, but only a minority of married couples have found abstinence both desirable and possible. Obviously, too, many persons are unwilling to accept abstinence until marriage.

STERILIZATION

Sterilization is an important method of preventing pregnancy which is growing in popularity. Over the years, the most common sterilization procedure for women has been the cutting and tying of the Fallopian tubes to prevent an ovum from becoming available to sperm. However, vasectomy, the male sterilization procedure, is simpler to perform, has less risk, and is being performed with increasing frequency both here and abroad. In 1970, there were 750,000 vasectomies performed in the United States. Small incisions are made in the sides of the scrotum and the spermatic cords (vas deferens) are cut and tied so that sperm cannot be ejaculated in the semen. The operation does not affect the ability to have intercourse or the sensations of intercourse; it neither lengthens nor shortens sexual life. For couples who have already had several children and desire no more, sterilization is an ideal method of preventing further pregnancies while allowing a normal sexual life free of contraceptive planning or worry. Furthermore, doctors are having increasing success with reversible vasectomies. (See also page 27, Chapter 3).

COITUS INTERRUPTUS

The most common method of contraception of all time, and probably even today, is coitus interruptus, or withdrawal. When the man feels that he is about to ejaculate, he withdraws his penis from the vagina, so that his semen is not ejaculated into the vagina. The method is far from 100 percent effective, for a few sperm may make their way into the vagina during the early part of intercourse, or the man may fail to withdraw in time, or he may ejaculate just outside the vagina and some sperm may make their way through the vagina into the uterus; any of these events may result in pregnancy. Furthermore, the withdrawal method involves substantial frustration for both men and women and is therefore not a particularly satisfying experience for either partner.

RHYTHM

Another method of contraception which uses no devices or medications is the rhythm method. The rhythm method is based on the fact that only near the time of ovulation can intercourse result in pregnancy. The ovum can be fertilized for only about 48 hours after it is released, and sperm can fertilize an ovum for only about 36 hours after ejaculation.

This system is unsatisfactory because the time of ovulation varies widely from person to person and even from month to month for some women. Most women ovulate about 14 days before the start of their next menstrual periods, with the usual range being from 12 to 16 days. The body temperature may rise a half degree or more at this time, and there may be minor cramps in the low abdomen because a tiny amount of blood is released with the ovum. However, women can become pregnant on any day of the menstrual cycle, including the days on which they are menstruating. This fact leads to the quip that couples who use the rhythm system of birth control are called *parents*.

Another group of birth-control methods is the use of physical or chemical means locally to prevent the sperm from reaching an ovum or to prevent a fertilized ovum from implanting in the uterus.

FOLK CONTRACEPTIVES

Old folk contraceptives included such ineffective methods as installations of tea leaves or lemon juice in the vagina; even today some women rely on the relatively ineffective use of a douche (flushing of the vagina with water or other liquids). A modern version of such methods is the use of spermicidal jellies and foams, discussed below.

CONDOMS

A more effective local method is the condom, male sheath, or prophylactic, which was known at least as long ago as the seventeenth century. Made of rubber, plastic, or some similar material, the condom is pulled onto the erect penis just before intercourse. In addition to preventing pregnancy in most cases, it prevents the spread of venereal disease when either partner is infected.

DIAPHRAGMS

The diaphragm is a device which fits loosely over the cervix of the uterus, and extends from the posterior portion of the vagina to the anterior portion just behind the pubic bone. Since the center of the diaphragm is soft and pliable, it does not interfere with intercourse. Many physicians advise that the diaphragm be used with a spermicidal jelly or foam for added protection.

Both the condom and the diaphragm are esthetically undersirable or bothersome to many people. Furthermore, occasionally they fail to be effective because of defects in the apparatus or in the method of use.

SPERMICIDAL JELLIES AND FOAMS

Spermicidal jellies and foams are widely used by themselves, and are often found more acceptable than the condom or diaphragm. They are more effective in preventing pregnancy than the rhythm system but slightly less effective than the condom or diaphragm. Like the condom but unlike the diaphragm, they are readily available in drugstores without prescription and without need for fitting. They are inserted into the vagina with an applicator before *each* sexual act.

INTRAUTERINE DEVICES

Intrauterine contraceptive devices (IUCDs or, more simply, IUDs) must be inserted into the uterus by a trained person, usually a physician. They remain in the uterus for extended periods, but may be removed at any time that their wearer wishes to become pregnant. Although most of them are entirely comfortable and effective, about 25 percent are either expelled (involuntarily) by the uterus or cause enough crampiness and bleeding that they must be removed. Rarely, a device will penetrate through the wall of the uterus into the general abdominal cavity and require abdominal surgery. On other rare occasions, pregnancy will occur even with a device in place. But since the IUD requires no action by either partner before

intercourse and no regular schedule of medication, it has some advantages over other methods of contraception. It has been used extensively in India and other underdeveloped countries in an effort to reduce the birth rate.

THE PILL

The adoption of oral contraceptives, collectively called "the pill," by the American public has been spectacular. Never in the history of mankind has so large a percentage of a population used a new drug so promptly. First readily available on prescription in 1960, the pill had been used by approximately a quarter of the women of childbearing age in its first half dozen years, and by 1970 three-quarters of all young women either had used, were using, or expected to use it. Effective, easy to use, esthetic, and relatively safe, the pill has seemed the answer to the contraceptive needs of the American people, and perhaps eventually the world. Its use has been followed by a significant reduction in birth rates, and the number of unplanned pregnancies has been significantly reduced.

The oral contraceptives work by suppressing ovulation. The chief agent in the pills is chemically similar to the progesterone hormones which are secreted in large amounts by the placenta during pregnancy; they make the body "think" it is pregnant. In their presence, the ovaries do not release ova.

The effectiveness of the pill is close to 100 percent. Occasional pregnancies have occurred among women taking the pill, but most if not all of these have occurred because the woman had forgotten to take one or more doses. Careful adherence to the instructions given at the time of prescription is necessary for effectiveness.

The pill appears safe. Clotting in the veins of the legs and occasionally elsewhere occurs rarely, and part of the clot can even break off and form an embolus to the lungs. But only 2 or 3 women out of 100,000 taking oral contraceptives have these complications; this is substantially safer than riding in an automobile regularly and is about twenty times as safe as being pregnant for 9 months. A few women have protracted nausea and even vomiting from the pill, which may or may not be relieved by switching to medication with a different formula. A rise in blood pressure rarely may necessitate discontinuance of medication. Weight gain and headaches are other relatively minor problems which affect a few women. No other serious complications are known; studies are under way to make sure that oral contraceptives do not increase the incidence of cancer. A woman receiving a prescription for the pill is given instructions on symptoms to look for which might indicate a complication due to her medication. It has been found that doses of hormone much lower than those originally given are still effective, so that the oral contraceptives in use in the 1970s are safer than those of the 1960s.

RESEARCH INTO NEW METHODS OF CONTRACEPTION

Present research on chemical methods to prevent pregnancy concentrates on three kinds of medications. First, a "morning-after" pill: medication which could be taken after intercourse exposure to an unwanted pregnancy. Even now, large doses of estrogen will often alter the lining of the uterus in such a way that implantation of a fertilized ovum cannot occur. Second, medication which would prevent the production of sperm, or at least sperm which are able to move under their own power through the uterus. Third, medication which will alter the chemical composition of semen or vaginal or uterine secretions in such a way as to immobilize sperm, to make sperm unable to fertilize an ovum, or to make a fertilized ovum unable to implant.

SOCIAL, ETHICAL, AND MORAL QUESTIONS IN CONTRACEPTION

It has become firmly established by law that contraception advice and prescriptions should be readily available. With this right and freedom established in most states, American couples now usually expect to use one or another method of birth control during parts of their married lives. Many will have had as many children as they feel they can or should bring up before they are out of their twenties; this means finding effective methods of birth control for another 20 or 30 years. Fortunately, this search is not difficult today. With the advent of oral contraceptives and the excellent work of Planned Parenthood associations throughout the country, the spread of birth-control practices throughout the population has been rapid.

FAMILY SIZE

The number of children in a family has become a major social issue as well as a matter of importance for individual families. Many environmental and political experts, as well as Zero Population Growth, an organization founded in 1969, have been calling for a cessation of any population growth in the United States. They urge that every married couple voluntarily refrain from having more than two children. The economics and dynamics of population growth are discussed in Chapter 3, Human Ecology.

The needs of the world for a restriction of population growth are clear enough. They place an obligation on each couple to consider how many children will be really beneficial to their society and their world. In recent years, about 12 percent of the families of the United States have had four or more children in contrast to only 6 percent in 1950. It will take determination by many couples to reverse this trend.

Even if a couple disclaim any responsibility to limit the size of their family for the benefit of society, they have an important decision to make about the number of children that they want, can afford, and can effectively raise. Some couples raise a large number of children with superb skill; their children are responsible, happy, and well-cared-for. In other families, a large number of children are an inordinate stress on the parents, particularly the mother, and the children themselves are poorly raised. The couple who want a home in absolute order, with all objects in their proper spot, cannot have a large family without being subjected to inordinate emotional strain. If neither partner is able to awaken easily at night to meet the needs of small children, they will not want to go through that period of child care often. Career plans and other interests must also be taken into consideration. Travel with small children is not usually pleasant.

As a group, children from large families do not prosper as well as children from smaller families, exclusive, that is, of the "only child." A child's emotional health is strongly affected by the number of brothers and sisters he has; his parents' attention, love, and commitment can be stretched just so far. Despite obvious exceptions of outstanding children from large families, the average youngster from a large family adjusts less readily, is smaller and less vigorous, and is more likely to have mental illness than the average youngster from a smaller family. Several studies of elementary and high school children have shown that the child from a small family gets along more happily with his brothers, sisters, and parents than the child from a large family. A survey of state hospitals in Maryland showed that mental illness among children in families with both parents present in the household increases with the number of children. About 70 percent of draftees rejected because of poor performance on tests of mental ability come from families of four or more children, and 47 percent of those rejected come from families with six or more children. Teen-age boys in the annual Westinghouse Talent Search rarely come from families with more than two children. Although babies born in large families have normal weights at birth, they are smaller when they reach school age. Babies in large families where the children are close together in age are less responsive and more lethargic than those in small families; these defects often persist into adulthood.

Some of the differences between small families and large families may be partly due to poverty. One study showed, however, that at any given level of poverty or wealth, children from small families outperformed children from large families intellectually.

The reasons for these differences are probably both psychological and physical. Mothers may not recover full physical strength and vigor between pregnancies. After the first child or two, each succeeding child is likely to receive less and less attention, and indeed, the care of younger children is likely to be relegated to older brothers and sisters after the number of children in the family passes four or five. A small child already second or third in the age hierarchy of the family often suffers severe deprivation when his mother has another baby; he goes from a modicum of attention as the reigning "baby of the family" to very little attention except for his immediate physical needs.

Furthermore, an increasing number of children may harm the relationship between the parents themselves. There is less time for parents to tend to each other's needs. As a result parents of large families suffer more mental and physical illness than parents of small families.

There are many exceptions to all these generalizations. Almost everyone knows outstanding large families or outstanding children or parents from large families, but this does not change the basic facts. A young couple who start out to have a large family are stacking the deck against themselves and against their children.

Similarly, unwanted children do not prosper as well as wanted children. In Sweden, children born of pregnancies during which the mothers requested but were denied an abortion were comprehensively studied over a long period and compared with a control group. Compared with the control group, the unwanted children were more likely to have an insecure childhood, to require psychiatric help, to be poorly educated, and to become juvenile delinquents—as well as being more likely to be born illegitimately and to be given out for adoption.

Little information is available on the effect of various amounts of spacing between children, but marriages in which the first child comes 2 or more years after the marriage have a lower divorce rate than marriages in which the first child arrives within 10 months of the marriage. Couples who wait to have children have a chance to strengthen their own relationship before taking on the responsibility of a child.

RAISING CHILDREN

Increasingly, babies are born to live and not to die. In the United States in 1900, 162 out of every 1,000 babies born alive died before their first birthdays; now only 20 babies out of every 1,000 fail to survive their first year. (See Figure 22.4.) In this country there is considerable concern about the fact that some thirteen countries, most of them in Western Europe, have lower infant death rates than the United States. However, Europe as a whole has a higher infant mortality rate than the United States.

A more challenging and relevant way of looking at infant mortality figures is to note that infant mortality is substantially higher in the impoverished areas of the cities and rural districts of the

Figure 22.4   Number of children reaching age 17 annually, 1950 to 1985 (anticipated). Source: Population Reference Bureau, Washington, D.C.

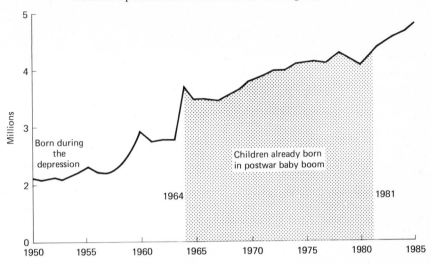

United States than in the more affluent parts of the country. An adequate diet for all pregnant women, adequate and readily accessible medical care during pregnancy, ready availability of effective contraception so that women who wish to avoid too many children can do so, and adequate housing for all would give the newborn babies who now die a reasonable chance for survival.

For the mother whose medical, dietary, and housing needs are well filled, the major concern may be the psychological nourishment of her child. She will as a matter of course see to it that he is well fed and obtains the desirable immunizations (see Chapter 17), but she may wonder about the desirability of breast feeding and about other factors that may affect his emotional health.

Bottle-fed and breast-fed babies are equal in physical and intellectual development, provided that the bottle-fed babies are picked up and cuddled as much as the breast-fed babies. However, as a group, nursing mothers are emotionally warmer to their babies and give them more attention than bottle-feeding mothers. Women who have misgivings about motherhood and about sexuality and who are excessively modest often do not attempt to nurse their babies. There have recently been movements toward natural childbirth (childbirth without anesthetics) and rooming-in (keeping the baby in the same hospital room as the mother

instead of in the hospital nursery). Probably the most beneficial effect of such practices has been to create an immediate, warm attitude by the mother toward the child.

From a psychological viewpoint, growing children need three things from their parents: love, attention, and discipline. Omitting any of the three is likely to give a child psychological difficulty as he grows older. It has become fashionable to criticize Dr. Benjamin Spock for advocating "permissiveness" with growing children. Dr. Spock was a major factor in helping American families get rid of the reliance on rules and schedules which some parents of the early decades of this century often used instead of love and attention. He gives such important advice as, "Love and enjoy your child for what he is, for what he looks like, for what he does, and forget about the qualities that he doesn't have." But his critics forget that he also has urged discipline and control of children's antisocial impulses: "He needs to feel that his mother and father, however agreeable, still have their own rights, know how to be firm, won't let him be unreasonable or rude. He likes them better that way."[1] This is still good advice.

The uses and misuses of experience are impor-

[1]Benjamin Spock, M.D.: *The Pocket Book of Baby and Child Care,* Cardinal Edition, Pocket Books, Inc., New York, 1951, p. 21, 256.

tant in parent-child relationships. Though young people often feel that the experience of older generations is useless, such experience does exist, is important, and may be relevant to the present and the future. Despite changing circumstances, human motives and human behavior remain remarkably similar—not predictable, perhaps, but similar. In many ways and every day, human beings give each other signals about their desires and intentions, signals which perceptive people learn to recognize better with experience. Experience becomes important not only in managing situations and people, but also in meeting the psychological and practical needs of other people and in avoiding doing them harm. Parents should consider experience, either direct or vicarious, as something which they have an obligation to pass on to their children and grandchildren, rather than something which gives them the right to make decisions for their children and grandchildren. There are some guidelines which can be useful. Experience should not be reserved for episodes of controversy or times of argument, to be used as a supposedly irrefutable bulwark to an adult position. Rather, periodic introduction of the young person to the experience of the older transmits events and knowledge as a vicarious experience as well as creating a greater bond between the two generations.

Next, the nature of past experience and its applicability to present circumstances should be carefully defined and discussed. It is useful for a man to say to his son, "Twenty-five years ago when I was in college, such and such happened to me. Perhaps your circumstances are similar in this way." It is not useful for him to say, "Twenty-five years ago such and such happened to me, and therefore you must do as I did (or as I didn't do)." The son may have less experience than his father, but he has an equal right to an opinion on the applicability to the present of what happened 25 years ago. When children are young, their actions are more subject to parental control than those of college students, but insofar as experience can be discussed between the generations, the discussion should be carried on with the rights of individuals in mind.

HAZARDS TO INFANTS AND CHILDREN

Modern medical and hospital care have reduced deaths among infants and children dramatically.

It is important, however, to remember that the primary responsibility for the care of the infant and child belongs to the parent. Not nearly all the improvement in infant mortality is due to hospital care. In the Netherlands, 70 percent of babies are delivered at home by general physicians and midwives, and that country has a lower infant mortality rate than the United States. The Dutch reduced infant mortality by half between 1900 and 1922, cut it in half again between 1923 and 1939, and again between 1948 and 1964. By 1964, of every 1,000 babies born alive, only 15 babies died. This success has been made possible by high standards of prenatal care and high standards of infant care in Dutch homes.

Most of the drop in infant mortality in Western society has been due to the decrease in infections and particularly in diarrheal and intestinal diseases. With sanitation, better general health, improved methods of infant feeding, and to some extent better medical care, diarrhea and intestinal disease are now rare causes of death in American infants.

It is important to recognize certain diseases early in the life of an infant in order to prevent or minimize the damage they can do. Phenylketonuria, a hereditary disease characterized by mental deficiency and by the excretion of a peculiar chemical, phenylketonuric acid, in the urine, can be detected shortly after birth by testing the urine and blood. When detected early, a diet very low in the amino acid phenylalanine prevents the mental deficiency. Similarly, a lack of thyroid hormone detected and treated in the first few months of life will prevent the mental deficiency and physical retardation called *cretinism*. (See page 296) Hyaline-membrane disease and cystic fibrosis are two diseases affecting the lungs of infants which respond partially to treatment.

A disease which causes jaundice in infants, erythroblastosis, used to cause many deaths among newborn infants, and some infants with the disease were born dead. A few years ago, it was discovered that this disease is caused by a certain incompatability in blood types. The terms *Rh negative* and *Rh postive* refer to a property of the red blood cells, with 85 percent of people being Rh positive. When a mother is Rh negative and her baby has inherited Rh-positive blood from the father, the mother becomes allergic to the baby's red blood cells. When a few of his cells get across the placenta into her bloodstream, an immunity is set up and the red blood cells of the baby are damaged, resulting in erythroblastosis. If many cells are damaged, the baby dies before birth. Fortunately this complication rarely occurs on the first pregnancy. In recent years, after an Rh-negative mother has given birth to an Rh-positive child, it has been possible to inject the mother with antibodies against the Rh factor which block her sensitivity to the Rh factor and keep her from starting to produce antibodies that would endanger children of future pregnancies. Unfortunately, however, if the mother is already a producer of antibodies, due to previous transfusion or pregnancy, the injection will be ineffective.

HEREDITY

Next to the physical and psychological care which parents give to children, heredity is the most important link between the generations. (See Figure 22.5.) Both physical and psychological characteristics are passed on from generation to generation by way of chromosomes. The ovum and the sperm have 23 chromosomes each, only half the normal number in human cells; the fertilized ovum, then, has the full human complement, 46, with half of the embryo's heredity (in the form of chromosomes) coming from the mother and half from the father. The sperm and the ovum each give twenty-two body chromosomes and one sex chromosome to the new person. Sex chromosomes can be either X or Y. All human beings have one X sex chromosome; if the other sex chromosome is also an X, the individual is female; if the other sex chromosome is a Y, the individual is male.

The chromosomes in each human cell contain perhaps 10 million genes, each of which is composed of the chemical molecule DNA. DNA has been called the tape recorder of life, storing, coding, and transmitting all hereditary information to the fertilized ovum and from cell to cell during division. In recent years, DNA has been synthesized in the laboratory, and scientists have even succeeded in putting together an entire gene. Mankind seems on the verge of being able to control heredity.

DNA, located in the nucleus of cells, is constantly sending out "messages" through a chemical intermediary, ribonucleic acid (RNA). In this way it controls cell development, growth, digestion, heartbeat, thinking, and feeling. There is no change in these chemical patterns or codes unless they are modified by influences from outside the cell, such as exposure to excessive radiation or other factors. Nothing that normally happens in the lives of either men or women alters the genes which their children receive, and the proportions and combinations of genes that are given to an individual ovum or sperm seem to be a matter of chance. For this reason, children of the same parents do not necessarily show identical hereditary patterns.

THE MENDELIAN LAW

Gregor Mendel, an Austrian monk of the nineteenth century, was the first to demonstrate the specific way heredity operates. His experimental materials were two varieties of peas, one tall and one dwarf. He fertilized the blossoms of the tall variety with pollen from the dwarf variety. The seeds which developed from the cross-pollinated plants were then planted. All the plants which grew from these seeds were of the tall variety. They were allowed to develop normally, fertilizing themselves, and the seeds they produced were planted. From these seeds there developed both tall and dwarf varieties, but there were three times as many of the tall as of the dwarf. When the self-pollinated seeds from this crop were planted, only dwarf peas grew from the seeds which had come from dwarf plants; but the seeds from the tall variety again produced both tall and dwarf plants, with five times as many of the tall as of the dwarf variety. This proportion continued generation after generation. However, by selection of plants, Mendel was able to obtain from among the tall variety certain plants, the seeds of which would produce only tall peas. From these observations was derived the rule that whenever a pure strain, either tall or dwarf variety, was fertilized from the same variety, the seeds which developed produced only the corresponding variety; but that cross fertilization between the pure tall and the pure dwarf varieties resulted in seeds which produced only the tall variety. From this it was concluded that, when hereditary elements which make for tallness or shortness are both present, the determinant for tallness always predominates. More specifically, there is a chromosome for tallness and a chromosome for dwarfness.

Figure 22.5 Chromosomes and genes.

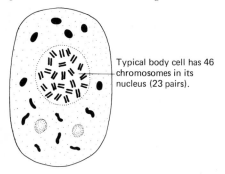

Typical body cell has 46 chromosomes in its nucleus (23 pairs).

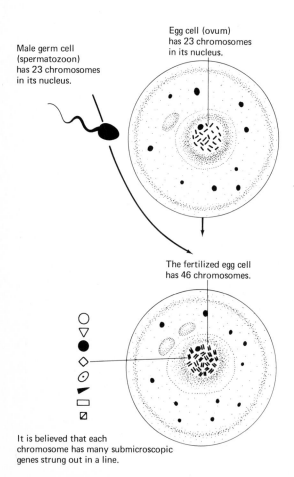

Male germ cell (spermatozoon) has 23 chromosomes in its nucleus.

Egg cell (ovum) has 23 chromosomes in its nucleus.

The fertilized egg cell has 46 chromosomes.

It is believed that each chromosome has many submicroscopic genes strung out in a line.

Each pea plant had two chromosomes. If both chromosomes were for dwarfness, the plant was dwarf, and if both chromosomes were for tallness, the plant was tall. But if the plant had one chromosome for tallness and one for dwarfness, the chromosome for tallness dominated and the plant was tall.

This phenomenon, which has been found to obtain in a large number of hereditary diseases and hereditarily transmitted characteristics, gave rise to the designation of certain traits as *dominant* and others as *recessive*. A simple example of this in human beings is the color of the eyes. It has been observed that brown eyes are dominant over blue. Consequently, if both parents have brown eyes, all the children's eyes will be brown, or if both parents have blue eyes, all the children's eyes will be blue. However, if one parent has pure brown eyes and the other pure blue eyes, the children will have brown eyes or a mixture of brown and blue, with brown predominating. On the other hand, if the parent has "mixed"—hybrid—brown eyes, the children may have either brown eyes or blue eyes. (Figure 22.6.)

Experimentally one can demonstrate the operation of the Mendelian law by breeding black rats with white rats. In this case black is predominant over white, with the result that the first generation of hybrid rats will all be black but hybrid, i.e., will carry the genes which make both for black and for white fur. If rats of this first generation of hybrid blacks are bred together the next generation will be one-fourth pure black, one-fourth pure white, and one-half hybrid black or mixed. Among small numbers of offspring these proportions may not hold, but in large numbers they will invariably hold true.

Among the more important human traits and conditions influenced or determined by heredity are:

1 Conditions the inheritance of which seems to follow the Mendelian pattern with the trait dominant in character: diabetes insipidus; telangiectasis (purple areas in the skin, frequently accompanied by serious nosebleeds); hypospadias (abnormal opening in male urethra); allergies; migraine headache; Huntington's chorea (progressive mental deterioration beginning about

middle age); mirror reading, cataract in young persons, glaucoma, optic-nerve atrophy, hereditary night blindness, drooping eyelids, opaque ring over iris, absence of iris; progressive inner-ear deafness; word deafness, absence of ear; defective enamel of teeth; stub fingers, extra fingers and toes, stiff joints, webbed fingers or toes; brittle bones; deformed spine; dwarfism; progressive muscular atrophy, muscle stiffness; Friedreich's ataxia; pigment spots on skin, lack of pigmentation in skin and hair, fatty growths in skin (frequently of eyelids); horny skin, cysts on scalp, baldness (men only); defective hair (beaded, infantile, excessively long, woolly, prematurely gray); defective nails; retinoblastoma

2 Conditions which are hereditary according to the Mendelian pattern but recessive in character—i.e., they develop only if inherited from both parents: diabetes mellitus; cystic fibrosis; jaundice of the newborn; certain types of feeblemindedness; nearsightedness and extreme farsightedness, complete colorblindness, blurred vision in strong light; albinism—skin and hair dead white and eyes pink; small fatty growths on face and scalp; skin sensitive to light; absent nails; phenylketonuria

3 Conditions which are transmitted according to the Mendelian patterns but are sex-linked—i.e., they act as dominant traits in males and as recessive in females, appearing in males if inherited from either parent but in females only if inherited from both parents: hemophilia (defective blood clotting, found in "bleeders"); red-green color-blindness; pink eyes without other albino characteristics; certain types of hernias

4 Conditions the inheritance of which is probably Mendelian in character but whose dominance is uncertain or imperfect: cleft palate, harelip; otosclerosis; double row of eyelashes; astigmatism; missing teeth, extra teeth, thick nails; imperfectly developed male sex organs; tendency to produce twins; lefthandedness; hypertension

5 Conditions which are hereditary but seem

Figure 22.6 Mendelian law and color of eyes.

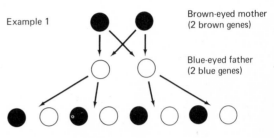

Brown gene (dominant)

Blue gene (recessive)

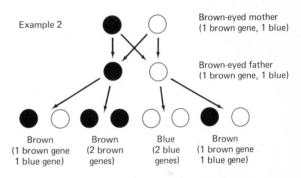

Example 1

Brown-eyed mother (2 brown genes)

Blue-eyed father (2 blue genes)

All the children are brown-eyed (1 dominant brown gene, 1 recessive blue)

Example 2

Brown-eyed mother (1 brown gene, 1 blue)

Brown-eyed father (1 brown gene, 1 blue)

Brown (1 brown gene 1 blue gene)   Brown (2 brown genes)   Blue (2 blue genes)   Brown (1 brown gene 1 blue gene)

to follow a pattern of blending of dominant and recessive characteristics: general body size, stature; weight; skin color; hair form; shape of head and facial proportions.

6 Conditions which apparently are influenced by heredity but the extent and manner of inheritance of which are uncertain: general mental ability, memory, temperament, musical ability, literary ability, artistic ability, mathematical ability, mechanical ability; longevity; liability to hernia; some types of epilepsy and insanity; high blood pressure; cancer; psoriasis; thick or shedding skin; deaf-mutism; gout; certain defects of the glands of internal secretion; pernicious anemia; paralysis agitans; birthmarks; resistance to disease

GENETIC COUNSELING AND EUGENICS

In most major medical centers, doctors who are particularly knowledgeable about genetic transmission of defects are now able to give expert advice to parents who have actual or potential problems in genetics. If one or both parents have diabetes, or epilepsy, or a family history of schizophrenia, for example, or if they have already had a child with a congenital defect, a genetic counselor can advise them on the chances that a prospective child will have the same problem. In many cases, the counselor can reassure them that the chances are small. A parent who has an abnormal hole between the two sides of the heart (a septal defect), for example, has only a very small chance of transmitting this defect to a child, provided that there are no such cases in his spouse's family. If the hole is in the upper part of heart (atrial septal defect), the possibility is 2.6 percent, and if the hole is between the two main chambers of the heart (ventricular septal defect), the possibility is 3.7 percent, but parents without such a history in their families have only one-twentieth that chance of producing a baby with a septal defect.

Eugenics is the practical application of the established principles of heredity to the improvement of the human race. In this sense, personal genetic counseling can contribute to eugenics. However, present knowledge of genetics is far from sufficient to allow controlling the genetic makeup of the race as the makeup of domestic animals has been controlled, even though Aldous Huxley considered the prospect as early as 1932 in *Brave New World*. The important aim for the present generation is to remember that heredity and genetics are essential parts of planning a family and being a parent.

QUESTIONS FOR DISCUSSION AND SELF-EXAMINATION

1 Describe the physiological forces which tend to favor pregnancy during a woman's lifetime.
2 What is the relationship of fertilization to implantation, and what is the role of each in pregnancy?
3 Describe the differences between identical and fraternal twins in their origin and in their development, both in the uterus and after birth.
4 What factors promote the chances of a healthy baby and a healthy mother at the end of pregnancy?
5 What were the two most common hazards of pregnancy and childbirth in the past, and what has led to their reduction?
6 Distinguish between the purposes and the results of contraception. How do they overlap?
7 How do the various contraceptive methods compare in effectiveness, in esthetic desirability, and in risk to health and life?
8 Discuss the effects upon children, adults, and society of (a) a large family and (b) a small family?
9 Is hospital delivery of babies essential to a low mortality rate among newborn infants? Document and explain your answer.
10 How is the principle of hereditary dominance important for human beings?

REFERENCES AND READING SUGGESTIONS

BOOKS

Beadle, George, and Muriel Beadle: *The Language of Life*, Doubleday & Company, Inc., Garden City, N.Y., 1966.

A Nobel Prize laureate and his journalist wife present a nontechnical explanation of the recently discovered genetic code and its significance to health and to the future of life on the earth.

Carson, Hampton L.: *Heredity and Human Life,* Columbia University Press, New York, 1963; paperback, 1965.

Latest scientific facts on man's origin, evolution, and heritage, and the implications they have on his life. A basic study of human evolution written for the literate layman.

Guttmacher, Alan F.: *Babies by Choice,* paperback, Avon Book Division, The Hearst Corporation, New York, 1961.

A forthright discussion of this important subject by a distinguished professor of obstetrics and gynecology who is president of the Planned Parenthood Federation of America.

PAMPHLETS AND PERIODICALS

Abraham, Willard: "Our Children—Our Problem," *Today's Health,* February 1966, p. 58.

Parental permissiveness has given rise to the nation's largest pressure group—our children. What can parents do about it?

Alk, Madelin (Ed.): *The Expectant Mother,* Trident Press, a division of Simon & Schuster, Inc., New York, 1967.

A reassuring guide to the special demands of pregnancy and childbirth. Prepared by *Redbook* magazine in cooperation with the American College of Obstetrics and Gynecology.

Apgar, V.: "What Every Mother-to-be Should Know about Pregnancy," *Today's Health,* March 1966, p. 6; April 1966, p. 8; and May 1966, p. 16.

Bergsma, Daniel, and James German: *New Directions in Human Genetics,* The National Foundation, New York, 1965.

A symposium presented by New York Hospital and Cornell University Medical Center.

"Birth Control—All the Methods That Work . . . and the Ones That Don't," Planned Parenthood of New York City, 1971.

Brody, Jane E.: "The Pill: Revolution in Birth Control," *The New York Times Magazine,* May 31, 1966, p. 1.

A splendid analysis of the medical, sociological, and ethical aspects of the use of "the pill" and certain other methods of birth control.

Carson, Ruth: *Nine Months to Get Ready: The Importance of Prenatal Care,* Public Affairs Pamphlet, New York.

"Drama of Life Before Birth," *Life,* Apr. 30, 1965, pp. 54–72.

A splendid explanation with remarkable and unique photographs of the development of a baby within the uterus of its mother.

"Genetics and Your Health," *World Health,* magazine of the World Health Organization, August-September 1966.

An excellent series of articles on genetics and its implication for human health.

23

AGING AND DYING

Youth, with its successes and its failures, its joys and its heartaches, is a thrilling, glorious adventure. But stores of exuberant energy, of hope and enthusiasm are not inexhaustible. It is important that this be understood and appreciated, because the years slip by quickly, and health in later years depends to a large extent on practices and habits begun in youth. Furthermore, most young people have associations with and frequently have responsibilities for older persons—parents, grandparents, other relatives, or friends—and should have some understanding of their health problems.

THE PROCESS OF AGING

Beginning at birth and continuing throughout life the cells of the various tissues and organs of the body are maturing, reproducing, aging, dying, and being replaced. Individual cells of the body live from a few days (9 days for white blood cells, about 20 days for the cells of the skin, and 120 days for red blood cells) to many years: in fact, muscle cells and nerve cells live throughout most if not all of one's life. The aging of the organs of the body likewise proceeds at different rates: e.g., visual acuity is greatest at about 10 years of age and declines gradually thereafter; hearing usually begins to decline during the twenties; and ovulation in women ceases with the menopause, usually in the forties or early fifties.

Recent studies of aging suggest that many of the changes characteristic of the aging process are hastened by habits of living and by the accumulation of injuries to tissues from disease and from the stresses, strains, and toxins to which we subject ourselves throughout life.

The rate of the aging process is influenced also by the genes inherited. Life insurance companies recognize this, and an application form for insurance requests information on the ages at death of one's brothers, sisters, parents, and grandparents. Although nothing can be done about heredity, much can be done to conserve and develop the physical and mental assets with which people are endowed. In fact, what one does in youth and early adult years not only influences but may well determine the condition of health in later years.

THE AGING POPULATION

As the diseases and conditions which cause death in the earlier years of life are brought under control, an increasing number of persons are reaching advanced years. In 1900 there were approximately 3 million persons in the United States over 65 years of age. In 1970 the corresponding number was 20 million, and it is estimated that by 1980 there will be 25 million over 65. Approximately 1,000 persons reach the age of 65 every day. Today the average life expectancy for 65-year-old men is 13 years and for 65-year-old women 16 years.

Many elderly or aging people are forced for financial or health reasons to live with younger family members. Such younger people therefore have daily contact with the elderly; the importance of understanding the physical and psychological difficulties experienced by the elderly is obvious.

Although 65 has become the widely accepted age for retirement, about 40 percent of the population continue employment beyond this age. Self-employed persons, such as physicians, lawyers, writers, small businessmen, and farmers, can continue to work as long as they wish and their health permits.

The increase in the proportion of older persons means an increase in the importance of health problems in advancing years. (See Figure 23.1.) There are physicians who specialize in geriatrics, although the term *geriatrics* was coined less than 50 years ago. Literally, from its Greek origin, it means "the medical care of aging persons." Closely allied to it is the term *gerontology*, which refers to the scientific study of the phenomena of aging and is often called the *science of aging*.

In a youth-oriented society, growing old gives rise to many difficult problems. Not only do the elderly often face failing health and financial pressures, but many also feel isolated from the mainstream of life. Some are fortunate enough to have their mates by their sides, or at least relatives and friends; but for many, old age is a time of loneliness. All these factors may start a downward spiral of emotional, social, and physical deterioration.

The customary image of old age as a time for rest and relaxation—a reward for years of toil—must be changed. Older persons are a social and economic asset if their value is seen in true perspective, if their great reservoir of wisdom and useful skills is utilized. A person can take pride in his family, his community, or his social group only if he feels himself a functioning part of the group and only to the degree that he can maintain his sense of personal worth and dignity within the group. One group whose aging members are still active and useful is an international organization for industrial consultation, formed several years ago by retired executives. These people are in great demand all over the world for advice on business. They are using their age to advantage.

With advancing age, physical strength and vigor decrease, but the same is not necessarily true of mental activity. Many people make their most significant achievements in their early years. However, studies show no decline in mental capacity in the fifties, and there is no evidence of decrease in memory, reasoning, and decision-making powers even in 60- and 70-year-olds. In fact, in one study, aging executives showed as much mental ability as 25-year-old medical students. It thus appears that most decline in mental power results from the brain's getting too little rather than too much work.

The chairman of the U.S. Senate Committee on Aging has said:

Senior citizens are not just some indefinable group separate and apart. They are our mothers and our

Figure 23.1 Sickness increases with age. Number of disability days per person per year, by age and sex. Source: National Health Survey, U.S. Public Health Service, Washington, D.C., June 1966.

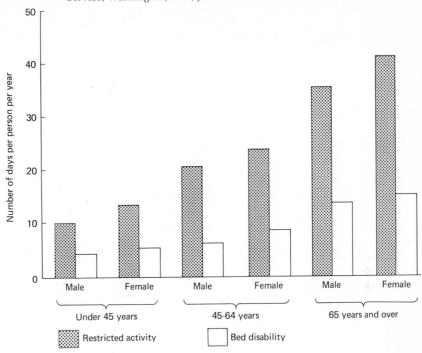

fathers. They are "ourselves" after a few short years. They are those of us who have made contributions to society and to our country. They are those who have given their energies, their skills,

and their children for the good of society. Society must not ignore them when their hair is grey and their shoulders bent.

SPECIAL HEALTH PROBLEMS

The number of chronic diseases, accidents, and disabilities increases with age. Heart disease, emphysema, arthritis and rheumatism, and accidents are the most common causes of disability among persons age 65 and over. Other common chronic conditions among older people are other respiratory diseases, visual impairments, defective hearing, hypertension, stroke, cancer, and mental and nervous degeneration.

In general, the factors that contribute to disease, disability, and good health in older persons differ only in degree and emphasis from those that affect younger persons.

NUTRITION

Basic nutritional needs for older persons are essentially the same as the requirements for good nutrition among younger persons. However, with decreased physical activity, fewer functioning body cells, and a lower rate of metabolism, fewer calories are required to maintain a desirable weight. Failure to recognize this can lead to overweight—a handicap which is especially serious for older people.

Various factors have a bearing on nutritional problems in the later years of life. The person living by himself finds it lonely to sit down to a meal

Figure 23.2 The aged frequently ignore their diet. (Photograph from U.S. Department of Agriculture.)

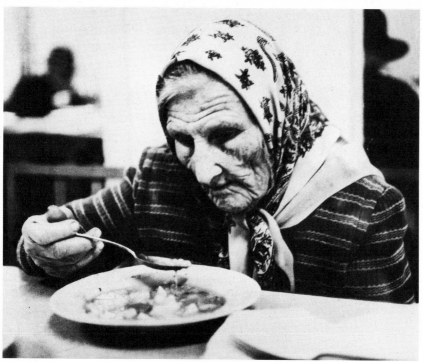

and consequently does not partake of good food even when it is available. Insufficient funds sometimes do not permit the purchase of foods which have been enjoyed in previous years. Often, because the older person is not physically able to prepare food, he eats a monotonous diet of foods which require very little preparation. The elderly person's diet is most commonly low in proteins, vitamins A and C, and iron. It is high in carbohydrates, which are cheaper and require less preparation than other foods. The elderly frequently eat only two meals a day, often deficient in nutrients and liquids. (See Figure 23.2.)

Older people have become the special target of many health swindles. The government estimates that each year Americans spend $500 million on vitamins, minerals, and "health foods" that they just don't need. Many of these dollars go for foods which promoters claim will prevent and cure ills ranging from arthritis to high blood pressure.

Most products which claim special health-giving properties contain the same nutritional properties found in more common, and much cheaper, foods. For example, yogurt may be recommended by a physician for certain intestinal conditions. Nutritionally, however, it is the same as milk, which is cheaper (though yogurt is fat-free, as skim milk is). The iodine in "kelp tablets" or "sea salt" is a costly substitute for the iodine in regular seafoods and iodized salt. And while wheat germ is a useful cereal food, it won't peform nutritional miracles. As for vitamins, older people can get all that they need from their everyday foods.

This does not mean that special diets may not be indicated for particular physical disabilities or diseases. If a physician prescribes some special type of diet, his instructions should be followed.

Pleasant surroundings and foods that are varied, carefully selected, and attractive in appearance are especially appreciated by the aging person for whom mealtime has become a real event in his or her daily routine. Some communities are rendering splendid services by providing "meals on wheels" for older persons who live alone and are unable to cook for themselves. Well-balanced and carefully planned meals are delivered at mealtime. These services are usually developed by volunteer groups. Some are affiliated with hospitals or private catering services. Others are operated in their entirety by the volunteers who sponsor them. Reports indicate that these programs, if well organized and managed, are meeting with great success and are making a tremendously valuable service to the health, welfare, and happiness of large numbers of handicapped elderly persons who want to live in their own homes but who without this service would have to be cared for in institutions.

There are also other programs which help the elderly with the difficult problem of eating well. Some provide reasonably priced meals and opportunities for socializing in high school cafeterias at hours when the students are in classes. Another type of program provides personal assistance in food shopping and preparation. The people it helps range from widowers who have never cooked for themselves to people who are faced with adapting to special diets prescribed by their physicians.

DENTAL PROBLEMS

Regular dental examinations and care are of great importance with advancing years. Peridontal disease and loss of teeth increase in frequency. Dentures which do not fit properly and the absence of teeth interfere with the proper mastication of food, thereby contributing to malnutrition. Most of these conditions can be prevented by good dental care.

WEIGHT

Lean men and women on the average live longer and remain active longer than men and women of average or overaverage weight. Excessive weight is disadvantageous to health and longevity throughout adult life, but its hazard becomes greater with increasing age. Weight control is discussed in Chapter 12.

EXERCISE

Physical fitness is important to a feeling of well-being and to good health in later as well as in earlier years. Muscles deteriorate rapidly with disuse; and flabby muscles predispose to fatigue, backache, painful feet, poor posture, constipation, and various other disabilities. It was the realization of this that led to the introduction of early ambulation

after surgical operations, i.e., having patients out of bed and physically active very soon following operations, instead of having them spend a week or two in bed as was the custom some years ago. The results are fewer complications, less disability, and more rapid convalescence.

Exercise should be continued in later years, but it should be regular and moderate rather than strenuous. Walking is enjoyed by most people, swimming and bicycling by many. In addition, simple setting-up exercises in the morning, as well as purposeful exercising of muscles throughout the day, will do much to keep the muscles in good tone and the figure trim.

VISION

Although the great majority of the aged have adequate vision, it is usually the onset of poor vision that makes one conscious of aging. It becomes increasingly difficult to focus on objects close by, necessitating reading glasses or bifocals. Bifocals, particularly during adjustment to their use, produce a new accident hazard: uncertainty about where one's feet are, especially when descending stairs. Decreasing fields of vision, particularly of side vision, contribute to accidents among aged pedestrians, who may be struck by turning cars when they are crossing streets at intersections.

Elderly persons also need greater illumination and have a decreased tolerance of glare. The aged driver exposed to oncoming headlights when driving at night is increasingly subject to accidents. Curtailment of night driving, therefore, may be indicated.

Cataracts and glaucoma, the most frequent causes of serious and progressive loss of vision with advancing age, can usually be treated succesfully, but proper treatment must be started early. Regular examinations of the eyes will detect both these conditions in their incipiency. (See also Chapter 14.)

HEARING

At least one person out of four over 65 years of age has loss of hearing to a degree that frequently leads to withdrawal from social contacts and contributes to the loneliness and depression of the aged. It also contributes to nervous tensions and irritations both in the one who is hard of hearing and in close associates. It is important that hearing loss be recognized early and alleviated or compensated for when the possibilities of success are greatest. (See Chapter 14.)

ACCIDENTS

Although old age is inevitable, accidents in old age are not. Yet, each year over 3.5 million persons 65 and over suffer accidental injuries, many resulting from falls in the home. Approximately half the deaths from home accidents occur among persons 65 years of age and over.

The older person is particularly liable to accidental injury because often he does not see, hear, or coordinate as well as younger persons. The only way to reduce the number and seriousness of injuries which occur to aged persons is to be constantly aware of where the danger lies. The elderly person must understand that he is particularly vulnerable to accidents and must be alert for dangers at all times; the family has the responsibility of seeing that hazards of the environment and equipment are corrected and maintained in a safe condition. Members of the family can do much to help the aged person to be aware of both present and potential accident hazards. Falls are the major accident hazard of the elderly; therefore, it is important that older persons realize and accept that their coordination is not so good as when they were younger.

Some important measures that can be taken to make life safer and easier for older persons are:

1 Provide "one-floor living" whenever possible.
2 Make living quarters convenient and free of obstructions.
3 Provide bright shadowfree lighting in all rooms used by older persons—with night lights in bedroom, hallway, and bath.
4 Provide strong handrails on all stairs.
5 Store commonly used household items in easily reached places so that climbing and overreaching are unnecessary.
6 Provide comfortable and safe footwear—nonslip shoes with medium or low heels.
7 Be sure that scatter rugs are of the nonskid variety.
8 Obtain an understanding escort for outside excursions if sight, hearing, or physical reactions are impaired.

Automobile accidents Elderly drivers are generally considered a high-risk group on the highways. Slow reflexes and poor vision are given as reasons for this. Yet, several studies indicate that drivers over 65 have fewer injury-producing accidents than other age groups. In fact, a study at the University of Denver covering thirty-one states reports that while older motorists represent about 7.5 percent of all drivers, they account for less than 5 percent of accidents. In view of this, several insurance companies assure older drivers that their automobile insurance will be continued as long as they meet basic eye, medical, and license requirements.

However, visual acuity in dim light and peripheral vision both decrease with age. Night driving by the elderly should therefore be avoided if possible, as should driving in bad weather, at peak traffic hours, and when overtired. Also, long trips should be interrupted by frequent periods of rest and of exercise outside the car.

HEART DISEASE

Heart disease, a leading cause of death and disability of the aged, increases progressively in frequency and in seriousness with age. (See Table 23.1.) For a consideration of heart diseases see Chapter 5.

STROKES

The frequency of strokes, often called *apoplexy* or *cerebrovascular accidents*, increases precipitously after the age of 60, until in persons 75 years of age and over they are second only to heart disease as a cause of death.

The basic reason that strokes occur is a reduction or complete stoppage of blood flow to an area of the brain. When this occurs that portion of the brain ceases to function, and if the loss of function continues for more than a few minutes the portion of the brain affected is seriously and often permanently damaged.

Warning signals of stroke are dizziness, blurred vision, numbness or weakness, slurred speech, changes in facial expression, disturbances of thought processes, and minute personality changes.

In most cases the person who has a stroke does not die in the initial attack. Some paralysis may occur, and there may be speech difficulties. The

Table 23.1 Leading causes of death in the United States, 1950 and 1965; by age groups—45 and over

Cause of death	No. of deaths, 1965	Death rate*	
		1965	1950
45–54:			
Heart diseases	56,915	258	293
Cancer	39,229	178	172
Accidents	11,968	54	57
Stroke	9,917	45	71
Cirrhosis of liver	7,015	32	23
Suicide	4,554	21	18
Influenza and pneumonia	3,329	15	19
Diabetes	2,624	12	12
Nephritis	1,582	7	15
Homicide	1,529	7	6
55–64:			
Heart diseases	119,407	704	783
Cancer	58,978	407	408
Stroke	21,700	128	191
Accidents	10,932	64	73
Cirrhosis of liver	6,800	40	32
Diabetes	6,130	36	44
Influenza and pneumonia	5,644	33	37
Emphysema	4,296	25	
Suicide	4,040	24	27
Ulcer of stomach and duodenum	2,148	13	17
65–74:			
Heart diseases	194,970	1,697	1,763
Cancer	86,409	752	703
Stroke	49,396	430	548
Influenza and pneumonia	10,866	95	75
Diabetes	10,636	93	95
Accidents	10,430	91	114
Emphysema	7,187	63	
Arteriosclerosis	5,982	52	128
Cirrhosis of liver	4,364	38	33
Ulcer of stomach and duodenum	2,841	25	25
75 and over:			
Heart diseases	317,621	4,763	5,200
Stroke	114,190	1,712	1,755
Cancer	77,248	1,158	1,295
Arteriosclerosis	30,139	452	592
Influenza and pneumonia	27,929	419	387
Accidents	17,704	265	437
Diabetes	11,672	175	204
Hypertension without heart mention	6,078	91	106
Emphysema	5,435	81	
Kidney Infections	4,140	62	25

*Rates per 100,000 population in age group.
SOURCE: U.S. Public Health Service.

rehabilitation of many persons who have had strokes can be accomplished with the help of members of the family and the family physician. Visiting nurses and public health nurses are among persons in the community who can give valuable help in the work of rehabilitation. However, to achieve maximum possible function, many people who have had strokes or other cerebrovascular diseases need the multiple services available in a rehabilitation center. (See page 87.) (For detailed consideration of strokes, see page 67.)

HYPERTENSION

In order to maintain a continuous and adequate flow of blood to the tissues that need oxygen and nourishment, the blood in the arteries is constantly under pressure. Adjustments by the mechanism which regulates this pressure are made to meet the body's needs. In hypertension this regulation is disturbed so that the pressure is maintained at an abnormally high level. This does not mean that circulation will be inadequate or that damage will necessarily result. The danger occurs when the pressure increases to such a degree that the heart is unable to maintain adequate circulation or when prolonged pressure damages the walls of the blood vessels, with resultant hemorrhages in the brain or with deficient circulation and excretion through the kidneys.

The cause or causes of hypertension are not completely understood. Heredity, nervous tension, and possibly salt intake are factors, but it is agreed that they are not the only causes. (See Chapter 5 for a further discussion.)

Many people with hypertension need little or no dietary or drug treatment. However, adequate and regular physical examinations are important so that the condition may be discovered and appropriate treatment may be instituted when necessary. Fortunately, the newer drugs and other methods of treatment provide much protection against the ravages of this disease. In fact, from 1952 to 1960, when "hypertensive drugs" first became generally available and used, the death rate from hypertension declined by 32 percent.

CANCER

Cancer also has been considered in Chapter 5, but its toll increases so greatly with advancing years that it demands further emphasis here. Preventive measures of greatest value for the general popula-

tion are the avoidance of cigarette smoking to prevent cancer of the lungs, which takes about 70,000 lives annually in this country, and the avoidance of excessive exposure to sunlight or ultraviolet light to prevent cancer of the skin. In addition, practically all the 9,000 deaths from cancer of the cervix of the uterus could be prevented if women would have annual pelvic examinations, including the Pap smear; and many of the 45,000 deaths from cancer of the colon and rectum could be prevented by annual proctosigmoidoscopic examinations and proper follow-up treatment when indicated. Women can examine their own breasts; if this is done regularly and followed up properly, it can lead to the discovery of many cancers of the breast at a stage in which they can be successfully and completely removed. Familiarity with and observance of the seven warning signals of cancer (page 76) will help to prevent suffering and save many lives.

PROSTATE TUMORS

The prostate gland is present only in males; it is the size of a small walnut and is located at the base of the urethra, the tube that carries the urine out of the body. (The function of the prostate is discussed on page 301.) Cancer of the prostate is the third most common form of cancer among men of all ages, and it is the most common form of cancer in men over 75. These cancers grow slowly at first and may not be detected early enough for cure. Because of the reluctance of men to discuss problems of the prostate, even with a doctor, many cancers go undiagnosed for years. Although some tumors of the prostate are malignant, many are not. It is extremely common for benign tumorlike growths to occur in men over 40. These growths block the passage of urine and may eventually cause infection. It is important that prostate tumors be diagnosed early, before complications can occur.

The usual treatment of a tumor of the prostate is surgery. In some cases, if the tumor is benign, this is a minor operation which may be done under local anesthetic. If, however, the tumor is malignant, and more important, if the tumor has gone undetected for a long time, the surgery may be considerably more extensive.

ARTHRITIS

Although arthritis is discussed in Chapter 6, the prevalence of arthritis among older people requires a special emphasis here. Arthritis occurs more frequently in women than in men. Since there is no uniformly effective treatment for this disease, arthritis has become a lucrative field for all sorts of irregular practitioners and for those who make fortunes by the promotion of preparations for self-medication. It is particularly important therefore that victims of arthritis, in order to avoid exploitation, understand the nature of the disease and follow sound medical advice. (See page 86.)

RESPIRATORY ILLNESSES

Respiratory illnesses (see also Chapter 18) occupy a position of major importance among the causes of illness and death in every age group but become increasingly important in the upper decades of life. With advancing years common colds become less frequent; but chronic bronchitis, emphysema, asthma, and pneumonia are more common and more serious. All too often they are accepted as an inevitable accompaniment of age, and the possibilities of obtaining relief are neglected. The cause of asthma frequently can be determined and eliminated. Bronchitis and emphysema are usually due to excessive smoking or to some remediable general condition. Occasionally a condition that is thought to be chronic bronchitis may be a low-grade chronic tuberculosis. Some elderly persons with tuberculosis are in reasonably good health themselves and yet a danger to others. No aged person with "chronic bronchitis" should be permitted in a home with young children unless it has been demonstrated that his condition is not tuberculosis.

Until recent years pneumonia was the most frequent cause of death among elderly persons. Sir William Osler said of it,

Pneumonia may well be called the friend of the aged. Taken off by it in an acute, short, and not often painful illness, the old escape those "cold gradations of decay" that make the last stage of all so distressing.

The antibiotic drugs and other life-prolonging measures have changed this—sometimes for the better, sometimes for the worse.

DIGESTIVE DISTURBANCES

Many digestive disturbances make their appearance or assume major importance in adult life. The effects of dietary indiscretion, nervous tension, indigestion, and ill-advised efforts to correct constipation accumulate over the years to produce distress and disability. (See also Chapter 12.)

DIABETES

Diabetes has already been considered (Chapter 19), but it becomes so much more important with advancing years that it should be mentioned again in this chapter. It is estimated that there are a million unknown diabetics in the nation. If this disease is discovered early, as it can be by examination of the urine and blood, its progress can be controlled and life prolonged by weight reduction, by restriction of carbohydrates in the diet, and by the use of insulin or one of the other drugs which control the amount of sugar in the blood.

PARKINSON'S DISEASE

Also called *paralysis agitans* or *shaking palsy,* Parkinson's disease is a crippling and little-understood disease of the nervous system which affects more than 1,500,000 Americans, most of whom are stricken after the age of 50. Symptoms usually begin with stiffness and tremor in a hand and arm. Other parts of the body gradually become affected, sometimes with an uncontrollable shaking of the head. Until recent years its victims faced years of suffering in which their productivity was progressively and significantly curtailed. Today, as a result of research and the development of new drugs, particularly L-Dopa, there is new hope for persons with this disease. Drugs, exercises, and in some cases brain surgery help many patients to continue useful and productive lives.

SEXUAL ADJUSTMENT

Most reproduction takes place during the first 20 or 30 years of adult life. During this period the sex glands are active and the sexual drive is prominent. Between ages 40 and 50 there is cessation of re-

productive life by women. This change, the "menopause," is anticipated with dread by many women. Such dread is unnecessary, as the symptoms which may accompany menopause are readily treated.

Physiologically what occurs is that the ovaries cease to discharge an ovum once each month and that menstruation ceases to occur. Simultaneously, the internal secretions related to sexual activity and reproduction decrease. During the period in which readjustments of glandular activities are taking place there may be physical and emotional disturbances. Irritability, jealousy, despondency, and self-pity may be bothersome. A severe type of depression can occur. Temporary though this stage is, sympathy and understanding are essential. Ordinarily no medical treatment is necessary for mild menopausal symptoms, but the counsel of the family physician may be helpful in obviating anxiety and unnecessary worry. Special treatment with estrogen, the hormone whose rapid diminish-

ment causes menopausal symptoms, is often helpful. Menopause may be followed by a stability and poise never before attained. The impetuous years of life are over; but the future holds broader interests, greater sympathy, and maturity of understanding. Sex life usually continues and with the burden of childbearing and the hazard of pregnancy removed, some women experience a more satisfactory sex life after menopause than before.

The reproductive life of men does not cease so abruptly as does that of women. No sharp change in secretion of sex hormones occurs. There is instead a gradual diminution of sexual urge and activity. Failure to recognize and adjust to this may give rise to serious emotional conflicts and psychological difficulties.

MENTAL HEALTH

Mental illnesses, particularly of the depressive types (Chapter 10), increase precipitously with age. Old people who have retired from the jobs that they held for years and whose children are grown and have left home tend to feel unneeded, useless, and frequently unwanted. (See Figure 23.3.) Feelings of this sort from time to time should not be considered abnormal or alarming because most older people experience them. It is important to recognize this and to make special efforts to pursue actively as many of one's interests as possible and to develop new interests to replace those from which one withdraws. Such feelings are often aggravated by poor physical health and other stresses characteristic of older people in our culture.

Although some older people become forgetful, irritable, or otherwise abnormal in their reactions as a result of degenerative conditions, there is no reason why most older persons cannot be mentally active. Family and friends can aid in maintaining the mental health and reducing the loneliness of aging relatives and acquaintances by encouraging

their interest and participation in a variety of activities. Nothing ages like boredom. Nothing perpetuates youth like an appetite and zest for living. To avoid boredom one should develop early in life hobbies and interests, intellectual and social, that will continue in later life. For those with an interest in the world and in the companions on their journey through life, living never becomes boring. Friendships are enriching both to those who give and to those who receive. For many people, pets are good therapy. In taking care of a pet's needs an elderly person may be taking care of his or her own needs. By exercising a dog, one is forced into activity that is good for health. When one buys food for a pet, he will also shop for himself. Moreover, an affectionate pet may lead to other interests and activities.

Our society must adjust to the increasing number of elderly persons in it. However, it is important also for the elderly to realize that they too must adjust if they are to live harmoniously with others.

MEDICAL CARE FOR THE AGED

Since the need for medical advice and medical care increases with advancing age, it is particularly important that elderly persons have personal

physicians in whom they feel confidence. The longer a physician knows a patient the better care he will be able to give. The choice of one's physi-

Figure 23.3 The elderly frequently feel unwanted and shut themselves away. (Photograph from U.S. Department of Agriculture.)

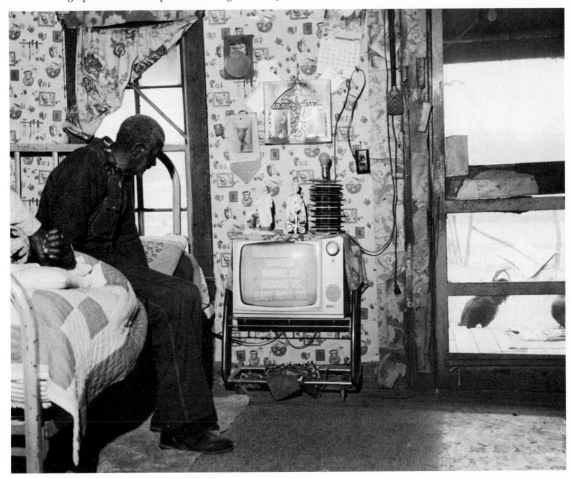

cian, therefore, should be made early and made with care. (Figure 23.4.)

The elderly, with their aches, pains, infirmities, and declining vigor, are frequently exploited by irregular medical practitioners and by the purveyors of gadgets, health foods, tonics, and other preparations publicly advertised.

For the almost 20 million persons eligible for social security benefits, the problem of paying for hospital care is greatly eased by the Medicare legislation that became effective July 1, 1966. (See also Chapter 26.) The optional supplement to this, at a cost of $7 per month, provides payment for additional hospital and nursing home care as well as for physician's services. For persons not eligible for this program, another federal law which also became effective in 1966 provides a wide range of medical and hospital services not only for the elderly but also for children and others receiving public assistance. In addition to these tax-supported programs, millions of elderly persons are covered by various types of hospital and medical care insurance. Together these programs eliminate the catastrophic financial burdens of serious illness for almost everyone.

The Social Security Administration reports

Figure 23.4   Physicians' visits, by age and sex of patients. Source: National Health Survey, U.S. Public Health Service.

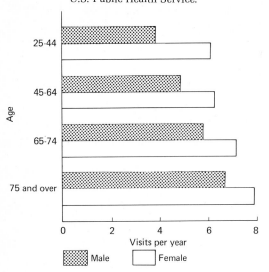

that in 1968 the per-capita medical expenditures of persons over 65 were three times as high as those of persons under 65: $590 as compared to $195. Medicare now pays about 70 percent of hospital and physician expenditures of senior citizens.

Remaining, however, are the problems of urgently needed hospital and outpatient clinic facilities, acceptable nursing homes, and above all, adequate personnel (physicians, dentists, nurses, technicians, etc.) to staff them. Planning by government—federal, state, and local—and by private voluntary groups of citizens is essential in this area in order to provide the services for the payment of which funds are now available.

Some communities have responded to the problems of their aged members by building apartment complexes, community centers, and mental health clinics particularly for the aged. Some of these developments are experimental but all represent possible solutions to a difficult problem.

DEATH AND DYING

Death is an inevitable experience. Yet until recent years discussion of it was rare. Even today many people try to ignore the fact that for everyone life will come to an end. This attitude subjects them and their loved ones to anxiety, anguish, and expense, much of which could be avoided by thoughtful consideration, discussion, and planning.

Many people fail to prepare wills for the distribution of their possessions and other assets after death. Everyone should make a will, with competent legal counsel, as soon as he or she has accumulated any assets and particularly when personal or family responsibilities are involved. To fail to do so may result in dissention and ill will and in court costs that can use up a large portion of the estate which one has accumulated and which is needed by his or her family. Husbands and wives should have separate wills, prepared after mutual discussion and consideration.

Another way to have one's own wishes carried out rather than to leave decisions to be made on the spur of the moment after one's death is to join one of the many so-called *memorial* or *funeral societies* that are being developed throughout the country.

These are nonprofit organizations frequently developed by a church, college, or other community group. There is usually a modest initial membership fee but no charge thereafter. Only the head of a family need join since his membership generally qualifies his dependents for the society's services. The society arranges with one of several respected funeral directors in the community to provide the necessary services after death at fees agreed upon in advance.

The members then indicate whether they wish to have their bodies embalmed or cremated. They choose the type of coffin desired, at the price indicated. They specify where they wish their bodies to be buried or what disposition should be made of the ashes if they are to be cremated. They specify the type of funeral or memorial service desired, where it shall be held, and whether the body should be available for viewing. One can request one's next of kin to authorize an autopsy (postmortem examination), if the physician wants it. (See page 47.) Also, the removal of tissues such as the cornea of the eye or of organs which may save the sight or the life of someone else may be authorized. Death certificates and obituary notices are taken care of by the funeral director in conference with the family.

Having such questions considered in advance by those concerned eliminates the necessity of emergency decisions in moments of emotional turmoil and grief. A great deal of anxiety, many unwise decisions, and much unnecessary expense can thus be avoided. Copies of one's specified wishes are given to the memorial society, to the funeral director, and to members of the family. Changes in or cancellation of the agreement can be made at any time.

The Minnesota Memorial Society, one of the earliest established, was founded in 1942. Any resident of Minnesota may join. Its purpose is "to promote dignity and simplicity of funeral rites, and to assist its members to arrange before death, for a funeral of the type and cost they desire for themselves and their families with a licensed funeral director. . . . It makes available services of the nearest reciprocating society for members who move to or travel through another state."

Sudden death usually involves little suffering for the victim but great heartaches for those who are left behind. Far greater problems are posed by the protracted illness and suffering caused by most of the major killers of today: cancer, heart disease, strokes, emphysema, etc.

Most patients when they realize that they have terminal illnesses tend, according to a study at the University of Chicago, to go through several stages: first, denial—"No, not me"; then anger—"Why me?"; then bargaining—"Give me just a little more time. There are things I want to do"; then depression—when the patient psychologically separates himself from his loved ones; and finally, acceptance—"My time is very close now and it's all right." This last stage is relatively devoid of feelings, but it is not resignation; is a real victory.[1] (See Figure 23.5.)

A question that always arises in the case of a patient with a serious fatal illness is whether the patient should be told of his condition. The answer is usually in the affirmative, but not infrequently a "conspiracy of silence" builds a wall of distrust among the patient, the doctor, and the family.

A woman was referred by her doctor to the Mayo Clinic for the possible removal of the adrenal glands because of generalized metastases from a cancer of the breast. After examination the doctor told her husband that the operation was indicated and asked whether he would give his permission for it. His reply was, "You have my permission to do anything that you feel will be of benefit to my wife. But," he said, "don't tell her about it." The doctor replied, "Do you mean that you have not talked together about this most important problem you have ever had to face?" "No," said the husband, "We have had 25 wonderful years together and she is a courageous woman, but I know that

[1] Jane E. Brody, "Dignity for the Dying and Those around Them Is Goal of Studies," *The New York Times*, May 3, 1971.

Figure 23.5 Stages of dying. Source: Adapted from *Medical World News*, May 21, 1971, p. 33.

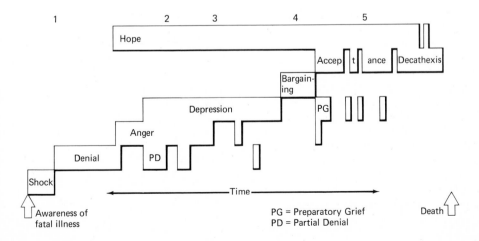

she couldn't stand the shock of knowing the seriousness of her condition." The doctor then went to the patient's room and said, "Do you know why you are here?" "Of course," she said. "I know that cancer has spread throughout my body and that the operation suggested may slow its growth." The doctor said, "Do we have your permission to go forward with the operation?" "Yes," she answered, "but don't tell my husband that my condition is serious. He just couldn't take it." The doctor then broke the "conspiracy of silence," and the couple faced the problem with mutual confidence and affection.

Another woman, 58 years of age, was dying of cancer. She had faced her illness with courage and dignity, maintaining a cheerful facade. But during her last hospital admission she became severely depressed. A conversation with a counselor revealed that she was prepared to die, but could not die in peace while her husband refused to accept the fact that her time had come. He pleaded with the doctors to prolong her life, and an operation toward that end was scheduled. As the day of surgery approached, the woman became increasingly upset, and in the operating room she began to show grossly psychotic symptoms; her screams led to cancellation of the surgery. Afterward she pleaded with the counselor to "talk to this man and make him understand." The counselor explained to the husband that his wife was prepared to die, that what he viewed as a rejection of himself after many years of happy marriage is a normal separation process, a sign that the dying person has found peace and is prepared to face death alone.[2]

Robert Anderson, the playwright, said of the protracted, ultimately fatal illness of his first wife, "I was advised not to tell Phyllis the truth. It would have been easier, far, far less lonely, if she had known. I would want to know. The complicated ruses, deceptions, explanations were incredible. The heartbreak of watching her thinking she was improving, while I knew that any improvement was temporary. I remember her saying as we woke up one morning, 'I've decided that I'm not going to make slow improvement. I am just going to wake up one morning completely well.'"

Then there was the reaction of Dr. William J. Mayo, the organizer of the world-famous Mayo Clinic, when he learned after an exploratory abdominal operation that a stomach cancer had spread to his liver. He said, "That is all I want to know. I do not want any palliative treatments, drugs, or intravenous feedings. I have had a good life and I want to spend the rest of it peacefully at home."

The above case reports are illustrative of the arguments for informing a patient of his or her condition. On the other hand, Dr. Elizabeth Kübler-Ross of the University of Chicago, renowned for her years of careful study and her writing about seriously ill and dying patients, says, "Never *ever* tell the patient he is dying, never. I have never seen one case where this was helpful. When he is ready to talk—and if he has one single person who can listen—he will tell you. The listener must allow the patient to say it in his own way. . . . Patients know, even children know. And most patients will talk about it if given a chance."[3]

The physician, the religous counselor (if there is one with whom the patient has good rapport), and the nearest of kin should jointly consider how best to give support to the patient during his or her last hours, days, or weeks of life.

Today, more than two-thirds of the 2 million Americans who die each year end their lives in hospitals or nursing homes, frequently after long illnesses. Instead of having his family at his bedside, the dying patient is surrounded by strangers and equipment. This is creating problems. Many patients would rather end their days at home than anywhere else, but at home it is not possible to provide them with the care they need. In hospitals, on the other hand, they are occupying beds that are needed by patients for whom much more can be done than for patients with terminal illnesses.

Another problem is that with modern resuscitation and supporting procedures hospitals are able to prolong the life, or—as some term it—to prolong the agony and isolation, of patients who would much prefer to go in peace. Sir George Pickering, Regius Professor of Medicine at Oxford University, summarized this problem as follows:

Society often overlooks the fact that death is as important and useful as life. . . . I know of nothing more tragic than the disruption of a happy and productive family life by a bedridden and con-

[2]Jane E. Brody, "Death: Making It Easier for Patient and Family," *The New York Times*, May 9, 1971.

[3]"Dealing with Death," *Medical World News*, May 21, 1971.

Figure 23.6 A "living will," stating the wishes of a person ill with a terminal disease. Source: Euthanasia Educational Fund, 250 West 57 Street, New York, N.Y. 10019 (copies available upon request), and Dr. David Starratt, Emmanuel Episcopal Church of Baltimore, Maryland.

To my family, my physician, my clergyman, my lawyer—

If the time comes when I can no longer take part in decisions for my own future, let this statement stand as the testament of my wishes:

If there is no reasonable expectation of my recovery from physical or mental disability, I, _____

request that I be allowed to die and not be kept alive by artificial means or heroic measures. Death is as much a reality as birth, growth, maturity and old age—it is the one certainty. I do not fear death as much as I fear the indignity of deterioration, dependence and hopeless pain. I ask that drugs be mercifully administered to me for terminal suffering even if they hasten the moment of death.

This request is made after careful consideration. Although this document is not legally binding, you who care for me will, I hope, feel morally bound to follow its mandate. I recognize that it places a heavy burden of responsibility upon you, and it is with the intention of sharing that responsibility and of mitigating any feelings of guilt that this statement is made.

Signed _____

Date _____

Witnessed by:

_____

_____

fused parent or grandparent. What might have been a respectful memory becomes a nightmare and a horror. Society is faced with a new issue, and it is important that society should look at it dispassionately from every angle. I would like once again to make a plea for the dignity of death, and that this should be regarded as a privilege earned by a long life.[4]

With many new miracle drugs, organ transplants, and other medical and surgical procedures, it is possible to postpone the termination of life of

[4]*Medical World News,* Sept. 20, 1968.

many patients. But when life has become a burden to all concerned, is postponement a blessing or an unkindness? This problem demands serious consideration not only by physicians and others in the health professions but even more by society as a whole. Prolongation of the process of dying puts added stress on patient and family. (See Figure 23.6.)

The death of a close and loved relative or friend causes grief. There is no virtue in ignoring this grief or in hiding it completely within oneself. Crying and speaking of the grief openly to close friends will help one to accept the loss and eventually to return to full participation in life.

HOW TO LIVE AFTER AGE 40

Health after 40 is determined largely by heredity and by what has occurred in the preceding years. The foundation has already been laid and the structure built, but much can be done to keep it in repair and to prevent unnecessary strain and wear

and tear. Periodic health examinations provide information concerning the state of health and make possible adjustments and the successful treatment of many major diseases before they become serious. Reduction of strenuous physical activity and emotional tension lessens the strain on the circulatory system and the danger of both functional and organic disorders. The limitation of the diet to the needs of the body removes the hazard of obesity. It is possible also that appropriate diets with liberal amounts of fresh fruits and vegetables will result in improvement in some degenerative diseases.

This is the time of life for intellectual interests, friendships, travel, recreation. Maturity and experience open new vistas of interests and pleasures which become richer as the years go by. An active physical and mental life may be continued, but now as never before it is essential to live intelligently.

QUESTIONS FOR DISCUSSION AND SELF-EXAMINATION

1 What cells live throughout a person's life? What cells are short-lived, being periodically replaced?
2 Discuss the interrelations of the physical, the intellectual, and the psychological aspects of incapacity in older people.
3 How does heredity affect longevity?
4 Compare the opportunities and the responsibilities of the individual himself on the one hand and society at large on the other in meeting the problems of old age.
5 How do the needs and the problems of nutrition in old age differ from those in younger years?

6 Why and in what specific ways are the safety problems of older people greater than those of younger people?
7 In what ways do diseases of old people differ from diseases of young people and diseases of middle-aged people?
8 What financial support for medical care is available for older people and not for younger people? Give details.
9 Discuss the place of psychological and intellectual stimuli in later life.
10 Why is the prostate gland of particular significance to older men?

REFERENCES AND READING SUGGESTIONS

BOOKS

Birren James E.: *The Psychology of Aging*, Prentice-Hall, Inc., Englewood Cliffs, N.J., 1964.

A useful discussion of the emotional problems which occur with advancing age.

Bortz, Edward L.: *Creative Aging*, The Macmillan Company, New York, 1963.

A distinguished student of aging and former president of the American Medical Association discusses with understanding and optimism the adjustments of advancing years.

Brim, Orville G., et al.: *The Dying Patient*, Russell Sage Foundation, New York, 1970.

Many authorities, physicians, sociologists, psychologists, anthropologists, lawyers, and clergymen discuss problems of impending death in this interesting and useful book.

Downey, A.B. (ed.): *Euthanasia and the Right to Death: The Case for Voluntary Euthanasia*, Humanities Press, New York, 1970.

Eleven essays by eminent authorities in the fields of medicine, law, theology, government, and philosophy present a strong case for allowing each person to have the freedom to choose "between a dignified and a squalid death."

Green, Betty R., and Trish, Donald P. (eds.): *Death Education: Preparation for Living*, Schenkman Publishing Co., Inc., Cambridge, Mass., 1971.

This is an unusually comprehensive, realistic, and helpful consideration of a subject that is of importance to everyone but is rarely discussed. It is based upon the concerns of children and youth instead of the aged. The value of this small book is immensely augmented by a well-selected bibliography.

May, Siegmund H. *The Crowning Years*, J. B.

Lippincott Company, Philadelphia, 1968.

A small book that is readable and full of reliable, sensible information and guidance for anyone facing middle age and the years beyond.

PAMPHLETS AND PERIODICALS

Dempsey, David: "Learning How to Die," *The New York Times Magazine*, Nov. 13, 1971, p. 58.

A well-written report of the studies of dying and of efforts to aid people to die in peace and with dignity, instead of impersonally with machines and apparatus.

Irwin, Theodore: "Neighbor to Neighbor Health Care," *Family Health*, January 1970, p. 25.

A story of an experimental neighborhood health center that offers tremendous possibilities for providing communities throughout the country with health care while maintaining the dignity of the individual.

Morison, Robert E.: "Death: Process and Event," and Leon R. Kass: "Death as an Event," comment on Robert Morison's article, *Science*, August 1971, pp. 694-702.

Philosophical and practical consideration of the meaning of death in this era when it is possible to keep the body functioning physiologically beyond the time when death would normally occur. The interests of the patient, of the family, and of society, and the responsibilities of physicians are considered.

Retirement Health Guide, American Association of Retired Persons, P.O. Box 199, Long Beach, Calif.

This 38-page booklet, available without charge, explains how many ailments of old age can be avoided by living sensibly and following a few simple rules of healthful living.

The Aging Skin, Committee on Cosmetics, American Medical Association, Chicago.

This pamphlet discusses the frequently unsightly skin changes which occur with age and makes suggestions as to what can be done about them.

24

COMMUNITY AND OCCUPATIONAL HEALTH

In 1629 in Digne, France, an epidemic of typhus started. The threat that the disease would spread to the provinces was so great that in June the gates of the city were closed. Troops placed around the city prevented anyone from leaving. When the gates were closed, 10,000 people lived in Digne; when the gates were reopened in June 1630, there were only 1,500 survivors, of whom all but 5 had had the disease and recovered.

In 1956 an official of the U.S. Public Health Service read in his morning newspaper of an outbreak of influenza in Hong Kong; local officials there suspected that it might be due to a new strain of the virus. Within 24 hours a United States expert was off to Hong Kong, where he gathered throat-washing samples from which he could grow the virus. From these samples he succeeded in growing a strain of influenza virus which came to be known as *Asian influenza,* and in a relatively short period

a vaccine was produced which protected several million Americans against the disease the next year when it swept across the United States.

During World War II, workers in a war industry began to sicken with cough and shortness of breath; a few died. Since they lived in different communities, it was some months before their common work suggested a common toxic substance—the fine dust of aluminum zinc silicate. Protective measures were taken and the use of this particular compound was abandoned.

These three stories illustrate two facts: first, that community action against disease is centuries old; and second, that modern community health demands close coordination of many people and the use of highly developed technology.

Though we think usually of the community as the area where we live, shop, and know people, sociologists define communities by their common characteristics, their common economic features, their reliance on the same means of transportation or the same trading area, and their joint activities. Making plans and taking action for an entire community requires a different approach from individual planning and action. Community planning helps the individual through a group program, while individual planning helps the community through individual actions usually focusing on a particular problem such as hospital facilities; immunizations; case finding for tuberculosis, diabetes, or some other disease; health education; or programs to make the environement safe and healthful.

LOOKING BACKWARD AND FORWARD

The progress which civilization has made has been dependent in large measure on man's ability to prevent and control the diseases which always before had taken a terrific toll of life and lowered the vitality of those who remained. The occurrence of epidemics, as in Digne, was dramatic and devastating, but diseases such as smallpox, typhoid fever, tuberculosis, and childbirth fever were present in every community and likely visitors to every household. In addition, there was malnutrition, usually unrecognized but omnipresent.

Progress in the control of contagious diseases was slow until about 100 years ago. Beginning early in human history, keen observers had noted that certain diseases were somehow related to food or drinking water and that some diseases were transmitted from one person to another. Thus originated the health codes of early Mosaic law, the emphasis of the Greeks on cleanliness, and the Roman aqueducts which carried relatively clean water to cities.

The discoveries of Robert Koch in Germany and Louis Pasteur in France a little less than 100 years ago established that microscopic forms of life commonly called *germs* cause many human diseases. Except for vaccination against smallpox (Chapter 17 this was the first solid foundation on which scientific measures for the control of communicable diseases could be based. Some of these control measures depend on individual citizen's activities, such as putting screens on houses to keep out flies, while others, such as provision of a good city water supply and sewerage system, obviously depend on community action. Other measures, such as immunizations, involve both individual initiative and community resources. (See Chapters 16 and 17.)

These were the initial community health services. The diseases against which they provide protection are rare today, but the possibility of serious epidemics remains; in fact, this possibility increases with the expanding population and the introduction into the environment of new substances that are hazardous to health.

Rapid increase in population in urban areas, particularly in large cities, creates community health problems of increasing complexity and seriousness. In addition, there has been a sharp increase in the per-capita production of pollutants. This involves automobiles, insecticides, electric power (much of which is produced by the burning of coal), fertilizers, nonreusable containers for foods, drinks, etc. (See Chapter 3.)

CONTROL OF COMMUNICABLE DISEASES

The possibility of serious outbreaks of communicable diseases will always be with us; and success in controlling such outbreaks will depend in the future, as it depended in the past, upon the contributions of many people: scientists to contribute new knowledge, public health specialists to plan and supervise community projects, physicians and nurses to apply knowledge and materials to the individual, and the individual to provide both cooperation and support.

The main initiative in this team effort must come from the health departments of local, state, and federal governments. Physicians report individual cases of communicable disease to these departments. The health departments note the changing incidence of each communicable disease and investigate both rising incidence and individual cases of threatening infections. For example, a report of a case of typhoid fever receives immediate attention to determine, if possible, the origin of the infection, the danger of spread to others either from the patient or from the original source, and the need for control measures. This type of specialized investigative service is called *epidemiology*.

Other contributions of health departments to control of communicable diseases include bacteriological and immunological laboratory services to assist physicians in diagnosis, vaccines for prevention, clinics for the administration of the vaccines to those unable to afford them privately, and information and publicity about the prevalence and seriousness of communicable diseases. The result of all these efforts has been the curtailment of many contagious diseases and the virtual elimination of a few. But each year needless deaths occur because of the failure of some people to take advantage of the facilities and vaccines available to them—or, what is worse, their failure to obtain them for their children, who become the victims of their parents' negligence.

CHRONIC DISEASES

Community concern for health have long since extended beyond communicable diseases alone. Most of the programs for therapeutic and preventive care involve mobilizing the community, financially and otherwise, to provide hospitals; medical, dental, and nursing education; school health services and industrial hygiene programs; special clinics for the handicapped and for mothers and children; and special programs for the mentally ill.

Early observations on the infectious diseases, long before mankind's knowledge of microorganisms, showed some of the patterns of spread of these diseases through a community and among mankind in general. This is part of the science of epidemiology. In recent years, the patterns of noninfectious disease in a community have come under study by the same methods. At present major efforts of epidemiology are devoted to the discovery of new knowledge about some of the serious disabling and killing diseases of modern man—heart disease, cancer, and mental illness, to name three of the most important.

Surveys of entire communities for the prevalence of certain chronic diseases have begun to give valuable information on the incidence and patterns of these diseases. One of the earliest was a survey of all the inhabitants of the town of Oxford, Massachusetts, for diabetes; it was discovered that 2 percent of the residents had diabetes, only half of whom knew that they had the disease. This discovery has been a major impetus to diagnostic and educational campaigns such as the "diabetes weeks" carried on in many communities, during which all citizens are encouraged to have free tests for diabetes.

In Framingham, Massachusetts, and Albany, New York, large groups of men have been studied over a period of time to determine the patterns of onset of heart disease in previously healthy men; such important facts as the double or triple incidence of heart attacks and of sudden death in cigarette smokers have been established.

The interest of physicians and laymen in community action against the chronic diseases led to the formation of the National Tuberculosis and Respiratory Disease Association in 1904, the American Cancer Society in 1912, and the American Heart Association in 1922, followed by the many other voluntary health agencies discussed in Chapter 27.

In recent years many state and some city health departments have established bureaus for the control of chronic diseases. These bureaus collect data concerning the occurrence of chronic diseases and cooperate with voluntary health agencies, medical societies, hospitals, and other health organizations to conduct control programs.

Community control measures are often educational and are directed toward helping people to understand the nature of these diseases, the possibilities of prevention, and the importance of securing proper medical care during the early stages when the chances of cures are greatest. Periodic medical examinations are urged as aids to early diagnosis.

Group action can be helpful in reducing these diseases by supporting voluntary campaigns for funds and by urging governmental appropriations for researches concerning their nature, prevention, and treatment. Sustained educational effort through group action will be helpful in reducing the disability and the lives lost unnecessarily through ignorance or procrastination.

An important part of community action against chronic disease is the provision of adequate facilities for care. For patients with chronic diseases who need institutional care, adequate medical and nursing services can be provided through specialized hospital facilities at lower cost than is possible in general hospital wards or rooms. Most such patients are not acutely ill and are therefore able to provide some self-care. Self-care improves patient morale and reduces the nursing and auxiliary services required. With high costs and shortages of hospital personnel the latter factors are exceedingly valuable, but important also is the happier situation for patients who, in cooperation with others in similar circumstances, are doing something for themselves and for their associates. Community interest and planning can provide specialized institutions or, better still, special wards or wings of general hospitals for this type of service.

Rehabilitation is important for those who suffer from chronic diseases. Chapter 6 discusses the opportunity of the community to help many persons disabled by chronic disease back to self-support or at least self-care.

MATERNAL AND CHILD HEALTH

Community responsibility for maternal and child health is now well established. Cities, towns, and states all provide clinical care and immunizations for mothers and children who cannot afford to obtain them privately. In addition, substantial efforts in health education and preventive medicine are aimed at better health for mothers and children.

Instruction on ways to improve the health of mother and child and to minimize the potential dangers of childbirth and infancy is contained in special pamphlets, bulletins, and monthly letters by health departments, by the United States Children's Bureau, and by other health agencies. To attain optimal effectiveness these printed materials need to be supplemented by personal instruction and medical supervision. Private physicians, public health nurses, special classes, and community clinics for mothers and children render these invaluable services. "Well-baby clinics" frequently offer not only instruction on child care and nutrition but also physical examinations and immunizations.

The health of mothers and children is of such great importance that both the federal government and the states have special bureaus or departments devoted to the health problems of these two groups. Chapter 26 considers these problems in some detail.

Statistics of births and infant deaths, and of deaths of mothers in childbirth are maintained by health departments. These statistics draw attention to increases in deaths or to rates which are above those of other communities, so that appropriate corrective action can be taken. Some health departments investigate every maternal death; in Massachusetts, for example, each such case is described anonymously in the *New England Journal of Medicine,* with an opinion given about whether the death could have been prevented or not.

As a result of improved medical care and these public health measures, dramatic reductions in childbirth deaths have occurred; in 1935, 9.8 mothers died in childbirth for every 10,000 live births, but by 1965 the rate was down to 2.5 for every 10,000 live births. Stated another way, approximately 8,500 mothers survived in 1965 who would have died had they been having their children in 1935. Even greater achievements are possible, however; in contrast to the national average of 3.3 deaths, one state has managed to lower its maternal death rate to 1.3 per 10,000 live births. (See Figure 24.1.)

Similar improvements have occurred in infant death rates. In 1915, 100 babies died during the first year of life for each 1,000 born alive, while in 1970 the rate was down to 20 per 1,000 live births; still in 1970 the rate varied considerably from state to state (see Figure 24.1); and thirteen countries in the world had lower mortality rates than the United States. For a baby, the time just before, during, and just after birth brings the greatest threat to life before old age.

Figure 24.1 (a) Maternal mortality by states, 1965. (b) Infant mortality rate by states, 1965. Source: U.S. Department of Health, Education, and Welfare.

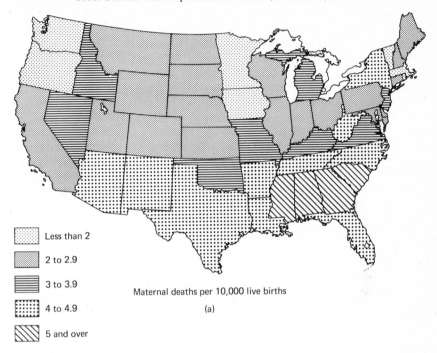

Less than 2

2 to 2.9

3 to 3.9

4 to 4.9

5 and over

Maternal deaths per 10,000 live births

(a)

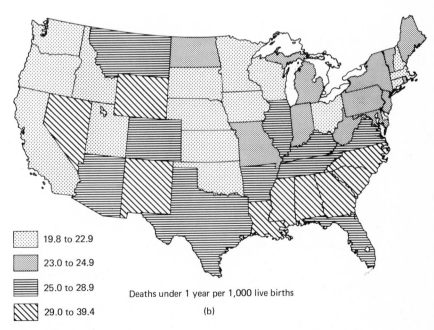

19.8 to 22.9

23.0 to 24.9

25.0 to 28.9

29.0 to 39.4

Deaths under 1 year per 1,000 live births

(b)

MENTAL HEALTH PROGRAMS

After centuries of relative neglect, the colossal problem of mental illness is finally beginning to receive adequate attention. In 1958 for the first time, the number of patients confined at any one time to mental hospitals in the United States was smaller than in the year before. Nevertheless, the overall direct cost of mental illness in the United States exceeds $3 billion yearly; statistics still indicate that nearly one out of ten people will spend some time in a mental hospital during his lifetime. (See Chapter 10.)

In good mental hospitals, new drugs and more effective methods of psychotherapy (including more use of open wards and of occupational therapy) have made hospital stays shorter. More extensive outpatient clinics have been effective in improving patients' conditions instead of allowing the increase in symptoms which would ordinarily lead to hospital admission. Emergency suicide-prevention squads have been organized in some cities so that a depressed patient or his relatives may call a number and receive immediate help. Some persons need hospitalization during the day but not at night, while others need the hospital at night but not during the day; many hospitals can now meet these needs.

Mental health clinics have become part of the hospital complex in a number of cities. These units operate mainly as outpatient centers. They service the community. At one community mental health center in New York, programs for the elderly, the young, and the mentally disturbed are community-initiated and largely community-run. A team of professionals—social workers, psychiatrists, psychologists, nurses, doctors, and community organizers—are constantly on call for any member of the community who needs help. This kind of cooperation and self-initiated action promises to be a major factor in improving the mental health of communities in the future.

Further progress in the fight against mental disease will depend on four types of community action:

1 Better facilities. Few mental hospitals in the United States have ideal buildings, equipment, and staffs.
2 Better prevention. Because of lack of facilities and because of old-fashioned unwillingness to recognize psychological problems for what they are, too many people fail to obtain professional help until it is too late to prevent hospitalization or suicide.
3 Research. Knowledge about serious mental illnesses is still in its infancy. Society must be willing to spend much larger sums of money for the investigation of mental disorders than it has been willing to spend up to now, either by governmental appropriation or by private donation.
4 Health education. Psychiatric illness has long suffered from a taboo which has interfered with diagnosis, treatment, and prevention. To admit that one has a mental problem has too often been regarded as a sign of weakness instead of as a sign of realism. Communities have been reluctant to take back patients who have improved during hospitalization, thereby making difficult continued improvement and even fostering relapse. Parents need to develop healthy attitudes toward child raising and to be willing to devote adequate time and emotional effort to their children.

Studies show that poverty, lack of education, and the conditions associated with them have as profound an influence upon mental as upon physical health. A much higher proportion of persons in poverty-stricken groups are under psychiatric care, both in and out of hospitals, than of persons in comfortable economic circumstances.

Many underprivileged people have a fatalistic attitude toward health and life. Preparation for the future plays little part in their thinking. Hence, even when public campaigns occur, as for the administration of a vaccine, many do not participate or give their children the advantages of participation. When it comes to individual action, such as obtaining periodic health checkups, they show little interest.

Obviously, therefore, future improvements in community health depend upon and must go hand in hand with efforts to raise all living standards, improve the education of underprivileged children, and educate everyone to the worth of making sacrifices for future goals.

OCCUPATIONAL HEALTH

The conditions under which the nation's millions of employed men and women work are of major importance both to personal and to community health. Pleasant, safe, and hygienic conditions of work minimize fatigue, reduce accidents, contribute to morale, and increase production.

The chief objective of occupational hygiene is to protect the health of the workers, whether in mines, factories, shops, stores, or offices, on construction sites or in transportation work, in farming, lumbering, or domestic work. Rarely is the individual employee, acting alone, able to change the conditions under which he is required to work. Such a change requires the interest and the cooperation of employers, of management, of supervisors, and of employees. These groups, working together, should identify health and accident hazards and institute protective, preventive, and remedial measures before damage occurs. In addition to general hygienic considerations—such as good nutrition, sanitation of the environment, and the value of rest and sleep, which have been discussed in previous chapters—there are certain special health problems, such as accident hazards, toxic gases, harmful dusts, and extremes of temperatures and air pressure, which occur in selected industries. A few of these problems merit special attention.

Industrial medical departments staffed by interested and competent physicians and nurses render preventive and emergency medical services and contribute to the health, well-being, and goodwill of the workers.

AIR PRESSURE

The human body adjusts to moderate changes in atmospheric pressure without difficulty, but marked increases or decreases in atmospheric pressure may seriously affect health. Conditions of increased pressure are found chiefly in mines or tunnels. Men can work under these increased atmospheric pressures provided they accustom themselves gradually to the change.

Greater pressure causes an increase in the amount of oxygen and nitrogen dissolved in the blood. This produces no ill effects in the high-pressure atmosphere but may have serious consequences if one returns quickly to an atmosphere of low pressure. With the reduction in atmospheric pressure the excess gasses dissolved in the blood are released. The oxygen causes no difficulty because it is immediately taken up by the tissues; but if the reduction in pressure is sudden, the nitrogen, which is not utilized by the body and which takes some time to pass through the membranes separating the blood vessels from the air sacs of the lungs, tends to form bubbles in the bloodstream, just as the carbon dioxide in a bottle of ginger ale forms bubbles when the cap is removed. These bubbles are carried along in the bloodstream and tend to plug some of the tiny blood vessels. This causes a disease commonly called *the bends* or *caisson disease*, the usual symptoms of which are nosebleed, abdominal pain, nausea, vomiting, dizziness, and unconsciousness. The prevention of caisson disease depends upon gradual decompression.

The health difficulties involved in high-altitude airplane flights are due primarily to the diminished amount of oxygen in the rarefied atmosphere. As a result of oxygen deprivation the pulse rate becomes higher, the respiratory rate increases, and mental disturbances develop, similar to those seen in alcoholic intoxication. Greater degrees of oxygen deprivation cause unconsciousness and eventual death. To prevent these conditions aeronautical engineers have designed sealed cabins with oxygen introduced from tanks in order to maintain the desired concentration and pressure. Combat pilots and crews have oxygen supplied to them from tanks by means of tubes and inhalation masks.

INDUSTRIAL ACCIDENTS

Although industrial accidents have been greatly reduced in recent years, they are still responsible for over 13,000 deaths and almost 2 million injuries each year. (See Table 24.1 and Figure 24.2.) Accidental deaths per 100,000 workers in manufacturing industries dropped from 25 in 1933 to 10 in 1964; in nonmanufacturing work, except for farming, substantial reductions in accidents also have occurred.

A study of fatal accidents in Pittsburgh showed that when it was possible to place responsibility, the victim or a fellow workman and the employer

Table 24.1   Working years lost by white males and females as a result of deaths under 65 years of age, 1960

Cause of death	White males			White females		
	No. of deaths during 1960	Average working years lost per death	Total working years lost	No. of deaths during 1960	Average working years lost per death	Total working years lost
Accidents	42,835	27.5	1,178,252	13,688	29.0	396,767
Heart disease	123,851	9.3	1,145,962	42,295	8.9	374,577
Cancer	56,011	11.4	637,164	52,194	12.9	674,994
Pneumonia and influenza	11,812	22.8	269,037	7,282	27.8	202,297
Apoplexy	15,222	9.4	142,975	12,476	10.0	125,155
Nephritis	1,935	18.5	54,212	1,957	19.0	37,205
Tuberculosis	3,239	11.4	37,049	1,138	18.2	20,657

SOURCE: American Cancer Society and U.S. Public Health Service.

were responsible with about equal frequency. Employees' contributions to accidents include emotional upsets, improper clothing or protective devices, carelessness, lack of knowledge, physical handicaps such as poor vision and defective hearing, intemperance, fatigue, certain illnesses such as epilepsy, and general unfitness for the job. The most important contributory factors to industrial accidents for which the employer is responsible are inadequate illumination, the lack of safeguards for machinery, working conditions which result in excessive fatigue, poor housekeeping in the plant, improper upkeep of the building, neglect of safety education of the employees, poor morale, and inadequate supervision. Employee and employer working together can do much to reduce the unnecessary toll which industrial accidents are still taking.

DUSTS

Most dusts are not harmful, because the body has natural mechanisms of protection. A few dusts, however, are dangerous either because they are irritating or because they may carry disease-producing organisms. Others, particularly those containing silica, are responsible for serious lung diseases. A disease commonly known as *silicosis* and easily mistaken for tuberculosis occurs among workmen in any occupation in which the inhalation of high concentrations of finely divided silica dust is continued over a long period of time. This is most frequent among granite workers, sandblasters, and miners of any type of ore that happens to be mixed with sandstone or granite. Frequently

silicosis does not produce symptoms for years; but once established, the disease is usually progressive and may be complicated by tuberculosis. Prevention depends on the use of adequate exhaust systems to remove the dust, appropriate masks, or water sprays or other means of preventing dust accumulation.

Asbestos   It has been known for some time that the continued inhalation of asbestos dust results in an increase in fibrous tissue in the lungs and a disease known as *asbestosis*. In addition, recent studies have shown that lung cancer is seven times as frequent among workers exposed to asbestos dust as among workers of the same age and the same smoking habits not so exposed. However, the risk of dying from lung cancer for asbestos workers who smoke cigarettes is 92 times as great as among nonsmokers of the same age and sex in the general population. This indicates that exposure to asbestos dust involves a small risk of lung cancer but that this risk is increased thirteenfold by cigarette smoking.

Black lung disease   The condition which has come to public attention in recent years under the name *black lung disease* was recognized in Scotland and Wales at least a century and a half ago and called *coal miners' black lung*.

Gradually, studies in this country and abroad concluded that coal dust, which frequently contains silica, produces a fibrosis of lung tissue, with loss of elasticity. This results in an increasing shortness of breath and may in time become com-

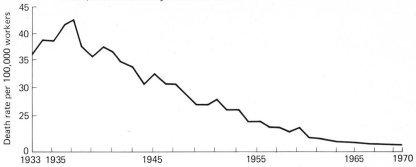

Figure 24.2 Trends of on-the-job accidental death rates, 1933 to 1965. Source: *Accident Facts*, National Safety Council, 1966.

pletely disabling. The medical term for this condition is *anthracosis*, or *pneumoconiosis* if dusts other than coal dust are involved.

Surveys in several states indicate that 10 to 35 percent of miners suffer from pneumoconiosis. The disease rate increases with the length of exposure —and with the type of mining—the risk is higher in deep mechanized mining than in the small so-called *household mines*. Pneumoconiosis also was found to occur more than twice as frequently among miners who smoke as among nonsmokers. This suggests that, as with asbestos workers, uranium miners, and city air pollution, the harmful effects of smoking are increased by the presence of other irritants.

In 1967 the Ninetieth Congress, after extensive consideration, designated anthracosis or pneumoconiosis as an occupational hazard subject to regulation and compensation under workmen's compensation laws.

POISONS

Lead poisoning In nearly all the industries using lead it is possible to prevent lead poisoning, but the cooperation of both employer and employee is necessary. Lead usually reaches the worker in the form of dust and fumes or is carried directly to the mouth by the hands. Hence, the prevention of inhalation of dust and fumes laden with lead by means of adequate ventilation and the use of masks will do much to protect the worker. In addition, workers must be instructed to wash their hands frequently (and always before eating), to take frequent baths, and to change clothing as soon as they have finished work.

The nature of lead poisoning and the high incidence of lead poisoning among children forced to live in debilitated housing in the inner cities are discussed in Chapter 3.

Other chemical poisons In various industries other chemical poisons may enter the body through inhalation (the most important route), through ingestion, and by absorption through the skin. Cadmium, arsenic, uranium, mercury, and beryllium are among the poisonous metals of particular significance. Lung cancer has been found to be five times as frequent among uranium miners as among workmen in other industries.

Recently, however, the U.S. Public Health Service reported that of 101 cases of lung cancer in uranium miners, 100 were cigarette smokers, and that lung cancer is practically nonexistent among Indian uranium miners, most of whom rarely smoke. Here again, cigarette smoke and dust from occupational exposure seem to act together to greatly increase the hazard of lung cancer.

The expression "mad as a hatter" had its origin in the days when mercury was used in making felt hats and the hatters sometimes developed mental symptoms. Laws forbidding the use of mercury in making felt hats have done away with this particular hazard. About 25 years ago attention was directed to the danger of beryllium in making fluorescent lamps, and its use was discontinued.

The hazards of mercury poisoning have been greatly increased by the careless dumping of mercury into waterways where it enters the human food web when fish ingest the wastes.

Figure 24.3   Accidental death rates in major industries. Source: *Accident Facts*, National Safety Council, 1966.

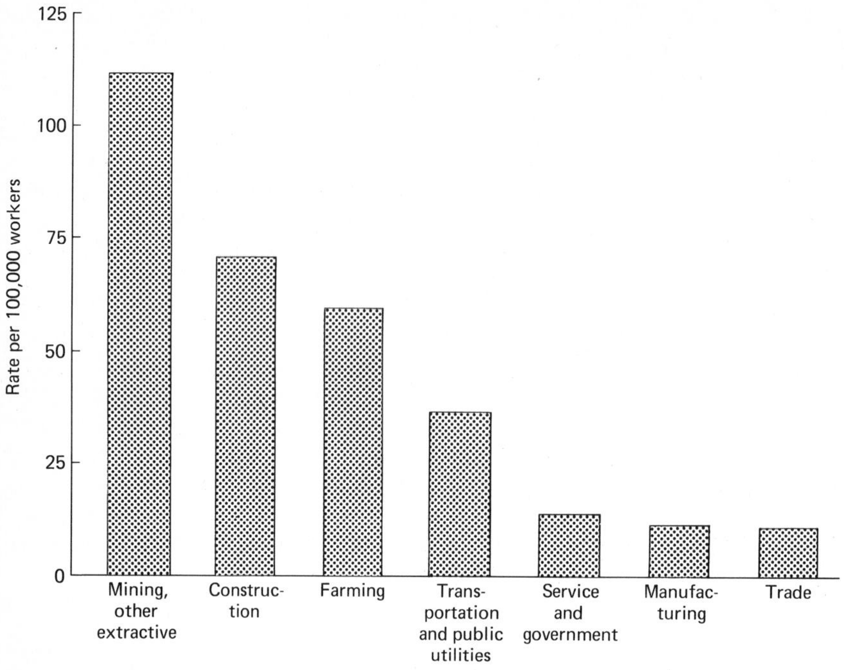

OCCUPATIONAL SKIN DISEASES

More than 50 percent of compensation cases due to occupational disease are concerned with skin conditions. Whether or not occupational dermatoses occur depends largely on how long a worker is exposed to the responsible agent and on the nature of that agent. Careful laboratory tests and clinical observation are necessary to determine the ability of a substance to cause skin disease. Provision of adequate facilities for washing, use of protective clothing, and application of ointments to the skin are methods which have proved helpful in the prevention of dermatitis.

CARBON MONOXIDE POISONING

Carbon monoxide is formed by the combustion of carbon compounds in an inadequate supply of oxygen. It is found in highest concentration in the burning of gasoline, coal, illuminating gas, coke, etc. This deadly gas can be neither seen nor smelled.

The poisonous effect of carbon monoxide is due to the fact that it forms a compound with hemoglobin which is from 100 to 200 times as stable as oxyhemoglobin. Therefore sufficient oxygen to sustain life is prevented from reaching the tissues when carbon monoxide "steals" sufficient hemoglobin. The chief sources of carbon monoxide poisoning are coal fires, leaky gas fixtures, and automobile exhausts. A running motor in a small closed garage will produce a sufficient concentration of carbon monoxide in a few minutes to cause death.

Most industries now provide their workers with protection against carbon monoxide poisoning, primarily by adequate ventilation. In domestic life the hazards have not been correspondingly reduced. Improperly adjusted "space heaters" and gas burners, leaky gas pipes, rubber hose connections, room or water heaters without proper exhaust outlets, inadequate drafts in coal stoves and furnaces, and automobiles running in closed garages are the chief sources of poisoning.

In recent years various studies have called attention to the potential danger from the inhalation of relatively low concentrations of carbon monoxide gas over a period of time. The exhaust gases from an automobile contain 5 to 15 percent carbon monoxide. Since carbon monoxide is heavier than air, it tends to concentrate near the ground, particularly in tunnels, garages, parking lots, and heavy traffic. Intake fans of automobiles may suck carbon monoxide into the car under such conditions, particularly if the intake vent is low. Leaks in the exhaust system between the motor and the tail pipe may result in dangerous accumulations of carbon monoxide within a car. Policemen after a day on duty in heavy traffic have been found to have as much as 35 percent of their hemoglobin combined with carbon monoxide.

Symptoms of carbon monoxide poisoning are headache, dizziness, blurring of vision, excessive fatigue, nausea, shortness of breath, pounding of the heart, and eventually unconsciousness and death. Symptoms usually begin when 20 to 30 percent of the hemoglobin is combined with carbon monoxide and increase progressively to unconsciousness and death at 60 percent or higher.

The highest concentration of carbon monoxide taken into the body is in the inhalation of cigarette smoke: 42,000 parts per million parts of air as compared with approximately 100 parts per million in garages, tunnels, and heavy city traffic.

Other irritant gases, such as the oxides of nitrogen, sulfur dioxide, hydrogen, sulfide, and carbon disulfide, occur in certain industries, but adequate systems of ventilation have removed any danger from them in most plants.

GOOD WORKING CONDITIONS

Adequate ventilation with temperature and humidity control, cleanliness, and a sufficient number of washstands and toilets are basic to good sanitation and hygiene in all places of employment. In addition, shower baths with adjacent dressing and locker rooms should be provided in industries where workers are exposed to excessive heat, dirt, or skin contamination with toxic or irritating materials. Proper lighting without glare, noise control, pleasant and sanitary eating facilities, and a well-planned nutrition program for large industries with cafeterias all contribute to worker efficiency, to the reduction of fatigue, and to alleviation of the monotony of the many jobs involved in mass production. The tempo of production and the lack of satisfaction in personal achievement which the skilled artisan of former days got from his work give rise to psychological problems which must be recognized and combatted if impaired morale and production are to be avoided.

RADIATION HAZARDS

The uses of x-rays in industry and for medical diagnosis and treatment have long constituted a hazard to workers employing them and occasionally also to patients. The increasing use of fluoroscopes and of radioactive chemicals in medicine has extended this danger. Concomitantly, improved safety measures and instruments for measuring radiation exposure have been developed. In spite of this, improper installations and the careless use of x-rays continue. In addition, the construction of atomic energy plants throughout the country has presented new problems. Proper engineering and the use of protective devices can prevent these hazards, but constant monitoring is essential. (See also page 38.)

DISEASES AFFECTING FARMERS

In addition to accidents to farm workers (page 83) and hazards from pesticides (page 36) several diseases affect farm workers.

Silo-fillers' disease A few years ago four men who entered corn silos within a day or two after the silos had been filled noticed irritating fumes and afterward developed respiratory symptoms of varying severity. Their condition remained stationary at first; but after 2 to 3 weeks deterioration set in, ending in death in two of the men.

Chemical analyses showed that surprisingly large amounts of nitrogen dioxide are formed during the first week of silage fermentation. This gas is known to be highly toxic on inhalation.

Prevention of silo-fillers' disease is simple; provision of adequate ventilation and prohibition of entrance into silos for 7 to 10 days after the silo is filled.

Farmer's lung Another lung disease peculiar to farmers has recently been described and given the name *farmer's lung*. The symptoms of this condition are shortness of breath, cough, fever, chills, weight loss, and occasionally the expectoration of blood. Apparently the cause is the inhalation of dust containing certain molds. Prevention depends on recognition of the hazard, the use of effective masks, and wetting down dry, dusty, or moldy hay before handling.

MEDICAL SERVICE IN INDSUTRY

It has long been considered good business practice to provide for the maintenance, repair, and depreciation of industrial plants and machines. In recent years real efforts have also been made to keep workers in good physical condition and to provide for their disability and retirement. Through the efforts of employers and labor unions and by the passage of state and federal laws, most employees now receive disability and retirement benefits; in addition most of the larger industries and some smaller ones now provide medical service.

Medical service in most industries began with the provision of emergency care for employees. Today in some industries it is still no more than that. In others, complete medical and hospital care are provided for the worker and the members of his family. In most industries the medical service is somewhere between these two extremes. Ninety-nine percent of all employers in this country have fewer than 500 persons on their payroll. This means that a large proportion of workers do not benefit from the services of full-time medical personnel within their company.

In general the illnesses and accidents of industrial workers are the same as those of other groups. Employment, however, provides unusual opportunities both for the reduction of these illnesses and for the improvement of health. The diseases and accidents directly due to the conditions of employment constitute only a small fraction of the total illnesses of industrial workers. These conditions, however, are practically all preventable as well as compensable by law.

Among the more general areas in which industrial medical service is able to make particularly valuable contributions are:

1 Preemployment examinations to ensure proper job placement.
2 Periodic examinations of all employees to discover early signs of disease, e.g., diabetes, tuberculosis, cancer, and heart disease; to note changes in general health or in specific physical defects; to provide a basis for recommendations concerning work assignments or personal habits, etc.
3 Periodic inspection of the plant to discover and eliminate unsafe practices and uses of hazardous materials.
4 Reduction of fatigue, employing methods to improve morale and provide incentive, rest periods, an optimum work week, reduction of unnecessary strain and repretitious movements, etc.
5 Improved nutrition, utilizing the services of a nutritionist to supervise the cafeteria, restaurant, and other eating facilities.
6 Employment of the physically handicapped, utilizing medical examinations and ability tests to determine physical and mental capacities and special skills and then giving workers special training and work assignments in accord with their capacities. In this way not only will employment be provided for a large number of handicapped persons but also, as experience has shown, industry can thus obtain many unusually competent and conscientious employees.
7 Psychiatry and psychology, utilizing modern testing techniques and counseling services to help workers to overcome problems which interfere with both personal lives and their ability to work, and to assist in the correct placement of employees at all levels.
8 Rehabilitation services for employees with special health problems such as alcoholism.
9 Health education, utilizing talks, conferences, posters, pamphlets, and movies. Industry has a unique opportunity to reduce the number of accidents and improve the health not only of employees but also, through them, of their families and the community.

The methods of providing occupational health services vary from having an individual physician or nurse employed on a fee or a part-time basis to supplying complete clinics, hospitals, and health centers with well-organized staffs of physicians, nurses, dentists, industrial hygienists, social workers, health educators, and technicians.

Some companies, such as the Kaiser Medical Care Foundation (page 52), make available to employees and their families complete preventive, diagnostic, outpatient, and hospital services on a prepaid basis. Other industries and employer groups contract for all or for some of these services with organizations such as the Health Insurance Program of New York or the Community Health

Association of Detroit. Still others contract with hospitals, clinics, or insurance companies to provide various types of services.

Financing industrial health services   The costs of health services in industry are borne sometimes completely by the employer, sometimes jointly by the employer and the employees, sometimes by voluntary or compulsory insurance plans, sometimes by insurance or other plans controlled by unions, and sometimes by adding the cost directly to the price of the product. In whatever way industrial medical service is financed, there is general agreement that it pays big dividends to all concerned. A survey of some 1,600 industries with good industrial medical services showed that as a result of the services a 63 percent reduction occurred in occupational diseases and a 30 percent reduction in absenteeism due to sickness.

INSURANCE PROGRAMS

Workmen's compensation   Until the middle of the nineteenth century, the accepted philosophy was that workers assumed the risks involved in their jobs. Gradually, however, employers and the community began to be concerned about the accidents and illnesses which occurred as the result of employment. This led to the enactment by states of compulsory workmen's compensation laws, the first of which was passed in Wisconsin in 1911. These provide for payment to the worker for loss of time due to illness or accident incurred in the course of his employment. Death benefits are also provided for the dependents. The employer then carries insurance to cover the claims that are evaluated and approved. The rate of premiums depends on the risks involved, thus providing an incentive to the employer to reduce the accident and health hazards to which his employees are exposed.

Subsequently, many other insurance plans have become available to workers. The coverage provided may be for medical and hospital services for a worker and members of his family, for death benefits, for disability, and for retirement. The federal social security system has the largest number of beneficiaries of any of these, but labor unions and private insurance companies provide additional coverage for many millions of employed men and women.

OTHER COMMUNITY HEALTH SERVICES

Many important health problems of today must have community interest, support, and involvement if progress is to be made in their solution. Drug and alcohol addiction, family planning, mental illnesses and suicide, emergency medical services, rehabilitation of the disabled and the aged, pollution of the environment, cigarette smoking, and the control of specific diseases such as heart disease, cancer, and the venereal diseases are examples of the problems currently claiming public attention.

To deal with some of these problems various national voluntary organizations and governmental agencies have been established. (See chapters 26 and 27.) Other problems are being attacked in local communities by groups of interested citizens, frequently with the cooperation of governmental agencies.

In some places air and water pollution are observed by concerned individuals and groups who make reports to responsible governmental agencies. Such groups also communicate with their representatives in government—local, state, and national—to urge better laws or more effective enforcement of existing laws relative to pollution.

Family planning centers not only provide family planning services but also give information by telephone concerning the availability of family planning centers, pregnancy testing, and legal abortion services.

Drug information centers provide counsel, both direct and by telephone, to youths who are becoming involved with drugs, to parents whose children are using drugs, and to drug addicts. These services are being developed under the leadership of concerned citizens with the cooperation of the medical profession, psychiatrists, psychologists, social workers, members of the clergy, departments of health, and others knowledgeable about the problems of addiction. Such centers not only render invaluable services to the individual at critical times of anxiety and panic but also can prevent irreparable damage to the victims and to their relationships with their families.

Alcoholics Anonymous offers similar services to alcoholics and their families. (See page 116.)

Confidential advisory services on venereal disease help victims to obtain proper treatment, and also aid health department efforts to control the spread of these diseases.

Mental health and suicide-control centers render valuable services to many depressed and otherwise disturbed persons.

Poison-control and drug or "bad-trip" telephone centers are able to save lives by advice about emergency measures that should be used.

In some communities interested groups are providing humanitarian services to lonely, elderly, and disabled persons to whom even a telephone call is an event in an otherwise dreary day.

These and other grass-roots community services are extremely important in our increasingly urbanized and impersonal society. Leadership in their organization and operation most frequently comes and should come from men and women concerned and disturbed about the problems of our society.

QUESTIONS FOR DISCUSSION AND SELF-EXAMINATION

1 Compare the purposes, functions, and scope of good industrial medical programs and good community health programs.
2 Which industrial diseases affect which parts of the body?
3 How has preventive medicine changed in emphasis over the last several centuries?
4 What are the most dangerous occupations and what are the dangers in each?
5 How do measures to combat the spread of tuberculosis compare with measures to combat the spread of syphilis?
6 What is the place of case finding in preventive medicine?
7 Describe the relationship of the different parts of a good program of community child care.
8 What factors have been effective in reducing the number of patients confined to mental hospitals?
9 Under what circumstances is carbon monoxide poisoning likely to occur?
10 What place does insurance have in industrial medical programs?

REFERENCES AND READING SUGGESTIONS

BOOKS

Baron, Robert Alex: The Tyranny of Noise, St. Martin's Press, Inc., New York, 1970.

A useful consideration of noise as it affects physical and mental health, and the quality of life, and what can be done about it. The author is head of Citizens for a Quieter City, New York's leading antinoise organization.

Health Is a Community Affair, Report of the National Commission on Community Health Services, Bethesda, Md., 1966.

A summary of a colossal nationwide 6-year study, with an analysis of findings and recommendations for action. The report contains the following chapters: (1) Position and Recommendations; (2) Health and the Community; (3) Comprehensive Personal Health Services; (4) Comprehensive Environmental Health Services; (5) The Consumer; (6) Health Manpower; (7) The Places for Personal Health Care; (8) Organization and Management of Resources; (9) Partners in Progress—The Government; (10) Partners in Progress—the Volunteers; (11) Action planning; (12) The Future.

Porterfield, John D. (ed.): *Community Health—Its Needs and Resources*, Basic Books, Inc., Publishers, New York, 1966.

A comprehensive consideration of all aspects of community health by recognized authorities in each field. Each chapter of this book was prepared and used by the Voice of America.

PAMPHLETS AND PERIODICALS

Gordon, James S.: "We are Poisoning Ourselves with Noise," *Reader's Digest*, February 1970, p. 187.

A practical consideration of the importance of noise as a hazard to health.

Rosenblatt, Daniel, and Levon Kabasakalian: "Evolution of Venereal Disease Information Campaign for Adolescents," *American Journal of Public Health*, vol. 56, p. 1104, July 1966.

An analysis of the effectiveness of various types of programs concerning venereal diseases which have been developed for adolescent groups in New York City.

Shilling, R. S. F.: "Changing Concepts in Occupational Health," *American Journal of Public Health*, vol. 59, p. 1367, August 1969.

Based on his experience over the past three decades, the author discusses how industrial medicine has developed into the broader and more challenging discipline of occupational health.

Tokuhata, George K., Paul Dessauer, Eugene P. Pendergrass, Thomas Hartmann, Edward Digon, and Wilda Miller: "Pneumoconiosis among Anthracite Coal Miners in Pennsylvania," *American Journal of Public Health*, March 1970, p. 441.

A 4-year study of a group of anthracite coal miners showed 9 to 34 percent to be suffering from pneumoconisis, much of which is frequently called *black lung disease*. It occurred much more frequently in smokers than in nonsmokers. In fact, it appears that smoking habits might be as important as the control of dust in preventing the disease. Studies needed to make control programs more effective are considered.

25

THE SCHOOLS AND HEALTH

The schools have come to perform a threefold service with regard to health in the United States. (1) Since the last part of the nineteenth century there has been a growing public commitment to health education in the schools, and (2) during the same period, schools have helped to maintain public health by providing certain kinds of health services. (3) More recently, there has been emphasis also on the necessity for creating a healthy environment within the school itself, and new concepts about what "healthy" means in that context have arisen. For example, many new schools are using carpeting in the halls and even in the classrooms, partly because of recent research that shows how harmful noise can be to human beings, both physiologically and psychologically, and partly so that students can study and concentrate better when the noise around them is diminished. Improved technology—such as the development of cheaper synthetic materials as in indoor-outdoor carpeting—has made feasible many changes of this kind.

HEALTH EDUCATION

Society's commitment to health education is relatively modern: only in the last century was there general acceptance of the idea that society should provide for the health and education of individuals. This was partly due to discoveries which elucidated the role of microorganisms (germs) in disease and helped people to recognize that control of certain disease was possible through proper sanitation and other public health measures. In 1850 Lemuel Shattuck published his *Report of the Sanitary Commission of Massachusetts,* and this is generally regarded as marking the beginning of the organized movement for public health in the United States.

It was some years before the schools became involved in health education of any kind, however. Horace Mann suggested in the middle of the nineteenth century that health should be taught, but not until the end of the century were basic anatomy and physiology commonly found in school curricula. Early in the twentieth century the schools also began to teach courses related to health habits, prevention of contagious diseases, and other aspects of hygiene.

Surprisingly enough, the temperance movement of 100 years ago contributed a great deal to the introduction of health education into the schools. Members of this movement naturally wished all children to be indoctrinated into the evils of alcohol. In many states and communities they succeeded in getting school districts committed to use of their programs, which included a large number of facts and psuedo-facts about the harmful effects of alcohol on health. They thus helped to establish the principle that it was desirable for schoolchildren to learn about health.

Another movement of the nineteenth century that helped lay the foundation for modern health education programs was the Turnverein movement. Little remembered by many Americans today, the Turnvereiners were exceedingly influential during the last half of the 1800s in the United States and Germany. The movement had originated in Germany in the wake of the defeats of the Napoleonic Wars, its aim being to reestablish national pride through gymnastics and the cultivation of health. Politically liberal, the Turnvereiners were devoted to the physical, moral, and mental development of young people. In the German revolutions of 1848 they backed the liberal elements who were defeated; as a result, many of them emigrated to the United States. There they were soon engaged in promoting gymnastic—physical fitness programs of personal development, which, they felt, promoted democracy and good citizenship. Physical education programs in the public schools were largely a result of the influence of this movement.

The first state law to require physical education was passed by Ohio in 1890. Not only was physical education largely a health-oriented program, but its teachers often taught other aspects of health. In some colleges, departments of "health and physical education" still exist.

Most schools today offer organized instruction in health within the regular curriculum, usually including sex education, which is increasingly thought to be an important responsibility of the school. Attention can also be paid to health and health issues in the social and natural sciences, and teachers often find themselves acting as informal advisers to students on health-related issues such as drugs, sex, and abortion. Most schools also offer occasional programs for the entire student body on drugs and similar topics.

SCHOOL HEALTH SERVICES

School health services began as inspection and screening stations for infectious diseases, at a time before immunizations, penicillin, and other drugs had reduced the threat of these diseases. Large numbers of schoolchildren suffered from communicable diseases and infections, and the school health services were among the control agents of the communities. Thus they were at first *contagion-centered.*

Later, greater interest developed in detecting physical and other defects in school children, and annual examinations were instituted, making the services *defect-centered.*

Since the next change of emphasis brought attention to focus on the child himself, the services were said to be *child-centered,* and finally it has become clear that the child cannot be divorced from his family in matters of health and development, and there has been interest in making school health services *family-centered.*

These approaches are not exclusive. As Harold Jacobziner has said:

Since maintenance of the child's health and development of his total personality are not isolated incidents but are significantly dependent on the health of the family and of the community, the school health services must become family-centered and family oriented. . . .

Preventive and curative services, and particularly health education, counseling, and guidance, must be focused on, and directed toward, the child as a member of the family unit and not merely on the child within the school.[1]

It is thought by educators that young children learn better when they feel that the school and their homes are related in some way. Thus, treating the child as a family member as well as a member of the school community has two important effects: not only does it promote his health, and perhaps that of his family as well, but it also makes his education more effective.

The aims of school health services, therefore, extend far beyond first aid for illness and injuries (important though that is). In the first place, a good program can help students develop an interest in and understanding of their own bodies and their health. Each examination can help establish the pattern of regular evaluation and respect for good health and for the positive efforts needed to promote and maintain it.

Sometimes, the health service can serve to interpret the child to his family or school. For example, if an athletic father is pushing his thin, uncoordinated son to complete in sports in which the father used to excel but in which the son has no interest, the health service personnel might try to point out to the father that his insistence could be harmful to the boy.

Or the health service may detect a hearing defect in a child which necessitates his being seated in a position in the classroom that allows him to hear. Other problems can arise that might necessitate the modification of a child's school athletic program, or even of his academic program for health reasons.

The school health services should detect or take note of defects, encourage the correction of remediable defects, and help plan the management of and adaptation to irremediable defects. They assess, note, and record growth, development, and changes in health status from time to time. They assess and encourage the maintenance of those im-

munizations known to be effective against serious contagious diseases. They should encourage the formation of good relationships between the child and physicians and dentists, with an appreciation of what good medicine and dentistry are. Finally, the school health services consult on and help plan the children's school environment, with the aim of making it contribute to their health.

Large school systems need a full-time physician to run a health program, whereas small systems need only part-time service. Full-time or part-time, the need is for a physician who will take genuine, conscientious interest in the school health program. The school dentist, if there is one, has a similar role.

Although the school psychologist often is not grouped with health professionals, to ignore his connection with them is unrealistic; the health of the mind and the health of the body are inseparable.

The school nurse becomes the key person in most programs. Most systems or schools have a full-time nurse who coordinates the efforts and knowledge of the doctor, dentist, teacher, family, and student—and should cooperate closely with the school psychologist. She provides first aid and makes the decision about whether an illness, injury, or chronic condition needs immediate medical attention, medical attention at a convenient time, or no medical attention at all unless the family desires it. She carries out ordinary nursing duties and any written standing orders for minor illness which have been given by the school physician. She alerts others to problems. She records growth, development, and the facts of illness on a record which remains with the child throughout his education.

But the person in the school who has the most contact with the children and who must be aware of their health status and health needs more than any other is the teacher. This does not mean that the teacher must become a nurse or physician, but rather must become familiar with whatever knowledge the school nurse and physician have about the children and must be constantly aware of developments that may represent small changes in the health of students.

The spirit of this approach, as well as some useful pointers on how to evaluate health at the beginning of the day, is expressed in this para-

[1] Harold Jacobziner, "Health Services for the School-age Child: A New Approach," *Journal of the American Medical Association*, vol. 165, pp. 1669–1677, Nov. 30, 1957.

graph by Wheatley and Hallock (see References and Reading Suggestions at the end of the chapter):

In informal morning inspections, the teacher observes each child as she says good morning. She stands with her back to the light and looks at the child unobtrusively, but with a purpose. Just as she notes whether his hair is combed and his face washed, so she makes a quick estimate of his facial expression? Is it happy and smiling? Or is it unusually pale or sad? Does he look tired or rested? Is his nose running? Are his eyes clear and bright? Or droopy-lidded? Or inflamed?

Wheatley and Hallock then go on to explain that occasionally children will need closer inspection and may then be referred to the school nurse. (It would be naive, of course, to assume that there are not schools in the country where, de facto, discipline is the teacher's major function and attention to small personal variations is next to impossible; similarly it would be naive to assume that there are not teachers who feel that discipline is their major problem, though it need not be, and are incompetent by personality to deal with personal variations. These unfortunate facts do not change the ideal, however.)

Most of the functions of a school health program which we have already discussed involve the good teacher; for example, one who is aware of family background, is aware of and responsible for safety planning, is of assistance to nurses, doctors, dentists, and psychologists when they deal with one of the pupils; and she must provide the supervision to meet the general classroom health needs of all the pupils and the specific needs as outlined by a physician. The teacher should serve as an example in health attitudes and practices insofar as possible, and, as we shall discuss shortly, be a health teacher.

We should not miss the opportunity to note the effect that attitudes of teachers and administrators have both on programs and on the individual child. The administrator and teacher who regard school health services and school health education as an integral part of the program, and who include the school nurse and school psychol-ogist (and school doctor if available) in the discussions of general curriculum planning and the handling of individual children, contribute to the success of these programs and make sure that the programs contribute properly to the school and its children. On the other hand, the teacher who feels that the personnel of the health program should be called in only when something goes wrong, limits their usefulness. The teacher who is interested in the whole child and his development (even though the teacher's primary responsibility is the child's intellectual development) helps the child much more than if he restricts his interest.

The school health program generally begins with the preschool requirement of immunizations: smallpox vaccination may be required and often immunization against measles, poliomyelitis, and diphtheria for protection of both individual and community, and tetanus for protection of the individual. The program includes the recording of pertinent medical information by the parents, and the discussion of possible health problems between parents and teachers. In addition, it includes periodic physical examinations, often every 2 to 3 years, yearly checks of eyesight and hearing, regular dental checks, and a careful, periodic tuberculin skin-testing program. Growth of height and weight should be recorded on some standard chart, such as the Wetzel grid,[2] and emotional development should be noted.

Provision for emergency care is essential, and the school usually requires the parents to provide not only a home telephone number but also a preference of physician and hospital in case of extreme need. (School accidents happen most frequently in organized athletics, next most frequently in auditoriums and classrooms, and third on playground equipment, according to the National Safety Council.)

Finally, the attitudes and health practices of teachers, administrators, nurses, and other school workers whom schoolchildren take as models are of paramount importance in determining the effectiveness of school health programs.

[2]Norman C. Wetzel, "Physical Fitness in Terms of Physique, Development, and Basal Metabolism," *Journal of the American Medical Association*, vol. 116, pp. 1187–1195, Mar. 22, 1941.

THE HEALTHFUL SCHOOL ENVIRONMENT

Planning for the healthful environment of a school begins with the design of the building. In the past care has been taken to provide such things as adequate lighting, safe stairways, ample space for classrooms, and perhaps a central, convenient location for the school nurse's office. More recently, educators and others interested in children's health have come to feel that the school should be constructed so as to help the child become aware that he is part of a school community he may feel comfortable in. A result is that some schools are being designed in the round, with play areas in the center or scattered outside classrooms. Sometimes movable furniture and even movable walls are provided to allow children greater physical activity and teachers greater versatility with the classroom. More and more, educators recognize the need for children to take an active part in planning and executing their own education, and the idea that young children should sit still all day in a classroom is being discarded. School construction has begun to reflect these ideas.

Other aspects of physical engineering are important in planning a school. Sanitation is an obvious requisite, involving bathrooms, cafeterias, kitchens, and ventilation or air conditioning. Adequate space for a physical fitness and physical education program should be provided, together with adequate locker and shower facilities. Recreational areas are essential.

Careful attention must be given also to providing temperatures and humidities appropriate for the various areas in the school. Temperatures in classrooms, where quiet sitting is the most common position, should be between 68 and 72°F; corridors where people are active, between 65 and 70°F; and the gymnasium, where vigorous activity will be taking place, from 60 to 70°F. The policy makers for the school system must anticipate any possible use of the school building for summer programs and provide for air conditioning accordingly.

The school has the added responsibility of organizing a healthful school day with proper length of classes, adequate break periods, adequate time for lunch. All such matters are health as well as administrative problems, though this does not mean that health personnel must make the decisions.

Provision of a hot lunch and in some schools, breakfast as well, is a significant contribution to health. The federal hot-lunch program was instituted in the 1930s to bring one adequate meal a day to children who had no adequate meals at home. Disgracefully, there are still children in the United States who do not get adequate nutrition—though a much smaller percentage of children are undernourished now than when the program was started. The lunch programs are usually carefully planned for balanced nutrition and can be used as a teaching instrument for nutrition.

Administrators must take the nature of the developing human organism into account when planning curricula. How long a span of attention can children of a given age be expected to have? What level of generalization or abstraction can they reach? School health professionals may be able to contribute to discussions of these subjects. The need of young children to have steady relationships with a very few adults bears upon the age at which team teaching and specialization of subject teaching should replace the self-contained classroom.

Printed materials, audio-visual aids, and other concrete resources for school health work are easy to come by; the resources of time and superior personnel are not so easily available. Devoted, skillful nurses are in scarce supply at best, and since school nurses must also have sensitivity about the growth, development, and adjustment of the child, the recruitment of topnotch school nurses is important. Doctors and dentists must be chosen for their skill and interest in the problems of schoolchildren, not for the amount of spare time they have available. School psychologists are perhaps more readily available, at least in urban areas, but equal care is needed in their selection. Obviously proper budgetary support is necessary in order to have good programs.

School health services are supervised by the administrations of the school and school systems, and directly or indirectly by state bodies. If this support is good, it can provide good materials for the health program, work on recruitment, and even furnish auxiliary personnel for special purposes (such as special health-education projects). In the federal government, the Office of Education, the Public Health Service, and the Children's Bureau (all within the U.S. Department of Health, Education, and Welfare) are concerned with school health programs and have substantial amounts of information, outlines and guides, and other printed aids for the program. The U.S. Department of Agriculture, through its Food Distribution Program,

gives support for school health programs. The catalog of the Superintendent of Documents, available in many libraries, list many low-cost pamphlets on this and many other subjects.

In addition, the great voluntary national organizations and the professional associations of physicians and dentists are often able to furnish materials, and on occasion even speakers, on health subjects (e.g., American Cancer Society, American Heart Association, American Medical Association) through their local offices, affiliates, and members.

QUESTIONS FOR DISCUSSION AND SELF-EXAMINATION

1 Compare the contributions to the individual and to the school community of the major parts of a good school health program.

2 How does a school health service compare with an industrial health service in organization and aims? (See also Chapter 24.)

3 Describe the health considerations which should be taken into consideration in planning a school building.

4 How should a school health service be related to a pupil's private physician and dentist?

5 In what ways can health professionals contribute to the planning of a school curriculum and a school organization?

6 What relationships between school health personnel and classroom teachers can contribute to community and individual pupil health?

7 What is the responsibility for health education of the teacher in the self-contained classroom?

8 Discuss the place of motivation in health education.

9 Compare the contributions of the several historical movements which influence the formation of health education.

10 How can the school environment be controlled or altered to affect health?

REFERENCES AND READING SUGGESTIONS

BOOKS

Grout, Ruth M.: *Health Teaching in Schools*, 4th ed., W. B. Saunders Company, Philadelphia, 1963.

Teachers and prospective teachers will find this practical book helpful in programs of health education.

Health Supervision of School Children, The Michigan University School of Public Health, Ann Arbor, Mich., 1961.

Moss, Bernice R., Warren H. Southworth, and John L. Reichert: *Health Education: Report of Joint Committee on Health Problems in Education of the National Education Association and the American Medical Association*, 5th ed., National Education Association, Washington, 1961.

A comprehensive, constructive analysis of health-education programs and potentialities from the kindergarten through the university.

Smolensky, Jack, and Robert Bonvechio: *Principles*

of School Health, Heath and Company, Boston, 1966.

A professor and associate professor of health education at San Jose State College, California, present practical suggestions based on successful experience in this field. The book considers such topics as child development, basic issues and problems, school health services, curriculum development, methods and materials, and legal aspects.

Turner, C. E., C. M. Sellery, and Sara Louise Smith: *School Health and Health Education*, 5th ed., The C. V. Mosby Company, St. Louis, 1966.

A revision of this respected overview of modern developments in school health programs.

PAMPHLETS AND PERIODICALS

A Dental Health Program for Schools, American Dental Association, Chicago, 1966.

Irwin, Theodore: "What Your Kids Don't Know about Health," *Today's Health*, May 1966, p. 19.

A nationwide survey provides strong evidence that many schools are falling down on the job of providing health education for their students.

Podair, S.: "Shall Our Schools Teach about Venereal Disease?" *Saturday Review*, Mar. 19, 1966, p. 72.

26

GOVERNMENT AND HEALTH

A mother takes her child's temperature but gives no thought to the accuracy of the thermometer. She does not know that the Food and Drug Administration has a program for sampling and testing the accuracy of clinical thermometers.

A doctor prescribes an antibiotic for a patient who is threatened with pneumonia. Neither the doctor nor the patient has any concern about the purity or the potency of the drug, because the Food and Drug Administration continuously tests and certifies the quality of all antibiotic drugs used on human patients in this country.

Accurate dosage of insulin is of life or death importance to several million diabetics in this country. Every batch of insulin that is manufactured is tested in the FDA laboratories to ensure that it has the exact strength stated on the label.

Today many chemicals known as *food additives* are used to make foods more attractive, better

tasting, and more economical. None of these may be used in foods unless it has been checked and cleared for safety by the Food and Drug Administration. (*Safe* in this context means that a drug is not harmful for the purposes intended and under the provisions outlined for its use. In a strict sense no drug is completely safe for all individuals or in any amount.)

The above illustrations are some of the ways in which a single agency of the federal government is related to the health of people throughout the nation. President Lincoln once said it should be the responsibility of government to do for its citizens things that they cannot do for themselves. Health protection and certain health services are in this category. In the early years of our country these services were relatively few, but as population increased and cities developed, as local health problems became national problems, and as medical services became increasingly complex and expensive, government at every level found it necessary to gradually expand its services both general and personal.

Concerted group action for any purpose can be attained only through some type of organization. Governmental bodies—local, state, national, and international—have been formed for this purpose, and in the field of public health their accomplishments have been magnificent. Much, however, remains undone, even in this country; in many areas of the world, health work is in its infancy.

OFFICIAL HEALTH AGENCIES

If a government is to function efficiently in the interests of public health, the following basic principles must always obtain:

1 Public health work must be in the hands of trained, competent personnel who have chosen and prepared themselves for careers in this field.
2 Political consideration must not be permitted to enter into appointments of public health personnel or into the determination of public health policies.
3 The public should be informed about what they have a right to expect in the way of public health services.
4 Public health programs should be planned so as to get the greatest possible returns for the money expended. Theoretically, it would be desirable to prevent every single case of typhoid fever, but to do so would be exceedingly expensive. In fact, the amount of money that would be required to prevent the few cases of typhoid fever which occur may be used to much better advantage for other health services.
5 Public health services must be adequately supported. Even though public health has long been recognized as one of the primary functions of government, it receives a relatively small share of local, state, and national appropriations, frequently only a few cents out of the tax dollar—much less than is spent for roads, military preparedness, relief, the custodial care of defective people, etc.

We might assume that the enactment of laws or regulations in the interest of the public health would receive the highest possible priority and support. Yet, frequently this is not the case, particularly if the proposed law or regulation infringes upon the business of an economically and politically powerful group, or if it will necessitate an increase in taxes, or if it is opposed by the antimedical fanatics who exist in surprising numbers throughout the country. For many years pasteurization of milk was opposed by people who owned a few cows and by the owners of small dairies who were unable or unwilling to afford pasteurization equipment and who claimed that a requirement that all milk sold commercially should be pasteurized was being promoted by big dairies in order to put the "little man" out of business.

The enactment of food and drug laws was bitterly opposed and was delayed for years by the "patent medicine" industry, commercial druggists, and the press that advertised these preparations. Early food and drug laws were very weak, but they have been gradually improved and strengthened by amendments. In order to pass these laws and amendments, however, various compromises with special-interest groups have been necessary; one example was provision that tobacco products shall not be subject to regulation by the Food and Drug Administration.

Until recently, the automobile industry resisted regulations to require safety belts, the reduction of exhaust fumes, and other measures to reduce the hazards to life and health caused by motor vehicles.

An example of how powerful business interests can influence health activities of government is the legislation relative to cigarette labeling and advertising. As noted earlier (page 166), an advisory committee of distinguished scientists, after 15 months of intensive study, reported to the Surgeon General that "cigarette smoking is a health hazard of sufficient importance in the United States to warrant appropriate remedial action." The report substantiated the fact that cigarette smoking is the principal cause of lung cancer in the United States and indicted cigarette smoking as an important factor contributing to coronary heart disease, emphysema, chronic bronchitis, and cancer of the mouth, throat, and larynx. No medical or health organization has disagreed with these conclusions.

The public concern about the harmful effects of smoking that followed this report caused the Eighty-ninth Congress in 1965 to pass a law requiring that beginning January 1, 1966, all cigarettes sold in this country must carry the label: "Warning: Cigarette smoking may be hazardous to your health." The Federal Trade Commission, the U.S. Public Health Service, the National Interagency Council on Smoking and Health, the American Cancer Society, the American Heart Association, the National Tuberculosis Association, the National Congress of Parents and Teachers, the American Association for Health, Physical Education, and Recreation, and other health groups urged a stronger warning and a requirement that the warning appear in cigarette advertising as well as on cigarette packages. The tobacco industry, sensing that some legislation was inevitable, decided to accept a weak label on cigarette packages provided that they could prevent any restriction of cigarette advertising. The tremendously powerful tobacco lobby then found members of Congress who could be prevailed upon to introduce legislation to this effect and corralled sufficient support to ensure its passage. The result was a law which indicated that Congress recognized that cigarette smoking is a health hazard, but provided that for a period of 4 years neither the Federal Trade Commission nor any state or local governmental agency could require any other label on cigarette packages or any warning on cigarette advertising.

During the next 4 years, as required by the 1965 law, annual reports were made to Congress relative to the smoking situation by the Public Health Service and by the Federal Trade Commission. These reports by the Public Health Service not only verified and extended the earlier conclusions but also presented further information about the mechanisms by which persistent cigarette smoking contributes to respiratory and to cardiovascular diseases. The reports by the Federal Trade Commission indicated no reduction in the extent of cigarette advertising or in its appeal to the American public, particularly youth, to take up or to continue the cigarette habit.

Since the provision in the 1965 law that prevented health warnings in cigarette advertising was due to expire on July 1, 1969, the tobacco industry promoted and the House of Representatives approved a bill to make a slight change in the warning on cigarette packages and to extend for 6 more years the prohibition of any regulation of cigarette advertising. The Senate passed a much stronger measure, most of the provisions of which were accepted by the Senate-House conference committee and approved by Congress. This 1970 law banned cigarette advertising on television and radio after January 1, 1971. However, it also directed the Federal Trade Commission not to take any action to regulate other cigarette advertising until July 1, 1971, and stated that no health warning could be required in cigarette advertising without 6 months' notice to Congress. This law was an improvement over the 1965 act, but it is still not strong enough. Action in the interest of health was impeded by commercial consideration.

This same Congress, while budgeting $2.6 million to educate the public about the harmful effects of smoking, appropriated more than $60 million to support smoking: $31.1 million to buy up surplus tobacco for shipment abroad under our Food for Peace Program; $27.9 million for tobacco export subsidies, and $240,000 for cigarette advertising abroad.

To prevent special interest or misguided pressure groups from influencing or controlling legislation, it is essential that citizens be intelligently informed about and interested in health problems and health legislation; that they communicate their wishes to their representatives in local, state, and national legislative bodies; and that they encourage other individuals and groups with which they are associated to do likewise.

HEALTH ACTIVITIES OF THE FEDERAL GOVERNMENT

The national government has only certain limited powers granted to it by the Constitution. The following are the more important of those related to public health.

1 Regulation of foreign and interstate commerce. Under this authority the federal government acts to prevent the introduction of communicable diseases from foreign countries and the spread of diseases between the states; it supervises the preparation of vaccines, serums, and certain medicinal products sold in interstate commerce, the working conditions in factories which manufacture materials sold in interstate commerce, and the sanitation of drinking water on interstate carriers.

2 Taxation. By levying special taxes the federal government can control the sale of such products as narcotics; it can also distribute funds raised by taxation to the states for public health work or other purposes on condition that the individual states meet the terms or requirements specified by the federal government. This is the method used for the development of health work throughout the states with the aid of complete or partial federal subsidies.

3 Education and research. Activities in these fields are based upon the power of the government to "provide for the common defense and general welfare of the United States." Public health work, health education, and scientific research are supported under this function of the government.

For 141 years the U.S. Public Service, the agency of the federal government concerned exclusively with health, was administratively under the Department of the Treasury. On July 1, 1939, it was transferred to the Federal Security Agency, which had been created in President Franklin D. Roosevelt's administration to bring together the federal government's activities in the fields of health, education, and welfare. In 1953 under President Dwight D. Eisenhower's administration, the Department of Health, Education, and Welfare was established with Cabinet status. The Public Health Service (established in 1798), the Children's Bureau (established in 1912), the Food and Drug Administration (established in 1906), and the Administration for Vocational Rehabilitation (established in 1943), were the major health agencies of this new department.

As the health programs of the federal government have been increased, the Department of Health, Education, and Welfare has been reorganized to meet its expanding responsibilities. Consideration is currently being given to the creation of a separate Department of Health. To coordinate the health activities of the department, the position of assistant secretary for health and scientific affairs has been created. The assistant secretary has deputy assistant secretaries for health and medical care, for science, for health manpower, for family planning and population, and for planning and program coordination.

Responsible to the office of the assistant secretary are the administrative officers of the health agencies of the department. Among these are the Surgeon General of the Public Health Service, the director of the National Institutes of Health, the commissioner of the Food and Drug Administration, the administrator of the Health Services and Mental Health Administration, the administrator of Social and Rehabilitation Services, the administrator of the Environmental Control Administration, and the commissioner of the National Air Pollution Control Administration.

Apart from the Department of Health, Education, and Welfare other departments of the government carry on important activities related to health. The Army, the Navy, and the Air Force all have major medical departments to provide health and medical services for their personnel, for certain dependents and civilian employees, and at times, for civilians of the countries in which they are serving. The Veterans Administration has as one of its major responsibilities the provision of medical care for the veterans of the various wars in which United States armed forces have been involved. The Department of Agriculture supervises many health activities relating to farm products, foods, and nutrition. The Bureau of Mines in the Department of the Interior is concerned with safety and health conditions of the mines of this country. The Department of Labor carries on many activities in the interest of the health of industrial workers. The Bureau of Narcotics and Dangerous Drugs in the Department of Justice regulates measures to control narcotic traffic. Foreign policies relating to health are dealt with in the Department of State. From these examples it is obvious that many agencies of the federal government are concerned with health matters.

PUBLIC HEALTH SERVICE

The Public Health Service, oldest of the organizations which composes the Department of Health, Education, and Welfare, is the principal health agency of the federal government. Through the Public Health Service, the federal government works with other groups to discover and apply knowledge that will help conquer disease and improve health. The programs of the service are conducted in close partnership with other agencies of the federal government, with the states and territories, and with many voluntary organizations, professional groups, institutions, and international agencies.

The U.S. Public Health Service began as the U.S. Marine Hospital Service in 1798, when an act of Congress providing for the care and relief of sick and injured seamen was signed by President John Adams. Since colonial days, the merchant fleet has been the nation's economic lifeline and a major element of its naval defense. The seaboard states and their local ports, therefore, called upon Congress to enact legislation giving the young federal government responsibility for the care of seamen put ashore by incoming vessels. The proponents of the act of 1798 argued that, in addition to humanitarian considerations, the national defense and the promotion of commerce demanded a nationwide system of hospitals and medical care for seamen. Since that time, the concept has prevailed that the federal government should play a part in the fields of civilian medical care and public health, which are closely related to national defense and the promotion of commerce.

The work of the U.S. Public Health Service falls into three major categories: research, medical and hospital services, and public health practice. The service also administers financial grants to the states for general and special public health services and for the construction of hospitals, health centers, and other medical facilities. Grants are also made to public and private nonprofit research institutions for medical research, and for the training of scientists and of health personnel.

The research programs of the Public Health Service include laboratory, clinical, epidemiologic, engineering, statistical, and administrative studies—all focused on contemporary health problems. Highly qualified scientists conduct the studies in facilities of the service, in the field, and in laboratories of other institutions under cooperative arrangements. The service also helps to increase the number of medical and public health scientists through fellowships and traineeships for qualified students.

The Public Health Service provides medical and hospital care only for certain groups of people whom Congress has made eligible to receive such care. Among these are the seamen of the American Merchant Marine, personnel of the United States Coast Guard, eligible American and Alaskan Indians and Eskimos, and civilian employees of the government (who receive care only for diseases and injuries contracted in connection with employment). The Public Health Service also provides medical personnel for the ships and shore establishments of the United States Coast Guard and the Maritime Administration, for the prisons and reformatories of the Department of Justice, for the health programs of the Agency for International Development (AID) (see page 400), and for several other federal agencies. It administers the nation's foreign quarantine laws and regulations and conducts medical and psychiatric examinations of immigrants seeking admission to the United States. Through its International Health Division, the Public Health Service concerns itself with official international health problems, particularly in connection with the programs of the World Health Organization of the United Nations.

In the field of public health practice, the service provides leadership and technical assistance to states and local communities. It develops and promulgates standards for the protection of the public from milk- and food-borne diseases. In cooperation with state and local health departments, it develops and tests new methods in the prevention and control of disease. It licenses the manufacture of biologics and assists states and communities in dealing with such special problems as water and air pollution and radiological contamination. It collects and distributes the nation's vital statistics and conducts special studies of health data. It provides teams of public health experts to help communities suppress epidemics and prevent the spread of disease in times of disaster. Broad responsibility for the health aspects of civilian defense programs is delegated to the service. In its cooperative programs with the states, the service helps communities through demonstration of new and improved methods, through the loan of personnel and equipment, and through the conduct of training programs for state and local health workers.

NATIONAL INSTITUTES OF HEALTH

The National Institutes of Health were developed by and, until the recent reorganization of the Department of Health, Education, and Welfare, were an integral part of the Public Health Service. The first of these institutes was the National Cancer Institute, created in 1937 as a part of the Public Health Service. Subsequently, Congress added the National Heart Institute, the National Institute of Neurological Diseases and Stroke, the National Institute of Mental Health, the National Institute of Arthritis and Metabolic Diseases, the National Eye Institute, the National Institute of Dental Research, the National Institute of Allergy and Infectious Diseases, the National Institute of Child Health and Human Development, and the National Institute of General Medical Sciences, all collectively known as the *National Institutes of Health* and located in Bethesda, Maryland.

Each year the Congress makes appropriations for the support of these institutes. Some of this money is used for research studies conducted by the institutes themselves; but most of it is distributed to universities and other research institutions to help train investigators and to support the research of scientists working in fields related to the interests of the institutes which make the grants.

FOOD AND DRUG ADMINISTRATION

After years of vigorous opposition the first Federal Pure Food and Drug Act was enacted by Congress in 1906. In 1912 it was amended to forbid false and fraudulent therapeutic claims on labels of patent-medicine containers, and in 1938 it was amended to include cosmetics and contrivances for diagnosis or treatment. In 1957 this act was again amended to ban any food containing a substance capable of producing cancer in man or animals. Further, the amendment shifted the responsibility for establishing the safety of an additive to the manufacturer. Previously, the Food and Drug Administration was required to prove an additive unsafe.

The Food and Drug Administration is the main federal organization which safeguards the quality of foods and drugs. The means employed in carry-

ing out this work are (1) inspecting factories where foods, drugs, and cosmetics are manufactured or processed, (2) testing samples of products, and (3) checking the results of such tests against the statements on the labels.

The law requires that drugs be pure and of good quality so that they are fully potent, and that drugs be licensed for sale only upon adequate evidence that they are safe and useful for the purposes stated.

The fact that 25 percent of the consumer's dollar is spent for items produced by industries regulated by the Food and Drug Administration clearly indicates the economic significance of the agency's activities. Even more significant is the direct impact on each individual in our society. Whether products are used to restore health or to enhance appearance, to increase agricultural productivity or merely to provide greater convenience, the responsibility for their purity, efficacy, and safety rests with the Food and Drug Administration.

Increasingly, pesticides are used to grow better crops and protect the health of livestock. Medicated feeds which enable animals to grow faster help keep down the cost of food production. But these potent chemicals must be carefully and correctly used. Scientists in this agency have the great responsibility for establishing what amount of residues may be safely permitted in foods going to market.

VETERANS ADMINISTRATION

The Bureau of Medicine and Surgery of the Veterans Administration operates a large system of hospitals, clinics, and domiciliary homes for sick or disabled war veterans whose illnesses or disabilities are "service-connected" or who have "non-service-connected" conditions which require medical care that the veterans are financially unable to provide for themselves. After World War II many Veterans Administration hospitals became affiliated with medical schools and have since contributed significantly to medical education, to specialty training, and to medical research, as well as to providing high-quality medical care for patients.

CHILDREN'S BUREAU

The U.S. Children's Bureau, which was initially in the Department of Labor, is concerned with the improvement of health services for mothers and children. Through federal grants to the states, funds have been provided to assist in such work. Of particular interest is the federal-state program of services for crippled children. In addition the Children's Bureau is making a nationwide effort to discourage cigarette smoking by children and is providing funds to state and local communities to support family planning programs and contraceptive services.

ADMINISTRATION FOR VOCATIONAL REHABILITATION

The U.S. Administration for Vocational Rehabilitation cooperates with states in rehabilitating persons who, as a result of accident, disease, or congenital defects, are permanently disabled and thus handicapped vocationally. (See page 87.)

DEPARTMENT OF AGRICULTURE

Of great importance to human health are many of the activities carried on by the Department of Agriculture. The Bureau of Animal Industry engages in research on animal diseases, many of which are transmissible to man; in cooperation with state officials and livestock organizations, it concerns itself with their control or eradication. An inspection service of meat sold in interstate or foreign commerce or for use by government agencies is under the Office of Production and Marketing Administration, which also controls insecticides, formulates standards for various food products, and, through its Labor branch, supports medical care and health services for seasonal workers who come from other countries. The Bureau of Dairy Industry and the Bureau of Human Nutrition and Home Economics represent still other activities of the Department of Agriculture. Both these agencies conduct research and educational programs of great value to human health.

DEPARTMENT OF STATE

In the field of international health the Department of State, through its Agency for International Development, is making an immense contribution to the improvement of health in the underdeveloped countries of the world.

Official recognition of the importance of this work was given several years ago by the establishment of a new position in the Department of State, with the rank of assistant secretary and the title assistant administrator of AID and director of the Division of Human Resources and Social Development. (See page 400.)

FEDERAL TRADE COMMISSION

The Federal Trade Commission is an independent agency of the government established by Congress in 1914. Its duties as they relate to health are to prevent false and deceptive advertising of drugs, foods, curative devices, cosmetics, and other products. It is constantly checking on advertising and ordering the discontinuance of any which the commission considers false or deceptive.

This is clearly in the public interest but frequently commercial interests attempt to prevent actions by the Commission which they believe would be harmful to their businesses. This may be done through political pressure, through the courts, or through congressional action. There have been many examples of this in the advertising of foods, non-prescription drugs, and cosmetics.

A recent illustration is the effort by the tobacco industry to prevent a proposed requirement by the Commission that all cigarette advertising carry a warning concerning the health hazards involved in smoking. A law passed by Congress in 1971 prohibits all advertising of cigarettes on television and radio. There is, however, no restriction on other types of cigarette advertising and promotion which have multiplied many times since the law went into effect.

FEDERAL COMMUNICATIONS COMMISSION

Another government agency that has become concerned with cigarette advertising is the Federal Communications Commission. It is the responsibility of this commission to ensure that the airways, which belong to the public, are used in the public interest. Concerning this the Honorable William E. Henry, chairman of the Federal Communications Commission in 1966, said in an address before the National Association of Broadcasters:

From the advertising presently being carried on radio and television no one would ever know that the great bulk of medical opinion, including a Surgeon General's Report, has concluded that there is an adverse causal relationship between cigarette smoking and health. Nor is there the slightest hint that the Congress of the United States last year passed a Cigarette Labeling Act which requires every pack to contain the warning—and I quote—"Caution: Cigarette Smoking May Be Hazardous to Your Health."

Despite all of this, the sign on broadcasting's door for cigarette advertisers reads: "Business as usual."

A startling anomaly is thus created. Television viewers in particular are led to believe that cigarette smoking is the key to fun and games with the opposite sex, good times at home and abroad, social success and virility. But as the individual approaches the tobacco stand and mystically changes from television viewer to cigarette customer, so the message changes. Life with cigarettes is no longer beautiful: the package warns that smoking may have ugly consequences indeed.

A year later the Communications Commission decided that it was not in the public interest for the airways to be used by radio and television to advertise cigarettes without warnings of the health hazards involved in smoking. The commission therefore ruled that radio and television stations which advertise cigarettes must give health agencies a "reasonable" amount of time to present information concerning the health damage caused by smoking. As a result of this ruling, many television and radio stations ran spot announcements about the hazards of smoking. The ruling, although attacked in the courts by the broadcasting and tobacco industries, has been upheld by the United States Supreme Court.

The law prohibiting cigarette advertising on television and radio, of course, negates the effect of this ruling. Some stations, however, still carry anticigarette "spots."

GOVERNMENT HEALTH LEGISLATION

"MEDICARE"

On July 30, 1965, President Johnson signed into law amendments to the Social Security Act which provide two kinds of health insurance for people 65 or older: a basic plan and a voluntary plan.

The *basic plan* pays most charges incurred within specified periods of time for hospital care and for posthospital care in a nursing facility or at home, after a $52 deductible is paid by the individual. Benefits for hospital care are similar in many respects to those of Blue Cross and other hospitalization plans. The basic plan is financed by the Medicare tax, with assistance from general revenues. Persons 65 years of age or older are eligible.

The *voluntary plan* reimburses most of the costs of doctor's bills and a number of other services and supplies not covered by the basic plan, whether the individual is in a hospital or not. It is similar in many respects to major medical insurance, reimbursing 80 percent of a wide range of expenses above a $50 deductible. The 20 percent "coinsurance" is paid by the individual. The voluntary plan is financed by contributions of $5.30 a month from each person enrolled in it ($10.60 for a couple over age 65), plus matching amounts from general tax revenues.

People aged 65 and over are eligible for the voluntary plan whether they have had any social security coverage or not. They have 7 months in which to sign up, starting 3 months before the first of the month in which they reach the age of 65.

Medicare benefits will be paid whether the covered person is working or not. There is no "work test," as there is for other social security benefits. The choice of physician, hospital, or other qualified medical person or institution to perform the covered services is made by the individual.

The scope of coverage   It is clear that everyone electing both parts of Medicare will have substantial protection against the heavy costs of serious illness or injury. In some respects Medicare goes beyond the limits of many health insurance plans. There are benefits for posthospital nursing home care, for a number of home health services, and for some out-of-hospital psychiatric care; and Medicare sets no overall dollar limit on a person's total benefits, as major medical plans do. On the other hand, Medicare has limits of its own, such as a time limit on benefits for hospital care. It also excludes a few important areas of expense that are presently insured by major medical plans; and Medicare requires the individual to pay deductibles and coinsurance.

MEDICAID

For persons not eligible for Medicare, a law commonly called *Medicaid* authorizes federal grants to the states under a matching formula for medical assistance to all persons receiving public assistance money payments and for certain other indigent persons. This includes the aged, the blind, the totally and permanently disabled, and needy families with children. It is estimated that at least 18 million children, living with their families or in foster homes or institutions, are aided. This program provides a complete system of tax-supported health care for all the needy, operated by the states and subsidized largely—50 to 83 percent—by the federal government.

ENVIRONMENTAL POLLUTION CONTROL

In 1899 Congress passed a Refuse Act that prohibits the discharge of refuse of all kinds into navigable waters. Had this law been enforced, the present sorry condition of most of our lakes, rivers, and offshore ocean areas would not have developed. But the law was ignored until recently, when some polluters have been found guilty in court of violating it.

In the past few years public concern about pollution of the environment has stimulated Congress to enact a number of laws to control it. Among these are:

The *Water Quality Act* of 1965, which established a program to set federal standards to prevent pollution of the country's lakes and streams.

The *Clean Waters Restoration Act* of 1960, which promised a federal contribution of up to 55 percent of the total cost for local construction of plants to treat sewage.

The 1970 *Clean Air Act*, which improved many of the provisions of its inadequate predecessors and set a 1975 deadline for a 90 percent reduction in auto emissions, speeds up federal enforcement procedures, and sets national standards for overall air quality. It sets deadlines for the states to implement and enforce these standards, and stipulates that state plans must include "emission standards" stating explicitly what and how much each plant may discharge from its stacks.

The *Solid Waste Disposal Act* of 1965, which sets up a Bureau of Solid Waste Management to do research and training and to provide information to state and local governments.

The *Resource Recovery Act* of 1970, which established a program of construction grants to local governments for projects with new technology in recycling or reuse of waste material. It directs establishment of Federal guidelines for waste disposal practices.

The *Environmental Protection Agency* was established in 1970 in the executive office of the President, to coordinate programs of the numerous agencies with responsibilities related to environmental pollution.

These are tremendously significant actions of the federal government, but what they will accomplish will depend upon adequate financial support, which to date has been lacking, upon competent and determined leadership, and upon strong backing by the administration for the enforcement of these laws. Such actions will occur only if concerned citizens insist upon them.

THE FAMILY PLANNING SERVICES AND POPULATION RESEARCH ACT

In 1970 Congress passed and the President signed the first comprehensive United States statute to provide funds and encouragement for family planning services and population research throughout the nation. The main objectives of this act are:

1 To make family planning fully available to the 5 million American women now lacking such services
2 To support research for new and better methods of family planning
3 To create an Office of Population Affairs in the Department of Health, Education, and Welfare, with full authority for family planning programs in the United States
4 To support training of personnel and preparation of information materials

This is a landmark piece of legislation. Its value, however, will depend upon the vigor and the imagination with which it is implemented and the vital appropriations which Congress will make for its support.[1]

[1]*The Family Planning Services and Research Act of 1970*, Population Crisis Committee, 1730 K Street N.W., Washington.

STATE HEALTH WORK

An official statement of the American Public Health Association regarding state health departments is as follows:

The states are sovereign units of government. Their authority in the health field is derived from the state's general powers to legislate for the protection of the public safety, health, and morals. Local governmental units, including county and municipal health departments, derive their authority and power from either primary local power or from the state constitution and laws. In most instances, health departments of county and municipal governments act as independent units, except for such advice and consultation as they may receive from the state through technical consultations, grant-in-aid programs, and cooperative agreements. In a few states, however, a more definitive relationship exists between the state and the local health departments in which the local health department may be, in fact, a branch of the state government and receive its direction and financial supervision directly from the state.

The theory and practice of public health have expanded to include not only the prevention of the onset of illness, but also, through the use of mass technics the prevention of the progress of disease, of associated complications and of disability and death. The sharp decrease in mortality and morbidity rates from infectious diseases has caused a marked change in the age distribution of the population and in the spectrum of our health problems, including greater emphasis on the attainment of optimal health. Consequently, the organization and functions of a state health department have undergone considerable change as a result of the advancement in science and in health practices.[2]

The state health department is composed of (1) the state health officer and his staff, which make up the administrative or executive section; and (2) the board of health, which comprises the advisory or policy-forming body. This board should be truly representative of the medical and other professional groups and of the public. Among its duties are reviewing plans, programs, budgets, and reports of the department; holding hearings; issuing licenses and permits; and promulgating regulations.

There are three general categories of activities of the state health department. They are:

1 Personal health services, such as diagnosis, care, and treatment of tuberculosis; immunization procedures; rehabilitation of the disabled; maternal and child health services; and discovering early cases of cancer.
2 Community health services, such as isolation of communicable disease; health education; fluoridation of water supplies; sanitary control of water, milk, and food, and disposal of sewage; and provision of laboratory or hospital facilities.
3 Administrative services, or those activities necessary for the operation of personal or community health services, such as budgeting, purchasing, and the operation of facilities, including basic program planning, coordination, and evaluation, which are essential to the operation of any such organized activity.

Some state health departments maintain special clinics and hospitals, particularly for patients with mental illnesses, tuberculosis, and cancer.

State health departments have responsibility also for the administration of programs of federal grants for hospital construction and for special programs of disease control and of new and improved methods for the provision of health and medical services. Such responsibilities are being extended from time to time by new federal legislation, such as the act of 1965 to improve the care of patients with heart disease, cancer, and stroke in local and regional hospitals. To discharge these new responsibilities adequately most state health departments are finding it necessary both to expand their staffs and to modify long-accepted philosophies of operation.

The enactment of laws in the interest of the public health is a responsibility of state legislatures. However, most of the health rules and regulations under which we live are formulated by state boards of health and, unless reversed by the legislature, have the force of law.

[2]The State Public Health Agency, *American Journal of Public Health*, vol. 55, pp. 2011, December 1965.

In addition to these rules and regulations, state legislatures enact certain laws concerned with the public health. These may relate to the environment, water supplies, air pollution, waste disposal, the use of insecticides, detergents, etc.; to medical and hospital services and the licensing of various types of health practitioners; to the control of certain diseases, for example, smallpox; or to personal health practices, such as family planning, voluntary sterilization, and abortion.

ABORTION LAWS

Public interest and legislative action currently are focused primarily upon protection of the environment, family planning, and abortion. Most controversial among these have been the efforts to change the pattern of long-standing state laws which permit the performance of abortions only to save the life of the mother. Since 1967, seventeen states have liberalized their abortion laws, but most of these limit the grounds for abortion to physical or mental health of the mother, rape, incest, or fetal deformity. Four states, Alaska, Hawaii, New York, and Washington, have made the question of abortion a matter of decision by a woman and her physician. Each of these states, however, has specified medical and hospital standards for abortions and has placed a limit upon the duration of pregnancy during which an abortion may be performed. (See References, page 402.)

In addition to these changes in laws, a considerable number of cases which challenge the constitutionality of restrictive abortion laws are pending in the courts. The first decision on this question came from California, where the State Supreme Court declared unconstitutional the state's law which permitted abortion only when necessary to preserve the life of the mother. Said the court: "The rights involved are the woman's right to life and to choose whether to bear children. . . . The fundamental right of the woman to choose whether to bear children follows the Supreme Court's and this court's repeated acknowledgment of a 'right to privacy' or 'liberty' in matters related to marriage, family, and sex." In states where the laws relative to abortion are found to be unconstitutional, the only restrictions on abortions are those that apply to other surgical procedures.

LOCAL HEALTH DEPARTMENTS

The local health department is responsible for providing its community with public health services. It obtains firsthand information concerning local health needs and should formulate plans for best meeting them.

For a local health department to be effective it should provide several types of service, including:

1 *Recording and analysis of health data* which are needed to define and locate local health problems and to ensure sound planning for optimum health.
2 *Health education and information,* which constitute the foundation for effective health services.
3 *Supervisory and regulatory responsibilities* covering various fields. These include "the protection of food, water, and milk supplies, the control of nuisances, the sanitary disposal of wastes and control of pollution, the prevention of occupational diseases and accidents, the control of human and animal sources of infection, the regulation of housing, and the inspection of hospitals, nursing homes, and other health facilities. In carrying out these functions, health departments use a variety of methods, of which probably the most important is public education and individual instruction. Others include the issuance of regulations, laboratory control, inspection and licensure, revocation of permits and, as a last resort, court action."
4 *Provision of direct environmental health services* when necessary in specific areas and under special conditions. For example, residual spraying of homes for insect control may be provided in some localities.
5 *Provision for, or administration of, a variety of personal health services.* These include immunization programs and other preventive measures, such as fluoridation programs; advisory health maintenance services (public health nursing visits, child

health conferences, etc.); case-finding programs; provision of laboratory services and consultation clinics as an aid to the physician; new programs, as in the fields of chronic diseases and mental hygiene.

6 *Provision of leadership in community health needs* by the coordination of activities and resources in the local community.[3]

[3]American Public Health Association, "The Local Health Department: Services and Responsibilities," official statement, *American Journal of Public Health*, vol. 54, pp. 131–139, January 1964.

INTERNATIONAL ORGANIZATIONS

THE WORLD HEALTH ORGANIZATION

The World Health Organization,[4] with headquarters in Geneva, Switzerland, is the only major agency through which the nations of the world can coordinate health action on an international scale. Membership is open to all nations. In 1970 the organization consisted of 131 member nations.

The creation of the World Health Organization in 1948 was the culmination of a long series of efforts made over the centuries to prevent the spread of disease from one country to another and to achieve international cooperation for better health throughout the world. During the last part of the nineteenth century, the United States began to participate in international programs directed primarily at reaching agreements on methods of preventing cholera and other plagues from spreading from nation to nation. These meetings culminated in a conference in Paris in 1903, where a convention was drawn up which consolidated earlier agreements and set up the first effective and comprehensive international pattern for foreign quarantine. The concept of international cooperation in controlling and preventing diseases grew out of these early sanitary conferences. Gradually these international health programs were broadened, and the International Office of Public Health was established in Paris in 1907.

The first major step toward broad international cooperation in the field of health came in 1920 when the League of Nations created an Epidemic Commission and, subsequently, a health

[4]*World Health Organization: What It Is, What It Does; How It Works*, WHO Regional Office, Washington.

Some county and city health departments have responsibilities also for the operation of public hospitals and clinics.

Further improvement of the public health urgently requires more adequate local, and particularly rural, health units. More trained personnel and more adequate health department budgets are essential, and these two requisites can be provided only by community interest and support under the leadership of informed and public-spirited citizens. This part of the job can be done only by the people themselves in their own homes and in their own communities.

organization that concerned itself not only with major diseases but also with studies on nutrition, housing, and the standardization of therapeutic substances.

When the Charter of the United Nations was drawn up in San Francisco in 1945, Brazil proposed that health be included in the United Nations Charter as one of the essential factors for international peace and stability. An international health conference held the following year in New York drew up a constitution for the new organization. Before the interim commission that launched the work of the WHO could be replaced by a permanent organization, it was necessary for twenty-six member nations of the United Nations to approve the constitution. It was ratified by the required number of countries on April 7, 1948. On that date the WHO constitution came into force and WHO was established as a permanent specialized agency of the United Nations. April 7 has since been observed throughout the world as World Health Day. The first World Health Assembly met in Geneva in June, 1948, and the permanent organization was established on September 1, 1948. The first time the World Health Assembly met in this country was in 1958 when Minneapolis was the site of the eleventh annual meeting. The twenty-second was held in Boston in 1969.

The World Health Organization is financed by its member governments. Each nation contributes to the budget according to its economic status. The budget for 1970, contributed by active member states, totals $70 million. Under the United Nations Technical Assistance program a further amount of almost $8 million is made available to WHO. As a member nation, the United States makes contributions to the regular budget and to special funds. The countries that are benefiting from international assistance are making a real effort to increase their financial support of health work. In 1966, for example, WHO from its regular and technical assistance budgets supported 1,276 health projects in 152 governments of the countries and territories. Toward these, national governments of the countries assisted contributed approximately $3.50 for every $1 supplied by WHO. These contributions were apart from their annual contributions to WHO.

The activities of the World Health Organization fall into three general groups:

1   Advisory service to governments, with special emphasis on control and eradication of communicable diseases, public health services, and training of public health workers for national public health service.

2   Central technical services in such fields as epidemiology, health statistics, standardization of therapeutic substances, health research, and population control. (See Figure 26.1.)

3   Emergency aid to governments (a) in dealing with epidemics, such as typhus fever, meningitis, malaria, and tuberculosis; (b) in meeting special health problems, such as the care of refugees in the Palestine area and the health problems in the Congo precipitated by its independence from Belgium.

The logic behind the establishment of WHO —and the reason for its support by the member

Figure 26.1   The World Health Organization sponsors health centers for mothers and children like this one in Indonesia. (Courtesy of the United Nations.)

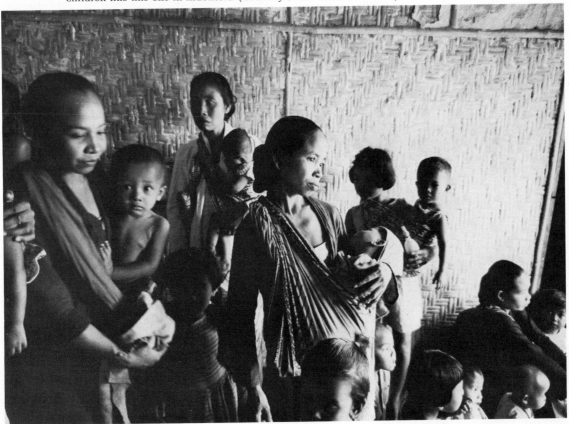

nations—is that today bad health conditions in one part of the world are almost certain to have an impact on the health of other areas. This may occur directly through the spread of communicable diseases or indirectly through the contribution of ill health to poverty and to the social and economic conditions that breed unrest and revolt. In addition to the World Health Organization, the following other organizations are conducting major programs in the field of international health:

FOOD AND AGRICULTURE ORGANIZATION

FAO. like WHO, is a specialized agency of the United Nations, supported by assessments upon member countries. Its purposes are to improve the nutrition of people of all countries, particularly where malnutrition is a major problem; to increase the efficiency of farming, fishing, and forestry, to better the condition of rural people; and through all these means to help raise standards of living. Thus FAO is making fundamental contributions to better health in the areas of the world where malnutrition, illness, and disease make economic, educational, social, and political progress almost impossible.

UNITED NATIONS CHILDREN'S FUND

Originally named and still frequently called *UNICEF*, this is still another specialized agency of the United Nations, but one which devotes its efforts to improving the health and welfare of children. Each year it assists about 500 projects in more than 100 countries and reaches more than 50 million mothers and children. Its programs include child feeding and other nutrition services; basic maternal, child welfare, and educational services; and programs in cooperation with WHO for the control of such major diseases as malaria, tuberculosis, yaws, trachoma, and leprosy. UNICEF is supported by contributions from governments and by private gifts. For every $1 allocated by UNICEF, the receiving countries are obligated to spend approximately $2.50 on the projects aided.

AGENCY FOR INTERNATIONAL DEVELOPMENT

AID is an agency in the State Department of the United States government that conducts and supports programs to aid other countries on a so-called *bilateral basis*—i.e., on the basis of programs formulated, subscribed to, and participated in by the government of the United States and the government of the other country concerned. This type of assistance was inaugurated under the Marshall Plan and the Point-four Program and administered successively by ECA (Economic Cooperation Administration), FOA (Foreign Operations Administration), ICA (International Cooperation Administration), and now by AID.

The programs of AID cover economic, industrial, scientific, educational, and social welfare activities as well as health activities. That our government considers the health work of AID of major importance is evidenced by the fact that last year some $50 million were expended for purposes through this agency, and several times that amount was expended by the governments of the countries assisted. Most of these programs were in the less well-developed countries of the world: South and Southeast Asia, the Near East, Africa, Latin America, and Southeastern Europe. In these regions there are more than twice as many people as in the better-developed regions of North America, Western and Southern Europe, Australia, and Japan.

The types of programs supported by this agency include practically all aspects of health and medical services. First priority, however, has been given to programs which afford rapid, recognizable, and appreciated results and affect large numbers of people at low cost per person—so low that the host country can practically always take over the maintenance job. Specifically, these programs include:

1 Mass campaigns against malaria, yaws, and nutritional deficiencies such as beri-beri, xerophthalmia, and goiter
2 Development of safe community water supplies
3 Demonstration through health centers of such community-wide services as sanitation, communicable-disease control, health records and statistics, home visiting, maternal and child health, nutrition, health education, and laboratory and general clinical service
4 Advice and assistance in strengthening and stabilizing the organization and oper-

ation of official public health services of the government

5 Advice and assistance in the planning and designing of hospitals, health centers, laboratories, and other health facilities

6 Development and support of the basic training of personnel for service in public health

7 Development of medical schools, including provision for training key medical school teachers, for necessary supplies and equipment, and for advisory and consultant services from schools in this country

8 Mass campaigns against other diseases of major importance, such as trachoma, smallpox, typhus, leprosy, and tuberculosis

9 Consultation on sanitary engineering or other specialized services

10 Special projects such as demonstration health centers, medical rehabilitation programs, and family planning and population control.

Over the past few years the increasing concern in this country with the rapid growth of the world's population has led to greatly increased appropriations, from $2.1 million in 1965 to $34.7 million in 1968, to AID for programs of family planning and population control in underdeveloped countries. In 1968 direct assistance was given to twenty-six countries, about half in East and Southeast Asia and half in Latin America. The programs supported, such as the training of personnel, the manufacture of contraceptive materials, and the development of education activities, are ones which the countries assisted can carry forward and expand with their own resources.

WORLD HEALTH FOR WORLD PEACE

Health is a subject in which all people of the world have a common interest. In fact, international cooperation in the field of health is proving to be a common ground for the development of cooperation and understanding that could well extend to more difficult and more controversial areas. This is a field in which the United States has the ability as well as the unique opportunity to assume world leadership. It is therefore important that citizens understand, support, and participate in these efforts. Such support and participation help protect the health of Americans at home and abroad; they further the progress of public health throughout the world; and probably most important of all, they are a potent force in the worldwide effort to build the conditions of peace.

QUESTIONS FOR DISCUSSION AND SELF-EXAMINATION

1 What has been the influence of private interests on the passage of laws governing public health matters?

2 How do the various official agencies in the field of public health compare in power and function?

3 What are the advantages and disadvantages of local autonomy in public health matters?

4 Describe the origin of the World Health Organization and the similarities and differences between the World Health Organization and the national public health agencies.

5 Describe the changing role, function, and structure of the U.S. Public Health Service.

6 How does the Food and Drug Administration protect the American public?

7 What legal powers does the federal government possess for combating pollution?
8 Compare the power and function of the various organizations active in international public health.
9 What diseases have been controlled by public health measures in the United States? In underdeveloped countries?
10 Apply the five basic principles of public health to two specific problems in public health or to two specific organizations.

REFERENCES AND READING SUGGESTIONS

BOOKS

Programs and Services, U.S. Department of Health, Education, and Welfare, Washington, D.C.

The federal government operates more than 200 separate programs to help people, most of them in cooperation with state and local governments, nongovernmental organizations, and individual Americans. This publication provides basic information about these programs and how they can be used.

Reiterman, Carl (ed.): *Abortion and the Unwanted Child,* Springer Publishing Co., Inc., New York, 1971.

A summary of what has happened in recent efforts to modify existing abortion laws, and current laws about who may get an abortion in the various states, for what reasons, where it may be performed, when and by whom, and who will pay for it.

PAMPHLETS AND PERIODICALS

Anderson, Oscar E., James H. Young, and Wallace F. Janssen: "The Government and the Consumer: Evolution of Food and Drug Laws," *Journal of Public Law,* vol. 13, no. 1, Emory University Law School, Atlanta, Ga., 1964.

A scholarly, comprehensive, and interesting report of the development and current operation of this important government service.

Deutsch, Albert: *The World Health Organization: Its Global Battle against Disease,* Public Affairs Pamphlet, New York.

Drew, Elizabeth B.: "The Quiet Victory of the Cigarette Lobby—How It Found the Best Filter Yet—Congress," *Atlantic,* September 1965, p. 76.

A behind-the-scenes story of the influence exerted on Congress relative to a warning label on cigarette packages.

The F.D.A.—What It Is and Does, Government Printing Office, 1966.

Harris, Richard: "Annals of Legislation: Medicare," *New Yorker,* July 2, 9, 16, and 23, 1966.

A detailed, illuminating political history of the Medicare legislation.

"Legal Abortion: How Safe? How Available? How Costly?" *Consumer Reports,* Mount Vernon, N.Y., July 1972.

A comprehensive report on the legal status of abortions in the United States, on the methods used, the risks, the costs, and sources of reliable information.

"World Health: The Work Goes On," *The Magazine of the World Health Organization,* Avenue Appia, 1211 Geneve, 27, Switzerland, May 1971.

This unusually interesting and significant issue is devoted entirely to highlights of the major health problems of the world today and what the World Health Organization is doing about them.

27

VOLUNTARY HEALTH ORGANIZATIONS

In late 1971, for the first time New York City reported a decline in the birth rate. The 1970 national census indicated that during the 1960–1970 decade there were 15 percent fewer children under 5 years of age in this country than there were in 1960. This means that the overall birth rate has declined and that the specter of overpopulation in the United States may be beginning to recede. What brought about this change?

One important factor has been the efforts of voluntary health organizations such as Planned Parenthood which through education and service helps hundreds of thousands of parents to control the size of their families. Such an example of what a health organization can do is dramatic and easily understood, but grants for investigation of obscure enzyme systems in body cells or of the conduct of electrical impulses in different kinds of tissues are equally or possibly even more important, for they may lead to practical preventive measures in heart disease, in cancer, and in other human disease problems in the years ahead.

In this country a vast amount of excellent health work is being done by organizations with no governmental connections. Some of these are voluntary health organizations supported by contributions or membership dues; others are endowed philanthropic foundations; others are professional organizations; other are large business enterprises, such as insurance companies and great corporations; and still others are local organizations of various types and purposes, such as hospitals, educational institutions, labor unions, group health organizations, and community chests. But much of the tremendous potential represented by such organizations is ineffectually used.

NATIONAL VOLUNTARY HEALTH ORGANIZATIONS

National voluntary health agencies are composed of individuals, both lay and professional, with a primary purpose of combating a particular disease, disability, or group of diseases and disabilities, or of improving the health of a particular group of people. They are supported largely by voluntary contributions from the public at large rather than from government sources or endowments. They engage in programs of research, education, and service to individuals and communities in their particular spheres of interest.

Among the health organizations supported by voluntary contributions or membership dues, the ones below are outstanding, most of them national organizations with state and local branches or chapters.

NATIONAL TUBERCULOSIS AND RESPIRATORY DISEASE ASSOCIATION

The National Tuberculosis Association, the first of the national health organizations, was started in 1904 when tuberculosis was the leading cause of death in this country. (See page 6.) Their largest public appeal for funds is made through the Christmas Seal sale. The association conducts a continuing campaign to educate people about tuberculosis; it supports some research and through its local associations it promotes early diagnosis and treatment and provides rehabilitation services for those who contract the disease. In recent years the association has concerned itself with other respiratory diseases, such as chronic bronchitis, emphysema, and asthma, and has publicized cigarette smoking and air pollution as major contributory causes of these diseases. In view of its expanded interests and activities, the association recently changed its name and became the National Tuberculosis and Respiratory Disease Association.

AMERICAN CANCER SOCIETY

This society, with its state divisions and more than 3,000 local units, is dedicated to finding cures or preventive measures for cancer. It collects funds by means of a well-organized nationwide campaign, and disburses the funds for cancer research, cancer education, and services to cancer patients.

The first suggestion for an organization to be concerned with cancer was made by a group of physicians in 1912. They were distressed by the large proportion of cancer patients in whom the disease was hopelessly advanced when first seen. The purpose of this initial organization was to inform the public about the possibilities of saving lives by early diagnosis and prompt and adequate treatment of cancer. This was a revolutionary idea because in those days cancer was considered a hopeless and loathsome disease, never mentioned in the public press and rarely in private conversation. In fact, many hospitals would not accept patients with cancer.

This new organization, the Society for the Control of Cancer, developed slowly, but eventually, with the cooperation of the Federation of Women's Clubs, its program became national in scope. Then in the early 1940s some business leaders became interested, reorganized the society, and obtained public support for research and expanded educational and service programs.

Today the American Cancer Society is governed by a board of directors of approximately 100 members, half physicians and scientists and half laymen, from all parts of the country. As components of the society there are 59 divisions, mostly statewide, and approximately 3,000 local units to carry out the society's programs.

Currently, the society is providing approximately $20 million a year for the support of cancer research in the medical schools, universities, research institutes, and hospitals of the country. This is less than half the amount of the research requests recommended for support by expert scientific review committees. The society also keeps the medical and allied health professions informed about new and improved methods for the prevention, diagnosis, and treatment of cancer. It conducts research concerning the cause and control of cancer. It supported the research that led to the development of the Pap smear for the early diagnosis of cancer of the cervix.

The society conducted the definitive epidemiologic studies that established the relationship between cigarette smoking and disease, particularly lung cancer, coronary heart disease, and emphysema. (See page 95.) Programs of information and education to inform the public about the prevention, early diagnosis, and proper treatment of cancer constitute an important and continuing activity of the society.

PLANNED PARENTHOOD—WORLD POPULATION

The Planned Parenthood Association has grown from a single birth-control clinic in Brooklyn in 1916 to a nationwide network of 181 affiliates with a total of 620 clinics, operating in 350 cities in 40 states and the District of Columbia. Through the International Planned Parenthood Federation, of which the American Federation is a member, Planned Parenthood helps family planning organizations in more than 100 countries around the world.

The principal goals of this organization are to help make information an effective means of family planning. This information includes contraception, voluntary abortion, and sterilization. They also stimulate relevant biomedical, socioeconomic, and demographic research to combat the world population crisis. The federation acts to stimulate government agencies and voluntary organizations and hospitals to provide birth-control information and services to all women who need and want them.

AMERICAN HEART ASSOCIATION

The national American Heart Association was organized in 1924 to stimulate, coordinate, and support programs of research and professional and public education relative to the prevention, diagnosis, and treatment of heart disease. The work of the association includes other diseases of the cardiovascular system, such as stroke, high blood pressure, and arteriosclerosis.

State heart associations, although locally incorporated, cooperate with the national organization in fund raising, the support of research, and educational programs.

AMERICAN RED CROSS

The American Red Cross provides an invaluable supplement to the medical services of the armed forces in wartime. In peacetime it is the agency best equipped and always called upon for disaster relief. During World War II and the wars in Korea and Vietnam, the American Red Cross collected and processed whole blood and blood plasma which saved the lives of thousands of American soldiers. Since the end of World War II the Red Cross has developed its "blood program" on a peacetime basis in order to make blood and blood products available for use when needed in civilian hospitals. The Red Cross is a leader also in teaching first aid and is active in improving nursing services and nutrition and health education of the public.

NATIONAL FOUNDATION

Formerly called the *National Foundation for Infantile Paralysis,* this foundation, which was started by President Roosevelt and is financed by the March of Dimes, has supported all aspects of research and service concerned with poliomyelitis. It supported the research that led to the development of a vaccine for the prevention of poliomyelitis. (See page 265.) In 1958 the National Foundation broadened its program to include arthritis, birth defects, and disorders of the central nervous system.

OTHER VOLUNTARY HEALTH ORGANIZATIONS

Prominent among the many other voluntary health organizations which operate in this country are the National Association for Mental Health; the National Association for Retarded Children; the United Cerebral Palsy Association; the Muscular Dystrophy Association; the National Council on Alcoholism; the American Social Health Association; the Arthritis and Rheumatism Foundation; the National Society for the Prevention of Blindness; and the National Society for Crippled Children and Adults, with its Easter seal sale.

Voluntary health organizations provide services, demonstrations, and experimentation and stimulate interest in and support for specialized programs. They are more free to try new procedures and to concentrate on special health problems than are governmental agencies. Almost without exception these agencies serve a valuable purpose in our overall health program and merit public support. However, if they are to function efficiently and make the best possible use of the money which is entrusted to them, public-spirited citizens must not only give them support but also participate in their activities and administration.

PHILANTHROPIC FOUNDATIONS

Most of the philanthropic foundations have been established and endowed by wealthy individuals. Some operate in local areas or in special fields; some are national or even international in scope. The larger ones have millions of dollars annually to spend or distribute. These foundations make large contributions each year for medical research, medical education, the training of public health personnel, the evaluation of public health measures, experimentation with new public health procedures, health education of the public, the support of actual public health services in special situations, etc. Below are examples of the better-known foundations operating in the health field.

ROCKEFELLER FOUNDATION

Supporting medical and public health education, research, and service over the world, the Rockefeller Foundation has pioneered in the establishment of schools of public health both in this country and abroad, has aided in the improvement of medical education, and has given support to medical research in all parts of the world. The International Health Division of this foundation played an important role in the control of yellow fever, malaria, and other epidemic diseases on a world-wide basis.

Currently the four principal areas of interest and support of the Rockefeller Foundation are (1) the conquest of hunger, (2) the problems of population, (3) university development, and (4) equal opportunity.

COMMONWEALTH FUND

For years the Commonwealth Fund has been supporting medical research and the improvement of medical education, particularly in special fields such as psychiatry and child guidance. It gave impetus to the improvement of health services by demonstrating in various parts of the country what an adequately supported and efficiently administered local health department, child guidance clinic, or rural hospital could accomplish. The Commonwealth Fund also has conducted a fellowship program to permit medical scientists of this country to study abroad and to bring health workers of other countries to America to study.

KELLOGG FOUNDATION

The Kellogg Foundation, of Battle Creek, Michigan, originally had as its primary interest the improvement of medical service in rural areas. Its funds have been used to improve local health departments, to construct and support hospitals, to provide special diagnostic services, such as x-ray departments and laboratories; and to make available to physicians, dentists, and nurses continuation study courses on the newer developments in medicine. This foundation for a number of years functioned exclusively in the state of Michigan but is now providing support for various types of health programs in other states and even in some Latin American countries.

FORD FOUNDATION

The largest of all philanthropic foundations, the Ford Foundation has as its stated purpose "to advance human welfare." This is a broad charter. As a matter of policy, however, the trustees have decided that, inasmuch as several other major foundations are devoting their resources largely to medicine and public health, the Ford Foundation should not support projects or programs in these same areas. They have, however, made one notable and important exception to this policy: namely, to support fundamental research on conception and to aid in the development of programs for population control throughout the world.

OTHER PHILANTHROPIC FOUNDATIONS

Other major foundations which devote their funds primarily to various aspects of medical and health work include the Markle Foundation, the Milbank Memorial Fund, the Macy Foundation, the Kress Foundation, and the Alfred Sloan Foundation.

PROFESSIONAL HEALTH ORGANIZATIONS

Various groups of professional workers in this country have formed organizations to promote the fields of their professional interests. Such organizations strive to improve the social and economic welfare of their members; to keep their members informed of changes and developments in professional practice; to set standards of ethical conduct and of professional practice and aid in the enforcement of these standards; to engage in research to improve practice and utilization of professional services; to speak for and on behalf of the profession in planning and action groups; to monitor government activities in health; to represent the profession in determination of public policy; to mediate for the profession with government and with other agencies; and to provide the public with information relative to the prevention of disease and the improvement of health. Examples of such organizations are the American Public Health Association and the American Medical Association.

AMERICAN PUBLIC HEALTH ASSOCIATION
Included in the membership of the American Public Health Association are the various professional workers in the field of public health, such as health officers, epidemiologists, public health engineers, sanitarians, public health nurses, health educators, and public health laboratory workers. The purpose of this association is to improve public health practice by the establishment of standards, by the support of research and experimentation, and by keeping its members informed through meetings and publications of new knowledge in their fields. In recent years the association has been studying possible ways to improve the provision of health care to the public. Other organizations with overlapping interests are the National League for Nursing; the American Epidemiological Society; the American College Health Association; the American Association for Health, Physical Education and Recreation; and the American School Health Association.

AMERICAN MEDICAL ASSOCIATION
An organization of licensed physicians, the American Medical Association is based upon local county units called *county medical societies*. The elected representatives of these county societies make up legislative bodies of state societies; and representatives from the state medical societies constitute the legislative body of the American Medical Association. The purpose of this association is to improve the quality of medical service to the American people. This is accomplished by insisting upon high standards in medical education; by aiding physicians to keep abreast of advances in medical knowledge and practice; by the support of research; by publishing the results of the investigations of medicines, foods, and appliances advertised and promoted for sale on the basis of alleged medical or health values; by education of the public on health matters; and by promoting special areas of health service, such as industrial hygiene, nutrition, emergency medical service, hospitals, and rural health.

OTHER PROFESSIONAL HEALTH ORGANIZATIONS
Other professional associations with similar purposes and types of organization are the Academy of Family Practice; the American College of Surgeons; the American College of Physicians; the American Dental Association; the American Nurses Association; the American Pharmaceutical Association; the American Society of Medical Technologists, the American Physical Therapy Association, and the American Occupational Therapy Association.

HOSPITALS

As medical science has progressed, the provision of medical care has become increasingly complex and involved. Two generations ago most patients were cared for in their own homes. The family physician called to make the diagnosis and to supervise treatment. The instruments and most of the drugs which he used were carried in his "little black bag." Members of the family or neighbors provided nursing care.

Today the situation is vastly different. The utilization of modern scientific procedures for diagnosis and for treatment requires facilities that are available only in doctors' offices or hospitals.

For example, generations ago when most patients with pneumonia were cared for at home, the physician based his diagnosis on symptoms and on his findings on examination of the patient. Treatment consisted of fresh air, good nursing care, and various drugs to relieve specific symptoms or to support the patient's general condition.

Today in making his diagnosis the physician still considers symptoms and physical findings, but in addition he asks for an x-ray examination to determine the exact location and the extent of the pneumonia and to observe from time to time its extension or recession. And he calls on the laboratory to find out what kind of microorganism is causing the pneumonia and to learn how the patient is reacting to the infection, as indicated by an increase or decrease in white blood cells. This information is important in deciding on treatment. In prescribing treatment the physician relies on the laboratory to help him decide how much of a drug should be given and perhaps whether or not the patient is in need of oxygen. To carry out these modern diagnostic and treatment procedures requires not only special facilities but also various types of specially trained personnel—radiologists, nurses, bacteriologists, medical technicians, x-ray technicians, pharmacists, dietitians, etc., who are available only in hospitals. Even if a patient is not admitted to a hospital the facilities and personnel of the hospital may be invaluable for his care.

Hospitals have existed since ancient times, but until modern times they were looked upon as places to be avoided. They were "pest houses," insane asylums, and places where people went to die. Until the last quarter of the nineteenth century, the chances were about one in two that persons entering a hospital would die of the disease with which they entered the hospital or of a disease which they contracted in the hospital. Today the situation is completely changed.

To the doctor, the hospital assumes a unique role. It aids him in practicing his art completely. It enables him to provide the best possible care of patients and to teach others what he has learned.

In a modern hospital an incredible array of skills, equipment, and therapies are available to the doctor. There are hundreds of new and experimental drugs, many developed and improved through hospital experience. There are machines that can measure the subtlest qualities of blood and other vital fluids. There are skills marshalled to provide more precise and successful diagnosis, surgery, and rehabilitation than ever before in human history. The hospital makes possible a high level of care for patients—and that is what the community expects and needs.

Today, as always, the patient in a hospital should not be merely a "case" with symptoms. He is a person with all the cares, worries, and anxieties of the ill, worries about family, about personal economics, about the future. And the hospital today brings into play all the professionals who can aid the physician in his efforts to restore the patient to society as a "total human being."

Increasingly, the general hospital is becoming the community medical center to which people go not only for the care of serious illnesses but also for diagnostic services and for short-term bed care.

In some areas, available hospitals are adequate to meet the needs; in other, additional hospitals should be built. Competent hospital authorities indicate that on a statewide basis there should be 4.5 beds in general hospitals and 5 beds in mental hospitals per 1,000 population. These figures are useful in estimating needs for hospitals over large areas, but they are not applicable to every community. In many situations better medical care will be provided by having patients driven to a hospital 25 or even 50 miles away than by attempting to build a small hospital in every community. For the best medical service a hospital must be large enough to provide all necessary facilities and equipment and in addition to have on its staff physicians, nurses, laboratory and x-ray technicians, and the other specially qualified personnel needed to utilize these facilities properly.

Hospitals are frequently classified according to ownership as *governmental* or *voluntary*. The federal government operates hospitals for personnel of the military services and the Public Health Service and their dependents, Indians, veterans, merchant seamen, special groups such as narcotic addicts, and patients with leprosy. State hospitals are primarily specialized hospitals for patients with mental illnesses or tuberculosis, or general hospitals associated with medical schools. City and county hospitals are usually general hospitals, frequently with facilities for the isolation of patients with communicable diseases.

Voluntary hospitals are mainly for general medical and surgical patients and are operated as nonprofit institutions. Some of them are established by church groups, some by interested individuals, and some by community effort. Responsible authority is vested in a governing board. This board, which represents the community, is responsible for the facilities, policies, financing, and management of the hospital, including the selection or approval of administrative and professional staffs.

Hospitals are community assets and community responsibilities. Citizens should be interested in the support and management of their community hospitals.

PHARMACIES AND PHARMACISTS

The manufacture and distribution of drugs is a big and exceedingly important business and public service. The discovery of insulin and penicillin would have been of no benefit to those who needed them if large and responsible drug manufacturers had not developed methods for their production in such quantities and of such quality that physi-cians everywhere could obtain them and use them with complete confidence in their purity and strength. The same is true concerning vaccines, serums, drugs, and all other types of pharmaceutical products.

For the protection of the public, drugs can be sold only by licensed pharmacists. Pharmacy is the science of preparing drugs and medicines. Pharmacists are educated in a school of pharmacy in a university. The modern trend of the so-called *drug-store* to offer for sale a varied line of merchandise, often specializing in soft drinks and light lunches, is a long way removed from the true meaning of the term "drugstore" and the original purpose of a pharmacy.

TEACHING AND RESEARCH INSTITUTIONS

Education for the health-service professions, such as medicine, dentistry, nursing, and public health, as well as research in the health fields, was inaugurated in this country by privately endowed and supported universities and research institutes. In recent years tax funds have come to play an increasingly important role in the support of medical research and in education for these professions, and because of the high costs involved, this trend will unquestionably continue.

BUSINESS AND LABOR ORGANIZATIONS

Business and industry, being concerned with production and efficiency, are giving increasing attention and support to medical and health programs for their employees. These programs include not only the provision of healthful conditions of employment but also health instruction and the provision of medical services. In some cases these services are provided not only for the workers but also for the members of their families. Experience has convinced leaders of industry that health services pay big dividends in efficiency, morale, and productivity.

Labor unions and some fraternal organizations are also becoming increasingly interested in the health of their members and are supporting or participating in various types of health and welfare programs.

INSURANCE COMPANIES

Life insurance companies spend large sums of money each year to support medical research, and to provide health information to the public, periodic health examinations to holders of certain types of policies, and nursing service to groups insured under industrial contracts. This is effective public health work, and the insurance companies can show that it represents a good invest-ment for them. They make money by prolonging the lives of their policyholders and, naturally, the policyholders do not object.

Some insurance companies make a contribution in the health field by offering insurance which provides cash payments in case of illnesses or accidents which require medical and hospital care and result in loss of time from employment.

Figure 27.1 Percentage of United States population with some form of health-insurance protection, 1940 to 1970. Source: Health Insurance Council.

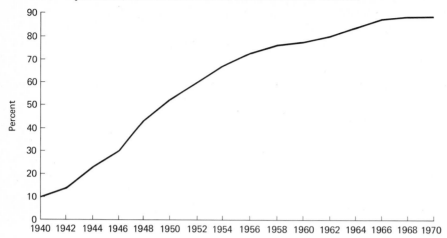

Policies are also being offered with special provisions to cover in whole or in part the costs of medical and hospital care.

By 1970 over 169 million persons, or more than 85 percent of the nation's population, were covered against the cost of hospital bills by some type of voluntary hospital insurance. A large number of the remaining population, such as members of the armed services and their dependents, veterans, and those in public institutions, had no need of it because hospital and medical care was provided for them. Also in 1968, 156 million were protected by surgical expense plans, 129 million by regular medical expense plans, and 55 million against loss of income due to disability. During 1968 insurance companies paid $7.1 billion in health and hospital insurance benefits. At the present rate of growth it will not be long before practically all people will have some type of insurance to protect themselves against the financial hardships occasioned by serious accidents or illnesses. (See Figure 27.1.)

Of special interest is the development by the hospitals of this country of the Blue Cross programs of hospital insurance. These are nonprofit enterprises, most of which are operated on a statewide basis. The national organization represents merely an affiliation of the state plans for cooperation and exchange of information. Allied with Blue Cross is the slightly newer Blue Shield which

provides insurance for the payment of medical and surgical fees when a patient is hospitalized. Some plans provide coverage only for surgical operations; others include all kinds of medical care. In some places Blue Cross and Blue Shield are combined in a single policy.

Although the vast majority of individuals who have hospital, surgical, and regular medical expense protection are covered by insurance company or Blue Cross-Blue Shield contracts, there are other types of independent plans which provide protection for the remainder. These include industrial plans, plans of private group clinics, etc. Great strides have been made in developing new forms of health insurance to fit various needs of the people of this country. The voluntary health insurance movement has had a tremendous growth in the past quarter of a century, both in the kinds of protection offered and in the number of persons who have sought this protection.[1]

MAJOR MEDICAL COVERAGE

A relatively new type of insurance now offered by certain insurance companies is comprehensive major medical coverage. This plan helps to take care of all reasonable, customary, and necessary medical expenses while a person is under the care of a physician. It covers expenses in or out of

[1]Data in this section are from *Source Book of Health Insurance Data*, 1970, Health Insurance Institute, New York.

the hospital, including physicians' fees, x-rays, laboratory charges, drugs, and often even nursing care in the hospital or home. These policies carry three special provisions (1) they limit the total benefits to a specified amount, usually up to $20,000 or even $100,000; (2) they provide, as in the case of automobile collision insurance, for a deductible amount; and (3) they include a coinsurance feature whereby the protected person pays a certain percentage of the expense above the deductible amount. The coinsurance provision is introduced for the purpose of letting the individual share in the expense of the services he orders, thus controlling, to some extent, the tendency on the part of some to demand almost unlimited health services. (See Figure 27.2.)

Minor medical expenses are a nuisance and at times create a financial hardship, but it is the catastrophic illness that may wreck the family finances. Comprehensive major medical coverage, therefore, is meeting a great need and is being purchased in increasing amounts both by individuals and by groups. Although it was first offered only about 20 years ago, over 67 million people were under major medical expense protection by the end of 1968. The optional portion B of the government's Medicare insurance program provides this type of comprehensive coverage.

When purchasing insurance to provide protection against loss of income from accidents or illnesses and against medical, surgical, and hospital expenses, the individual must read and study carefully the provisions and the costs of the policies offered and select those best suited to his needs.

Figure 27.2 Growth of nongovernmental hospital-expense protection in the United States. Source: Health Insurance Council.

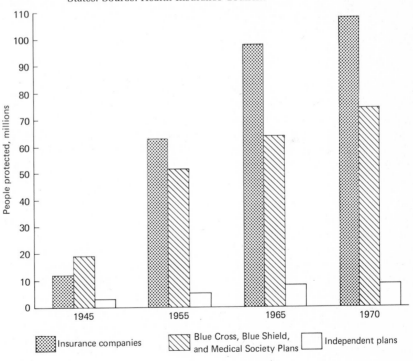

Totals: Not adjusted for
duplication

THE NATIONAL HEALTH COUNCIL

As these various types of health organizations developed throughout the country, the need to provide for an exchange of ideas and for the coordination of certain services of general interest became obvious. This led to the formation of the National Health Council, an organization "to aid in the promotion of health throughout the nation through joint planning and, where indicated, joint action."[2]

All major voluntary health agencies, all major professional societies concerned with health, and all major units of the federal government con-

[2]From the constitution of the National Health Council, New York.

cerned with health are members of the National Health Council. Among its activities are the conduct of an annual forum devoted to the consideration of some major health problem of concern to citizens of the United States, the improvement of basic local community health services, and the conduct of a nationwide program to interest young people in careers in the health field.

As national health agencies have grown in number and in scope of activities, the role and importance of the National Health Council have increased and will continue to increase in the years ahead.

NATIONAL INTERAGENCY COUNCIL ON SMOKING AND HEALTH

The National Interagency Council is a voluntary association of health, education, and youth leadership organizations vitally concerned with the problem of cigarette smoking and its effects on human health. Council membership consists of professional, private, voluntary, and governmental organizations. It seeks to provide a unified, coordinated force to inform the public regarding the harmful effects of tobacco use, especially cigarette smoking. (For membership see the list below.) The council operates under its own constitution with a directorate of representatives of member organizations and elected officers.

MEMBERS
American Academy of Pediatrics
American Association of Health, Physical Education and Recreation
American Cancer Society
American College of Chest Physicians
American College Health Association
American College of Physicians
American College of Radiology
American College of Surgeons
American Dental Association
American Heart Association
American Hospital Association
American Medical Association
American Nurses' Association
American Pharmaceutical Association
American Public Health Association

American School Health Association
Association of Classroom Teachers of the NEA
Association of State and Territorial Health Officers
Boys' Clubs of America
National Board of Young Men's Christian Associations
National Board of Young Women's Christian Association
National Congress of Parents and Teachers
National Jogging Association
National League of Nursing
National Medical Association
National Student Nurses' Association
National Tuberculosis and Respiratory Disease Association
Public Health Cancer Association of America
Student American Medical Association
U.S. Department of Defense
U.S. Office of Child Development
U.S. Office of Education
U.S. Public Health Service
U.S. Veterans Administration

MEMBERS-AT-LARGE
Emerson Foote
Luther L. Terry, M.D.

The principal objective of the National Interagency Council is to join the resources and energies of many organizations in the achievement of a single goal. By establishing a cooperative body, the council seeks to avoid duplication, to serve as a medium for the exchange of information, to plan when indicated for coordinated and cooperative action, and to provide a mechanism for stimulating new programs on smoking and health and evaluating existing programs.

A PLACE FOR ALL

Some people ask, since federal, state, and some local governments are appropriating money for medical research and for the control of many diseases, whether voluntary health organizations are any longer necessary, whether their functions could not be better carried out by government.

The answers to such questions are many, but prominent among them are: (1) that voluntarism is an essential element of a free, democratic society; (2) that nongovernmental organizations are best able to deal with many controversial problems and to experiment with new ideas and programs; and (3) that research scientists should have more than one possible source of support. No one speaks more positively concerning this than those who administer the huge federal programs of medical research support.

In the modern public health program, which has as its objective the prevention of disease, the prolongation of life, and the improvement of physical and mental health and efficiency, there is a place and a need for these many different types of health organizations. They can succeed, however, only if and when they have the intelligent interest, support, and participation of the citizens whom they are attempting to serve.

QUESTIONS FOR DISCUSSION AND SELF-EXAMINATION

1 Describe the similarities and dissimilarities among the major foundations active in the health field.
2 Describe the similarities and dissimilarities among the major voluntary health organizations active in the health field.
3 What is the relationship between the various voluntary health organizations and research in specific diseases?
4 Compare the purposes and membership of the American Public Health Association and the American Medical Association.
5 How has the role of the hospital in human disease changed in the past?
6 How do hospitals differ in purpose and function?
7 With what organization do the different health professionals relate? Be inclusive.
8 What is the importance of the development of health insurance?
9 How is major medical coverage related to other insurance and how does it differ?
10 What coordination of voluntary health activities exists?

REFERENCES AND READING SUGGESTIONS

BOOKS
Carter, Richard: *The Gentle Legions*, The Curtis Publishing Company, Philadelphia, 1959.

An intimate, personalized story of the work of the American Red Cross, the National Tuberculosis Association, the National Foundation for Infantile Paralysis, the American Cancer Society, and the American Heart Association.

Proceedings of Second National Voluntary Health Conference, American Medical Association, Chicago, 1966.

Discussion of the role of national voluntary

health agencies in the changing social, economic, and political environment.

Source Book of Health Insurance Data, Health Insurance Institute, New York. Published annually.

The extent to which nongovernmental insurance offsets health-care expenses and income loss resulting from illness and injury; and an analysis of medical-care costs in the United States.

PAMPHLETS AND PERIODICALS

Diehl, H.S.: "Relationship of Voluntary Health Agencies to College Health Programs," *Journal of the American College Health Association,* vol. 13, no. 3, p. 299, Apr. 15, 1964.

National Voluntary Health Agencies, American Medical Association, Chicago, 1967.

This booklet describes the purpose, organizational pattern, financing, and programs of the major national voluntary health agencies.

Pamphlets are available from many government agencies discussed in this chapter.

Voluntarism and Health, National Health Council, New York, 1962.

A concise but comprehensive view of the origin of, development of, role of, and need for a national voluntary health organization.

28

CRITICAL HEALTH PROBLEMS OF THE FUTURE

The advances in science, in technology, and in social organization have provided for the more fortunate of the world's population a standard of living previously undreamed of. Yet these same advances are creating serious health problems. The environment is becoming dangerously polluted; cities, large and small, are overcrowded; the needs for health services, for education, for housing, and even for food are increasing more rapidly than the rate of supply.

The public has become aware that disease does not have to be endured, that many hazards to health can be eliminated, and that good health is a requisite of a vigorous, progressive society. Furthermore, individuals now believe themselves entitled to health and medical services, just as they expect education and police and fire protection.

Continuing progress in the improvement of health and in the reduction of illnesses and pre-ventable deaths is clearly possible, but it will be more difficult to attain than the brilliant achievements of the past. However, we can lengthen and enrich the lives of millions of persons by the control of population, by the elimination of malnutrition, by improved housing, by reducing the pollution of the environment, and by better control of cardiovascular diseases, cancer, mental illnesses, respiratory diseases, and other serious chronic and disabling conditions.

In considering the possibilities of further improvement in health, we tend to think first of improved and expanded public health and medical services and of research to provide new methods for the prevention and treatment of disease. These are all essential elements in a program for better health. But much more is necessary. The public must be better informed on matters of personal and public health; and people everywhere, acting as individuals and as groups, must make better use of available information concerning the improvement of health and the prevention of accidents and of diseases. Other factors, too, such as good housing and income adequate to provide the essentials of healthful living, are in many instances more important than more medical services for the improvement of health.

POPULATION CONTROL

Prior to and during World War II, women who had large families in Hitler's Germany and in Stalin's Russia were financially rewarded by the government. Today students of the social, economic, and health situation of the world consider the population increase, at a rate more rapid than the production of food and other necessities of life, as the most dangerous threat which civilization faces.

The decreasing birth rate in the United States over the past several years is encouraging (Table 28.1). If this trend were to continue, it might be possible to achieve zero population growth within the present century. However, at present the number of births exceeds the number of deaths by approximately 100,000 per month. Furthermore, the number of women of prime childbearing age is expected to increase by 30 percent by 1980. The current trend, therefore, could easily be reversed.[1]

ON THE BRINK OF GLOBAL FAMINE

Dr. Norman E. Borlang, whose development of new wheat strains to aid the fight against world hunger won him the 1970 Nobel Peace Prize, says, "My life has been devoted to food production, but population growth transcends all other problems. Increases in food production provide the human race with time, possibly thirty years, to get the world's birth rate under control. Unless this is done, population growth will one day wipe us from the earth's surface."

WORLD POPULATION YEAR

The United Nations' Economic and Social Council has declared 1974 to be World Population Year. The purpose is to emphasize the importance of population control measures if there is to be avoidance of a catastrophe which is imminent with the present growth of world population of at least 100 million every year. At this rate the population of the world may double in just 30 years; however, the availability of food and other needs cannot be provided in quantities double the present amount, which even now are meager and poorly distributed among nations.[2]

Increasing recognition of and concern about this problem by individuals, by voluntary groups, by governments, and by the World Health Organization are heartening. But a mere beginning has been made. For example, despite the great increase in Planned Parenthood clinics and the expansion of public health services in this field, four out of five women in the United States still do not have access to such family planning services in their home communities. More than half the nation's counties have no such clinics. More than 4,000 hospitals provide no family planning services. Only about half of the nation's local health departments which provide maternal and child care also offer birth-control services. And the most neglected consist primarily of women of low incomes.

The various aspects of this problem and methods for dealing with it are considered in Chapter 3, pages 22 to 27. Strong statements are being made

[1] *American Medical News,* July 17, 1972, p. 6

Table 28.1 Birth rates and fertility rates in the United States, 1964–1971.

Year	Birth rate*	Fertility rate†
1964	21.0	105.0
1965	19.4	96.6
1966	18.4	91.3
1967	17.8	87.6
1968	17.5	85.7
1969	17.7	85.5
1970	18.2	87.6
1971	17.3	83.3

* Births per 1,000 population
† Births per 1,000 women aged 25–44
SOURCE: National Center for Health Statistics.

[2] *Journal of the American Medical Association,* July 31, 1972, p. 517.

Table 28.2   World population in 1970

Area	Population, mid-1970s (estimated)	Annual growth rate (estimated), percent
Industrial countries of Europe and the Soviet Union Japan and North America	1,000,000,000	1
Mainland China	775,000,000	2 (+ or −)
India	550,000,000	2½
Latin America, Africa, and the parts of Asia not listed above	1,375,000,000	2½ (+)
The world	3,700,000,000	2

by leading national and international personages, resolutions are passed, and laws are even enacted. Yet progress is slow.

In 1971 a new group, the Coalition for a National Population Policy, was organized to lobby for federal policies aimed at halting population growth in the United States. Dr. Milton Eisenhower, former president of Johns Hopkins University, and former United States Senator Joseph Tydings of Maryland are co-chairmen. Concerning the purpose of this coalition Senator Tydings said that the organization will work to inform the public that

... A rapidly growing population is guaranteeing human misery and degradation, inadequate education, poor health facilities, political instability and a lack of human progress. ... Either we must act now to develop rational voluntary policies and programs to stabilize population size or face the possibility of a drastic deterioration in the quality of national life and the collapse of many of our cherished institutions under the sheer weight of human numbers. ... In the long run continued population growth will pose an enormous threat to our ability to survive as a democratic nation characterized by well-being rather than want.

The coalition's executive committee includes representatives of fifteen major environmental and population planning groups, ranging from the Sierra Club and Friends of the Earth to Planned Parenthood and Zero Population Growth.

Organizations such as this can be influential but the young people of the country more than any other group will determine the future of population growth. Therefore, concern, action, and leadership of youth are essential in this exceedingly important but highly personal area.

POLLUTION OF THE ENVIRONMENT

The current situation relative to environmental pollution has been considered in Chapter 3, pages 27 to 39. A widespread awakening and concern about the deterioration of the environment are developing. However, effective action to reduce pollution or even to prevent continuing pollution is exceedingly difficult. Substantial progress is almost impossible because of opposition by economic interests; unwillingness by individuals and by groups to forego personal conveniences or desires; the failure both of government—federal, state, and local—and of industry to provide adequate funds to implement laws and regulations to reduce pollution; and a general apathy about the problem.

Concerning this progress, René Dubois, distinguished student of population and pollution, says,

Man is not on his way to extinction. He can adapt to most anything. ... That is the real tragedy. ... As we become adapted we accept worse and worse conditions without realizing that a child born and raised in this environment has no chance of developing his total physical and mental potential. It is essential that we commit ourselves to such problems as societies and as nations, not because we are threatened with extinction, but because if we do not understand what the environment is doing to us, something perhaps worse than extinction will take place—a progressive degradation of the quality of human life.[3]

To overcome these obstacles will require dedicated and determined effort. In many places youth groups, who have the biggest stake in the conditions of life in the future, are taking leadership roles in efforts to safeguard and improve the environment.

[3]*Population Pollution and Affluence,* selection no. 36, Population Reference Bureau, Inc., Washington, March 1971.

IMPROVEMENT OF NUTRITION AND HOUSING, AND THE REDUCTION OF POVERTY

At the recent White House Conference on Foods, Nutrition, and Health, surveys were reported that revealed an unbelievable amount of hunger and serious malnutrition in many areas of this country. Similar surveys of housing show that the conditions under which millions of families live are way below minimum standards of healthful housing. Most of these are in the slim areas of urban centers and in Appalachia and the rural South, but they exist in essentially every community, particularly for those who live in ghetto areas or on the "wrong side of the tracks." (See Figure 28.1.)

Figure 28.1   Poor housing in this mining community contributes to poor health. (U.S. Department of Agriculture.)

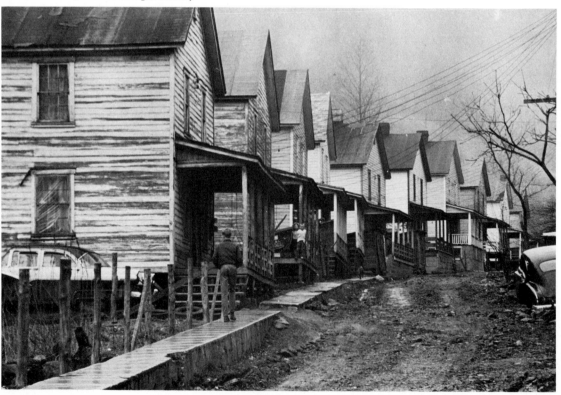

Poverty is the basic cause of these conditions and of the excessive rates of illness and disability which result. The reduction of poverty, therefore, becomes a most important health measure for millions of people. Employment for those who are able to work and for all families incomes adequate to provide the essentials of healthful living may not seem to be health problems, but without them the improvement of medical and health services will accomplish little.

ADEQUATE HEALTH SERVICES FOR ALL

In Chapter 4, Modern Medical Services, on pages 47 to 53, the present status of medical services in this country is considered: what these services offer to the individual, the unavailability of such services to a substantial portion of the population; and experiments with various methods of organizing and paying for medical care.

The quality of medical care received by the more affluent and better-educated portion of the population of the United States is the best in the world. But for vast numbers of people quality medical care or even any medical care is unavailable. This must be changed. How to make good medical care available to all is an urgent health problem.

A rigid, impersonal government-operated or government-controlled plan, such as exists in some countries, would be unacceptable here. This country is too diverse, the people too individualistic to be satisfied with that. Experimental programs, such as those in progress, must be continued, and other types of programs under imaginative and resourceful leadership should be undertaken. Government financing, at least in part, is necessary, but personal interest, responsibility, and iniative are essential.

But adequate health services for all means much more than the provision of medical care. The prevention of disease offers much greater potentialities for contributing to good health than does even the best of medical care. The 300,000 deaths and the colossal amount of illness and disability attributable to cigarette smoking can be prevented by not smoking, while medical care can do little to cure the diseases attributable to this habit. The amount of illness, disability, and premature death attributable to alcoholism and to drug abuse is staggering. The avoidance of obesity will reduce the likelihood of developing many diseases such as diabetes, heart disease, high blood pressure, and arthritis. The avoidance of excessive exposure to sunlight will prevent most of the 75,000 cases of skin cancer diagnosed each year in this country.

Vaccination against measles, poliomyelitis, whooping cough, diphtheria, German measles, tetanus, and so on (see pages 259 to 269) will prevent many thousands of cases of illness and a considerable number of deaths each year. Breast self-examination, Pap smears, and proctosigmoidoscopic examinations of adults will detect many thousands of beginning cancers when they can be cured. Likewise, regular physical examinations will discover many abnormal conditions or incipient diseases before they produce symptoms. Family planning services will prevent unwanted and many illegitimate children.

The provision of adequate medical care and of preventive health services for all is an important and, with the increasing number of older persons in the population, a constantly increasing health problem.

RESEARCH—MEDICAL, PSYCHOLOGICAL, AND SOCIAL

Medical research has made possible the prevention and control of many of the age-old scourges of mankind—smallpox, typhoid fever, yellow fever, malaria, diphtheria, poliomyelitis, tuberculosis, rickets, scurvy, beriberi, cholera, typhus, and bubonic plague. It has made possible the successful treatment of many diseases that in the past took a heavy toll of life and health—diabetes, pernicious anemia, pneumonia, syphilis, and appendicitis.

In spite of all this progress, however, the unknown in medicine still exceeds the known. Much is yet to be learned before the diseases which are the major causes of death today can be prevented or successfully treated—heart disease, cancer, stroke,

Medical science has not yet achieved the successful control of other diseases that greatly reduce people's effectiveness and pleasure in living—arthritis, the common cold, and mental illness. It does not yet know the causes for many diseases, such as multiple sclerosis, Parkinson's disease, and diabetes: it does not yet understand the physiological reasons for the changes of aging.

Difficult, challenging problems remain to be solved. A scientific discovery or development which would make possible the prevention or cure of any one of the leading causes of illness would contribute more to the welfare of the people of this country than flights to the moon, or even the building of hospitals or the extension of medical services. Clearly, then, in planning for the future, high priority must be given to providing the funds necessary to train research workers and to provide able scholars and scientists with the time, facilities, and support for investigative work.

The total funds currently available for medical research—mostly from government sources—are greater than ever before, but they are only a small fraction of the amount spent for the exploration of outer space or for the development of new military weapon systems.

And research is needed not only on direct health and medical problems, but also in the related fields of psychology and sociology.

Why do people continue to smoke cigarettes, to take mind-altering and habit-forming drugs, to use alcohol to excess, to become overweight, to fail to take the examinations that will detect cancer and other diseases when they are still in the curable state? The information about what can and should be done is available. Why do not all people know what they need to know to maintain good health? And why do many people fail to act upon what they do know? What good does it do for medical science to make available ways to prevent disease and to improve health if little or no use is made of them?

These are questions upon which vastly more psychological and behavioral research needs to be done. Here and there isolated studies are in progress, but major research attacks upon these problems remain for the future.

More studies and experimental programs are also needed to provide information about effective ways to make adequate medical and health services available to all people in a manner that they will accept and at a cost that they can afford. This is an important area in which dogmatic opinions are expressed and penaceas proposed, but relatively little information upon which sound planning for the future could be based is currently available.

It is hoped that before the end of the twentieth century more information will be available concerning the prevention and treatment of disease, and that people will be making greater use of currently available information to prevent and to cure many of the diseases which today cause unnecessary illness, disability, and premature death.

QUESTIONS FOR DISCUSSION AND SELF-EXAMINATION

1 How are population control, pollution, nutrition, housing, and poverty related one to the other?

2 "Government financing, at least in part, is necessary, but personal interest, responsibility, and initiative are essential." Discuss how this sentence from the text could be implemented.

3 What is the relationship of preventive medicine to therapeutic medicine in improving the health of the country?

4 In which area of medicine, or in which disease, do you think research offers the most (a) opportunity and (b) challenge for improving health and lengthening life? Defend your answer.

REFERENCES AND READING SUGGESTIONS

BOOKS

Allison, Anthony: *Population Control*, Penguin Books, Inc., Baltimore, 1970.

In an attempt to place human population problems in their biological perspective, thirteen essays by behavioral and natural scientists deal with the food-population equation and methods of birth control in sophisticated and primitive societies.

Bryant, John: *Health and the Developing World*, Cornell University Press, Ithaca, N.Y. 1970.

A book of fascinating "case presentations" of the important factors—social, cultural, economic, and biological—which influence health in developing countries, together with consideration of what can be done to improve health and national vitality in various situations.

DeBell, Garrett: *The Environmental Handbook: Prepared for the First Environmental Teach-in*, paperback, Ballantine Books, Inc., New York, 1970.

This fascinating book consists of discussions of the major aspects of the pollution of our environment by eminent and experienced scholars of the subject. It is invaluable to any individual or group that is concerned about the deterioration of the environment and wants to do something about it.

Editors of the Progressive Division and the College Division: *The Crisis of Survival*, Scott, Foresman and Company, Glenview, Ill. 1970.

As a contribution to student involvement in academic environmental programs, twenty-one scholars in the social sciences discuss the major demographic, political, economic, and ecological threats facing man today, offering some prospects and hopes for the future.

Leach, Gerald: *Biocrats*, McGraw-Hill Book Company, New York, 1971.

A remarkable book by a British journalist about advances in medicine as they relate to important problems today and in the future. Among these are transplant surgery, the postponement of death in hopelessly ill patients, possibilities of eugenic improvements in our human stock, abortion, the prevention of deformed and mentally deficient infants and other problems which need consideration both by physicians and by laymen.

Population and Family Planning in the People's Republic of China, The Victor-Bastrom Fund and The Population Crisis Committee, 1730 K St., N.W., Washington.

Exceedingly interesting and significant reports by foreign experts about what China is doing to deal with its population and food problem.

PAMPHLETS AND PERIODICALS

Annual Report, Population Reference Bureau, Washington.

Ehrlich, Paul R.: "World Population: Is the Battle Lost?" springboard for discussion, *Reader's Digest*, February 1969.

A distinguished student of population problems and professor at Stanford University "raises some profoundly disturbing problems on whether, and how man can survive his own biggest error."

Galton, Lawrence: "The New Mystery—Maybe Miracle—Drug," *The New York Times Magazine*, Dec. 5, 1971, p. 46.

A fascinating story of an observation first made 40 years ago that has become a major medical research effort. The substances upon which this research is centered are called prostaglandins. They are present in varying amounts in many tissues and secretions of the human body as well as in various other animals. They can now be produced also in the chemical laboratory. They hold potential for more effective population control measures than are now available and for the treatment and prevention of hypertension, the formation of blood clots in small arteries, asthma, emphysema, and arthritis.

This is a story of tremendously important ongoing research which no one interested in the present methods and the future possibilities of medical research should fail to read.

Maddon, John: *The Doomsday Syndrome*; McGraw-Hill Book Company, New York, 1972. A distinguished English scientist takes issue with the pessimistic view of man's ability to deal effectively with population, pollution, food and water shortages, etc. His aim is not to deny these problems but to encourage people to attack them.

APPENDIX: NUTRITIVE VALUE OF FOODS

CONTENTS

Dairy Products	424–425
Eggs	425
Fats and Oils	443
Fruit and Fruit Products	432–438
Grain Products	438–443
Meat, Cooked, per Pound of Raw Meat	446
Meat, Poultry, Fish, etc.	425–428
Miscellaneous	444–445
Nuts, Beans, Peas, etc.	428–429
Sugar and Sweets	444
Vegetables and Vegetable Products	429–432

The following self-explanatory table lists important constituents of most foods currently consumed in the United States. To read it, hold a ruler under the item for which information is desired, and then find in the proper column the information desired (whether water percentage, food energy in the form of calories, or one of the specific nutriments).

Most of the foods listed are in ready-to-eat form; a few are basic products widely used in food preparation, such as flour, fat, and cornmeal.

Measurements are in cups, ounces (oz), pounds (lb), grams (g), milligrams (mg), a piece of a certain size, or some other well-known unit.

A special note about niacin is desirable. Nearly all foods contain some tryptophan, an amino acid which the body converts to niacin. The average diet in the United States, which contains a generous amount of protein, provides enough tryptophan to increase the niacin value of the diet by about one-third.

Additional technical information about this table is available in the Bulletin of the Department of Agriculture.

EQUIVALENTS BY WEIGHT

1 LB (16 OZ)	= 453.6 G
1 OZ	= 28.35 G
3½ OZ	= 100 G

EQUIVALENTS BY VOLUME (ALL MEASUREMENTS LEVEL)

1 QT	= 4 CUPS
1 CUP	= 8 FL OZ
	= ½ PINT
	= 16 TBSP
2 TBSP	= 1 FL OZ
1 TBSP	= 3 TSP
1 LB BUTTER OR MARGARINE	= 4 STICKS
	= 2 CUPS
	= 64 PATS OR SQUARES
1 STICK BUTTER OR MARGARINE	= ½ CUP (APPROXIMATELY)
	= 16 PATS OR SQUARES

TABLE 1 NUTRITIVE VALUES OF THE EDIBLE PART OF FOODS

[Dashes show that no basis could be found for imputing a value although there was some reason to believe that a measurable amount of the constituent might be present.]

FOOD, APPROXIMATE MEASURE, AND WEIGHT		GRAMS	WATER, %	FOOD ENERGY, CALORIES	PROTEIN, G	FAT (TOTAL LIPID), G	FATTY ACIDS SATURATED (TOTAL), G	UNSATURATED OLEIC	UNSATURATED LINOLEIC	CARBOHYDRATE, G	CALCIUM, G	IRON, G	VITAMIN A VALUE, INTERNATIONAL UNITS	THIAMINE, G	RIBOFLAVIN, G	NIACIN, G	ASCORBIC ACID, G
MILK, CREAM, CHEESE; RELATED PRODUCTS																	
MILK, COW'S:																	
FLUID, WHOLE (3.5% FAT)	1 CUP	244	87	160	9	9	5	3	TRACE	12	288	0.1	350	0.08	0.42	0.1	2
FLUID, NONFAT (SKIM)	1 CUP	246	90	90	9	TRACE	—	—	—	13	298	.1	10	.10	.44	.2	2
BUTTERMILK, CULTURED, FROM SKIM:																	
MILK	1 CUP	246	90	90	9	TRACE	—	—	—	13	298	.1	10	.09	.44	.2	2
EVAPORATED, UNSWEETENED, UNDILUTED	1 CUP	252	74	345	18	20	11	7	1	24	635	.3	820	.10	.84	.5	3
CONDENSED, SWEETENED, UNDILUTED	1 CUP	306	27	980	25	27	15	9	1	166	802	.3	1,090	.23	1.17	.5	3
DRY, WHOLE	1 CUP	103	2	515	27	28	16	9	1	39	936	.5	1,160	.30	1.50	.7	6
DRY, NONFAT, INSTANT	1 CUP	70	3	250	25	TRACE	—	—	—	36	905	.4	20	.24	1.25	.6	5
MILK, GOAT'S: FLUID, WHOLE	1 CUP	244	88	165	8	10	6	2	TRACE	11	315	.2	390	.10	.27	.7	2
CREAM:																	
HALF-AND-HALF (CREAM AND MILK)	1 CUP	242	80	325	8	28	16	9	1	11	261	.1	1,160	.08	.38	.1	2
	1 TBSP	15	80	20	TRACE	2	1	1	TRACE	1	16	TRACE	70	TRACE	.02	TRACE	TRACE
LIGHT, COFFEE OR TABLE	1 CUP	240	72	505	7	49	27	16	1	10	245	.1	2,030	.07	.36	.1	2
	1 TBSP	15	72	30	TRACE	3	2	1	TRACE	1	15	TRACE	130	TRACE	.02	TRACE	TRACE
WHIPPING, UNWHIPPED (VOLUME ABOUT DOUBLE WHEN WHIPPED):																	
LIGHT	1 CUP	239	62	715	6	75	41	25	2	9	203	.1	3,070	.06	.30	.1	2
	1 TBSP	15	62	45	TRACE	5	3	2	TRACE	1	13	TRACE	190	TRACE	.02	TRACE	TRACE
HEAVY	1 CUP	238	57	840	5	89	49	29	3	7	178	.1	3,670	.05	.26	.1	2
	1 TBSP	15	57	55	TRACE	6	3	2	TRACE	TRACE	11	TRACE	230	TRACE	.02	TRACE	TRACE
CHEESE:																	
BLUE OR ROQUEFORT TYPE	1 OZ	28	40	105	6	9	5	3	TRACE	1	89	.1	350	.01	.17	.1	0
CHEDDAR OR AMERICAN:																	
UNGRATED	1-IN. CUBE	17	37	70	4	5	3	2	TRACE	TRACE	128	.2	220	TRACE	.08	TRACE	0
	1 CUP	112	37	445	28	36	20	12	1	2	840	1.1	1,470	.03	.51	.1	0
GRATED	1 TBSP	7	37	30	2	2	1	1	TRACE	TRACE	52	.1	90	TRACE	.03	TRACE	0
CHEDDAR, PROCESS	1 OZ	28	40	105	7	9	5	3	TRACE	TRACE	219	.3	350	TRACE	.12	TRACE	0
CHEESE FOODS, CHEDDAR	1 OZ	28	43	90	6	7	4	2	TRACE	2	162	.2	280	.01	.16	TRACE	0
COTTAGE CHEESE, FROM SKIM MILK:																	
CREAMED	1 CUP	225	78	240	31	9	5	3	TRACE	7	212	0.7	380	0.07	0.56	0.2	0
	1 OZ	28	78	30	4	1	1	TRACE	TRACE	1	27	.1	50	.01	.07	TRACE	0
UNCREAMED	1 CUP	225	79	195	38	1	TRACE	TRACE	—	6	202	.9	20	.07	.63	.2	0
	1 OZ	28	79	25	5	TRACE	—	—	—	1	26	.1	TRACE	.01	.08	TRACE	0
CREAM CHEESE	1 OZ	28	51	105	2	11	6	4	TRACE	1	18	.1	440	TRACE	.07	TRACE	0
	1 TBSP	15	51	55	1	6	3	2	TRACE	TRACE	9	TRACE	230	TRACE	.04	TRACE	0
SWISS (DOMESTIC)	1 OZ	28	39	105	8	8	4	3	TRACE	1	262	.3	320	TRACE	.11	TRACE	0

Food, approximate measure																	
MILK BEVERAGES:																	
COCOA . . . . 1 CUP	242	79	235	9	11	6	4	TRACE	26	286	.9	390	.09	.45	.4	2
CHOCOLATE-FLAVORED MILK DRINK (MADE WITH SKIM MILK) . . . 1 CUP	250	83	190	8	6	3	2	TRACE	27	270	.4	210	.09	.41	.2	2
MALTED MILK . . . . . 1 CUP	270	78	280	13	12	—	—	—	32	364	.8	670	.17	.56	.2	2
MILK DESSERTS:																	
CORNSTARCH PUDDING, PLAIN (BLANC MANGE) . . . 1 CUP	248	76	275	9	10	5	3	TRACE	39	290	.1	390	.07	.40	.1	2
CUSTARD, BAKED . . . 1 CUP	248	77	285	13	14	6	5	1	28	278	1.0	870	.10	.47	.2	1
ICE CREAM, PLAIN, FACTORY PACKED:																	
SLICE OR CUT BRICK, 1/8-QT BRICK . . 1 SLICE OR CUT BRICK	71	62	145	3	9	5	3	TRACE	15	87	.1	370	.03	.13	.1	1
CONTAINER . . . . . 3½ FL OZ	62	62	130	2	8	4	3	TRACE	13	76	.1	320	.03	.12	.1	1
CONTAINER . . . . . 8 FL OZ	142	62	295	6	18	10	6	1	29	175	.1	740	.06	.27	.1	1
ICE MILK . . . . . . 1 CUP	187	67	285	9	10	6	3	TRACE	42	292	.2	390	.09	.41	.2	2
YOGHURT, FROM PARTIALLY SKIMMED MILK . . . . . 1 CUP	246	89	120	8	4	2	1	TRACE	13	295	.1	170	.09	.43	.2	2
EGGS																	
EGGS, LARGE, 24 OZ PER DOZ:																	
WHOLE, WITHOUT SHELL . . 1 EGG	50	74	80	6	6	2	3	TRACE	TRACE	27	1.1	590	.05	.15	TRACE	0
WHITE OF EGG . . . 1 WHITE	33	88	15	4	TRACE	—	—	—	TRACE	3	TRACE	0	TRACE	.09	TRACE	0
YOLK OF EGG . . . . 1 YOLK	17	51	60	3	5	2	2	TRACE	TRACE	24	.9	580	.04	.07	TRACE	0
SCRAMBLED, WITH MILK AND FAT . . 1 EGG	64	72	110	7	8	3	3	TRACE	1	51	1.1	690	.05	.18	TRACE	0
MEAT, POULTRY, FISH, SHELLFISH; RELATED PRODUCTS																	
BACON, BROILED OR FRIED, CRISP. . 2 SLICES	16	8	100	5	8	3	4	1	1	2	.5	0	.08	.05	.8	—
BEEF, TRIMMED TO RETAIL BASIS,[a] COOKED:																	
CUTS BRAISED, SIMMERED, OR POT-ROASTED:																	
LEAN AND FAT . . . 3 OZ	85	53	245	23	16	8	7	TRACE	0	10	2.9	30	.04	.18	3.5	—
LEAN ONLY . . . . 2.5 OZ	72	62	140	22	5	2	2	TRACE	0	10	2.7	10	.04	.16	3.3	—
HAMBURGER (GROUND BEEF), BROILED:																	
LEAN . . . 3 OZ	85	60	185	23	10	5	4	TRACE	0	10	3.0	20	.08	.20	5.1	—
REGULAR . . . 3 OZ	85	54	245	21	17	8	8	TRACE	0	9	2.7	30	.07	.18	4.6	—
ROAST, OVEN-COOKED, NO LIQUID ADDED:																	
RELATIVELY FAT, SUCH AS RIB:																	
LEAN AND FAT . . . 3 OZ	85	40	375	17	34	16	15	1	0	8	2.2	70	.05	.13	3.1	—
LEAN ONLY . . . 1.8 OZ	51	57	125	14	7	3	3	TRACE	0	6	1.8	10	.04	.11	2.6	—
RELATIVELY LEAN, SUCH AS HEEL OF ROUND:																	
LEAN AND FAT . . . 3 OZ	85	62	165	25	7	3	3	TRACE	0	11	3.2	10	.06	.19	4.5	—
LEAN ONLY . . . 2.7 OZ	78	65	125	24	3	1	1	TRACE	0	10	3.0	TRACE	.06	.18	4.3	—
STEAK, BROILED:																	
RELATIVELY FAT, SUCH AS SIRLOIN:																	
LEAN AND FAT . . . 3 OZ	85	44	330	20	27	13	12	1	0	9	2.5	50	.05	.16	4.0	—
LEAN ONLY . . . 2.0 OZ	56	59	115	18	4	2	2	TRACE	0	7	2.2	10	.05	.14	3.6	—
RELATIVELY LEAN, SUCH AS ROUND:																	
LEAN AND FAT . . . 3 OZ	85	55	220	24	13	6	6	TRACE	0	10	3.0	20	.07	.19	4.8	—
LEAN ONLY . . . 2.4 OZ	68	61	130	21	4	2	2	TRACE	0	9	2.5	10	.06	.16	4.1	—

[a] Outer layer of fat on the cut was removed to within approximately ½ in. of the lean. Deposits of fat within the cut were not removed.

SOURCE: *Nutritive Value of Foods*, Home and Garden Bulletin No. 72, A177, U.S. Department of Agriculture, Washington, 1964.

TABLE 1 NUTRITIVE VALUES OF THE EDIBLE PART OF FOODS (Cont.)

[Dashes show that no basis could be found for imputing a value although there was some reason to believe that a measurable amount of the constituent might be present.]

FOOD, APPROXIMATE MEASURE, AND WEIGHT	GRAMS	WATER, %	FOOD ENERGY, CALORIES	PROTEIN, G	FAT (TOTAL LIPID), G	FATTY ACIDS SATURATED (TOTAL), G	UNSATURATED OLEIC	UNSATURATED LINOLEIC	CARBOHYDRATE, G	CALCIUM, G	IRON, G	VITAMIN A VALUE, INTERNATIONAL UNITS	THIAMINE, G	RIBOFLAVIN, G	NIACIN, G	ASCORBIC ACID, G
MEAT, POULTRY, FISH, SHELLFISH (Cont.)																
BEEF, CANNED:																
CORNED BEEF .... 3 OZ	85	59	185	22	10	5	4	TRACE	0	17	3.7	20	.01	.20	2.9	—
CORNED BEEF HASH .... 3 OZ	85	67	155	7	10	5	4	TRACE	9	11	1.7	—	.01	.08	1.8	—
BEEF, DRIED OR CHIPPED .... 2 OZ	57	48	115	19	4	2	2	TRACE	0	11	2.9	—	.04	.18	2.2	—
BEEF AND VEGETABLE STEW .... 1 CUP	235	82	210	15	10	5	4	TRACE	15	28	2.8	2,310	.13	.17	4.4	15
BEEF POTPIE, BAKED: INDIVIDUAL PIE, 4¼-IN. DIAMETER, WEIGHT BEFORE BAKING ABOUT 8 OZ .... 1 PIE	227	55	560	23	33	9	20	2	43	32	4.1	1,860	.25	.27	4.5	7
CHICKEN, COOKED:																
FLESH ONLY, BROILED .... 3 OZ	85	71	115	20	3	1	1	1	0	8	1.4	80	0.05	0.16	7.4	—
BREAST, FRIED, ½ BREAST:																
WITH BONE .... 3.3 OZ	94	58	155	25	5	1	2	1	1	9	1.3	70	.04	.17	11.2	—
FLESH AND SKIN ONLY .... 2.7 OZ	76	58	155	25	5	1	2	1	1	9	1.3	70	.04	.17	11.2	—
DRUMSTICK, FRIED:																
WITH BONE .... 2.1 OZ	59	55	90	12	4	1	2	1	TRACE	6	.9	50	.03	.15	2.7	—
FLESH AND SKIN ONLY .... 1.3 OZ	38	55	90	12	4	1	2	1	TRACE	6	.9	50	.03	.15	2.7	—
CHICKEN, CANNED, BONELESS .... 3 OZ	85	65	170	18	10	3	4	2	0	18	1.3	200	.03	.11	3.7	3
CHICKEN POTPIE. SEE POULTRY POTPIE.																
CHILE CON CARNE, CANNED:																
WITH BEANS .... 1 CUP	250	72	335	19	15	7	7	TRACE	30	80	4.2	150	.08	.18	3.2	—
WITHOUT BEANS .... 1 CUP	255	67	510	26	38	18	17	1	15	97	3.6	380	.05	.31	5.6	1
HEART, BEEF, LEAN, BRAISED .... 3 OZ	85	61	160	27	5	—	—	—	1	5	5.0	20	.21	1.04	6.5	1
LAMB, TRIMMED TO RETAIL BASIS,[a] COOKED:																
CHOP, THICK, WITH BONE, 1 CHOP, BROILED .... 4.8 OZ	137	47	400	25	33	18	12	1	0	10	1.5	—	.14	.25	5.6	—
LEAN AND FAT .... 4.0 OZ	112	47	400	25	33	18	12	1	0	10	1.5	—	.14	.25	5.6	—
LEAN ONLY .... 2.6 OZ	74	62	140	21	6	3	2	TRACE	0	9	1.5	—	.11	.20	4.5	—
LEG, ROASTED:																
LEAN AND FAT .... 3 OZ	85	54	235	22	16	9	6	TRACE	0	9	1.4	—	.13	.23	4.7	—
LEAN ONLY .... 2.5 OZ	71	62	130	20	5	3	2	TRACE	0	9	1.4	—	.12	.21	4.4	—
SHOULDER, ROASTED:																
LEAN AND FAT .... 3 OZ	85	50	285	18	23	13	8	1	0	9	1.0	—	.11	.20	4.0	—
LEAN ONLY .... 2.3 OZ	64	61	130	17	6	3	2	TRACE	0	8	1.0	—	.10	.18	3.7	—
LIVER, BEEF, FRIED .... 2 OZ	57	57	130	15	6	—	—	—	3	6	5.0	30,280	.15	2.37	9.4	15
PORK, CURED, COOKED: HAM, LIGHT CURE, LEAN AND FAT, ROASTED .... 3 OZ	85	54	245	18	19	7	8	2	0	8	2.2	0	.40	.16	3.1	—

LUNCHEON MEAT:																	
BOILED HAM, SLICED	2 OZ	57	59	135	11	10	4	4	1	0	6	1.6	0	.25	.09	1.5	—
CANNED, SPICED OR UNSPICED	2 OZ	57	55	165	8	14	5	6	1	1	5	1.2	0	.18	.12	1.6	—
PORK, FRESH, TRIMMED TO RETAIL BASIS,ᵃ COOKED:																	
CHOP, THICK, WITH BONE	1 CHOP, 3.5 OZ	98	42	260	16	21	8	9	2	0	8	2.2	0	.63	.18	3.8	—
LEAN AND FAT	2.3 OZ	66	42	260	16	21	8	9	2	0	8	2.2	0	.63	.18	3.8	—
LEAN ONLY	1.7 OZ	48	53	130	15	7	2	3	1	0	7	1.9	0	.54	.16	3.3	—
ROAST, OVEN-COOKED, NO LIQUID ADDED:																	
LEAN AND FAT	3 OZ	85	46	310	21	24	9	10	2	0	9	2.7	0	.78	.22	4.7	—
LEAN ONLY	2.4 OZ	68	55	175	20	10	3	4	1	0	9	2.6	0	.73	.21	4.4	—
CUTS, SIMMERED:																	
LEAN AND FAT	3 OZ	85	46	320	20	26	9	11	2	0	8	2.5	0	.46	.21	4.1	—
LEAN ONLY	2.2 OZ	63	60	135	18	6	2	3	1	0	8	2.3	0	.42	.19	3.7	—
POULTRY POTPIE (BASED ON CHICKEN POTPIE). INDIVIDUAL PIE, 4¼-IN. DIAMETER	1 PIE	227	57	535	23	31	10	15	3	42	68	3.0	3,020	.25	.26	4.1	5
SAUSAGE:																	
BOLOGNA, SLICE, 4.1 IN. BY 0.1 IN.	8 SLICES	227	56	690	27	62	—	—	—	2	16	4.1	—	.36	.49	6.0	—
FRANKFURTER, COOKED	1 FRANKFURTER	51	58	155	6	14	—	—	—	1	3	.8	—	.08	.10	1.3	—
PORK, LINKS OR PATTY, COOKED	4 OZ	113	35	540	21	50	18	21	5	TRACE	8	2.7	0	.89	.39	4.2	—
TURKEY POTPIE. SEE POULTRY POTPIE.																	
VEAL, COOKED:																	
CUTLET, WITHOUT BONE, BROILED	3 OZ	85	60	185	23	9	5	4	TRACE	—	9	2.7	—	.06	.21	4.6	—
ROAST, MEDIUM FAT, MEDIUM DONE; LEAN AND FAT	3 OZ	85	55	230	23	14	7	6	TRACE	0	10	2.9	—	.11	.26	6.6	—
FISH AND SHELLFISH:																	
BLUEFISH, BAKED OR BROILED	3 OZ	85	68	135	22	4	—	—	—	0	25	.6	40	.09	.08	1.6	—
CLAMS:																	
RAW, MEAT ONLY	3 OZ	85	82	65	11	1	—	—	—	2	59	5.2	90	.08	.15	1.1	8
CANNED, SOLIDS AND LIQUID	3 OZ	85	86	45	7	1	—	—	—	2	47	3.5	—	.01	.09	.9	—
CRABMEAT, CANNED	3 OZ	85	77	85	15	2	—	—	—	1	38	.7	—	.07	.07	1.6	—
FISH STICKS, BREADED, COOKED, FROZEN; STICK, 3.8 IN. BY 1.0 IN. BY 0.5 IN.	10 STICKS OR 8-OZ PACKAGE	227	66	400	38	20	5	4	10	15	25	.9	—	.09	.16	3.6	—
HADDOCK, FRIED	3 OZ	85	66	140	17	5	1	3	TRACE	5	34	1.0	—	0.03	0.06	2.7	2
MACKEREL:																	
BROILED, ATLANTIC	3 OZ	85	62	200	19	13	—	—	—	0	5	1.0	450	.13	.23	6.5	—
CANNED, PACIFIC, SOLIDS AND LIQUIDᵇ	3 OZ	85	66	155	18	9	—	—	—	0	221	1.9	20	.02	.28	7.4	—
OCEAN PERCH, BREADED (EGG AND BREAD-CRUMBS), FRIED	3 OZ	85	59	195	16	11	—	—	—	6	28	1.1	—	.08	.09	1.5	—
OYSTERS, MEAT ONLY:																	
RAW, 13–19 MEDIUM SELECTS	1 CUP	240	85	160	20	4	—	—	—	8	226	13.2	740	.33	.43	6.0	—
OYSTER STEW, 1 PART OYSTERS TO 3 PARTS MILK BY VOLUME, 3–4 OYSTERS	1 CUP	230	84	200	11	12	—	—	—	11	269	3.3	640	.13	.41	1.6	—

ᵃOuter layer of fat on the cut was removed to within approximately ½ in. of the lean. Deposits of fat within the cut were not removed.

ᵇVitamin values based on drained solids.

TABLE 1 NUTRITIVE VALUES OF THE EDIBLE PART OF FOODS (Cont.)

[Dashes show that no basis could be found for imputing a value although there was some reason to believe that a measurable amount of the constituent might be present.]

FOOD, APPROXIMATE MEASURE, AND WEIGHT	GRAMS	WATER, %	FOOD ENERGY, CALORIES	PROTEIN, G	FAT (TOTAL LIPID), G	FATTY ACIDS SATURATED (TOTAL), G	UNSATURATED OLEIC	LINOLEIC	CARBOHYDRATE, G	CALCIUM, G	IRON, G	VITAMIN A VALUE, INTERNATIONAL UNITS	THIAMINE, G	RIBOFLAVIN, G	NIACIN, G	ASCORBIC ACID, G
MEAT, POULTRY, FISH, SHELLFISH (Cont.)																
SALMON, PINK, CANNED . . 3 OZ	85	71	120	17	5	1	1	TRACE	0	c167	.7	60	.03	.16	6.8	—
SARDINES, ATLANTIC, CANNED IN OIL, DRAINED SOLIDS . . 3 OZ	85	62	175	20	9	—	—	—	0	372	2.5	190	.02	.17	4.6	—
SHAD, BAKED . . 3 OZ	85	64	170	20	10	—	—	—	0	20	.5	20	.11	.22	7.3	—
SHRIMP, CANNED, MEAT ONLY . . 3 OZ	85	70	100	21	1	—	—	—	1	98	2.6	50	.01	.03	1.5	—
SWORDFISH, BROILED WITH BUTTER OR MARGARINE . . 3 OZ	85	65	150	24	5	—	—	—	0	23	1.1	1,750	.03	.04	9.5	—
TUNA, CANNED IN OIL, DRAINED SOLIDS . . 3 OZ	85	61	170	24	7	—	—	—	0	7	1.6	70	.04	.10	10.1	—
MATURE DRY BEANS AND PEAS, NUTS, PEANUTS; RELATED PRODUCTS																
ALMONDS, SHELLED . . 1 CUP	142	5	850	26	77	6	52	15	28	332	6.7	0	.34	1.31	5.0	TRACE
BEANS, DRY: COMMON VARIETIES, SUCH AS GREAT NORTHERN, NAVY, AND OTHERS, CANNED:																
RED . . 1 CUP	256	76	230	15	1	—	—	—	42	74	4.6	TRACE	.13	.10	1.5	—
WHITE, WITH TOMATO SAUCE:																
WITH PORK . . 1 CUP	261	71	320	16	7	3	3	1	50	141	4.7	340	.20	.08	1.5	5
WITHOUT PORK . . 1 CUP	261	68	310	16	1	—	—	—	60	177	5.2	160	.18	.09	1.5	5
LIMA, COOKED . . 1 CUP	192	64	260	16	1	—	—	—	48	56	5.6	TRACE	.26	.12	1.3	TRACE
BRAZIL NUTS . . 1 CUP	140	5	915	20	94	19	45	24	15	260	4.8	TRACE	1.34	.17	2.2	—
CASHEW NUTS, ROASTED . . 1 CUP	135	5	760	23	62	10	43	4	40	51	5.1	140	.58	.33	2.4	—
COCONUT:																
FRESH, SHREDDED . . 1 CUP	97	51	335	3	34	29	2	TRACE	9	13	1.6	0	.05	.02	.5	3
DRIED, SHREDDED, SWEETENED . . 1 CUP	62	3	340	2	24	21	2	TRACE	33	10	1.2	0	.02	.02	.2	0
COWPEAS OR BLACKEYE PEAS, DRY, COOKED . . 1 CUP	248	80	190	13	1	—	—	—	34	42	3.2	20	.41	.11	1.1	TRACE
PEANUTS, ROASTED, SALTED:																
HALVES . . 1 CUP	144	2	840	37	72	16	31	21	27	107	3.0	—	.46	.19	24.7	0
CHOPPED . . 1 TBSP	9	2	55	2	4	1	2	1	2	7	.2	—	.03	.01	1.5	0
PEANUT BUTTER . . 1 TBSP	16	2	95	4	8	2	4	2	3	9	.3	—	.02	.02	2.4	0
PEAS, SPLIT, DRY, COOKED . . 1 CUP	250	70	290	20	1	—	—	—	52	28	4.2	100	.37	.22	2.2	—
PECANS:																
HALVES . . 1 CUP	108	3	740	10	77	5	48	15	16	79	2.6	140	.93	.14	1.0	2
CHOPPED . . 1 TBSP	7.5	3	50	1	5	TRACE	3	1	1	5	.2	10	.06	.01	.1	TRACE

WALNUTS, SHELLED:																	
BLACK OR NATIVE, CHOPPED	1 CUP	126	3	790	26	75	4	26	36	19	TRACE	7.6	380	.28	.14	.9	—
ENGLISH OR PERSIAN:																	
HALVES	1 CUP	100	4	650	15	64	4	10	40	16	99	3.1	30	.33	.13	.9	3
CHOPPED	1 TBSP	8	4	50	1	5	TRACE	1	3	1	8	.2	TRACE	.03	.01	.1	TRACE
VEGETABLES AND VEGETABLE PRODUCTS																	
ASPARAGUS:																	
COOKED, CUT SPEARS	1 CUP	175	94	35	4	TRACE	—	—	—	6	37	1.0	1,580	.27	.32	2.4	46
CANNED SPEARS, MEDIUM:																	
GREEN	6 SPEARS	96	92	20	2	TRACE	—	—	—	3	18	1.8	770	.06	.10	.8	14
BLEACHED	6 SPEARS	96	92	20	2	TRACE	—	—	—	4	15	1.0	80	.05	.06	.7	14
BEANS:																	
LIMA, IMMATURE, COOKED	1 CUP	160	71	180	12	1	—	—	—	32	75	4.0	450	.29	.16	2.0	28
SNAP, GREEN:																	
COOKED:																	
IN SMALL AMOUNT OF WATER, SHORT TIME	1 CUP	125	92	30	2	TRACE	—	—	—	7	62	.8	680	.08	.11	.6	16
IN LARGE AMOUNT OF WATER, LONG TIME	1 CUP	125	92	30	2	TRACE	—	—	—	7	62	0.8	680	0.07	0.10	0.4	13
CANNED:																	
SOLIDS AND LIQUID	1 CUP	239	94	45	2	TRACE	—	—	—	10	81	2.9	690	.08	.10	.7	9
STRAINED OR CHOPPED (BABY FOOD)	1 OZ	28	92	5	TRACE	TRACE	—	—	—	1	9	.3	110	.01	.02	.1	TRACE
BEAN SPROUTS. SEE SPROUTS.																	
BEETS, COOKED, DICED	1 CUP	165	91	50	2	TRACE	—	—	—	12	23	.8	40	.04	.07	.5	11
BROCCOLI SPEARS, COOKED	1 CUP	150	91	40	5	TRACE	—	—	—	7	132	1.2	3,750	.14	.29	1.2	135
BRUSSELS SPROUTS, COOKED	1 CUP	130	88	45	5	1	—	—	—	8	42	1.4	680	.10	.18	1.1	113
CABBAGE:																	
RAW:																	
FINELY SHREDDED	1 CUP	100	92	25	1	TRACE	—	—	—	5	49	.4	130	.05	.05	.3	47
COLESLAW	1 CUP	120	83	120	1	9	2	2	5	9	52	.5	180	.06	.06	.3	35
COOKED:																	
IN SMALL AMOUNT OF WATER, SHORT TIME	1 CUP	170	94	35	2	TRACE	—	—	—	7	75	.5	220	.07	.07	.5	56
IN LARGE AMOUNT OF WATER, LONG TIME	1 CUP	170	94	30	2	TRACE	—	—	—	7	71	.5	200	.04	.04	.2	40
CABBAGE, CELERY OR CHINESE:																	
RAW, LEAVES AND STALK, 1-IN. PIECES	1 CUP	100	95	15	1	TRACE	—	—	—	3	43	.6	150	.05	.04	.6	25
CABBAGE, SPOON (OR PAKCHOY), COOKED	1 CUP	150	95	20	2	TRACE	—	—	—	4	222	.9	4,650	.07	.12	1.1	23
CARROTS:																	
RAW:																	
WHOLE, 5½ IN. BY 1 IN. (25 THIN STRIPS)	1 CARROT	50-	88	20	1	TRACE	—	—	—	5	18	.4	5,500	.03	.03	.3	4
GRATED	1 CUP	110	88	45	1	TRACE	—	—	—	11	41	.8	12,100	.06	.06	.7	9
COOKED, DICED	1 CUP	145	91	45	1	TRACE	—	—	—	10	48	.9	15,220	.08	.07	.7	9

ᶜBased on total contents of can. If bones are discarded, value will be greatly reduced.

TABLE 1 NUTRITIVE VALUES OF THE EDIBLE PART OF FOODS (Cont.)

[Dashes show that no basis could be found for imputing a value although there was some reason to believe that a measurable amount of the constituent might be present.]

FOOD, APPROXIMATE MEASURE, AND WEIGHT	GRAMS	WATER, %	FOOD ENERGY, CALORIES	PROTEIN, G	FAT (TOTAL LIPID), G	SATURATED (TOTAL), G	OLEIC	LINOLEIC	CARBOHYDRATE, G	CALCIUM, G	IRON, G	VITAMIN A VALUE, INTERNATIONAL UNITS	THIAMINE, G	RIBOFLAVIN, G	NIACIN, G	ASCORBIC ACID, G
VEGETABLES AND VEGETABLE PRODUCTS (Cont.)																
CANNED, STRAINED OR CHOPPED (BABY FOOD) . . . . . 1 OZ . . .	28	92	10	TRACE	TRACE	—	—	—	2	7	.1	3,690	.01	.01	.1	1
CAULIFLOWER, COOKED, FLOWERBUDS . . . 1 CUP . . .	120	93	25	3	TRACE	—	—	—	5	25	.8	70	.11	.10	.7	66
CELERY, RAW:																
STALK, LARGE OUTER, 8 IN. ABOUT 1½ IN. AT ROOT END . . . 1 STALK . . .	40	94	5	TRACE	TRACE	—	—	—	2	16	.1	100	.01	.01	.1	4
PIECES, DICED . . . 1 CUP . . .	100	94	15	1	TRACE	—	—	—	4	39	.3	240	.03	.03	.3	9
COLLARDS, COOKED . . . 1 CUP . . .	190	91	55	5	1	—	—	—	9	289	1.1	10,260	.27	.37	2.4	87
CORN, SWEET:																
COOKED, EAR 5 IN. BY 1¾ IN.[d] . . . 1 EAR . . .	140	74	70	3	1	—	—	—	16	2	.5	[a]310	.09	.08	1.0	7
CANNED, SOLIDS AND LIQUID . . . 1 CUP . . .	256	81	170	5	2	—	—	—	40	10	1.0	[a]690	.07	.12	2.3	13
COWPEAS, COOKED, IMMATURE SEEDS . . . 1 CUP . . .	160	72	175	13	1	—	—	—	29	38	3.4	560	.49	.18	2.3	28
CUCUMBERS, 10-OZ; 7½ IN. BY ABOUT 2 IN.:																
RAW, PARED . . . 1 CUCUMBER . . .	207	96	30	1	TRACE	—	—	—	7	35	.6	TRACE	.07	.09	.4	23
RAW, PARED, CENTER SLICE ⅛-IN. THICK . . . 6 SLICES . . .	50	96	5	TRACE	TRACE	—	—	—	2	8	.2	TRACE	.02	.02	.1	6
DANDELION GREENS, COOKED . . . 1 CUP . . .	180	90	60	4	1	—	—	—	12	252	3.2	21,060	.24	.29	—	32
ENDIVE, CURLY (INCLUDING ESCAROLE) . . . 2 OZ . . .	57	93	10	1	TRACE	—	—	—	2	46	1.0	1,870	.04	.08	.3	6
KALE, LEAVES INCLUDING STEMS, COOKED . . . 1 CUP . . .	110	91	30	4	1	—	—	—	4	147	1.3	8,140	—	—	—	68
LETTUCE, RAW:																
BUTTERHEAD, AS BOSTON TYPES; HEAD, 4-IN. DIAMETER . . . 1 HEAD . . .	220	95	30	3	TRACE	—	—	—	6	77	4.4	2,130	.14	.13	.6	18
CRISPHEAD, AS ICEBERG; HEAD, 4¾-IN. DIAMETER . . . 1 HEAD . . .	454	96	60	4	TRACE	—	—	—	13	91	2.3	1,500	.29	.27	1.3	29
LOOSELEAF, OR BUNCHING VARIETIES, LEAVES . . . 2 LARGE . . .	50	94	10	1	TRACE	—	—	—	2	34	.7	950	.03	.04	.2	9
MUSHROOMS, CANNED, SOLIDS AND LIQUID . . . 1 CUP . . .	244	93	40	5	TRACE	—	—	—	6	15	1.2	TRACE	.04	.60	4.8	4
MUSTARD GREENS, COOKED . . . 1 CUP . . .	140	93	35	3	1	—	—	—	6	193	2.5	8,120	.11	.19	.9	68
OKRA, COOKED, POD 3 IN. BY ⅝ IN. . . . 8 PODS . . .	85	91	25	2	TRACE	—	—	—	5	78	.4	420	.11	.15	.8	17
ONIONS:																
MATURE:																
RAW, ONION 2½-IN. DIAMETER . . . 1 ONION . . .	110	89	40	2	TRACE	—	—	—	10	30	0.6	40	0.04	0.04	0.2	11
COOKED . . . 1 CUP . . .	210	92	60	3	TRACE	—	—	—	14	50	.8	80	.06	.06	.4	14
YOUNG GREEN, SMALL, WITHOUT TOPS . . . 6 ONIONS . . .	50	88	20	1	TRACE	—	—	—	5	20	.3	TRACE	.02	.02	.2	12
PARSLEY, RAW, CHOPPED . . . 1 TBSP . . .	3.5	85	1	TRACE	TRACE	—	—	—	TRACE	7	.2	300	TRACE	.01	TRACE	6

Food, approximate measure																
PARSNIPS, COOKED ... 1 CUP	155	82	100	2	1	—	—	—	23	70	.9	50	.11	.13	.2	16
PEAS, GREEN:																
COOKED ... 1 CUP	160	82	115	9	1	—	—	—	19	37	2.9	860	.44	.17	3.7	33
CANNED, SOLIDS AND LIQUID ... 1 CUP	249	83	165	9	1	—	—	—	31	50	4.2	1,120	.23	.13	2.2	22
CANNED, STRAINED (BABY FOOD) ... 1 OZ	28	86	15	1	TRACE	—	—	—	3	3	.4	140	.02	.02	.4	3
PEPPERS, HOT, RED, WITHOUT SEEDS, DRIED (GROUND CHILI POWDER, ADDED SEASONINGS) ... 1 TBSP	15	8	50	2	2	—	—	—	8	40	2.3	9,750	.03	.17	1.3	2
PEPPERS, SWEET:																
RAW, MEDIUM, ABOUT 6 PER LB: GREEN POD WITHOUT STEM AND SEEDS ... 1 POD	62	93	15	1	TRACE	—	—	—	3	6	.4	260	.05	.05	.3	79
RED POD WITHOUT STEM AND SEEDS ... 1 POD	60	91	20	1	TRACE	—	—	—	4	8	.4	2,670	.05	.05	.3	122
CANNED, PIMIENTOS, MEDIUM ... 1 POD	38	92	10	TRACE	TRACE	—	—	—	2	3	.6	870	.01	.02	.1	36
POTATOES, MEDIUM (ABOUT 3 PER LB RAW): BAKED, PEELED AFTER BAKING ... 1 POTATO	99	75	90	3	TRACE	—	—	—	21	9	.7	TRACE	.10	.04	1.7	20
BOILED:																
PEELED AFTER BOILING ... 1 POTATO	136	80	105	3	TRACE	—	—	—	23	10	.8	TRACE	.13	.05	2.0	22
PEELED BEFORE BOILING ... 1 POTATO	122	83	80	2	TRACE	—	—	—	18	7	.6	TRACE	.11	.04	1.4	20
FRENCH-FRIED, PIECE 2 IN. BY ½ IN. BY ½ IN.																
COOKED IN DEEP FAT ... 10 PIECES	57	45	155	2	7	2	2	4	20	9	.7	TRACE	.07	.04	1.8	12
FROZEN, HEATED ... 10 PIECES	57	53	125	2	5	1	1	2	19	5	1.0	TRACE	.08	.01	1.5	12
MASHED:																
MILK ADDED ... 1 CUP	195	83	125	4	1	—	—	—	25	47	.8	50	.16	.10	2.0	19
MILK AND BUTTER ADDED ... 1 CUP	195	80	185	4	8	4	3	TRACE	24	47	.8	330	.16	.10	1.9	18
POTATO CHIPS, MEDIUM, 2-IN. DIAMETER ... 10 CHIPS	20	2	115	1	8	2	2	4	10	8	.4	TRACE	.04	.01	1.0	3
PUMPKIN, CANNED ... 1 CUP	228	90	75	2	1	—	—	—	18	57	.9	14,590	.07	.12	1.3	12
RADISHES, RAW, SMALL, WITHOUT TOPS ... 4 RADISHES	40	94	5	TRACE	TRACE	—	—	—	1	12	.4	TRACE	.01	.01	.1	10
SAUERKRAUT, CANNED, SOLIDS AND LIQUID ... 1 CUP	235	93	45	2	TRACE	—	—	—	9	85	1.2	120	.07	.09	.4	33
SPINACH:																
COOKED ... 1 CUP	180	92	40	5	1	—	—	—	6	167	4.0	14,580	.13	.25	1.0	50
CANNED, DRAINED SOLIDS ... 1 CUP	180	91	45	5	1	—	—	—	6	212	4.7	14,400	.03	.21	.6	24
CANNED, STRAINED OR CHOPPED (BABY FOOD) ... 1 OZ	28	88	10	1	TRACE	—	—	—	2	18	.2	1,420	.01	.04	.1	2
SPROUTS, RAW:																
MUNG BEAN ... 1 CUP	90	89	30	3	TRACE	—	—	—	6	17	1.2	20	.12	.12	.7	17
SOYBEAN ... 1 CUP	107	89	40	6	2	—	—	—	4	46	.7	90	.17	.16	.8	4
SQUASH:																
COOKED:																
SUMMER, DICED ... 1 CUP	210	96	30	2	TRACE	—	—	—	7	52	.8	820	.10	.16	1.6	21
WINTER, BAKED, MASHED ... 1 CUP	205	81	130	4	1	—	—	—	32	57	1.6	8,610	.10	.27	1.4	27
CANNED, WINTER, STRAINED AND CHOPPED (BABY FOOD) ... 1 OZ	28	92	10	TRACE	TRACE	—	—	—	2	7	.1	510	.01	.01	.1	1

d Measure and weight apply to entire vegetable or fruit including parts not usually eaten.

e Based on yellow varieties; white varieties contain only a trace of cryptoxanthin and carotenes, the pigments in corn that have biological activity.

TABLE 1 NUTRITIVE VALUES OF THE EDIBLE PART OF FOODS (Cont.)

[Dashes show that no basis could be found for imputing a value although there was some reason to believe that a measurable amount of the constituent might be present.]

FOOD, APPROXIMATE MEASURE, AND WEIGHT	GRAMS	WATER, %	FOOD ENERGY, CALORIES	PROTEIN, G	FAT (TOTAL LIPID), G	SATURATED (TOTAL), G	OLEIC	LINOLEIC	CARBOHYDRATE, G	CALCIUM, G	IRON, G	VITAMIN A VALUE, INTERNATIONAL UNITS	THIAMINE, G	RIBOFLAVIN, G	NIACIN, G	ASCORBIC ACID, G
VEGETABLES AND VEGETABLE PRODUCTS (Cont.)																
SWEET POTATOES:																
COOKED, MEDIUM, 5 IN. BY 2 IN., WEIGHT RAW ABOUT 6 OZ:																
BAKED, PEELED AFTER BAKING . . . . 1 SWEET POTATO	110	64	155	2	1	—	—	—	36	44	1.0	8,910	0.10	0.07	0.7	24
BOILED, PEELED AFTER BOILING . . . 1 SWEET POTATO	147	71	170	2	1	—	—	—	39	47	1.0	11,610	.13	.09	.9	25
CANDIED, 3½ IN. BY 2¼ IN. . . . . 1 SWEET POTATO	175	60	295	2	6	2	3	1	60	65	1.6	11,030	.10	.08	.8	17
CANNED, VACUUM OR SOLID PACK . . 1 CUP	218	72	235	4	TRACE	—	—	1	54	54	1.7	17,000	.10	.10	1.4	30
TOMATOES:																
RAW, MEDIUM, 2 IN. BY 2½ IN. ABOUT 3 PER LB . . . . 1 TOMATO	150	94	35	2	TRACE	—	—	—	7	20	.8	1,350	.10	.06	1.0	34
CANNED . . . . 1 CUP	242	94	50	2	TRACE	—	—	—	10	15	1.2	2,180	.13	.07	1.7	40
TOMATO JUICE, CANNED . . . . 1 CUP	242	94	45	2	TRACE	—	—	—	10	17	2.2	1,940	.13	.07	1.8	39
TOMATO CATSUP . . . . . . 1 TBSP	17	69	15	TRACE	TRACE	—	—	—	4	4	.1	240	.02	.01	.3	3
TURNIPS, COOKED, DICED . . . . 1 CUP	155	94	35	1	TRACE	—	—	—	8	54	.6	TRACE	.06	.08	.5	33
TURNIP GREENS:																
COOKED:																
IN SMALL AMOUNT OF WATER, SHORT TIME . . . . . . 1 CUP	145	93	30	3	TRACE	—	—	—	5	267	1.6	9,140	.21	.36	.8	100
IN LARGE AMOUNT OF WATER, LONG TIME . . . . . . 1 CUP	145	94	25	3	TRACE	—	—	—	5	252	1.4	8,260	.14	.33	.8	68
CANNED, SOLIDS AND LIQUID . . . 1 CUP	232	94	40	3	1	—	—	—	7	232	3.7	10,900	.04	.21	1.4	44
FRUITS AND FRUIT PRODUCTS																
APPLES, RAW, MEDIUM, 2½-IN. DIAMETER, ABOUT 3 PER LB[d] . . . . 1 APPLE	150	85	70	TRACE	TRACE	—	—	—	18	8	.4	50	.04	.02	.1	3
APPLE BROWN BETTY . . . . . 1 CUP	230	64	345	4	8	4	3	TRACE	68	41	1.4	230	.13	.10	.9	3
APPLE JUICE, BOTTLED OR CANNED . . 1 CUP	249	88	120	TRACE	TRACE	—	—	—	30	15	1.5	—	.01	.04	.2	2
APPLESAUCE, CANNED:																
SWEETENED . . . . 1 CUP	254	76	230	1	TRACE	—	—	—	60	10	1.3	100	.05	.03	.1	3
UNSWEETENED OR ARTIFICIALLY SWEETENED . . . . . . 1 CUP	239	88	100	TRACE	TRACE	—	—	—	26	10	1.2	100	.04	.02	.1	2
APPLESAUCE AND APRICOTS, CANNED, STRAINED OR JUNIOR (BABY FOOD) . . 1 OZ	28	77	25	TRACE	TRACE	—	—	—	6	1	.1	170	TRACE	TRACE	TRACE	1

Food, approximate measure	Weight (g)	Water (%)	Food energy (cal.)	Protein (g)	Fat (g)	Saturated fatty acids (total)	Unsaturated: Oleic	Unsaturated: Linoleic	Carbohydrate (g)	Calcium (mg)	Iron (mg)	Vitamin A (I.U.)	Thiamin (mg)	Riboflavin (mg)	Niacin (mg)	Ascorbic acid (mg)
APRICOTS:																
RAW, ABOUT 12 PER POUND[d] . . . . 3 APRICOTS	114	85	55	1	TRACE	—	—	—	14	18	.5	2,890	.03	.04	.7	10
CANNED IN HEAVY SIRUP:																
HALVES AND SIRUP . . . . . 1 CUP	259	77	220	2	TRACE	—	—	—	57	28	.8	4,510	.05	.06	.9	10
HALVES (MEDIUM) AND SIRUP . . . 4 HALVES; 2 TBSP SIRUP	122	77	105	1	TRACE	—	—	—	27	13	.4	2,120	.02	.03	.4	5
DRIED:																
UNCOOKED, 40 HALVES, SMALL . . . 1 CUP	150	25	390	8	1	—	—	—	100	100	8.2	16,350	.02	.23	4.9	19
COOKED, UNSWEETENED, FRUIT AND LIQUID . . . . . 1 CUP	285	76	240	5	1	—	—	—	62	63	5.1	8,550	.01	.13	2.8	8
APRICOT NECTAR, CANNED . . . . 1 CUP	250	85	140	1	TRACE	—	—	—	36	22	.5	2,380	.02	.02	.5	7
AVOCADOS, RAW:																
CALIFORNIA VARIETIES, MAINLY FUERTE:																
10-OZ AVOCADO, ABOUT 3⅓ IN. BY 4¼ IN., PEELED, PITTED . . . ½ AVOCADO	108	74	185	2	18	4	8	2	6	11	.6	310	.12	.21	1.7	15
½-IN. CUBES . . . . . 1 CUP	152	74	260	3	26	5	12	3	9	15	.9	440	.16	.30	2.4	21
FLORIDA VARIETIES:																
13-OZ AVOCADO, ABOUT 4 IN. BY 3 IN., PEELED, PITTED . . . ½ AVOCADO	123	78	160	2	14	3	6	2	11	12	.7	360	.13	.24	2.0	17
½-IN. CUBES . . . . . 1 CUP	152	78	195	2	17	3	8	2	13	15	.9	440	.16	.30	2.4	21
BANANAS, RAW, 6 IN. BY 1½ IN., ABOUT 3 PER LB[d] . . . . 1 BANANA	150	76	85	1	TRACE	—	—	—	23	8	.7	190	.05	.06	.7	10
BLACKBERRIES, RAW . . . . . 1 CUP	144	84	85	2	1	—	—	—	19	46	1.3	290	.05	.06	.5	30
BLUEBERRIES, RAW . . . . . 1 CUP	140	83	85	1	1	—	—	—	21	21	1.4	140	.04	.08	.6	20
CANTALOUPS, RAW; MEDIUM, 5-IN. DIAMETER, ABOUT 1⅓ LB[d] . . . ½ MELON	385	91	60	1	TRACE	—	—	—	14	27	.8	6,540[g]	.08	.06	1.2	63
CHERRIES:																
RAW, SWEET, WITH STEMS[d] . . . 1 CUP	130	80	80	2	TRACE	—	—	—	20	26	.5	130	.06	0.07	0.5	12
CANNED, RED, SOUR, PITTED, HEAVY SIRUP . . . . . 1 CUP	260	76	230	2	1	—	—	—	59	36	.8	1,680	.07	.06	.4	13
CRANBERRY JUICE COCKTAIL, CANNED . . . 1 CUP	250	83	160	TRACE	TRACE	—	—	—	41	12	.8	TRACE	.02	.02	.1	^[h]
CRANBERRY SAUCE, SWEETENED, CANNED, STRAINED . . . . . 1 CUP	277	62	405	TRACE	1	—	—	—	104	17	.6	40	.03	.03	.1	5
DATES, DOMESTIC, NATURAL AND DRY, PITTED, CUT . . . . . 1 CUP	178	22	490	4	1	—	—	—	130	105	5.3	90	.16	.17	3.9	0
FIGS:																
RAW, SMALL, 1½-IN. DIAMETER, ABOUT 12 PER LB[d] . . . . 3 FIGS	114	78	90	1	TRACE	—	—	—	23	40	.7	90	.07	.06	.5	2
DRIED, LARGE, 2 IN. BY 1 IN. . . . 1 FIG	21	23	60	1	TRACE	—	—	—	15	26	.6	20	.02	.02	.1	0
FRUIT COCKTAIL, CANNED IN HEAVY SIRUP, SOLIDS AND LIQUID . . . 1 CUP	256	80	195	1	1	—	—	—	50	23	1.0	360	.04	.03	1.1	5

[d] Measure and weight apply to entire vegetable or fruit including parts not usually eaten.

[f] Year-round average. Samples marketed from November through May average around 15 mg per 150-g tomato; from June through October, around 39 mg.

[g] Value based on varieties with orange-colored flesh; for green-fleshed varieties value is about 540 IU per ½ melon.

[h] About 5 mg per 8 fl oz is from cranberries. Ascorbic acid is usually added to approximately 100 mg per 8 fl oz.

TABLE 1 NUTRITIVE VALUES OF THE EDIBLE PART OF FOODS (Cont.)

[Dashes show that no basis could be found for imputing a value although there was some reason to believe that a measurable amount of the constituent might be present.]

FOOD, APPROXIMATE MEASURE, AND WEIGHT	GRAMS	WATER, %	FOOD ENERGY, CALORIES	PRO-TEIN, G	FAT (TOTAL LIPID), G	FATTY ACIDS SATU-RATED (TOTAL), G	UNSATURATED OLEIC	LINOLEIC	CARBO-HY-DRATE, G	CAL-CIUM, G	IRON, G	VITA-MIN A VALUE, INTER-NATIONAL UNITS	THIA-MINE, G	RIBO-FLAVIN, G	NIACIN, G	ASCOR-BIC ACID, G
FRUITS AND FRUIT PRODUCTS (Cont.)																
GRAPEFRUIT:																
RAW, MEDIUM, 4¼-IN. DIAMETER, SIZE 64:																
WHITE^d . . . ½ GRAPEFRUIT	285	89	55	1	TRACE	—	—	—	14	22	.6	10	.05	.02	.2	52
PINK OR RED^d . . . ½ GRAPEFRUIT	285	89	60	1	TRACE	—	—	—	15	23	.6	640	.05	.02	.3	52
RAW SECTIONS, WHITE . . . 1 CUP	194	89	75	1	TRACE	—	—	—	20	31	.8	20	.07	.03	.3	72
CANNED, WHITE:																
SIRUP PACK, SOLIDS AND LIQUID . . . 1 CUP	249	81	175	1	TRACE	—	—	—	44	32	.7	20	.07	.04	.5	75
WATER PACK, SOLIDS AND LIQUID . . . 1 CUP	240	91	70	1	TRACE	—	—	—	18	31	.7	20	.07	.04	.5	72
GRAPEFRUIT JUICE:																
FRESH . . . 1 CUP	246	90	95	1	TRACE	—	—	—	23	22	.5	‡	.09	.04	.4	92
CANNED, WHITE:																
UNSWEETENED . . . 1 CUP	247	89	100	1	TRACE	—	—	—	24	20	1.0	20	.07	.04	.4	84
SWEETENED . . . 1 CUP	250	86	130	1	TRACE	—	—	—	32	20	1.0	20	.07	.04	.4	78
FROZEN, CONCENTRATE, UNSWEETENED:																
UNDILUTED, CAN, 6 FL OZ . . . 1 CAN	207	62	300	4	1	—	—	—	72	70	.8	60	.29	.12	1.4	286
DILUTED WITH 3 PARTS WATER, BY VOLUME . . . 1 CUP	247	89	100	1	TRACE	—	—	—	24	25	.2	20	.10	.04	.5	96
FROZEN, CONCENTRATE, SWEETENED:																
UNDILUTED, CAN, 6 FL OZ . . . 1 CAN	211	57	350	3	1	—	—	—	85	59	.6	50	.24	.11	1.2	245
DILUTED WITH 3 PARTS WATER, BY VOLUME . . . 1 CUP	249	88	115	1	TRACE	—	—	—	28	20	.2	20	.08	.03	.4	82
DEHYDRATED:																
CRYSTALS, CAN, NET WEIGHT 4 OZ . . . 1 CAN	114	1	430	5	1	—	—	—	103	99	1.1	90	.41	.18	2.0	399
PREPARED WITH WATER (1 LB YIELDS ABOUT 1 GAL) . . . 1 CUP	247	90	100	1	TRACE	—	—	—	24	22	.2	20	.10	.05	.5	92
GRAPES, RAW:																
AMERICAN TYPE (SLIP SKIN), SUCH AS CONCORD, DELAWARE, NIAGARA, CATAWBA, AND SCUPPERNONG^d . . . 1 CUP	153	82	65	1	1	—	—	—	15	15	.4	100	.05	.03	.2	3
EUROPEAN TYPE (ADHERENT SKIN), SUCH AS MALAGA, MUSCAT, THOMPSON SEEDLESS, EMPEROR, AND FLAME TOKAY^d . . . 1 CUP	160	81	95	1	TRACE	—	—	—	25	17	.6	140	.07	.04	.4	6
GRAPE JUICE, BOTTLED OR CANNED . . . 1 CUP	254	83	165	1	TRACE	—	—	—	42	28	.8	—	.10	.05	.6	TRACE

Food, approximate measure		Grams	Water (%)	Food energy	Protein	Fat				Carbohydrate	Calcium	Iron	Vitamin A	Thiamine	Riboflavin	Niacin	Ascorbic acid
LEMONS, RAW, MEDIUM, 2⅛-IN. DIAMETER, SIZE 150[d]	1 LEMON	106	90	20	1	TRACE	—	—	—	6	18	.4	10	.03	.01	.1	38
LEMON JUICE:																	
FRESH	1 CUP	246	91	60	1	TRACE	—	—	—	20	17	.5	40	.08	.03	.2	113
	1 TBSP	15	91	5	TRACE	TRACE	—	—	—	1	1	TRACE	TRACE	TRACE	TRACE	TRACE	7
CANNED, UNSWEETENED	1 CUP	245	92	55	1	TRACE	—	—	—	19	17	.5	40	.07	.03	.2	102
LEMONADE CONCENTRATE, FROZEN, SWEETENED:																	
UNDILUTED, CAN, 6 FL OZ	1 CAN	220	48	430	TRACE	TRACE	—	—	—	112	9	.4	40	.05	.06	.7	66
DILUTED WITH 4⅓ PARTS WATER, BY VOLUME	1 CUP	248	88	110	TRACE	TRACE	—	—	—	28	2	.1	10	.01	.01	.2	17
LIME JUICE:																	
FRESH	1 CUP	246	90	65	1	TRACE	—	—	—	22	22	0.5	30	0.05	0.03	0.3	80
CANNED	1 CUP	246	90	65	1	TRACE	—	—	—	22	22	.5	30	.05	.03	.3	52
LIMEADE CONCENTRATE, FROZEN, SWEETENED:																	
UNDILUTED, CAN, 6 FL OZ	1 CAN	218	50	410	TRACE	TRACE	—	—	—	108	11	.2	TRACE	.02	.02	.2	26
DILUTED WITH 4⅓ PARTS WATER, BY VOLUME	1 CUP	248	90	105	TRACE	TRACE	—	—	—	27	2	TRACE	TRACE	TRACE	TRACE	TRACE	6
ORANGES, RAW:																	
CALIFORNIA, NAVEL (WINTER), 2⅛-IN. DIAMETER, SIZE 88[d]	1 ORANGE	180	85	60	2	TRACE	—	—	—	16	49	.5	240	.12	.05	.5	75
FLORIDA, ALL VARIETIES, 3-IN. DIAMETER[d]	1 ORANGE	210	86	75	1	TRACE	—	—	—	19	67	.3	310	.16	.06	.6	70
ORANGE JUICE:																	
FRESH:																	
CALIFORNIA, VALENCIA (SUMMER)	1 CUP	249	88	115	2	1	—	—	—	26	27	.7	500	.22	.06	.9	122
FLORIDA VARIETIES:																	
EARLY AND MIDSEASON	1 CUP	247	90	100	1	TRACE	—	—	—	23	25	.5	490	.22	.06	.9	127
LATE SEASON, VALENCIA	1 CUP	248	88	110	1	TRACE	—	—	—	26	25	.5	500	.22	.06	.9	92
CANNED, UNSWEETENED	1 CUP	249	87	120	2	TRACE	—	—	—	28	25	1.0	500	.17	.05	.6	100
FROZEN CONCENTRATE:																	
UNDILUTED, CAN, 6 FL OZ	1 CAN	210	58	330	5	TRACE	—	—	—	80	69	.8	1,490	.63	.10	2.4	332
DILUTED WITH 3 PARTS WATER, BY VOLUME	1 CUP	248	88	110	2	TRACE	—	—	—	27	22	.2	500	.21	.03	.8	112
DEHYDRATED:																	
CRYSTALS, CAN, NET WEIGHT 4 OZ	1 CAN	113	1	430	6	2	—	—	—	100	95	1.9	1,900	.76	.24	3.3	406
PREPARED WITH WATER, 1 LB YIELDS ABOUT 1 GAL.	1 CUP	248	88	115	1	TRACE	—	—	—	27	25	.5	500	.20	.06	.9	108
ORANGE AND GRAPEFRUIT JUICE:																	
FROZEN CONCENTRATE:																	
UNDILUTED, CAN, 6 FL OZ	1 CAN	209	59	325	4	1	—	—	—	78	61	.8	790	.47	.06	2.3	301
DILUTED WITH 3 PARTS WATER, BY VOLUME	1 CUP	248	88	110	1	TRACE	—	—	—	26	20	.2	270	.16	.02	.8	102

[d] Measure and weight apply to entire vegetable or fruit including parts not usually eaten.

[i] For white-fleshed varieties value is about 20 IU per cup; for red-fleshed varieties, 1,080 IU per cup.

435

TABLE 1 NUTRITIVE VALUES OF THE EDIBLE PART OF FOODS (Cont.)

[Dashes show that no basis could be found for imputing a value although there was some reason to believe that a measurable amount of the constituent might be present.]

FOOD, APPROXIMATE MEASURE, AND WEIGHT	GRAMS	WATER, %	FOOD ENERGY, CALORIES	PROTEIN, G	FAT (TOTAL LIPID), G	SATURATED (TOTAL), G	OLEIC	LINOLEIC	CARBOHYDRATE, G	CALCIUM, G	IRON, G	VITAMIN A VALUE, INTERNATIONAL UNITS	THIAMINE, G	RIBOFLAVIN, G	NIACIN, G	ASCORBIC ACID, G
FRUITS AND FRUIT PRODUCTS (Cont.)																
PAPAYAS, RAW, 1/2-IN. CUBES . . . . . 1 CUP	182	89	70	1	TRACE	—	—	—	18	36	.5	3,190	.07	.08	.5	102
PEACHES:																
RAW:																
WHOLE, MEDIUM, 2-IN. DIAMETER, ABOUT 4 PER LB . . . 1 PEACH	114	89	35	1	TRACE	—	—	—	10	9	.5	ʲ1,320	.02	.05	1.0	7
SLICED . . . . . 1 CUP	168	89	65	1	TRACE	—	—	—	16	15	.8	2,230	.03	.08	1.6	12
CANNED, YELLOW-FLESHED, SOLIDS AND LIQUID:																
SIRUP PACK, HEAVY:																
HALVES OR SLICES . . . . . 1 CUP	257	79	200	1	TRACE	—	—	—	52	10	.8	1,100	.02	.06	1.4	7
HALVES (MEDIUM) AND SIRUP . . . 2 HALVES AND 2 TBSP SIRUP	117	79	90	TRACE	TRACE	—	—	—	24	5	.4	500	.01	.03	.7	3
WATER PACK . . . . . 1 CUP	245	91	75	1	TRACE	—	—	—	20	10	.7	1,100	.02	.06	1.4	7
STRAINED OR CHOPPED (BABY FOOD) . . . 1 OZ	28	78	25	TRACE	TRACE	—	—	—	6	2	.1	140	TRACE	.01	.2	1
DRIED:																
UNCOOKED . . . . . 1 CUP	160	25	420	5	1	—	—	—	109	77	9.6	6,240	.02	.31	8.5	28
COOKED, UNSWEETENED, 10–12 HALVES AND 6 TBSP LIQUID . . . 1 CUP	270	77	220	3	1	—	—	—	58	41	5.1	3,290	.01	.15	4.2	6
FROZEN:																
CARTON, 12 OZ, NOT THAWED . . . 1 CARTON	340	76	300	1	TRACE	—	—	—	77	14	1.7	2,210	.03	.14	2.4	ᵏ135
CAN, 16 OZ, NOT THAWED . . . 1 CAN	454	76	400	2	TRACE	—	—	—	103	18	2.3	2,950	.05	.18	3.2	ᵏ181
PEACH NECTAR, CANNED . . . . . 1 CUP	250	87	120	TRACE	TRACE	—	—	—	31	10	.5	1,080	.02	.05	1.0	1
PEARS:																
RAW, 3 IN. BY 2½-IN. DIAMETERᵈ . . . 1 PEAR	182	83	100	1	1	—	—	—	25	13	.5	30	.04	.07	.2	7
CANNED, SOLIDS AND LIQUID:																
SIRUP PACK, HEAVY:																
HALVES OR SLICES . . . . . 1 CUP	255	80	195	1	1	—	—	—	50	13	0.5	TRACE	0.03	0.05	0.3	4
HALVES (MEDIUM) AND SIRUP . . . 2 HALVES AND 2 TBSP SIRUP	117	80	90	TRACE	TRACE	—	—	—	23	6	.2	TRACE	.01	.02	.2	2
WATER PACK . . . . . 1 CUP	243	91	80	TRACE	TRACE	—	—	—	20	12	.5	TRACE	.02	.05	.3	4
STRAINED OR CHOPPED (BABY FOOD) . . . 1 OZ	28	82	20	TRACE	TRACE	—	—	—	5	2	.1	10	TRACE	.01	.1	1
PEAR NECTAR, CANNED . . . . . 1 CUP	250	86	130	1	TRACE	—	—	—	33	8	.2	TRACE	.01	.05	TRACE	1

Food	Measure	Grams	Water (%)	Food energy	Protein (g)	Fat (g)	Saturated	Oleic	Linoleic	Carbohydrate (g)	Calcium (mg)	Iron (mg)	Vitamin A (IU)	Thiamine (mg)	Riboflavin (mg)	Niacin (mg)	Ascorbic acid (mg)
PERSIMMONS, JAPANESE OR KAKI, RAW, SEEDLESS, 2½-IN. DIAMETER [d]	1 PERSIMMON	125	79	75	1	TRACE	—	—	—	20	6	.4	2,740	.03	.02	.1	11
PINEAPPLE: RAW, DICED	1 CUP	140	85	75	1	TRACE	—	—	—	19	24	.7	100	.12	.04	.3	24
CANNED, HEAVY SIRUP PACK, SOLIDS AND LIQUID: CRUSHED	1 CUP	260	80	195	1	TRACE	—	—	—	50	29	.8	120	.20	.06	.5	17
SLICED, SLICES AND JUICE	2 SMALL OR 1 LARGE AND 2 TBSP JUICE	122	80	90	TRACE	TRACE	—	—	—	24	13	.4	50	.09	.03	.2	8
PINEAPPLE JUICE, CANNED	1 CUP	249	86	135	1	TRACE	—	—	—	34	37	.7	120	.12	.04	.5	22
PLUMS, ALL EXCEPT PRUNES: RAW, 2-IN. DIAMETER, ABOUT 2 OZ [d]	1 PLUM	60	87	25	TRACE	TRACE	—	—	—	7	7	.3	140	.02	.02	.3	3
CANNED, SIRUP PACK (ITALIAN PRUNES): PLUMS (WITH PITS) AND JUICE [d]	1 CUP	256	77	205	1	TRACE	—	—	—	53	22	2.2	2,970	.05	.05	.9	4
PLUMS (WITHOUT PITS) AND JUICE	3 PLUMS AND 2 TBSP JUICE	122	77	100	TRACE	TRACE	—	—	—	26	11	1.1	1,470	.03	.02	.5	2
PRUNES, DRIED, "SOFTENIZED," MEDIUM: UNCOOKED [d]	4 PRUNES	32	28	70	1	TRACE	—	—	—	18	14	1.1	440	.02	.04	.4	1
COOKED, UNSWEETENED, 17-18 PRUNES AND ⅓ CUP LIQUID [d]	1 CUP	270	66	295	2	1	—	—	—	78	60	4.5	1,860	.08	.18	1.7	2
PRUNES WITH TAPIOCA, CANNED, STRAINED OR JUNIOR (BABY FOOD)	1 OZ	28	77	25	TRACE	TRACE	—	—	—	6	2	.3	110	.01	.02	.1	1
PRUNE JUICE, CANNED	1 CUP	256	80	200	1	TRACE	—	—	—	49	36	10.5	—	.02	.03	1.1	4
RAISINS, DRIED	1 CUP	160	18	460	4	TRACE	—	—	—	124	99	5.6	30	.18	.13	.9	2
RASPBERRIES, RED: RAW	1 CUP	123	84	70	1	1	—	—	—	17	27	1.1	160	.04	.11	1.1	31
FROZEN, 10-OZ CARTON, NOT THAWED	1 CARTON	284	74	275	2	1	—	—	—	70	37	1.7	200	.06	.17	1.7	59
RHUBARB, COOKED, SUGAR ADDED	1 CUP	272	63	385	1	TRACE	—	—	—	98	212	1.6	220	.06	.15	.7	17
STRAWBERRIES: RAW, CAPPED	1 CUP	149	90	55	1	1	—	—	—	13	31	1.5	90	.04	.10	1.0	88
FROZEN, 10-OZ CARTON, NOT THAWED	1 CARTON	284	71	310	1	1	—	—	—	79	40	2.0	90	.06	.17	1.5	150
FROZEN, 16-OZ CAN, NOT THAWED	1 CAN	454	71	495	2	1	—	—	—	126	64	3.2	150	.09	.27	2.4	240
TANGERINES, RAW, MEDIUM, 2½-IN. DIAMETER, ABOUT 4 PER LB [d]	1 TANGERINE	114	87	40	1	TRACE	—	—	—	10	34	.3	350	.05	.02	.1	26
TANGERINE JUICE: CANNED, UNSWEETENED	1 CUP	248	89	105	1	TRACE	—	—	—	25	45	.5	1,040	.14	.04	.3	56
FROZEN CONCENTRATE: UNDILUTED, CAN, 6 FL OZ	1 CAN	210	58	340	4	1	—	—	—	80	130	1.5	3,070	.43	.12	.9	202

[d] Measure and weight apply to entire vegetable or fruit including parts not usually eaten.

[i] Based on yellow-fleshed varieties; for white-fleshed varieties value is about 50 IU per 114-g peach and 80 IU per cup of sliced peaches.

[k] Average weighted in accordance with commercial freezing practices. For products without added ascorbic acid, value is about 37 mg per 12-oz carton and 50 mg per 16-oz can; for those added with ascorbic acid, 139 mg per 12 oz and 186 mg per 16 oz.

TABLE 1 NUTRITIVE VALUES OF THE EDIBLE PART OF FOODS (Cont.)

[Dashes show that no basis could be found for imputing a value although there was some reason to believe that a measurable amount of the constituent might be present.]

FOOD, APPROXIMATE MEASURE, AND WEIGHT	GRAMS	WATER, %	FOOD ENERGY, CALORIES	PROTEIN, G	FAT (TOTAL LIPID), G	FATTY ACIDS SATURATED (TOTAL), G	FATTY ACIDS UNSATURATED OLEIC	FATTY ACIDS UNSATURATED LINOLEIC	CARBOHYDRATE, G	CALCIUM, G	IRON, G	VITAMIN A VALUE, INTERNATIONAL UNITS	THIAMINE, G	RIBOFLAVIN, G	NIACIN, G	ASCORBIC ACID, G
FRUITS AND FRUIT PRODUCTS (Cont.)																
DILUTED WITH 3 PARTS WATER, BY VOLUME ... 1 CUP	248	88	115	1	TRACE	—	—	—	27	45	.5	1,020	.14	.04	.3	67
WATERMELON, RAW, WEDGE, 4 IN. BY 8 IN. (1⁄16 OF 10 IN. BY 16-IN. MELON, ABOUT 2 LB WITH RIND) ... 1 WEDGE	925	93	115	2	1	—	—	—	27	30	2.1	2,510	.13	.13	.7	30
GRAIN PRODUCTS																
BARLEY, PEARLED, LIGHT, UNCOOKED ... 1 CUP	203	11	710	17	2	TRACE	1	1	160	32	4.1	0	0.25	0.17	6.3	0
BISCUITS, BAKING POWDER WITH ENRICHED FLOUR, 2½-IN. DIAMETER ... 1 BISCUIT	38	27	140	3	6	2	3	1	17	46	.6	TRACE	.08	.08	.7	TRACE
BRAN FLAKES (40% BRAN) ADDED THIAMINE ... 1 OZ	28	3	85	3	1	—	—	—	23	20	1.2	0	.11	.05	1.7	0
BREADS:																
BOSTON BROWN BREAD, SLICE, 3 IN. BY ¾ IN. ... 1 SLICE	48	45	100	3	1	—	—	—	22	43	.9	0	.05	.03	.6	0
CRACKED-WHEAT BREAD:																
LOAF, 1-LB, 20 SLICES ... 1 LOAF	454	35	1,190	39	10	2	5	2	236	399	5.0	TRACE	.53	.42	5.8	TRACE
SLICE ... 1 SLICE	23	35	60	2	1	—	—	—	12	20	.3	TRACE	.03	.02	.3	TRACE
FRENCH OR VIENNA BREAD:																
ENRICHED, 1-LB LOAF ... 1 LOAF	454	31	1,315	41	14	3	8	2	251	195	10.0	TRACE	1.26	.98	11.3	TRACE
UNENRICHED, 1-LB LOAF ... 1 LOAF	454	31	1,315	41	14	3	8	2	251	195	3.2	TRACE	.39	.39	3.6	TRACE
ITALIAN BREAD:																
ENRICHED, 1-LB LOAF ... 1 LOAF	454	32	1,250	41	4	TRACE	1	2	256	77	10.0	0	1.31	.93	11.7	0
UNENRICHED, 1-LB LOAF ... 1 LOAF	454	32	1,250	41	4	TRACE	1	2	256	77	3.2	0	.39	.27	3.6	0
RAISIN BREAD:																
LOAF, 1-LB, 20 SLICES ... 1 LOAF	454	35	1,190	30	13	3	8	2	243	322	5.9	TRACE	.24	.42	3.0	TRACE
SLICE ... 1 SLICE	23	35	60	2	1	—	—	—	12	16	.3	TRACE	.01	.02	.2	TRACE
RYE BREAD:																
AMERICAN, LIGHT (⅓ RYE, ⅔ WHEAT):																
LOAF, 1-LB, 20 SLICES ... 1 LOAF	454	36	1,100	41	5	—	—	—	236	340	7.3	0	.81	.33	6.4	0
SLICE ... 1 SLICE	23	36	55	2	TRACE	—	—	—	12	17	.4	0	.04	.02	.3	0
PUMPERNICKEL, LOAF, 1 LB ... 1 LOAF	454	34	1,115	41	5	—	—	—	241	381	10.9	0	1.05	.63	5.4	0
WHITE BREAD, ENRICHED:																
1-2% NONFAT DRY MILK:																
LOAF, 1-LB, 20 SLICES ... 1 LOAF	454	36	1,225	39	15	3	8	2	229	318	10.9	TRACE	1.13	.77	10.4	TRACE
SLICE ... 1 SLICE	23	36	60	2	1	TRACE	TRACE	TRACE	12	16	.6	TRACE	.06	.04	.5	TRACE

Food	Weight (g)	Water (%)	Food energy (calories)	Protein (g)	Fat (g)	Fatty acids — Saturated (total) (g)	Fatty acids — Unsaturated oleic (g)	Fatty acids — Unsaturated linoleic (g)	Carbohydrate (g)	Calcium (mg)	Iron (mg)	Vitamin A (IU)	Thiamine (mg)	Riboflavin (mg)	Niacin (mg)	Ascorbic acid (mg)
3–4% NONFAT DRY MILK:[l]																
LOAF, 1-LB . . . 1 LOAF	454	36	1,225	39	15	3	8	2	229	381	11.3	TRACE	1.13	.95	10.8	TRACE
SLICE, 20 PER LOAF . . . 1 SLICE	23	36	60	2	1	TRACE	TRACE	TRACE	12	19	.6	TRACE	.06	.05	.6	TRACE
SLICE, TOASTED . . . 1 SLICE	20	25	60	2	1	TRACE	TRACE	TRACE	12	19	.6	TRACE	.05	.05	.6	TRACE
SLICE, 26 PER LOAF . . . 1 SLICE	17	36	45	1	1	TRACE	TRACE	TRACE	9	14	.4	TRACE	.04	.04	.4	TRACE
5–6% NONFAT DRY MILK:																
LOAF, 1-LB, 20 SLICES . . . 1 LOAF	454	35	1,245	41	17	4	10	2	228	435	11.3	TRACE	1.22	.91	11.0	TRACE
SLICE . . . 1 SLICE	23	35	65	2	1	TRACE	TRACE	TRACE	12	22	.6	TRACE	.06	.05	.6	TRACE
WHITE BREAD, UNENRICHED:																
1–2% NONFAT DRY MILK:																
LOAF, 1-LB, 20 SLICES . . . 1 LOAF	454	36	1,225	39	15	3	8	2	229	318	3.2	TRACE	.40	.36	5.6	TRACE
SLICE . . . 1 SLICE	23	36	60	2	1	TRACE	TRACE	TRACE	12	16	.2	TRACE	.02	.02	.3	TRACE
3–4% NONFAT DRY MILK:[l]																
LOAF, 1-LB . . . 1 LOAF	454	36	1,225	39	15	3	8	2	229	381	3.2	TRACE	.31	.39	5.0	TRACE
SLICE, 20 PER LOAF . . . 1 SLICE	23	36	60	2	1	TRACE	TRACE	TRACE	12	19	.2	TRACE	.02	.02	.3	TRACE
SLICE, TOASTED . . . 1 SLICE	20	25	60	2	1	TRACE	TRACE	TRACE	12	19	.2	TRACE	.01	.02	.3	TRACE
SLICE, 26 PER LOAF . . . 1 SLICE	17	36	45	1	1	TRACE	TRACE	TRACE	9	14	.1	TRACE	.01	.01	.2	TRACE
5–6% NONFAT DRY MILK:																
LOAF, 1-LB, 20 SLICES . . . 1 LOAF	454	35	1,245	41	17	4	10	2	228	435	3.2	TRACE	.32	.59	4.1	TRACE
SLICE . . . 1 SLICE	23	35	65	2	1	TRACE	TRACE	TRACE	12	22	.2	TRACE	.02	.03	.2	TRACE
WHOLE-WHEAT BREAD, MADE WITH 2% NONFAT DRY MILK:																
LOAF, 1-LB, 20 SLICES . . . 1 LOAF	454	36	1,105	48	14	3	6	3	216	449	10.4	TRACE	1.17	.56	12.9	TRACE
SLICE . . . 1 SLICE	23	36	55	2	1	TRACE	TRACE	TRACE	11	23	.5	TRACE	.06	.03	.7	TRACE
SLICE, TOASTED . . . 1 SLICE	19	24	55	2	1	TRACE	TRACE	TRACE	11	22	.5	TRACE	.05	.03	.6	TRACE
BREADCRUMBS, DRY, GRATED . . . 1 CUP	88	6	345	11	4	1	2	1	65	107	3.2	TRACE	.19	.26	3.1	TRACE
CAKES:[m]																
ANGELFOOD CAKE; SECTOR, 2-IN. (1/12 OF 8-IN. DIAMETER CAKE) . . . 1 SECTOR	40	32	110	3	TRACE	—	—	—	24	4	.1	0	TRACE	.06	.1	0
CHOCOLATE CAKE, CHOCOLATE ICING; SECTOR, 2-IN. (1/16 OF 10-IN. DIAMETER LAYER CAKE) . . . 1 SECTOR	120	22	445	5	20	8	10	1	67	84	1.2	"190	0.03	0.12	0.3	TRACE
FRUITCAKE, DARK (MADE WITH ENRICHED-FLOUR); PIECE, 2 IN. BY 2 IN. BY 1/2 IN. . . . 1 PIECE	30	18	115	1	5	1	3	1	18	22	.8	"40	.04	.04	.2	TRACE
GINGERBREAD (MADE WITH ENRICHED FLOUR); PIECE, 2 IN. BY 2 IN. BY 2 IN. . . . 1 PIECE	55	31	175	2	6	1	4	TRACE	29	37	1.3	50	.06	.06	.5	0
PLAIN CAKE AND CUPCAKES, WITHOUT ICING:																
PIECE, 3 IN. BY 2 IN. BY 1½ IN. . . . 1 PIECE	55	24	200	2	8	2	5	1	31	35	.2	"90	.01	.05	.1	TRACE
CUPCAKE, 2¾-IN. DIAMETER . . . 1 CUPCAKE	40	24	145	2	6	1	3	TRACE	22	26	.2	"70	.01	.03	.1	TRACE
PLAIN CAKE AND CUPCAKES, WITH CHOCOLATE ICING:																
SECTOR, 2-IN. (1/16 OF 10-IN. LAYER CAKE) . . . 1 SECTOR	100	21	370	4	14	5	7	1	59	63	.6	"180	.02	.09	.2	TRACE
CUPCAKE, 2¾-IN. DIAMETER . . . 1 CUPCAKE	50	21	185	2	7	2	4	TRACE	30	32	.3	"90	.01	.04	.1	TRACE

[l] When the amount of nonfat dry milk in commercial white bread is unknown, values for bread with 3 to 4 percent nonfat dry milk are suggested.

[m] Unenriched cake flour and vegetable cooking fat used unless otherwise specified.

[n] If the fat used in the recipe is butter or fortified margarine, the vitamin A value for chocolate cake with chocolate icing will be 490 IU per 2-in. sector, 100 IU for fruitcake, for plain cake without icing, 300 IU per piece, 220 IU per cupcake, for plain cake with icing, 440 IU per 2-in. sector, 220 IU per cupcake, and 300 IU for poundcake.

TABLE 1 NUTRITIVE VALUES OF THE EDIBLE PART OF FOODS (Cont.)

[Dashes show that no basis could be found for imputing a value although there was some reason to believe that a measurable amount of the constituent might be present.]

FOOD, APPROXIMATE MEASURE, AND WEIGHT	GRAMS	WATER, %	FOOD ENERGY, CALORIES	PROTEIN, G	FAT (TOTAL LIPID), G	FATTY ACIDS: SATURATED (TOTAL), G	FATTY ACIDS: UNSATURATED: OLEIC	FATTY ACIDS: UNSATURATED: LINOLEIC	CARBOHYDRATE, G	CALCIUM, G	IRON, G	VITAMIN A VALUE, INTERNATIONAL UNITS	THIAMINE, G	RIBOFLAVIN, G	NIACIN, G	ASCORBIC ACID, G
GRAIN PRODUCTS (Cont.)																
POUNDCAKE, OLD-FASHIONED (EQUAL WEIGHTS FLOUR, SUGAR, FAT, EGGS); SLICE, 2¾ IN. BY 3 IN. BY ⅝ IN. . . . 1 SLICE	30	17	140	2	9	2	5	1	14	6	.2	[n]80	.01	.03	.1	0
SPONGE CAKE; SECTOR, 2-IN. (½ OF 8-IN. DIAMETER CAKE) . . . 1 SECTOR	40	32	120	3	2	1	1	TRACE	22	12	.5	180	.02	.06	.1	TRACE
COOKIES:																
PLAIN AND ASSORTED, 3-IN. DIAMETER . . . 1 COOKY	25	3	120	1	5	—	—	—	18	9	.2	20	.01	.01	.1	TRACE
FIG BARS, SMALL . . . 1 FIG BAR	16	14	55	1	1	—	—	—	12	12	.2	20	.01	.01	.1	TRACE
CORN, RICE AND WHEAT FLAKES, MIXED, ADDED NUTRIENTS . . . 1 OZ	28	3	110	2	TRACE	—	—	—	24	11	.5	0	.11	—	.9	0
CORN FLAKES, ADDED NUTRIENTS:																
PLAIN . . . 1 OZ	28	4	110	2	TRACE	—	—	—	24	5	.4	0	.12	.02	.6	0
SUGAR-COVERED . . . 1 OZ	28	2	110	1	TRACE	—	—	—	26	3	.3	0	.12	.01	.5	C
CORN GRITS, DEGERMED, COOKED:																
ENRICHED . . . 1 CUP	242	87	120	3	TRACE	—	—	—	27	2	[o].7	[p]150	[o].10	[o].07	[o]1.0	0
UNENRICHED . . . 1 CUP	242	87	120	3	TRACE	—	—	—	27	2	.2	[p]150	.05	.02	.5	0
CORNMEAL, WHITE OR YELLOW, DRY:																
WHOLE GROUND, UNBOLTED . . . 1 CUP	118	12	420	11	5	1	2	2	87	24	2.8	[p]600	.45	.13	2.4	0
DEGERMED, ENRICHED . . . 1 CUP	145	12	525	11	2	TRACE	1	1	114	9	[o]4.2	[p]640	[o].64	[o].38	[o]5.1	0
CORN MUFFINS, MADE WITH ENRICHED DEGERMED CORNMEAL AND ENRICHED FLOUR; MUFFIN, 2¾-IN. DIAMETER . . . 1 MUFFIN	48	33	150	3	5	2	2	TRACE	23	50	.8	[q]80	.09	.11	.8	TRACE
CORN, PUFFED, PRESWEETENED, ADDED NUTRIENTS . . . 1 OZ	28	5	110	1	TRACE	—	—	—	26	3	.5	0	.12	.05	.6	0
CORN, SHREDDED, ADDED NUTRIENTS . . . 1 OZ	28	3	110	2	TRACE	—	—	—	25	1	.7	0	.12	.05	.6	0
CRACKERS:																
GRAHAM, PLAIN . . . 4 SMALL OR 2 MEDIUM	14	6	55	1	1	—	—	—	10	6	.2	0	.01	.03	.2	0
SALTINES, 2-IN. SQUARE . . . 2 CRACKERS	8	4	35	1	1	—	—	—	6	2	.1	0	TRACE	TRACE	.1	0
SODA:																
CRACKER, 2½-IN. SQUARE . . . 2 CRACKERS	11	4	50	1	1	TRACE	1	TRACE	8	2	.2	0	TRACE	TRACE	.1	0
OYSTER CRACKERS . . . 10 CRACKERS	10	4	45	1	1	TRACE	1	TRACE	7	2	.2	0	TRACE	TRACE	.1	0
CRACKER MEAL . . . 1 TBSP	10	6	45	1	1	TRACE	1	TRACE	7	2	.1	0	.01	TRACE	.1	0
DOUGHNUTS, CAKE TYPE . . . 1 DOUGHNUT	32	24	125	1	6	1	4	TRACE	16	13	[r].4	30	[r].05	[r].05	[r].4	TRACE
FARINA, REGULAR, ENRICHED, COOKED . . . 1 CUP	238	90	100	3	TRACE	—	—	—	21	10	[o].7	0	[o].11	[o].07	[o]1.0	0

MACARONI, COOKED:																
ENRICHED:																
COOKED, FIRM STAGE (8–10 MIN; UNDERGOES ADDITIONAL COOKING IN A FOOD MIXTURE)	1 CUP	130	64	190	6	1	—	—	—	39	14	[o]1.4	0	[o]0.23	[o]0.14	[o]1.9	0
COOKED UNTIL TENDER	1 CUP	140	72	155	5	1	—	—	—	32	11	[o]1.3	0	[o].19	[o].11	[o]1.5	0
UNENRICHED:																
COOKED, FIRM STAGE (8–10 MIN; UNDERGOES ADDITIONAL COOKING IN A FOOD MIXTURE)	1 CUP	130	64	190	6	1	—	—	—	39	14	.6	0	.02	.02	.5	0
COOKED UNTIL TENDER	1 CUP	140	72	155	5	1	—	—	—	32	11	.6	0	.02	.02	.4	0
MACARONI (ENRICHED) AND CHEESE, BAKED	1 CUP	220	58	470	18	24	11	10	1	44	398	2.0	950	.22	.44	2.0	TRACE
MUFFINS, WITH ENRICHED WHITE FLOUR;																
MUFFIN, 2¾-IN. DIAMETER	1 MUFFIN	48	38	140	4	5	1	3	TRACE	20	50	.8	50	.08	.11	.7	TRACE
NOODLES (EGG NOODLES), COOKED:																
ENRICHED	1 CUP	160	70	200	7	2	1	1	TRACE	37	16	[o]1.4	110	[o].23	[o].14	[o]1.8	0
UNENRICHED	1 CUP	160	70	200	7	2	1	1	TRACE	37	16	1.0	110	.04	.03	.7	0
OATS (WITH OR WITHOUT CORN) PUFFED, ADDED NUTRIENTS	1 OZ	28	3	115	3	2	TRACE	1	1	21	50	1.3	0	.28	.05	.5	0
OATMEAL OR ROLLED OATS, REGULAR OR QUICK-COOKING, COOKED	1 CUP	236	86	130	5	2	TRACE	1	1	23	21	1.4	0	.19	.05	.3	0
PANCAKES (GRIDDLECAKES), 4-IN. DIAMETER:																
WHEAT, ENRICHED FLOUR (HOME RECIPE)	1 CAKE	27	50	60	2	2	TRACE	1	TRACE	9	27	.4	30	.05	.06	.3	TRACE
BUCKWHEAT (BUCKWHEAT PANCAKE MIX, MADE WITH EGG AND MILK)	1 CAKE	27	58	55	2	2	1	1	TRACE	6	59	.4	60	.03	.04	.2	TRACE
PIECRUST, PLAIN, BAKED:																
ENRICHED FLOUR:																
LOWER CRUST, 9-IN. SHELL	1 CRUST	135	15	675	8	45	10	29	3	59	19	2.3	0	.27	.19	2.4	0
DOUBLE CRUST, 9-IN. PIE	1 DOUBLE CRUST	270	15	1,350	16	90	21	58	7	118	38	4.6	0	.55	.39	4.9	0
UNENRICHED FLOUR:																
LOWER CRUST, 9-IN. SHELL	1 CRUST	135	15	675	8	45	10	29	3	59	19	.7	0	.04	.04	.6	0
DOUBLE CRUST, 9-IN. PIE	1 DOUBLE CRUST	270	15	1,350	16	90	21	58	7	118	38	1.4	0	.08	.07	1.3	0
PIES (PIECRUST MADE WITH UNENRICHED FLOUR); SECTOR, 4-IN., 1/7 OF 9-IN.-DIAMETER PIE:																
APPLE	1 SECTOR	135	48	345	3	15	4	9	1	51	11	.4	40	.03	.02	.5	1
CHERRY	1 SECTOR	135	47	355	4	15	4	10	1	52	19	.4	590	.03	.03	.6	1
CUSTARD	1 SECTOR	130	58	280	8	14	5	8	1	30	125	.8	300	.07	.21	.4	0
LEMON MERINGUE	1 SECTOR	120	47	305	4	12	4	7	1	45	17	.6	200	.04	.10	.2	4
MINCE	1 SECTOR	135	43	365	3	16	4	10	1	56	38	1.4	TRACE	.09	.05	.5	1
PUMPKIN	1 SECTOR	130	59	275	5	15	5	7	1	32	66	.6	3,210	.04	.13	.6	TRACE

[o] Iron, thiamine, riboflavin, and niacin are based on the minimum levels of enrichment specified in standards of identity promulgated under the Federal Food, Drug, and Cosmetic Act.

[p] Vitamin A value based on yellow product. White product contains only a trace.

[q] Based on recipe using white cornmeal; if yellow cornmeal is used, the vitamin A value is 140 IU per muffin.

[r] Based on product made with enriched flour. With unenriched flour, approximate values per doughnut are iron, 0.2 mg; thiamine, 0.01 mg; riboflavin, 0.03 mg; niacin, 0.2 mg.

TABLE 1 NUTRITIVE VALUES OF THE EDIBLE PART OF FOODS (Cont.)

[Dashes show that no basis could be found for imputing a value although there was some reason to believe that a measurable amount of the constituent might be present.]

FOOD, APPROXIMATE MEASURE, AND WEIGHT	GRAMS	WATER, %	FOOD ENERGY, CALORIES	PROTEIN, G	FAT (TOTAL LIPID), G	FATTY ACIDS SATURATED (TOTAL), G	UNSATURATED OLEIC	LINOLEIC	CARBOHYDRATE, G	CALCIUM, G	IRON, G	VITAMIN A VALUE, INTERNATIONAL UNITS	THIAMINE, G	RIBOFLAVIN, G	NIACIN, G	ASCORBIC ACID, G
GRAIN PRODUCTS (Cont.)																
PIZZA (CHEESE); 5½-IN. SECTOR; ⅛ OF 14-IN. DIAMETER PIE ... 1 SECTOR	75	45	185	7	6	2	3	TRACE	27	107	.7	290	.04	.12	.7	4
POPCORN, POPPED, WITH ADDED OIL AND SALT ... 1 CUP	14	3	65	1	3	2	TRACE	TRACE	8	1	.3	—	—	.01	.2	0
PRETZELS, SMALL STICK ... 5 STICKS	5	8	20	TRACE	TRACE	—	—	—	4	1	0	0	TRACE	TRACE	TRACE	0
RICE, WHITE (FULLY MILLED OR POLISHED), ENRICHED, COOKED:																
COMMON COMMERCIAL VARIETIES, ALL TYPES ... 1 CUP	168	73	185	3	TRACE	—	—	—	41	17	*1.5	0	*.19	*.01	*1.6	0
LONG GRAIN, PARBOILED ... 1 CUP	176	73	185	4	TRACE	—	—	—	41	33	*1.4	0	*.19	*.02	*2.0	0
RICE, PUFFED, ADDED NUTRIENTS (WITHOUT SALT) ... 1 CUP	14	4	55	1	TRACE	—	—	—	13	3	.3	0	.06	.01	.6	0
RICE FLAKES, ADDED NUTRIENTS ... 1 CUP	30	3	115	2	TRACE	—	—	—	26	9	0.5	0	0.10	0.02	1.6	0
ROLLS:																
PLAIN, PAN; 12 PER 16 OZ:																
ENRICHED ... 1 ROLL	38	31	115	3	2	TRACE	1	TRACE	20	28	.7	TRACE	.11	.07	.8	TRACE
UNENRICHED ... 1 ROLL	38	31	115	3	2	TRACE	1	TRACE	20	28	.3	TRACE	.02	.03	.3	TRACE
HARD, ROUND; 12 PER 22 OZ ... 1 ROLL	52	25	160	5	2	TRACE	1	TRACE	31	24	.4	TRACE	.03	.05	.4	TRACE
SWEET, PAN; 12 PER 18 OZ ... 1 ROLL	43	32	135	4	4	1	2	TRACE	21	37	.3	30	.03	.06	.4	TRACE
RYE WAFERS, WHOLE-GRAIN, 1⅞ IN. BY 3½ IN. ... 2 WAFERS	13	6	45	2	TRACE	—	—	—	10	7	.5	0	.04	.03	.2	0
SPAGHETTI:																
COOKED, TENDER STAGE (14–20 MIN):																
ENRICHED ... 1 CUP	140	72	155	5	1	—	—	—	32	11	*1.3	0	*.19	*.11	*1.5	0
UNENRICHED ... 1 CUP	140	72	155	5	1	—	—	—	32	11	.6	0	.02	.02	.4	0
SPAGHETTI WITH MEAT BALLS IN TOMATO SAUCE (HOME RECIPE) ... 1 CUP	250	70	335	19	12	4	6	1	39	125	3.8	1,600	.26	.30	4.0	22
SPAGHETTI IN TOMATO SAUCE WITH CHEESE (HOME RECIPE) ... 1 CUP	250	77	260	9	9	2	5	1	37	80	2.2	1,080	.24	.18	2.4	14
WAFFLES, WITH ENRICHED FLOUR, ½ IN. BY 4½ IN. BY 5½ IN. ... 1 WAFFLE	75	41	210	7	7	2	4	1	28	85	1.3	250	.13	.19	1.0	TRACE
WHEAT, PUFFED:																
WITH ADDED NUTRIENTS (WITHOUT SALT) ... 1 OZ	28	3	105	4	TRACE	—	—	—	22	8	1.2	0	.15	.07	2.2	0
WITH ADDED NUTRIENTS, WITH SUGAR AND HONEY ... 1 OZ	28	3	105	2	1	—	—	—	25	7	.9	0	.14	.05	1.8	0
WHEAT, ROLLED; COOKED ... 1 CUP	236	80	175	5	1	—	—	—	40	19	1.7	0	.17	.06	2.1	0

WHEAT, SHREDDED, PLAIN (LONG, ROUND, OR BITE-SIZE) . . 1 OZ	28	7	100	3	1	—	—	—	23	12	1.0	0	.06	.03	1.2
0															
WHEAT AND MALTED BARLEY FLAKES, WITH ADDED NUTRIENTS . . 1 OZ	28	3	110	2	TRACE	—	—	—	24	14	.7	0	.13	.03	1.1
WHEAT FLAKES, WITH ADDED NUTRIENTS . . 1 OZ	28	4	100	3	TRACE	—	—	—	23	12	1.2	0	.18	.04	1.4
WHEAT FLOURS:															
WHOLE-WHEAT, FROM HARD WHEATS, STIRRED . . 1 CUP	120	12	400	16	2	TRACE	1	1	85	49	4.0	0	.66	.14	5.2
ALL-PURPOSE OR FAMILY FLOUR:															
ENRICHED, SIFTED . . 1 CUP	110	12	400	12	1	TRACE	TRACE	TRACE	84	18	°3.2	0	.48	°.29	°3.8
UNENRICHED, SIFTED . . 1 CUP	110	12	400	12	1	TRACE	TRACE	TRACE	84	18	.9	0	.07	.05	1.0
SELF-RISING, ENRICHED . . 1 CUP	110	11	385	11	1	TRACE	TRACE	TRACE	82	292	°3.2	0	°.49	°.29	°3.9
CAKE OR PASTRY FLOUR, SIFTED . . 1 CUP	100	12	365	8	1	TRACE	TRACE	TRACE	79	17	.5	0	.03	.03	.7
WHEAT GERM, CRUDE, COMMERCIALLY MILLED . . 1 CUP	68	11	245	18	7	1	2	4	32	49	6.4	0	1.36	.46	2.9

FATS, OILS

BUTTER, 4 STICKS PER LB:															
STICKS, 2 . . 1 CUP	227	16	1,625	1	184	101	61	6	1	45	0	[b]7,500	—	—	—
STICK, ⅛ . . 1 TBSP	14	16	100	TRACE	11	6	4	TRACE	TRACE	3	0	[b]460	—	—	—
PAT OR SQUARE (64 PER LB) . . 1 PAT	7	16	50	TRACE	6	3	2	TRACE	TRACE	1	0	[b]230	—	—	—
FATS, COOKING:															
LARD . . 1 CUP	220	0	1,985	0	220	84	101	22	0	0	0	0	0	0	0
LARD . . 1 TBSP	14	0	125	0	14	5	6	1	0	0	0	0	0	0	0
VEGETABLE FATS . . 1 CUP	200	0	1,770	0	200	46	130	14	0	0	0	—	0	0	0
VEGETABLE FATS . . 1 TBSP	12.5	0	110	0	12	3	8	1	0	0	0	—	0	0	0
MARGARINE, 4 STICKS PER LB:															
STICKS, 2 . . 1 CUP	227	16	1,635	1	184	37	105	33	1	45	0	[c]7,500	—	—	—
STICK, ⅛ . . 1 TBSP	14	16	100	TRACE	11	2	6	2	TRACE	3	0	[c]460	—	—	—
PAT OR SQUARE (64 PER LB) . . 1 PAT	7	16	50	TRACE	6	1	3	1	TRACE	1	0	[c]230	—	—	—
OILS, SALAD OR COOKING:															
CORN . . 1 TBSP	14	0	125	0	14	1	4	7	0	0	0	—	0	0	0
COTTONSEED . . 1 TBSP	14	0	125	0	14	4	3	7	0	0	0	—	0	0	0
OLIVE . . 1 TBSP	14	0	125	0	14	2	11	1	0	0	0	—	0	0	0
SOYBEAN . . 1 TBSP	14	0	125	0	14	2	3	7	0	0	0	—	0	0	0
SALAD DRESSINGS:															
BLUE CHEESE . . 1 TBSP	16	32	80	1	8	2	2	4	1	13	TRACE	30	TRACE	0.02	TRACE
COMMERCIAL, MAYONNAISE TYPE . . 1 TBSP	15	41	65	TRACE	6	1	1	3	2	2	TRACE	30	TRACE	TRACE	TRACE
FRENCH . . 1 TBSP	15	39	60	TRACE	6	1	1	3	3	2	.1	—	.01	.03	.03
HOME COOKED, BOILED . . 1 TBSP	17	68	30	1	2	1	1	TRACE	3	15	.1	80	TRACE	.01	.01
MAYONNAISE . . 1 TBSP	15	15	110	TRACE	12	2	3	6	TRACE	3	.1	40	TRACE	TRACE	TRACE
THOUSAND ISLAND . . 1 TBSP	15	32	75	TRACE	8	1	2	4	2	2	.1	50	TRACE	TRACE	TRACE

Ascorbic acid column (rightmost): 0 for all wheat and flour items and wheat germ; 0 for butter and lard; — for vegetable fats; 0 for margarine and oils; salad dressings: TRACE, —, TRACE, —, TRACE, TRACE.

° Iron, thiamine, riboflavin, and niacin are based on the minimum levels of enrichment specified in standards of identity promulgated under the Federal Food, Drug, and Cosmetic Act.

[a] Iron, thiamine, and niacin are based on the minimum levels of enrichment specified in standards of identity promulgated under the Federal Food, Drug, and Cosmetic Act. Riboflavin is based on unenriched rice. When the minimum level of enrichment for riboflavin specified in the standards of identity becomes effective the value will be 0.12 mg per cup of parboiled rice and of white rice.

[b] Year-round average.

[c] Based on the average vitamin A content of fortified margarine. Federal specifications for fortified margarine require a minimum of 15,000 IU of vitamin A per pound.

TABLE 1 NUTRITIVE VALUES OF THE EDIBLE PART OF FOODS (Cont.)

[Dashes show that no basis could be found for imputing a value although there was some reason to believe that a measurable amount of the constituent might be present.]

FOOD, APPROXIMATE MEASURE, AND WEIGHT	GRAMS	WATER, %	FOOD ENERGY, CALORIES	PROTEIN, G	FAT (TOTAL LIPID), G	FATTY ACIDS SATURATED (TOTAL), G	UNSATURATED OLEIC	UNSATURATED LINOLEIC	CARBOHYDRATE, G	CALCIUM, G	IRON, G	VITAMIN A VALUE, INTERNATIONAL UNITS	THIAMINE, G	RIBOFLAVIN, G	NIACIN, G	ASCORBIC ACID, G
SUGARS, SWEETS																
CANDY:																
CARAMELS . . . . 1 OZ	28	8	115	1	3	2	1	TRACE	22	42	.4	TRACE	.01	.05	TRACE	TRACE
CHOCOLATE, MILK, PLAIN . . . 1 OZ	28	1	150	2	9	5	3	TRACE	16	65	.3	80	.02	.09	.1	TRACE
FUDGE, PLAIN . . . . . . 1 OZ	28	8	115	1	3	2	1	TRACE	21	22	.3	TRACE	.01	.03	.1	TRACE
HARD CANDY . . . . . . 1 OZ	28	1	110	0	TRACE	—	—	—	28	6	.5	0	0	0	0	0
MARSHMALLOWS . . . . . 1 OZ	28	17	90	1	TRACE	—	—	—	23	5	.5	0	0	TRACE	TRACE	0
CHOCOLATE SIRUP, THIN TYPE . 1 TBSP	20	32	50	TRACE	TRACE	TRACE	TRACE	TRACE	13	3	.3	—	TRACE	.01	.1	0
HONEY, STRAINED OR EXTRACTED 1 TBSP	21	17	65	TRACE	0	—	—	—	17	1	.1	0	TRACE	.01	.1	TRACE
JAMS AND PRESERVES . . . 1 TBSP	20	29	55	TRACE	TRACE	—	—	—	14	4	.2	TRACE	TRACE	.01	TRACE	TRACE
JELLIES . . . . 1 TBSP	20	29	55	TRACE	TRACE	—	—	—	14	4	.3	TRACE	TRACE	.01	TRACE	1
MOLASSES, CANE:																
LIGHT (FIRST EXTRACTION) . . 1 TBSP	20	24	50	—	—	—	—	—	13	33	.9	—	.01	.01	TRACE	—
BLACKSTRAP (THIRD EXTRACTION) 1 TBSP	20	24	45	—	—	—	—	—	11	137	3.2	—	.02	.04	.4	—
SIRUP, TABLE BLENDS (CHIEFLY CORN), LIGHT AND DARK) . . 1 TBSP	20	24	60	0	0	—	—	—	15	9	.8	0	0	0	0	0
SUGARS (CANE OR BEET):																
GRANULATED . . . . . . 1 CUP	200	TRACE	770	0	0	—	—	—	199	0	.2	0	0	0	0	0
. . . . 1 TBSP	12	TRACE	45	0	0	—	—	—	12	0	TRACE	0	0	0	0	0
LUMP, 1⅛ IN. BY ¾ IN. BY ⅜ IN. 1 LUMP	6	TRACE	25	0	0	—	—	—	6	0	TRACE	0	0	0	0	0
POWDERED, STIRRED BEFORE . 1 CUP	128	TRACE	495	0	0	—	—	—	127	0	.1	0	0	0	0	0
MEASURING . . . . . . 1 TBSP	8	TRACE	30	0	0	—	—	—	8	0	TRACE	0	0	0	0	0
BROWN, FIRM-PACKED . . . 1 CUP	220	2	820	0	0	—	—	—	212	187	7.5	0	.02	.07	.4	0
. . . . 1 TBSP	14	2	50	0	0	—	—	—	13	12	.5	0	TRACE	TRACE	TRACE	0
MISCELLANEOUS ITEMS																
BEER (AVERAGE 3.6% ALCOHOL BY WEIGHT) . . . . . . 1 CUP	240	92	100	1	0	—	—	—	9	12	TRACE	—	.01	.07	1.6	—
BEVERAGES, CARBONATED:																
COLA TYPE . . . . . . 1 CUP	240	90	95	0	0	—	—	—	24	—	—	0	0	0	0	0
GINGER ALE . . . . . . 1 CUP	230	92	70	0	0	—	—	—	18	—	—	0	0	0	0	0
BOUILLON CUBE, ⅝ IN. . . . 1 CUBE	4	4	5	1	TRACE	—	—	—	TRACE	—	—	—	—	—	—	—
CHILI POWDER. see VEGETABLES, PEPPERS.																
CHILI SAUCE (MAINLY TOMATOES) 1 TBSP	17	68	20	TRACE	TRACE	—	—	—	4	3	.1	240	.02	.01	.3	3
CHOCOLATE:																
BITTER OR BAKING . . . . 1 OZ	28	2	145	3	15	8	6	TRACE	8	22	1.9	20	.01	.07	.4	0
SWEET . . . . 1 OZ	28	1	150	1	10	6	4	TRACE	16	27	.4	TRACE	.01	.04	.1	TRACE
CIDER. see FRUITS, APPLE JUICE.																

Food	Measure	Grams	Water (%)	Food energy (cal.)	Protein (g)	Fat (g)	Saturated fat (g)	Oleic (g)	Linoleic (g)	Carbo-hydrate (g)	Calcium (mg)	Iron (mg)	Vitamin A (I.U.)	Thiamine (mg)	Riboflavin (mg)	Niacin (mg)	Ascorbic acid (mg)
GELATIN, DRY:																	
PLAIN	1 TBSP	10	13	35	9	TRACE	—	—	—	0	—	—	—	—	—	—	—
DESSERT POWDER, 3-OZ PACKAGE	1/2 CUP	85	2	315	8	0	—	—	—	75	—	—	—	—	—	—	—
GELATIN DESSERT, READY-TO-EAT:																	
PLAIN	1 CUP	239	84	140	4	0	—	—	—	34	—	—	—	—	—	—	—
WITH FRUIT	1 CUP	241	82	160	3	TRACE	—	—	—	40	—	—	—	—	—	—	—
OLIVES, PICKLED:																	
GREEN	4 MEDIUM OR 3 EXTRA LARGE OR 2 GIANT	16	78	15	TRACE	2	TRACE	2	TRACE	TRACE	8	.2	40	—	—	—	—
RIPE: MISSION	3 SMALL OR 2 LARGE	10	73	15	TRACE	2	TRACE	2	TRACE	TRACE	9	.1	10	TRACE	TRACE	—	—
PICKLES, CUCUMBER:																	
DILL, LARGE, 4 IN. BY 1¾ IN.	1 PICKLE	135	93	15	1	TRACE	—	—	—	3	35	1.4	140	TRACE	.03	TRACE	8
SWEET, 2¾ IN. BY ¾ IN.	1 PICKLE	20	61	30	TRACE	TRACE	—	—	—	7	2	.2	20	TRACE	TRACE	TRACE	1
POPCORN. see GRAIN PRODUCTS.																	
SHERBET, ORANGE	1 CUP	193	67	260	2	2	—	—	—	59	31	TRACE	110	.02	.06	TRACE	4
SOUPS, CANNED; READY-TO-SERVE (PREPARED WITH EQUAL VOLUME OF WATER):																	
BEAN WITH PORK	1 CUP	250	84	170	8	6	2	2	1	22	62	2.2	650	.14	.07	1.0	2
BEEF NOODLE	1 CUP	250	93	70	4	3	1	1	1	7	8	1.0	50	.05	.06	1.1	TRACE
BEEF BOUILLON, BROTH, CONSOMME	1 CUP	240	96	30	5	0	0	0	0	3	TRACE	.5	TRACE	TRACE	.02	1.2	TRACE
CHICKEN NOODLE	1 CUP	250	93	65	4	2	1	1	1	8	10	.5	50	.02	.02	0.8	TRACE
CLAM CHOWDER	1 CUP	255	92	85	2	3	—	—	—	13	36	1.0	920	.03	.03	1.0	—
CREAM SOUP (MUSHROOM)	1 CUP	240	90	135	2	10	5	3	5	10	41	.5	70	.02	.12	.7	—
MINESTRONE	1 CUP	245	90	105	5	3	1	1	1	14	37	1.0	2,350	.07	.05	1.0	—
PEA, GREEN	1 CUP	245	86	130	6	2	1	1	1	23	44	1.0	340	.05	.05	1.0	7
TOMATO	1 CUP	245	90	90	2	2	1	1	1	16	15	.7	1,000	.06	.05	1.1	12
VEGETABLE WITH BEEF BROTH	1 CUP	250	92	80	3	2	1	1	1	14	20	.8	3,250	.05	.02	1.2	—
STARCH (CORNSTARCH)	1 CUP	128	12	465	TRACE	TRACE	—	—	—	112	0	0	0	0	0	0	0
	1 TBSP	8	12	30	TRACE	TRACE	—	—	—	7	0	0	0	0	0	0	0
TAPIOCA, QUICK-COOKING	1 CUP	152	13	535	1	TRACE	—	—	—	131	15	.6	0	0	0	0	0
GRANULATED, DRY, STIRRED BEFORE MEASURING	1 TBSP	10	13	35	TRACE	TRACE	—	—	—	9	1	TRACE	0	0	0	0	0
VINEGAR	1 TBSP	15	—	2	0	—	—	—	—	1	1	.1	—	—	—	—	—
WHITE SAUCE, MEDIUM	1 CUP	265	73	430	10	33	18	11	1	23	305	.5	1,220	.12	.44	.6	2
YEAST:																	
BAKER'S: COMPRESSED	1 OZ	28	71	25	3	TRACE	—	—	—	3	4	1.4	TRACE	.20	.47	3.2	TRACE
DRY ACTIVE	1 OZ	28	5	80	10	TRACE	—	—	—	11	12	4.6	TRACE	.66	1.53	10.4	TRACE
BREWER'S, DRY, DEBITTERED	1 TBSP	8	5	25	3	TRACE	—	—	—	3	17	1.4	TRACE	1.25	.34	3.0	TRACE
YOGHURT. see MILK, CREAM, CHEESE; RELATED PRODUCTS.																	

TABLE 2   YIELD OF COOKED MEAT PER POUND OF RAW MEAT

MEAT AS PURCHASED	MEAT AFTER COOKING (LESS DRIPPINGS)	
	PARTS WEIGHED	APPROXIMATE WEIGHT OF COOKED PARTS PER POUND OF RAW MEAT PURCHASED, OZ
CHOPS OR STEAKS FOR BROILING OR FRYING:		
WITH BONE AND RELATIVELY LARGE AMOUNT OF FAT, SUCH AS PORK OR LAMB CHOPS; BEEF RIB, SIRLOIN, OR PORTERHOUSE STEAKS	LEAN, BONE, FAT	10–12
	LEAN AND FAT	7–10
	LEAN ONLY	5–7
WITHOUT BONE AND WITH VERY LITTLE FAT, SUCH AS ROUND OF BEEF, VEAL STEAKS	LEAN AND FAT	12–13
	LEAN ONLY	9–12
GROUND MEAT FOR BROILING OR FRYING, SUCH AS HAMBURGER, LAMB, OR PORK PATTIES	PATTIES	9–13
ROASTS FOR OVEN COOKING (NO LIQUID ADDED):		
WITH BONE AND RELATIVELY LARGE AMOUNT OF FAT, SUCH AS BEEF RIB, LOIN, CHUCK; LAMB SHOULDER, LEG; PORK, FRESH OR CURED	LEAN, BONE, FAT	10–12
	LEAN AND FAT	8–10
	LEAN ONLY	6–9
WITHOUT BONE	LEAN AND FAT	10–12
	LEAN ONLY	7–10
CUTS FOR POT-ROASTING, SIMMERING, BRAISING, STEWING:		
WITH BONE AND RELATIVELY LARGE AMOUNT OF FAT, SUCH AS BEEF CHUCK, PORK SHOULDER	LEAN, BONE, FAT	10–11
	LEAN AND FAT	8–9
	LEAN ONLY	6–8
WITHOUT BONE AND WITH RELATIVELY SMALL AMOUNT OF FAT, SUCH AS TRIMMED BEEF, VEAL	LEAN WITH ADHERING FAT. .	9–11

Index

A Glossary has been incorporated into this index. Glossary terms, in **boldface**, are followed by their definitions and any Subject Index page references, subentries, and/or cross-references.

Abdominal pain, 178–179
Abortion. Expulsion of product of conception during the first 3 months of pregnancy (*See also* **Fetal death**). 25–27, 318–319, 397
  chemical means, 318
  denied, 336
  illegal, 318
  risk, 26
  safety, 26
  smoking, 99
  therapeutic, 318–319
Abrasions, 265
Abscess. A collection of pus in the body, localized by surrounding tissue, usually painful, and occasionally causing serious illness.
  apical, 224
Absorption. The transfer into the blood of materials such as water and food

from the intestinal tract, toxins from an area of infection, and drugs from mucous membranes. 176
Accidents, 6–8, 83, 79ff., 350, 351
  athletic, 82–83
  automobile, 350
  cerebrovascular (*see* Stroke)
  home, 80
    decline, 82
  industrial, 369–370
  occupational, 82
  public, 82–83
  rates, 80
  school, 382
  smoking, 99
  traffic, and alcohol, 112
  in transportation, 80
  work, 82
Achievement, 131

Acid, lactic, 197
  (*See also* LSD)
Acidosis. A condition in which circulating acids increase and circulating alkalis diminish. May be potentially fatal in severe cases, as in diabetic acidosis (*See also* Diabetes).
Acne, 228
Acromegaly, 297
ACTH in arthritis, 85
Actinomycin D, 332
Activity, 61
  physical, 174
Addiction, 110
  nicotine, 94
  treatment, 120
Addicts, narcotic, 265
Addison's disease, 296
Adenitis. Inflammation of a lymph node.

Adenoids, 214, 215
Adenoviruses, 274
Adolescence, 12
Adrenal (suprarenal). Two glands of internal secretion which lie just above the kidneys (*See also* **Adrenal hormones**).
Adrenal hormones, 94
Adrenalin (*see* Epinephrine)
Age:
  life expectancy with, 4
    at 1 year, 4
  risks of air pollution, 35
Age-adjusted death rate. The computed death rate which would have resulted if the age distribution of the population had remained constant.
Agency for International Development, 400–421
Aggression, 133
  and traffic, 14
Aging, 191, 345ff.
Agranulocytosis. An acute disease with a marked decrease in number of white blood cells in the blood.
Agriculture, Department of, 393
  mechanization, 27
  (*See also* Farmers; Nutrition)
Air, fresh, 187–190
  (*See also* Pollution)
Air pressure, 369
Air sacs, 187, 285
Airlines and railroads, smoking, 102
Albumin. A protein found in nearly every animal tissue and fluid.
Albuminuria. The occurrence of albumin in the urine; usually denotes some disturbance of the kidneys.
Alcohol, 110ff.
  accidents, 112
  costs, 112
  diseases of, 111
  drinking patterns, 113–114
  drinking types, 113–114
  effects, 111
  metabolism, 111
  traffic accidents, 14
  wood, 205
Alcoholics Anonymous, 116, 376
Alcoholism:
  chronic, 114ff.
    causes, 114–115
    patterns and development, 114
  legal aspects, 116–117
  personality and culture, 115
  prevention and treatment, 116
Aldosterone, 290, 291
Alkaline. Having the properties of an alkali; the opposite of acid.

Allergies, 275
Allergy. Hypersensitiveness of an individual to some chemical substance called an antigen, usually protein in nature. 286
Alopecia, 235
Alum, 29
Aluminum, 29
Alveoli, 187
American Board, specialty certification, 48
American Cancer Society, 72, 76, 88, 101, 285, 404
American College Health Association, 412
American Heart Association, 405
American Medical Association, 82, 407
  Council on Medical Education, 45
American Public Health Association, 407
American Red Cross, 405
American Social Health Association, 314, 405
Amino acids, 158, 166
Amnion. The innermost membrane covering the embryo.
Amnionic sac, 318
Amphetamines, 118, 119, 177, 198
Amygdala, 133
Anaerobic. Referring to bacteria which thrive best in the absence of free oxygen or air.
Analgesic. A drug to relieve pain.
Anatomy of the personality, 126ff.
Anderson, Robert, 358
Anemia. Deficient quantity of hemoglobin reducing its capacity to carry oxygen. 75
  pernicious, 164
Anger, 133
Angina. From the Latin word "to throttle." Most often used in angina pectoris, the term for a heart condition in which attacks of constricting chest pain occur (*See also* Coronary heart disease). Also, a painful, constricting throat infection.
Angina pectoris, 61
Animals (*see* Zoonoses)
Ankylosis. Abnormal immobility of a joint.
Anomaly. Something which is out of the ordinary; an irregularity.
Anonymity of the highway, 14
Anorexia. Loss of appetite.
Anoxia, 188
Anthrax, 249, 252
Antibiotic. A drug effective against microorganisms.

Antibiotics, 3, 60, 246, 281
  in colds, 279
Antibodies, 243
  specific, 244
Antidepressants, 142
Antigens, 244
Antihistamines, 217
Antimony, 180
Antiperspirants, 235
Antiseptics, 243, 278
Anus, 156
Anxiety, 133
Aorta in syphilis, 315
Aortic aneurysm, 98
Apoplexy, 6, 350
  (*See also* Strokes)
Appendicitis, 184
Appendix, 156
Appetite and amphetamines, 119
Armed Forces, health, 8
Arousal, sexual, 305
Arsenic, 371
Arteries, 66
  coronary, 60
Arteriosclerosis, 6, 60, 351
Artery. A blood vessel which conveys blood away from the heart.
Arthralgia, 83
Arthritis, 83ff., 352
  definition, 83
  degenerative, 12
    or osteoarthritis, 84
  rheumatoid, 79, 83–85, 146
    treatment, 85
  treatment, 85–86
Arthritis and Rheumatism Foundation, 405
Arthropods, 248
Artificial respiration, 83
Asbestos, 71, 370
Ascorbic acid, 165–166
Asepsis. Aseptic state; free from harmful organisms, as in surgery.
Asphyxia. Unconsciousness or death from lack of oxygen in the blood.
Aspirin, 55, 56, 278–279
  in arthritis, 85
  poisoning, 81
Assimilation. The process of absorption of nourishment and transformation of it into tissues.
Association of American Medical Colleges, 45
Asthma, 128–129, 286
  treatment, 286–287
Astigmatism, 208
Astringent. A substance which causes contraction of tissues and decreases discharges.
Atabrine, 246

Atelectasis. Partial collapse or incomplete expansion of the lungs.
Atherosclerosis. A type of arteriosclerosis (hardening of the arteries) in which the artery's wall contains plaques (streaks) of fatty materials. Afflicts the coronary arteries, causing heart disease. 60, 67
(*See also* Heart disease)
Athletes, 193
  performance, 192
  superior, 192
Athletic programs, 192–193
Athletics, skills, 12
Atomic Energy Commission, 38, 39
Atrophy. Wasting or diminution in size.
Atropine, 207
Attention, 337
  span, 383
Attenuated. Weakened.
Attitudes toward self, 126
Automobiles:
  effect on pollution, 40
  exhaust, 35
  pollution-free, 36
  (*See also* Pollution; Traffic)
Autonomic nervous system. That portion of the nervous system which regulates the action of involuntary muscles, blood vessels, and the organs and glands of the body.
Autonomy, 126
Autopsy. Dissection of a dead body to learn the cause, seat, or nature of disease, or the cause of death; postmortem examination. 356

Babies:
  bottle-fed, 337
  breast-fed, 337
  newborn, 4
Bacilli, 240
Back, 196–197
Backaches, 196
Bacteremia. The presence of bacteria in the bloodstream.
Bacteria (bacterium). One-celled microorganisms that multiply by simple division and occur in three main forms: cocci (spherical), bacilli (rod-shaped), and spirilla (spiral-shaped). 18, 240
  arthritis, 86
  and caries, 220
  gram-negative, 246
  nitrogen fixing, 157
Bacteriophages, 240
Bags, inflatable, 15
Baldness, 236

Banting, F. G., 294
Baptists and alcohol, 115
Barbiturates, 118
Barium carbonate, 180
Barium meal. A suspension of barium that is drunk in order to show by x-ray the passage of food in the digestive tract.
Baths for colds, 278
BCG (bacillus Calmette-Guérin) vaccine, 284
Beef, 182
Behavior therapy, 149
Belts, seat, 15
Bends, the (*see* Caisson disease)
Benign. Harmless. Not cancerous.
Beriberi, 164–165
Beryllium, 371
Best, C. H., 294
Bifocals, 348
Bile ducts, 156
Bill of rights for athletes, 82
Biochemistry, cellular, 292
Biopsy. The excision of a piece of living tissue for microscopic examination.
Birds, 252
Birth, vision at, 207
Birth control, 24–25
  (*See also* Contraception; Population)
Birth rate, 22
Birthmarks, 228
Bisexuals, 309
Black Death, 252
Blackheads, 228
Bladder, urinary, cancer, 74–75
Bleeding, cancer, 74
Blindness, 202
  color, 208–209
Bloating, 183
Blood, 187
  plasma, 8
Blood cells:
  red, 188
  white, 243
Blood pressure, high, 172
  (*See also* Hypertension)
Blood sugar, low, 205
Blood vessels, 160
  alcohol and, 111
  exercise and, 12
Bloodstream, 177
Blue babies, 65
Blue Cross-Blue Shield, 50
  (*See also* Insurance)
Body and mind, 127
Body temperature, 226–227
Boiling, water supplies, 30
Boils, 228
Bombs, atomic and hydrogen, 39
Booster shot, 265

Borlong, Norman E., 416
Botulism, 179
Bovine. Pertaining to cows.
Bowel, 183
Brain, 188, 251
  damage in heart attack, 67
  and diet, 167
  in syphilis, 315
Brave New World, 342
Breast:
  cancer, 70
    prevention, 73
    prognosis, 73
    treatment, 73
  in pregnancy, 330
  self-examination, 72
Breast feeding, 337
Breath, bad, 226
Breathing, obstructions to, 214
Breatholater, 14
Bright's disease (*see* Nephritis)
Bronchi, 94, 281
Bronchitis. Inflammation of the bronchi. 6, 267
  chronic, 34, 284, 285
  smoking, 98
Bronchopneumonia, 281
Bronchoscope. An instrument for looking into the bronchi.
Bronchus (bronchi). A bronchial tube, one of the divisions, large or small, of the trachea (wind pipe) in the lungs.
Brouha step test, 11
Brucellosis, 182, 248, 249
Buboes, 252
Buerger's disease, 97
Bureau of Census, 87
Bureau of Narcotics and Dangerous Drugs, 121
Burkitt's lymphoma, 76

Cabins, pressurized, 188
Cadmium, 180, 371
Caffeine, 119, 122
Caisson disease, 188, 369
Calcium, 162, 220
Calculus, 224
California, abortion, 26
Calories:
  definition and sources, 159
  empty, 167, 169
Canada, 51
Cancer. A collection of body tissue cells which reproduce rapidly and without limit until they destroy life; a malignant tumor, which usually gives rise to secondary growths (metastases). 6–8, 68ff., 184, 351, 352
  and age, 12

in asbestos workers, 370
basal-cell, 233
breast, 70–73
causes and nature, 69
death rates, 3
digestive, 70
digestive organs, 74
epidemiology, 69
epidermoid, 233
genes and heredity, 70
larynx, rehabilitation, 86
lung, 70
  and air pollution, 34
    versus cigarettes, 35
oral, smoking, 96
penis, 76
prevention, 77
  and control, 75–76
quackery, 77
seven warning signals, 76
sites, 68
of skin, 75, 93, 232ff.
  diagnosis, prevention, and
    treatment, 233
smoking pipe and cigars, 100
tobacco, smoking, 95
treatment, 76–77
uterus, 73–74
Cannabis (see Marijuana)
Capillaries, 187
Capillary. A tiny blood vessel
  connecting artery and vein. Transfer
  of oxygen, carbon dioxide, and
  nutriments between blood and
  tissue occurs through the walls of
  capillaries, for the most part.
Carbohydrates, 158–160, 174–175,
  297
  in fruits and vegetables, 168
Carbon dioxide, 157, 187, 188
Carbon monoxide, 34, 93, 372
Carboxyhemoglobin, 34
Carcinogen. A substance that produces
  cancer.
Carcinoma. Cancer arising from
  epithelial tissue.
Cardiovascular system, 192
Care, medical: financing, 50
  prepayment, 52
Caries, 220
Carious. Affected with caries (decay).
  Usually used of teeth.
Carrier of disease, 241
Cars (see Traffic)
Carson, Rachel, 180
Case finding, 317
Cataract. Opacity of the lens of the eye.
Cataracts, 204, 348
Catharsis, 148
Cathartic. A medicine which causes
  emptying of the bowels. 185

Cecum. A pouch which forms the first
  part of the large intestine.
Cell. A minute mass of protoplasm
  which is the structural and
  functional unit of plants and
  animals.
Cells:
  in cancer, 69
  Leydig, 302
Cementum, 219
Cereals, 159
Cerebellum. A division of the brain
  located in the base of the skull just
  above the neck. It is particularly
  important for coordination of
  motion.
Cerebral. Pertaining to the cerebrum,
  the larger part of the brain.
Cerebral cortex, 290
Cerumen, 212
Cervix. A neck or neck-like part.
  Usually applies to the entrance to
  the uterus. 303
  (See also Uterus)
Cesarean section, 330
Cesspool. A pit dug in the ground,
  usually lined with stone and capped
  with some solid cover, into which
  the sewage of a household is
  drained. Inferior to a septic tank
  if a public sewer is not available
  (See also **Septic tank**). 32
Chagas' disease, 249
Chancre, 314
  soft, 316
Chapping, 227
Character:
  development, 13
  disorders, 146
Cheating, 127
Checkup (see Examinations)
Chemicals in food, 180
Chemotherapy of cancer, 76
Chicago, air pollution, 34
Chicken pox, 247
Child-rearing, 336–338
Children:
  emotionally sick, 147
  food poisoning, 37
  number of, 22
  raising, 336–338
  unwanted, 336
Children's Bureau, 392
Chill, wind, 190
Chilling, 274
  and colds, 17
Chiropractic, 53–54
Chlorine, 30
Chlorophyll, 157
Chloroquine, 246, 254–255
Cholera, 29

Cholesterol. A crystalline fatlike
  substance found in all animal fats;
  in bile, blood, brain tissue, nerve
  fibers; in milk and yolk of egg; in
  liver, kidneys, and adrenal glands.
  It constitutes a large part of most
  gallstones and occurs in atheroma
  of the arteries. 161
Choriocarcinoma, 76, 332
Choroid, 202
Chromosomes. That part of cells which
  carry hereditary characteristics;
  composed largely of genes. 328, 339
  sex, 339
Cigarettes, 91ff.
  advertising, 388–389
  and cancer, 70–71
  filter-tip, 103
  length, 103
  less harmful, 103
  in pregnancy, 330
  and traffic accidents, 15
  (See also Smoking)
Cigars, 95
Cilia, 94, 276
Ciliary muscle. A muscle which
  regulates the thickness of the lens
  of the eye.
Cinder, 205
Circulation, smoking, 93, 94
Circulatory system diseases, 59ff.
  (See also Blood vessels; Heart;
  Hypertension)
Cirrhosis. Hardening of an organ,
  especially of the liver, due to
  excessive formation of connective
  tissue as a result of inflammation.
  111–112
  smoking, 98
  (See also Liver)
Clams, 180
Clean Air Act, 395
Clean Air Amendments Act of 1970, 35
Clean Waters Restoration Act, 395
Cleanliness:
  of hair, 235
  of teeth, 224, 225
Climate, 274
Clinics, mental health, 368
Clitoris, 301, 302
Clomiphene, 329
Clostridium, 179
Clostridium botulinum, 179
Clothing, 334
Clots (see Thrombosis)
Clotting, 164
Coalition for a National Population
  Policy, 417
Cobalt therapy in cancer, 76
Cocaine. A drug which comes from the
  leaves of the coca tree and is a

local anesthetic; cocaine addicts refer to the drug as "snow." 110, 119–120
Cocarcinogens, 93
Cocci, 240
Cochlea, 213
Cocoa, 122
Codeine-papaverine, 279
Coffee, 109, 122
Coitus interruptus, 333
Coitus reservatus, 305
Cola, 110, 122
Colchicine, 85
Cold:
  causes, 17
  common, 17, 214, 273–279
    complications, 275
    epidemiology, 275
    prevention, 275–277
    treatment of, 278–279
Colitis, 7
  arthritis, 86
  mucous, 183
  spastic, 183
  ulcerative, 129, 146
College:
  counseling services, 13
  health patterns, 19
  health services, 19
  life, 19
  psychiatric services, 13
  years, 11
  (*See also* Students)
Colon, 156, 183, 184
  cancer, 74
  irritable, 183
Colorado, abortion, 26
Common cold (*see* Cold)
Commonwealth Fund, 406
Communists, 308
Community health, 363ff.
Companionship, 131
Conditioning, physical, 193
Condom, 316, 333–334
Conductors, bus, London, 193
Conflicts, psychological, 131ff.
Congenital. Present at birth; literally, "born with."
Congenital anomalies. Malformations, anomalies, or deformities present when a person is born; sometimes congenital anomalies may not be evident or may not be noticed at the time of birth.
Congestion. Overfullness of capillaries or other blood vessels in any locality or organ.
Conjunctiva. The mucous membrane which covers the front of the eyeball and lines the eyelids.
Conjunctivitis, 205

granular, 203
of newborn, 204
Connecticut, accident death rate, 80
Conscience and superego, 127
Consistency in personal goals, 12
Constipation, 182, 183
Contact, 317
Contagions, 240ff.
Contamination (*see* Pollution)
Construction, accidents, 82
Contraception, 25, 332–336, 395
  as national policy, 27
  results of, 332
Contraceptives:
  folk, 333
  oral, 334
  techniques, 332
Contraction, 330
Contributions to society, 4
Cornea. The transparent portion of the front of the eyeball. 202, 208
Corona, 301
Coronary (*see* Arteries; Heart disease; Infarction; Thrombosis)
Coronary heart disease, 60ff.
  (*See also* Heart disease)
Coronary thrombosis. Development of obstruction due to a clot formed in the coronary arteries of the heart.
Corpsmen, medical, 44
Corpus luteum. The yellow mass in an ovary in the place of a discharged ovum; produces an internal secretion. 303, 304
Cortex. The external layer of an organ.
Cortisone, 19, 231, 291
  in arthritis, 85
Coryza. Acute cold in the head with watery discharge.
Cosmetics, 233–234
Costs, medical, 43, 50
Cough, 284
Coughing in tuberculosis, 282
Counseling in the healthy, 13
  (*See also* Psychiatry)
Course, medical, 46–47
  duration, 46
  organization, 46
Cowpox, 45, 262
Cox, Rachel Dunaway, 126
Cramps:
  heat, 191
  menstrual, 303
Creams:
  face, 233–234
  vanishing, 234
Creighton, Michael, 43
Cremation, 356
Cretinism, 136, 296, 338
Cretins, 296

Cross-eye, 207–208
Crowding, 28
Crown, 219
Cryptococcosis, 253
Cults, healing, 53
Culture in alcoholism, 115
Curie, Marie, 38
Curie, Pierre, 38
Cuspids, 220
Cytoplasm. The substance of the cell outside the nucleus.

Dame, Donald, 59
Dandruff, 235
Darwin, Charles, 5, 39
Dating, 319–320
  decline of, 320
Daydreaming, 132
Daytop (drug rehabilitation community), 120
DDT, 8, 36–37, 254, 256
Deaf, employment, 88
Deafness, 212
  conduction, 212
  services for, 213–214
Death, 356–359
  changes of causes of, 6
  preventable causes of, 5
  rates, 22
  from strokes, 67
Decay, dental, 220
Decision-making, 346
Defecation. Discharge of the feces.
Defects:
  birth, 268
  congenital, 328
  hereditary, 204
  septal, 342
  visual, 206
Deglutition. Swallowing.
Delirium. A disordered mental state in which there may be hallucinations, illusions, or delusions.
Delirium tremens, 110, 112
Delusion. An erroneous belief or idea held by an individual even when sound evidence is presented to prove it is false, such as "delusions of grandeur." 140
Demerol, 110
Demyelination, 86
Dengue, 257
Denial, 134
Dental decay, 220
  fluorosis, 223
Dentin, 219
Dentist, 44, 226
  school, 383
Deodorants, 235, 253
Department of Health, 181

Dependency:
 in alcoholism, 115
 amphetamines, 119
 barbiturates, 119
 cycle of, 22
 to drugs, 110
 (*See also* Addiction)
Depilatories, 234
Depression, 13, 136, 142ff., 143–144, 354
 in alcoholics, 115
Dermatitis. Inflammation of the skin.
Detergents, 32
Dextrose. Glucose; a single sugar.
Diabetes, 6, 160, 172, 293, 351, 353, 365
 boils in, 228
 complications, 294
 diabetic acidosis, 294
 familial, 295
 incidence and occurrence, 295
 longevity, 294
 treatment, 294–295
Diabetes insipidus, 293
Diaphragm. The muscular band which separates the chest and abdominal cavities from each other. On contraction it moves down, drawing air into the lungs.
Diaphragms, 334
 (*See also* Contraception)
Diarrhea, 5, 6, 18, 128–129, 178, 179, 182, 183
Diastole. The rest period of the heart between beats during which expansion takes place.
Dieldrin, 36
Diet, 5
 for athletes, 167–168
 and caries, 220
 in heart disease, 63
 pills for, 119
 social, 176
Dieting, 168
Dietitians, 44
Differences, international, in longevity, 4
Digestion, 156
Digestive tract, cancer, 74
Digitalis, 180
Dihydroxyacetone, 234
Diphtheria, 6, 261, 263–264
Diplococci, 240
Dirt from air pollution, 34
Disability, 8, 87
 in the elderly, 347
 from smoking, 99
Discipline, 337
Disease:
 Addison's, 296
 animal, 248
 black lung, 370
 chronic, 365
 chronic degenerative, 6

communicable, 5, 239ff.
 control of, 364–365
 endemic, 240
 endocrine, 176
 epidemic, 240
 heart, 6, 192, 350
 insect-borne, 2
 pandemic, 240
 pulmonary, 284
 related to soil, 33
 resistance to, 242–243
 respiratory, 353
 silo-filler's, 373
 sporadic, 240
 venereal, 313ff.
 (*See also* specific diseases)
Disinfection. The destruction of all organisms and their products capable of producing disease. 243
 of air, 276
Disorders:
 mental, 354
 treatment, 142, 147–148
Disorientation, 140
 from drugs, 118
Disposal of wastes, 31
Disturbances:
 digestive, 353
 mental, 139ff.
Disulfiram, 116
Diuretic pills, 177
Diving and hearing, 213
DNA (deoxyribonucleic acid). A nucleoprotein which occurs in the chromosomes of cells and is responsible for their effects upon growth, reproduction, and other cellular processes and activities. Occurs also in some viruses. 69, 292, 328, 339, 251
Dole, Vincent, 121
Dollar, consumer, 51
Dominance, 340
Dominant trait. The stronger of mutually antagonistic parental characters.
Donora, Pennsylvania, air pollution, 34
Dreams, wet, 305
Drinking (*see* Alcohol)
Driving (*see* Traffic)
Drugs, 109ff., 375
 addiction, habituation, and dependence, 110
 in communicable diseases, 246
 definitions, 110
 escalation, 117
 legal aspects, 121–122
 mind-affecting and therapeutic, 142
 terminology, 110
 (*See also* Addiction; Alcohol; Psychedelics; Narcotics; *and* specific medications and drugs)
Dryness of hair, 235

DT's (*see* Delirium tremens)
Dubois, René, 417
Duodenum, 156, 183
 ulcer of, 351
Dust, 205
 and colds, 276
 in industry, 370
Dysentery, 29
 amebic, 182
 bacillary, 182
Dysmenorrhea. A painful or otherwise abnormal menstruation.

Ear:
 canal, 213
 in measles, 267
 structure and anatomy, figure, 213
 (*See also* Deafness; Hearing)
Eardrum, 213
Ebstein-Barr virus, 18
Eclampsia. A disease of pregnancy characterized by convulsions.
Ecology, human, 21ff.
Ectomorph, 175
Ectopic pregnancy. Pregnancy outside of the uterus, as in the fallopian tube or in the abdomen.
Eczema. An inflammatory itching disease of the skin. 128–129, 146
Edema. Swelling due to watery fluids in the body tissues.
Edison, Thomas, 5
Education:
 health, 20, 379–380
 medical, 45
 physical, 380
 (*See also* College; Students)
Effluent, septic tank, 32
Ego defenses, 133
Ego identity, stabilizing, 13
Ego strengths, 126
Ejaculation, 301
 premature, 323
Electricity, 40
Electrolysis, 234
Embalming, 356
Embolus. A piece of blood clot or other material, such as a particle of fat, which is carried by the bloodstream and causes obstruction when it lodges in a blood vessel too small for it to pass through. 61, 334
Embryo. The fetus in the early stage of its development, especially before the end of the second month. 328
 development, 329
Emerson, Ralph Waldo, 135
Emissions, nocturnal, 305
Emmetropia, 206
Emotions (*see* Psychiatry; Psychology)

Emphysema, 6, 34, 86, 93, 284, 285, 351
  smoking, 98
Empirical. Based solely on experience.
Emulsify. To divide fat in solution into
  minute particles.
Enamel, 219
  mottled, 223
Encephalitis, 249, 253
  equine, 253
  measles, 267
Encounter groups, 149
Endemic. A disease present continuously
  in an area.
Enders, Dr. John F., 266
Endocrine gland. A gland producing a
  chemical substance which passes
  directly into the bloodstream and
  affects various functions and
  organs.
  and exercise, 12
Endocrine system, smoking, 94
Endocrines, 128
Endogenous. Originating within the
  organism.
Endometrium. The mucous membrane
  which lines the uterus. 303
Endomorph, 175
Energy, 155–156, 158–160, 192
Engel, George L., 146
Engineering, 2
  sanitary, 8
Enteric. Relating to the intestine.
Enteritis. Inflammation of the intestine.
  5–7
Environment, 21
  and health, 39
  healthy school, 383–384
  pollution control, 395
  relationship to, 126
  (See also Ecology)
Environmental Protection Agency, 36
Enzyme. A chemical ferment.
Ephedrine. A synthetic drug similar in
  its effects to epinephrine.
Epidemic Commission, 398
Epidemics, 241
  measles, 268
Epidemiologists, 44
Epidemiology. The science of the study
  of the conditions under which
  diseases occur.
Epididymis. An elongated mass at the
  back of the testicle; consists of
  tortuous tubes leading from the
  testicle. 301, 314
Epilepsy, 151–152
Epinephrine, 128, 291
Episiotomy, 330
Epithelioma, 233
Epithelium. The cellular tissue which
  covers surfaces and lines cavities
  of the body.

Equine encephalitis, 253
Erection, 301, 305
Erlich, Paul, 36
Erysipelas, 247
Erythroblastosis, 339
Erythrocyte. A red blood corpuscle.
Escalation phenomenon in psychedelics,
  117
Esophagus, 156
  cancer, 74
Estrogen, 235, 303
Ethanol (see Alcohol)
Ethmoid. Referring to the bone located
  at the front part of the base of the
  skull which forms part of the walls
  and septum of the nasal cavity.
Ethyl alcohol (see Alcohol)
Eugenics. The science of improving the
  human race through control of
  offspring. 342
Eustachian tube. A tube between the
  middle ear and the pharynx.
Evaporation, 189
Examinations:
  health, 50
  physical, 50
  recommended frequency, 50
  in tuberculosis, x-ray, 283
Excreta, 31
Exercise, 19, 177, 191–195, 198
  and adrenals, 297
  in aging, 348
  for colds, 278
  eye, 208, 210
  goals, 12
  and health, 11
  and illness, 193
  and mononucleosis, 19
  tests, 11
  in weight loss, 175, 177
Exertion, physical, 198
Exhaustion, heat, 191
Expectations, 307
Experiences, uses and misuses of,
  337–338
Extinguishment, 126
Eye, 201ff., 205
  anatomy, 202
  care of, 210–212
  drops, 207
  foreign body or particle in, 205
  injuries, 204–205
  pain in, 204
  specialists, 209–210
    (See also Ophthalmologists)
  types, 203
    (See also Vision)
Eyeball in visual defects, 208
Eyewashes, 205–206

Faith, 131
Fallopian tubes, 302, 304, 314

Fallout, radioactive, 39
Falls, 350
Family:
  large, 335–336
  and mental health, 126
  planning, 395
    (See also Contraception)
  size, 24, 335
  smaller, 335–336
Famine, future, 416
Farmers, hazards, 373
Farsightedness, 206, 208
Fat, 160–162, 173, 174, 177
  in atherosclerosis, 60
  saturated versus unsaturated,
    160–161
Fatality. Rate percent of patients who
  die from a particular disease.
Fate, 9
Fatigue, 197–198
  in mononucleosis, 18
  smoking, 94
Fatty acids. Chemical compounds
  whose base is a "chain" of carbon
  atoms; they combine with glycerine
  to form fats.
Fearfulness in alcoholism, 115
Federal Communications Commission,
  393
Federal Trade Commission, 389, 393
Feet, 196–197
Feiron, Bernard Charles, 116
Fertility, 302
Fertilizer, 169
Fetal death. The loss of the developing
  baby during pregnancy, labor, or
  delivery. The term "fetal death,"
  as now used, includes abortions,
  miscarriages, and stillbirths.
Fetish, 149
Fetus. The unborn offspring.
  damage to, 328
Fever:
  jungle yellow, 256
  in mononucleosis, 18
  puerperal, 247, 331
  Q, 249
  relapsing, 257
  rheumatic, 60, 64
  Rocky Mountain spotted, 257
  scarlet, 213, 247
  spotted, 249
  trench, 257
  typhoid, 6, 179, 268–269
  typhus, 249, 256
  yellow, 249, 255–256
    (See also specific diseases)
Fibrositis, 83
Field, absorption, septic tank, 32
Filters, 29
Fire patients, 43
Fires, 81

Fish, 182
    meal, 166
Fitzgerald, Edward, 9
Flaccid. Soft, weak.
Floc, 29
Flourine, 221
Flu, 17
    (*See also* Influenza)
Fluids, 177
Fluoride, 163
    and caries, 220–221
Fluoroscope. A device used in making
    x-ray examinations.
Focus of eye, 206–207
Fog, 34
Follicle, 303, 304
Food, 155ff., 173–174
    chemicals in, 180
    daily food guide, 167–168
    handlers, 179
    hazards, 31
    organic, 169
    poisoning, 178–181
        bacterial, 178–180
        clostridial, 179
        staphylococcal, 178
    quackery, 169
    safe, 2
Food and Agriculture Organization, 400
Food and Drug Administration, 110,
    180, 387, 392
    (*See also* United States)
Foot, athlete's, 228
Ford Foundation, 406
Foreplay, 323
Foreskin, 301
Foundations, 406
Fovea. A cup-shaped depression. 209
Foxglove, 180
Franklin, Benjamin, 5, 322
Fredrickson, Donald T., 105
Freud, Sgimund, 125, 127
Fruits, carbohydrates in, 168
Frustration in alcoholism, 115
Fulminating. Sudden, severe.
Fumigation, 243
Fungus. A class of vegetable organisms
    of low order, e.g., molds and
    mushrooms. 229
Furuncles, 228

Gallbladder, 156
Gallstones, 184
Gamma globulin, 184, 245, 247, 267
Ganglia, 305
Gangrene. The dying of tissue due to
    interference with local nutrition,
    e.g., cutting off blood supply.
    smoking, 93
Garbage, 33
Gargles, 278

Gastric. Pertaining to the stomach.
Gastritis. Inflammation of the stomach.
    7
Gastroenteritis, 18
Gaudenzia, 120
Gay liberation, 300
General paresis. A degenerative disease
    which involves the cells of the
    cerebral cortex; due to chronic
    syphilitic infection.
Genes. The basic elements which
    transmit hereditary characteristics
    and of which chromosomes are
    composed. 328
    recessive, 295
Genetic counseling, 342
Genetics:
    criminal behavior, 134, 147
    radiation, 38
Genitalia, anatomy, 300–304
Geography, accidents, 80
Geriatrics, 346
Germ plasm. The substance of repro-
    ductive cells.
Germicide. An agent that destroys germs.
Germs, 240
Gerontology, 346
Gibson, Althea, 132
Gigantism, 297
Gingivitis, 224–225
Glands:
    adrenal, 291
    endocrine, 289ff.
    swollen, 290
    (*See also* Endocrines)
Glare, 211–212
Glaucoma, 204, 210, 348
Glenn, John, 77
Globulin, gamma, 184, 245, 247, 267
Glycosuria. Sugar in the urine.
Godber, Sir George, 105
Goethe, Johann, 5
Goggles, 210
Goiter, 162, 296
    toxic, 296
Gonads. The ovaries and testicles; the
    organs which produce the
    reproductive cells, the ova and
    spermatazoa.
    radiation, 38
Gonococci, 314
Gonorrhea, 202, 314
    arthritis, 86
    symptoms of, 314
Goofballs (see Barbiturates)
Gout, 85
Government and health, 387ff.
Goya, 68
Graafian follicle. One of the small
    spherical bodies in the ovary, each
    of which contains an ovum.
Grand mal epilepsy, 151

Grand Rapids, Michigan, fluoridation
    of water, 222
Granulomatous. Consisting of small
    masses of new fleshy tissue.
Graves' disease, 296
Gravid. Pregnant; with child.
Great Britain, traffic accidents, 14
Grief, 359
Grippe, 17, 279–280
    (*See also* Influenza)
Group clinics, 48
Group reinforcement, 177
Groups, socioeconomic, 173
Growth, need for minerals, 162
Guidance, 131
Gynecology. The science of the diseases
    peculiar to women.

Habits, health, 9
Habituation, 110
Hair, 219, 227, 234
    care of, 235
    dryness and oiliness, 235
    dyes, 236
Halitosis, 226
Hallucination. Perception of objects or
    sounds which are not present.
Hallucinations, 140, 197
    due to drugs, 118
Hallucinogens, 142
Handicapped, employment, 88
Handrails, 81
Hansen, Dr. G. A., 248
Hansen's disease, 248
Happiness, 135
Harrison Narcotic Act, 121
Harvard Medical School, 53
Harvard Step Test, 11
Hashish, 117
Hawaii, 80
    abortion, 26
Hay fever, 216
Hazards, food, 31
Headache, 204
    tension, 145
    from visual defect, 207
Health, 1ff.
    agencies, 388ff.
    community services, 375–377
    critical problems of future, 415
    Department of Health, Education,
        and Welfare, 390
    and diet, 166
    education, 20, 379–380
    educators, 44
    and exercise, 11
    future of services, 419
    insurance, 409–412
    legislation, 394–396
    local departments, 397
    maternal and child, 366

mental, 125
   characteristics, 126
   promotion, 135
national institutes of, 392
personal and community, 19
practices and habits, 9
problems in college years, 11ff.
professional organizations, 406ff.
public, 2
school services, 380–382
in schools, 379ff.
services, 374
   in college, 19
state efforts, 396
voluntary organizations, 403ff.
Hearing, 212–214, 348
   aids, 214
      conduction type of, 212
   loss, 212
      due to noise, 28
      sensorineural, 213
Heart:
   artificial, 66
   coronary disease, 60ff.
   exercise and, 12
   in syphilis, 315
Heart attacks (see Infarction;
   Thrombosis)
Heart disease, 6, 7, 59ff., 192
   age, 61
   cholesterol, 61, 63
   chronic emotional stress, 64
   cigarettes, 61, 62
   congenital, 65
   diabetes, 61
   diet, 63
   exercise, 64
   and fats, 160–161
   gout, 61
   heredity, 61, 62
   high-risk factors, 61–64
   hypertension, 61–63
   hypertensive, 352
   hypothyroidism, 61–63
   obesity, 63
   prevention of heart attacks, 60–64
   rheumatic, 64
   sex, 61
   smoking, 97ff.
   surgery, 65–66
Heat, 160
   (See also Chill; Cold; Cramps;
   Exhaustion; Humidity; Stroke)
Height, 172–173
Helmholtz, Hermann, 202
Helminth. A worm or wormlike parasite,
   especially of the intestines.
Hemoglobin. The red pigment of the
   blood, which transports oxygen
   from lungs to organs and tissues.
   162, 165, 188, 372
Hemolytic. Causing destruction of red
blood corpuscles with liberation
of hemoglobin into surrounding
fluids or tissues.
Hemophilia. A condition in which the
   clotting time of the blood is
   prolonged, producing a strong
   tendency to bleeding, usually
   hereditary.
Hemorrhage. The escape of blood from
   the blood vessels. Bleeding of any
   extent. 63, 75, 184, 319
Hemorrhoid. A pile; a swelling formed
   by dilation of blood vessels at the
   anus.
Hepatitis, 180, 184, 246–247
   infectious, 182, 184
   serum, 247
Herbicides, 37, 169
Heredity:
   breast cancer, 72
   and diabetes, 295
Hernia. A protrusion of a part or organ
   through the walls of its cavity; a
   rupture. 7
Heroin, 110, 120–121
   (See also Addiction)
Herpes simplex, 204, 230
Herpes zoster. A virus disease with a
   blisterlike rash on the skin that
   follows the course of the nerves
   involved; commonly called
   "shingles." 230, 247
Highways (see Traffic)
H.I.P. (Health Insurance Plan), 53
Hippocrates, 45, 49, 241
Hogs, 33
Holmes, Oliver Wendell, 331
Homatropine, 202
Home accidents, 80ff.
Homicide, 6–8, 351
Homosexuality, 134, 309
Honeybee, 286
Hooker, Evelyn, 309
Hookworm, 33, 241–242
Hormone. A chemical substance
   produced in one organ and carried
   in the blood to another organ or
   part of the body where it stimulates
   functional activity.
Hormones, 133, 192, 289ff.
   androgenic, 291
   glucorticoids, 291
   male, 110
   mineralcorticoid, 291
   sex, 292
Horn, Daniel, 101
Hospitalization, mental, 148
Hospitals, 47, 407–408
   psychiatric, 148
Host. An animal or plant which harbors
   or nourishes another organism.
Hostility, 133

Hotels, 31
Housing, 27, 418
Hudson River, 29
Humidity, 189
Hunger, 177
Huxley, Aldous, 342
Hybrid. An animal or plant bred from
   two species or races.
Hydatidosis, 249
Hydrogen cyanide, 93
Hydrophobia, 251
Hygiene, occupational, 369ff.
Hymen, 302
Hyperkinesis, 147
Hyperkinetic state, 133
Hyperopia, 206–207
Hyperparathyroidism, 297
Hypertension, 6, 62–63, 67, 128–129,
   146, 172, 350–352
   racial incidence, 63
   and salt, 163
Hyperthyroidism, 296
Hypertrophy. Increase in the size of an
   organ.
Hypochondria. A mental disorder
   characterized by morbid anxiety as
   to one's health.
Hypodermic. Applied beneath or
   situated under the skin.
Hypoglycemia, 160, 293, 295–296
Hypotension. Lowered blood pressure,
   found in shock and in Addison's
   disease. Lower-than-average blood
   pressure is usually not productive
   of symptoms.
Hypothalamus. An area within and
   towards the base of the brain;
   believed to be the most important
   part of the limbic system (See also
   Limbic system). 174, 290
Hypothyroidism, 296

Id, 127
Identity (see Ego identity)
Idiosyncrasy. A peculiarity of constitu-
   tion or temperament.
Ileum. The third, last, and longest
   division of the small intestine.
   156
Illegitimacy, 317
Illness, 8
   in children of smokers, 102
   mental, 139ff., 354
   in smokers versus nonsmokers, 102
Illuminating Engineering Society, 211
Illumination, 211
Immunity:
   active, 244
   passive, 244
Immunization, 242, 259ff., 419

artificial, 244
  school, 382
Impetigo contagiosa, 230
Implantation, 304, 328
Impotence. Lack of power, strength, or vigor; chiefly, inability to attain or maintain an erection of the penis. 327
Incidence. The rate of occurrence of a disease.
Incisors, 220
Incubation. Period of development of an infectious disease.
Incubation period, 241
  extrinsic, 256
Independence, 130
India, population, 22
Indigestion, nervous, 182–183
Industrialization, 4
Infancy, diseases of, 6
Infanticide, 333
Infarct, myocardial, 61
Infarction, myocardial, 60ff.
Infections, 178, 240ff.
  drug-resistance, 246
  kidney, 351
  middle ear, 267
  reservoirs of, 241
  sinus, 215
  in students, 16
Inferiority, feelings of, 132
  in alcoholism, 115
Infestation. An invasion by animal parasites.
Influenza, 6–8, 17, 279–281, 351, 363
  Asian, 280–281
  epidemics, 17
  Hong Kong, 280
  vaccines, 280–281
Infrared, 190
Inheritence (see Genetics)
Inoculation. The introduction of substances into the body for the purpose of immunization; the term is also used in the field of bacteriology for the implantation of materials in a culture medium.
Insanity, 315
Insect-borne diseases, 2
Insecticides, 8
Insects, 286
Insecurity, 133
Insight, 148–149
Insomnia, 145, 197
Insulation, body, 174
Insulin, 159, 174, 176, 293, 294
Insurance:
  health, 375
  medical, 49, 51
Insurance companies and health, 409–412

Integration, 126
Intercourse:
  frequency, 12
  sexual, 292
Interests, 13
Interferon, 245
Internists, 48
Intoxication, alcoholic versus anoxia, 188
Intrauterine devices, 334
  (See also Contraception)
Inversion, atmospheric, 34
Iodine, 30, 162–163, 297
Ion. An atom or group of atoms having a charge of electricity.
IPV (inactivated poliovirus vaccine), 266
Iris. The pigmented contractile diaphragm of the eyeball, perforated by the pupil. 202, 209
Iron, 162, 348
Isolation, 242
Isometric. Of equal measure. Isometric exercises are those in which the muscles are exerted against a force but do not change in their length.
Itch (see Scabies; Swimmer's itch)
IUD, 334
  (See also Contraception)
Ivy, poison, 230–231

James, William, 143
Japan:
  atomic bomb effects, 38
  population, 25
Jaundice. The presence of bile in the blood, producing a yellow pigmentation of the skin. 111, 180, 184, 246–247
  in mononucleosis, 18
Jefferson, Thomas, on colds, 17
Jejunum. The second portion of the small intestine, between the duodenum and the ileum. 156
Jenner, Edward, 45, 262
Jesuits, 308
Joint, pains, 83
  (See also Arthritis)
Joint Commission on Mental Illness and Health, 126

Kaiser Medical Care Foundation, 52, 374
Keller, Helen, 201
Kellogg Foundation, 406
Keratin. The nitrogenous base of such tissues as horn, hair, and feathers.
Keratosis, 232
Kidney stones, 177

Kingston, New York, fluoride study, 222
Kissing and mononucleosis, 18
Korsakoff's syndrome, 111, 112
Kwashiorkor, 166
Kyphosis. Humpback or hunchback.

L-Dopa, 87, 353
Label, medication, 55
Labia, 302
Labor, 330
Laboratory technologists, 44
Lactation. The secretion of milk.
  need for calcium, 162
Lake Erie, water pollution, 29
Langerhans, islets of, 294
Larva. An immature stage in the development of an animal in which it is unlike the parent, e.g., the first stage in the development of an insect after it leaves the egg.
Laser. A light beam of single wavelength, of greater intensity than any previous light source and one that can be finely focused on a small point. It is very destructive to animal tissues, especially to certain malignant growths.
Latent. Inactive but ready to be made manifest.
Latin America, population, 24
Law:
  and alcoholism, 116
  and drugs, 121
  industrial compensation, 82
Laxatives, 185
Lead:
  industrial, 81
  in pipes, 180
  poisoning, 37, 81, 371
Legalization of marijuana, 121
Leguminous. Plants the seeds of which are in pods, as peas and beans.
Lens, 202, 204, 206, 208
  in astigmatism, 208
  contact, 210–211
  impact-resistant, 210
Lepers, 241
Leprosy, 247–248
Leptospirosis, 249
Lesion. Any local abnormality: bruise, wound, inflammation, tumor, cavity, etc.
Leukemia, 75
  treatment, 75
Leukocyte. A white blood corpuscle.
Leukocytosis. An increase in the number of white blood cells.
Leukopenia. A decrease in the number of white blood cells.
Leukoplakia, 232

Lexington Hospital, 120
Licensing, medical, 47
Life:
    biological limits to the span of, 5
    expectancy, 2–4
    family, 4
    length of, 1
Lighting, home, 81
Limbic system. A series of areas in the interior of the brain believed to function together and to be important in the appreciation of and expression of emotions. It includes the hypothalamus, which controls the pituitary. 290
Limestone, 30
Lincoln, Abraham, 143
Lip, cancer, 96
Lipase. A ferment which breaks down or digests fats.
Lipstick, 234
Liquids for colds, 278
Liver, 156
    cirrhosis of, 6, 7, 351
    (*See also* Cirrhosis; Hepatitis)
Llamas, 146
London, air pollution, 34
Longevity:
    international differences, 4
    smoking, 100
Lordosis. Abnormal forward curvature of the spine, usually in the lumbar region.
Los Angeles, California, air pollution, 34
Lotions, suntan, 234
Love, 129, 337
LSD (lysergic acid diethylamide). Also known as "acid," the most potent psychedelic agent yet known. 117–118
Lunch, school, 383
Lung:
    cancer, 70, 95
    farmer's, 373
Lupus erythematosus, 86
Lymph. The fluid contained in the lymphatic vessels or spaces.
Lymph node. Any one of the nodules occurring along the course of lymphatic vessels; they act as filters for infection and become swollen when inflamed.
Lymph nodes, 290
    in mononucleosis, 18
Lymphatic. Pertaining to lymph, or to a lymphatic node or vessel.
Lymphocyte. One form of white blood corpuscle.
Lymphogranuloma, 316
Lysergic acid diethylamide (*see* LSD)

Maidenhead, 302
Major Medical Insurance, 410–412
Malaise. A vague feeling of bodily discomfort.
Malaria, 36, 246, 254
    antimalarial drugs, 8
Malformations, congenital, 6–8
Malignant. Dangerous; tending to produce death. Often used as synonym for "cancerous."
Malignant melanoma, 232–233
Malnutrition, 155ff.
    effect on brain, 167
    in U.S., 166
    (*See also* Beriberi; Kwashiorkor; Xerophthalmia)
Mammography, 73
Man-years. The total number of years represented by the experience of a group of individuals, e.g., two persons over a period of 50 years or 100 persons over a period of one year each would represent 100 man-years.
Manhattan, New York City, mental illness study, 140
Manic-depressive disorders, 142ff.
Mann, Horace, 380
Manuals, marriage, 309
Marasmus, 166
Marijuana, 117–118
    classification and legal status, 121
Marijuana Commission, 121
Marine transportation, 82
Marriage, 4, 308, 320–324
    definitions of, 322
    number, 24
    and sex, 308
    success of, 322–323
    tastes in, 322–323
Maryland, abortion, 26, 27
Masochism, 306
Massage, closed chest heart, 59, 66
Mastectomy. Surgical removal of a breast. 73
Mastoid. The nipple-shaped bone behind the lower part of the ear.
Masturbation, 308
Maxilla (maxillary bone). The upper jawbone.
May, Rollo, 306
Mayo, Dr. William J., 358
"Meals on wheels," 348
Measles, 213, 261, 267
    German, 151, 203–204, 267–268
Medicaid, 51, 394
Medical education (*see* Course, medical; Education; Specialists)
Medical expenditures in aging, 356
Medical service in industry, 373
Medicare, 51, 355, 394

Medications, 55
    specific, 56
    in weight loss, 177
Medicine-osteopathic (*see* Osteopathy)
Melancholia. A state of marked depression of spirits. 143
Melanin. Dark brown or black pigment in the body.
Melanoma, 233
Memory, 346
Men:
    mortality of, 173
    ratio to women, 2
    traffic deaths, 14
Mendel, Gregor, 339
Mendelian law, 339
Meniere's disease, 213
Meninges. The three membranes covering the brain and spinal cord.
Meningitis. Inflammation, usually due to infection, of the meninges; this is a dangerous disease. 6, 7
Menopause, 292, 308, 354
Menstrual cycle, 303
Menstruation, 303
    in pregnancy, 330
Mental health (*see* Disturbances; Health; *and* specific problems)
Mental health programs, 368
Mental power, 346
Mercury, 31, 371
Mescoline, 117
Mesomorph, 175
Metabolic, 192
Metabolism. The processes in the body of the building up and the destruction of materials that are used for the production of energy, for growth, and for the replacement of worn-out tissues.
    intermediary, 292
Metastasis. The transfer of disease from one organ to another; usually applied to the spread of cancer. 69
Methadone, 110
    treatment of addiction, 121
Methedrine, 119
Methotrexate, 76, 332
Meuse Valley, France, pollution, 34
Mexico City, 188
Microorganism. An organism that can be seen only with a microscope.
Migraine. A periodic sick headache.
Military (*see* Armed Forces)
Milk, 31, 158, 181
Mind and body, 127
Minerals, 162–164, 168
    trace, 163
Mining, 82
Minnesota Memorial Society, 357
Modern medical services, 43ff.

Molars, 220
Moles, 232
Money in marriage, 322
Mononucleosis, infectious, 18–19
Morbid. Sick or sickly.
Morbidity, 2
Mormons and alcohol, 115
Morris, Desmond, 27
Mortality, 2
  infant, 338
  in tuberculosis, 282
  (*See also* Death)
Mortality ratio. The ratio of one
  mortality (or death) rate to another.
  For example, if we consider the
  mortality rate of nonsmokers as 1
  and the mortality rate of pipe
  smokers as 20 percent higher, the
  mortality ratio is 1:2; also, if the
  mortality rate of cigarette smokers
  is 2½ times as high as that of
  nonsmokers, the mortality ratio is
  2:5.
Mosquito:
  Aedes Aegypti, 255
  anopheles, 254
Motion in pregnancy, 330
Motorcycles, 16
  (*See also* Traffic)
Mouth, 156, 159
  cancer, 74
Mouthwashes, 226, 278
Mucosa. A membrane lining the cavities
  and tubes communicating with the
  surface of the body and secreting
  a mucous fluid.
Mucous. Pertaining to or resembling
  mucus.
Mucus. The sticky watery secretion of
  the glands in a mucous membrane
  that is moistened and protected by
  it. 94, 183, 286
  of nose, 275
Mueller, Paul, 36
Multiple sclerosis, 86
Mumps, 213, 261, 268, 302
Murmurs, heart, 64
Muscle, 173, 192
  oxidation in, 160
Mushrooms, 180
Mutant, virus in influenza, 280
Mutation. A sudden change in the
  hereditary, genetically determined
  characteristics of an individual.
  The change occurs as a result of a
  change in a gene, due to radiation,
  chemical influence, or unknown
  influence. The individual produced
  is a *mutant* (*See also* Fetus, damage
  to).
Mutations, radiation, 38

Mycoplasma, 316
  pneumoniae, 281, 282
Myopia, 208
Myxedema, 296

Nail, 264
Narcotic. A drug that induces sleep and
  relieves pain; in large doses causes
  coma and then death. Use
  commonly restricted to addicting
  drugs.
Narcotics, 120–122
  legal aspects, 121
Nasal catarrh, 215, 216
Nasal polyps, 216
National Academy of Sciences, 38
National Association for Mental Health,
  405
National Clearinghouse for Smoking
  and Health, 101
National Foundation, 88, 405
National Health Council, 412
National Interagency Council on
  Smoking and Health, 412
National Safety Council, 16
National Society for Crippled Children
  and Adults, 88, 405
National Society for the Prevention of
  Blindness, 204
National Tuberculosis and Respiratory
  Disease Association, 404
Nausea in pregnancy, 330
Nearsightedness, 208
Necrosis. The decay of body cells or
  tissues.
Needs, emotional, 129
Neoplasm. A new, abnormal growth;
  a tumor. May be cancerous or
  benign.
Nephritis. One of several types of
  inflammatory disease of the
  kidneys. 6, 351
  chronic, 61
Nerve, optic, 202
Nervous system, 111
  autonomic, 128–129
  parasympathetic, 182
  smoking, 94
  sympathetic, 182
Neuralgia. Nerve pain; pain of a severe,
  throbbing character along the
  course or path of a nerve.
Neurasthenia. A term which has been
  used for nervous debility from
  prolonged mental strain, worry, etc.
Neuritis. Inflammation of a nerve.
Neuroleptics, 142
Neuroses, 145–147
Neurotic. One who suffers from a
  functional nervous disorder.

Newark, New Jersey, air pollution
  survey, 34
Newburgh, New York, fluoride study,
  222
New York, New York:
  abortion, 25
  air pollution, 34
  pollution and death rates, 35
  water supplies, 29
Nicotine, 93, 94
Nitrogen, 188
Nitrogen cycle, 157
Nitrogen dioxide, 34, 373
Nits. The eggs of lice.
Nixon, Richard M., 121
Noise, 28–29, 213
Normality, 125–126
Nose, 190, 214–216
  anatomy, 215
Nuclear power, 39
Nucleus. A small body within a cell;
  the vital part of the cell.
Nurses, 44
  school, 381–382
Nutrition, 2, 19, 155ff., 418
  in the elderly, 347
Nyswander, Marie, 121

Obesity, 63, 172ff., 192
Obstruction, 184
Occupation, 3
Occupational health, 363ff.
Occupational therapists, 44
O'Connor, John, 43
Oculist, 209
OD (*see* Overdose)
Office of Vocational Rehabilitation, 87
Oiliness of hair, 235
Oils, 161
Onchocerciasis, 203
Ophthalmologists, 44, 209, 210
Opium, 55, 110
  poppy, 120
Optician, 209
Optics of eye, 206–207
Optometrist, 209, 210
OPV (oral poliovirus vaccine), 266
Orchitis. Inflammation of the testis.
Organic. Pertaining to or derived from
  living organisms; in chemistry,
  pertaining to compounds containing
  carbon; in disease, affecting the
  structure.
Orgasm, 303, 305
Orthopedics. Correction or prevention
  of deformities in children or
  persons of any age.
Osler, Sir William, 353
Ospreys, 36
Osteoarthritis, 84, 172

Osteopathy, 49
Otosclerosis, 212, 213
Ova, 292
Ovaries, 292, 302, 304
  (See also Gonads)
Overdose, 121
Overpopulation, 22ff.
Overweight, 172, 297
  causes of, 173ff.
Ovum, 303, 328
Oxford, Massachusetts, chronic
  diseases survey, 365
Oxidation. Combining with oxygen;
  burning. 177
Oxygen, 33, 157, 187, 188
  in flight, 369
Oxygenation, 160
Oysters, 180
Ozone, 34

Pacemakers, 65
Pain, 183
  abdominal, 179
    appendicitis, 184–185
Palm Beach shores, air pollution, 35
Palsy, shaking, 353
Pancreas, 156, 293
Pandemic. A disease that is worldwide.
Pap smear, 404
Pap test, 74
Papanicolaou, George, 74
Paper, pollution, 40
Papillae, 119
Papyrus, Ebers, 294
Paracelsus, 239
Paralysis. Loss of power of voluntary
  motion. 6, 67
  agitans, 353
  infantile (see Poliomyelitis)
Paranoid, 197
  misuse of term, 140
  schizophrenic, 141
Parasite. A plant or animal living on or
  in some other living organism from
  which it obtains its food and
  shelter.
Parasites, 241
  plant, 240
Paregoric, 18
Parenteral. Not through the intestinal
  tract, e.g., subcutaneous, intrave-
  nous, and intramuscular.
Parkinsonism, 86
Parkinson's disease, 353
Parotid. A salivary gland on the side of
  the head, situated below and in
  front of the ear. 156
Particulate matter in air, 35
Pasteur, Louis, 68, 251
Pasteurization, 31, 182

Pathogenic. Literally, "causing suffer-
  ing"; hence, causing disease, or
  having the ability to cause disease,
  as in "pathogenic bacteria."
Pathogens, 240
Pathological. Pertaining to or due to
  disease.
Pathologists, 44
Pauling, Linus, 277
Peace and health, 401
Pediatrics. A medical specialty dealing
  with children.
Pediculosis, 230
  pubis, 316
Pellagra, 164–165
Penicillin, 60, 245, 246, 281
  in colds, 279
  in rheumatic fever, 64
Penis, 301
  cancer, 76
People, older, 6
Perfectionists, 305
Perforation, 184
Period, latency, 308
Periodontal. Around a tooth.
Periodontitis, 224–225
Peristalsis. Rhythmical contraction of
  the stomach or intestines.
Peritoneum. Membrane lining the
  abdomen.
Peritonitis, 184
Personality:
  alcoholism, 115
  anatomy and structure, 126–127
  development, 13
  sociopathic and psychopathic, 146
Pertussis, 265
Pesticides, 36–37, 169, 180
Petechia. A small spot formed by the
  escape of blood into tissues such
  as the skin.
Petit mal epilepsy, 151
Pets, 354
Pharmacies, 409
Pharynx, 156
  cancer, 96
Phenols, 93
Phenylalanine, 338
Phenylketonuria, 338
Phenylpyruvic, oligophrenia, 136
Philanthropic foundations, 404ff.
Phosphates, 32
Phosphorus, 162, 220
Photosynthesis, 157
Physiatrist. Specialist in physical
  medicine and rehabilitation.
Physical fitness, 191–193
Physical therapists, 44
Physicians, 47–50
  assistants and associates, 44
  choice of, 47–48

  expectations of, 49
  family, 48
  numbers, 45–46
  personal, 354–355
  schools, 383
  specialist (see Specialists; and
    specific type of specialty)
Physiology. The study of the function
  of the organs and parts of the body.
Pickering, Sir George, 358
Pill:
  birth control, 297, 334
  "morning-after," 335
  pep, 198
  sleeping, 197
Pipe smoking, 95
  Pipes, lead water, 180
Pituitary, 291
  adrenal, 192
Placenta. The vascular structure attached
  to the uterus, through which the
  fetus is nourished, usually about 7
  inches in diameter and 1 inch in
  thickness, and weighing about 16
  ounces; known also as the "afterbirth." 328, 329
Plague, 249, 251–252
  bubonic, 251
  pneumonic, 251
Planned Parenthood associations, 335
  world population, 405, 416
Plaques, dental, 224
Plasma. The fluid portion of the blood.
  blood, 8
Plastic:
  contact lens, 211
  for teeth, 224
Plateau, 305
Platelet. A formed element of the
  blood associated with the clotting
  of the blood; also called
  "thrombocyte."
Pleura. Serous membrane lining the
  chestcavity and covering the lungs.
Pleurisy. Inflammation of the pleura.
Plutonium, 210
Pneumonia, 3, 5–8, 189, 267, 281–282,
  353
  mycoplasmal, 282
  pneumococcal, 281
  primary atypical, 282
  streptococcal, 281
  virus, 281
Pneumothorax. Presence of air or gas
  in the pleural cavity, causing
  collapse of the lung.
Poison, 180, 205
  industrial, 371–375
  ivy, 230–231
Poisoning, food, 178–181
  (See also specific agents)

Poliomyelitis, 261, 265–266
Pollen. The male fertilizing element of plants and trees.
Pollens, 216
Pollution:
  air, 33–36, 39, 95, 189, 285
    lung cancer, 71
  of the environment, 417–418
  law and, 35
  varied, 39
  of water, 29
  (See also Environment)
Polyp. A grapelike outgrowth of a mucous membrane.
Population, 22ff., 395
  control, 416–417
  cycle of dependency, 22
  of U.S., 22
  world increase, 22
Pork, 182, 249
Postmortem examinations, 47
Posture:
  good, 193
  varied, 196
Potassium, 163
Potency, 302
  sexual, 27
Pott, Percival, 75, 232
Poverty and mental health, 368
Powders, face, 234
Powell case, 116
Precancerous skin conditions, 232
Pregnancy, 327ff.
  duration of, 330
  fear of, 332
  hazards of, 331–332
  illegitimate, 317
  need for calcium, 162
  smoking, 99
  symptoms and care, 330–331
  toxemia of, 332
Prematurity, smoking, 99
Presbyopia, 208
Pressure, 188
  blood: diastolic, 63
    systolic, 62
    (See also Hypertension)
  intraocular, 204
Prevention, 1
  of communicable disease, 242–243
  of skin cancer, 233
Princeton University, 19, 25
Privies, 32
Problems, dental, 348
Professional health organizations, 406ff.
Progesterone, 297
Prohibition, 111, 121
Prolongation (see Life; Longevity)
Promiscuity, 318
Prophylactic. Pertaining to the prevention of disease.

Prostate. A gland surrounding the neck of the bladder and urethra in the male. 301, 314
  gland, 301
Prostheses, 88
Prostitution, addicts and, 120
Proteins, 158, 166–167, 292, 348
  malnutrition, 168
Pruritus. Itching.
Protoplasm. The substance of cells.
Psittacosis, 249, 252–253
Psoriasis, 86
Psychedelics, 117, 142
Psychiatrists, 44, 150
Psychiatry. The branch of medicine concerned with emotional illness and asocial behavior and including origin, diagnosis, prevention, and treatment of such conditions. (Readers interested in the meanings of words most frequently used in psychiatry are referred to "A Psychiatric Glossary," prepared by the Committee on Public Information of the American Psychiatric Association and obtainable from the Mental Health Materials Center, 1760 Broadway, New York, New York, 10019.)
  community, 136
  disorders, 52
  preventive, 136
  treatment, 13
Psychoanalysts, 308
Psycholeptics, 142
Psychologists, 44, 150
  school, 381
Psychology, problems in youth, 12
Psychoneurosis. A synonym for neurosis.
Psychoses, 140ff.
  varied causes, 144
Psychosomatic disorders, 146
Psychostimulants, 142
Psychotherapy. Treatment of functional nervous disorders by psychologic methods, including psychoanalysis. 148–149
  group, 149
  results, 149
  professionals practicing, 150
Ptyalin. A ferment in saliva which acts on starches. 159
Puberty. The earliest age at which one can beget or bear children, the age of sexual maturation. 292, 305
Public health, engineers, 44
Public Health Service (see United States Public Health Service)
Puerperium. The period between the termination of labor (childbirth)

and the return to normal of the uterus.
Pulmonary. Pertaining to the lungs.
Pulp, 219
Pulses, 192
Pupil, 202
Pus. The creamy matter produced by an infection; consists chiefly of leukocytes in a serous exudate. 243
Pustule. An elevation of the skin filled with pus or serum.
Pylorus. Opening from the stomach into the intestines. 184
Pyorrhea, 225
Pyridoxine, 165

Quackery:
  in arthritis, 86
  in medicine, 54
Quadruplets, 329
Quarantine, 241, 242
Quickening, 330
Quinine, 55, 205, 246

Rabbits, 252
Rabies, 3, 249–250, 261
Race and hypertension, 63
Radiation hazards, 38, 373
Radiologists, 44
Radium. A chemical element which gives off emanations similar to x-rays.
Rash, 315
  drug, 231–232
Rat flea, 251
Ratio of men to women, 2
Rationalization, 134
Rats and alcohol, 114
Reaction formation, 134
Reading in bed, 210
Reality, perceptions of, 126
Reasoning, 346
Rebellion, 133
Recessive. The weaker of mutually antagonistic inherited characteristics.
Recessiveness, 340
Recreation, 198
Rectum, 156, 184
  cancer, 74
Red Cross, American, 405
Reflex. An action produced by stimulation without any intervention of consciousness.
Refraction. The determination of refractive errors of the eye and correction of same by glasses.
Registration area. The states in which the reporting and recording of

births, deaths, etc., meet the standards established by the U.S. Bureau of Census.
Regurgitation. A reverse flow of food or blood.
Rehabilitation, 79, 86ff.
  Administration for Vocational, 393
  economics, 88
  employment, 88
  needs for, 86
Reinforcement, 126
Relations, sexual (*see* Sex)
Relationships:
  and maturity, 13
  stereotyped, 13
Religion:
  and alchol, 115
  and mental health, 131
Renal. Pertaining to the kidneys.
Repression, 132
Reproduction, radiation, 38
Research, 419–420
Reservoir of venereal disease, 316
Residues (*see* Pesticides)
Respiration, artificial, 83
Respiratory disease, smoking, 94
Respiratory infections, 17ff.
  bacteria versus viruses, 18
  (*See also* specific infections)
Respiratory system, smoking, 94
Restaurants, 31
Resuscitation units, 67
Retardation, mental, 150–151
Retina. The innermost coat lining the eyeball; contains the nerve endings of vision that are stimulated by light. 202, 206
Retinoblastoma, 70
Revolution, green, 36
Rh negative, 339
Rh positive, 339
Rheumatism (*see* Arthritis, rheumatoid)
Rhinitis. Inflammation of the nasal mucous membrane.
Rhode Island, accident death rate, 80
Rhythm, 333
Riboflavin, 165
Rickets, 164, 191
Ricketts, Dr. Howard Taylor, 256
Rickettsia, 256
Rickettsiae, 240
Rickettsialpox, 257
Ringworm, 228
RNA (ribonucleic acid). A chemical substance that acts as an intermediary between DNA and the cytoplasm of the cell, thought to be associated with protein synthesis. Occurs also in some viruses. 292, 339
Roads (*see* Traffic)

Rockefeller Foundation, 406
Rocky Mountain spotted fever, 257
Rodenticide. An agent for destroying rodents.
Roentgenologist. A physician who specializes in the application of x-rays for diagnosis or treatment. A widely used synonym is "radiologist."
Root, 219
  dental, 224
Rouge, 234
Rubáiyát of Omar Khayyam, The, 9
Rubella, 261, 267–268
Rugs, 81
Rural areas, 46

Sabin, Dr. Albert, 266
Sadism, 306
Safety (*see* Traffic)
Safety devices, 15
Salk, Dr. Jonas, 266
Salmonella, 179
Salmonellosis, 249
Salt, 163
  in hypertension, 63
Sanitation, school, 383
Saprophytes, 240
Saprophytic. Obtaining nourishment from decaying vegetable matter; not disease-producing.
Sarcoma. Cancer arising from connective tissues.
Scabies, 230
Scandinavia, abortion, 26
Schick test, 264
Schistosome dermatitis, 230
Schistosomiasis, 249
Schizophrenia, 13, 136, 140–142
  causes, 141
    treatment, 141–142
    types, 141
Schools and health, 379ff.
Sclera, 202
Screens, sun, 191
Scrotum, 232, 301, 333
  cancer, 75
Scurvy, 165
Security, 130–131
Sedative. An agent that promotes sleep and relaxation, and hence combats nervous tensions.
Sedatives, 118–120, 142, 145, 197
Sedimentation basin, 29
Seepage, 30
Self-fulfillment, 126
Self-medication, 56
Semen, 301
Semicircular canal. Organ of the inner ear that controls equilibrium.

Seminal vesicles, 301
Seminiferous tubules, 301
Senility, 144
Sensations, 226
Sensitivity training, 149
Sensitization, 245
Sepsis. Presence of pathogenic organisms or their products in the blood.
Septic. Relating to or caused by sepsis.
Septicemia. Presence of pathogenic organisms or their toxins in the blood; also called "blood poisoning."
Septic tank. A prefabricated metal tank into which the sewage of a household is drained. The wastes ferment in the tank and lose much, but not all, of their unpleasant and dangerous characteristics. 32
Septum. A thin wall dividing two cavities or masses of tissue.
of nose, 214, 215
Serous. Like serum.
Serum. Clear liquid which may be separated from the clot and corpuscles of the blood.
Services, modern medical, 2, 43ff.
Sewage, 31
Sewerage, 31
Sex, 131, 299ff.
  in aging, 353–354
  characteristics, secondary, 305
  conflicts, 134
  cookbook, 323
  decision making about, 323–324
  hormones, 292
  in marriage, 322, 323
  during pregnancy, 330
  sexual activity 12
  social and emotional aspects, 313ff.
Sexual performance, 308
Sexual play, 308
Sexual roles, 299
Sexuality, 299, 300
Shattuck, Lemuel, 380
Sheldon, Edward, 175
Shellfish, contamination, 29
Shingles, 247
Shoes, 196
Shubik, Phillippe, 101
Siecus, 300
Sigmoidoscope (proctosigmoidoscope). A tubelike instrument for inspecting the inside of the rectum and lower colon. A proctoscope examines only the rectum.
"Silence, conspiracy of," 357–358
Silent Spring, 180
Silicosis, 370
Silo-filler's disease, 34, 373

Simulium fly, 203
Sinus. A hollow space or cavity. Applies particularly to paranasal sinuses.
  paranasal, 215
Sinusitis, 215, 273
Skin, 219, 226ff.
  anatomy and structure, 227
  cancer, 75, 232
  care of, 227
  functions of, 226–227
  occupational diseases, 372
  precancerous, 232
  psychologic effects on, 128–129
  tanning, 187
Sleep, 19, 197
Sleeplessness, 197
Sludge, 32
Smallpox, 45, 259–263
Smog, 34
Smoking:
  accidents, 99
  aortic aneurysm, 98
  beginning, 93, 95
  bronchitis and emphysema, 98
  causing cancers, 93–96
  cessation, 95
  characteristics, 104
  cigar and pipe, 100
  cigarette, 285
  circulation, 94
  cirrhosis, 98
  deaths, 92
  dogs and cancer, 96
  effect of: on children, 102
    on nonsmokers studies, 92
  endocrine system, 94
  fatigue, 94
  heart disease, 97
  illness and disability, 99–100
  immediate effects, 93
  incidence, 101
  inhalation, 95
  longevity, 100
  loss of teeth, 98
  nervous system, 94
  and periodontitis, 225
  personal characteristics, 104
  by physicians, 101
  versus pollution in lung cancer, 95
  pregnancy, 99
  rate, 95
  reasons for, 101
  reducing the hazard, 102
  respiratory system, 94
  stopping, 103–105
    heart disease, 97
  stroke, 98
  ulcers, 94
  (See also Cigarettes; Cigars; Pipe smoking)

Snacking, 168–169
Sociability in alcoholism, 115
Social class, death rates according to, 3
Social Security Administration, 355–356
Social workers, 44
Societies:
  county medical, 47
  funeral, 356
  memorial, 356
Sodium, 163
Soil and disease, 33
Somatotyping, 175
Spasm. A sudden violent involuntary contraction, e.g., a contraction of the muscles.
Spasmophilia. A tendency to convulsive seizures.
Specialists, 44, 48
Speed (see Amphetamines; Methedrine)
Sperm, 292, 301, 328
Spermatazoa, 301
Spermatic cord, 301, 333
Spermatogenesis. The formation of sperm.
Spermicidal jellies and foams, 334
Spine, subluxation, 54
Spirochete. A spiral-shaped germ; one type causes syphilis.
Spock, Dr. Benjamin, 337
Spondylitis, 85
Spore. The reproductive element of one of the lower organisms; bacterial spores; inactive or resistant forms produced with the body of a bacterium.
Sprays, nasal, 278
Squints, 207
Stapes, 212
Staphylococci, 240, 246
Staphylococcus, 178
Starch. A carbohydrate made of multiple units of glucose.
State, Department of, 393
Steapsin. A fat-digesting ferment of the pancreas.
Sterility. Inability to produce young. Also, absence of microorganisms (See also **Microorganism**).
Sterilization, 26, 243, 333
  legality, 27
Steroids, 291
Sterol. A chemical related to the facts.
Still, Andrew, 49
Stimulants, 118–120, 122, 142
Stirrup, 212
Stomach, 156, 183
  cancer, 74
  ulcer of, 351
Stones, kidney, 177
Strabismus, 207–208

Strabo, 207
Strep throat, 247
Streptococci, 244
  henolytic, 247
  and rheumatic fever, 64
Stress, 230
Stroke, 7, 67ff. 350–352
  causes, 67
  heat, 189, 191
  prognosis, 68
  rehabilitation, 68
  and salt, 163
  smoking, 98
  (See also Apoplexy)
STS (serological tests for syphilis), 316
Student councils, 13
Students:
  common infections, 16
  suicide in, 143
  traffic deaths, 14
Sublimation, 132, 134
Sugars (see Carbohydrates)
Suicide, 6–8, 143–144, 351
  prevention, 144
Sulfonamides in colds, 279
Sunglasses, 212
Sunshine, 190
Suntan protection, 234
Superego, 127
Support, psychological, 148
Suppression, 132
Suppurative. Producing pus.
Surgeon General's Report on Smoking and Health, 91
Surgeons, 44
  (See also Physicians)
Surgery:
  breast cancer, 73
  heart, 64–66
Sweat gland, 227
Sweating, 177
Sweden, traffic accidents, 14
Swimmer's itch, 230
Swimming and hearing, 213
Swordfish, 31
Symptoms, psychosomatic and psychogenic, 127
Synanon (drug rehabilitation center), 120
Syndrome. A set of symptoms which occur together.
Synergistic. Working together.
Synovia, 85
Synthesis. Processes of building up a compound by union of simpler compounds or its elements.
Synthetic. Relating to or made by synthesis.
Syphilis, 60, 136, 144, 246, 314–316
  serological tests for, 316

Systole. Contraction of the heart, or the period of contraction of the heart; used in contradistinction to diastole, the period of relaxation.

T groups, 149
Tachardia lacca, 286
Tachycardia. Excessively rapid rate of the heart.
Tapeworm, 182, 251
Tar, 93
Tartar, 224
Tea, 110, 122
Teamwork in rehabilitation, 87
Teeth, 219ff.
    care of, 226
    smoking and loss, 98
Temperance movement, 380
Temperature, 189–190
    body, 226–227
Tensions, 135
Testicles, 292, 301, 302
    (See also Gonads)
Tests, exercise, 11
Tetanus, 33, 261, 264
Tetracyclines, 249, 282
Thalidomid, 248
Theft, addicts and, 120
Theobromine, 122
Therapeutic. Curative; pertaining to the treatment of disease.
Therapists, 44
Therapy. Treatment of disease.
    new forms, 45
    (See also Psychotherapy)
Thermography, 73
Thiamine, 164–165
Thinness, 177
Thoracic. Pertaining to the thorax or chest.
Throat, 190, 214–216
    sore, in mononucleosis 18
Thrombi (see Thrombosis)
Thromboangiitis obliterans, 97
Thrombosis:
    arterial, 61
    cerebral, 61, 67ff.
    coronary, 60ff.
Thrombus. A clot which forms in a blood vessel and remains at its site of formation.
Thyroid, 176, 296
Titian, 5
Tobacco, 91ff.
    cancer, 95
    harmful components, 92–93
    tar, 93
    and vision, 205
    (See also Cigarettes; Smoking)
Toilets, chemical, 32

Tongue, cancer, 96
Tonometer, 204
Tonsils, 210, 211
Toothbrush, 225
Toothpastes, 226
TOPS (Take off pounds), 177
Toscanini, 5
Toxin. A poison; used as the term for the poisonous substance produced by pathogenic organisms.
Toxoid. A modified toxin used for the purpose of immunization.
Toxoids, 244, 263
Trachea. The windpipe; the air tube extending from the larynx to the bronchi. 296
Trachoma, 203, 210
Traffic:
    alchohol and accidents, 14
    anonymity, 14
    causes of accidents, 14
    cigarettes and accidents, 15
    defensive driving, 16
    driving education, 15–16
    driving skills, 15
    highways, 16
    implied consent laws, 14
    Interstate System, 16
    laws, 14
    preventable accidents, 14
    prevention of accidents, 15
    psychology, 14
    risks, 14
    safe cars: car size, 16
        door latches, 16
        headrest, 16
        tires, 16
        windshield glass, 16
        windshield wipers, 16
    safety, 15
    seat belts, 15
    slowness and accidents, 15
    speed and accidents, 15
Tranquilizers, 18, 142, 145
Transmission:
    biological of disease, 253
    mechanical of disease, 253
Transplantation, heart, 65
Transplants:
    arterial, 66
    pancreas, 294
    venous, 66
Transport, 175
Transportation, accidents, 80
Travel, 269
Treatment:
    new forms, 45
    Pasteur, 251
    (See also specific diseases)
Tremor, 86
Treponema pallidum. A spirochete

which causes syphilis (See also **Spirochete**).
Trichinella spiralis, 182
Trichinosis, 33, 182, 249
Triplets, 329
Trudeau, Dr. Edward Livingston, 188
Trypanosomiasis, 257
Trypsin. The principal protein-digesting enzyme (ferment) of the pancreatic juice.
Tube, Eustachian, 213
Tuberculin tests, 283
Tuberculosis, 5, 6, 182, 188, 249, 282–284
    bovine, 249
    in students, 283
    treatment, 283–284
    vaccination, 84
Tularemia, 249, 252
Tumor: Swelling; an abnormal mass of tissue, especially one due to morbid growth of tissue not normal to a part.
Tumors, 69
    prostate, 352
Tuna, 31
Turbinates. Small bones in the nasal passageways; also known as "conchae." 215
Turnverein, 380
Twins:
    fraternal, 329
    identical, 329
Tympanic membrane. The eardrum.
Tympanoplasty, 212
Typhoid, 6, 261
    fever, 29, 33, 179
Typhus:
    endemic, 256
    epidemic, 256
    fever, 8, 36
    flea-borne, 256
    louse-borne, 256
    mite-borne, 257
    scrub, 257

Ulcer. An open sore, other than a wound.
    peptic, 128–129, 146, 183
    smoking, 94
Ultraviolet, 190, 191
    light, 229
Ultraviolet rays. The invisible rays of light beyond the violet of the visible spectrum.
Umbilical cord. The cord which connects the fetus to the placenta; includes the blood vessels which carry nourishment and oxygen to the fetus.

Umbilicus. The navel; the point of entrance of the umbilical cord into the fetus.
Unconsciousness, 67
Underactivity, 174
Underprivileged groups, 26
Underweight, 177
UNICEF, 400
United Nations, food and agriculture programs, 36
United States:
  birth and death rates, 23
  physicians in, 46
  population, 22
U.S. Department of Agriculture, 182
U.S. Food and Drug Administration, 31
U.S. Public Health Service, 32, 262, 363, 391–392
  Bureau of Water Hygeine, 30
Uppsala, Sweden, 119
Uranium, 71, 371
Urbanization, 27
Ureter. The duct that carries urine from a kidney to the bladder.
Urethra. The duct through which urine is discharged from the bladder; in the male it also conveys the semen.
Urethral, 301
Urethritis, nonspecific, 316
Uric acid, 85
Urticaria. Hives; an allergic eruption of itching wheals. 230
Uterus. The womb; the organ which contains the developing baby. 292, 302, 314, 319
  cancer, 73–74
    prevention, 74
    prognosis, 74
    treatment, 74
  cervix, 74

Vaccination. The process of using a vaccine for the purpose of producing active immunity; the term originally referred to the introduction of cowpox virus to prevent smallpox, but it is now used in a broader sense. 45, 263
Vaccine. A substance which consists of living, attenuated, or killed organisms used for the purpose of producing active immunity.
Vaccines, 8, 244, 266–269
  for colds, 277–278
  inactivated poliovirus, 266
  influenza, 17
  oral poliovirus, 266
  smallpox, 244
  in tuberculosis, 284

  typhoid, 244
Vaccinia. Cowpox; the disease, usually local and limited to the site of inoculation, induced in man by the inoculation of cowpox virus.
Vagina, 302, 314
Value systems and alcohol, 115
Valves, 13
  heart, 64
Varicose. Unnaturally swollen, applied especially to veins.
Vas deferens, 301, 314
Vasectomy, 333
Veganism, 168
Vegetables, carbohydrates in, 168
Vegetarianism, 168
Vein. A blood vessel which conveys blood toward the heart.
Veins, 66
Venereal. Relating to or resulting from sexual intercourse. From Venus, the goddess of love.
Venereal disease, 313ff.
Ventilation, 276
  at work, 373
Verruca accuminata, 316
Vesicular. Composed of small saclike bodies.
Veterans Administration, 392
Viable. Capable of living.
Vibrissae, 275
Violence, 133, 147
Viremia. The presence of viruses in the blood.
Virile. Having the qualities of an adult man; capable of procreation.
Virulence, 245
Viruses, 240, 243, 246, 247, 250, 253, 260, 266, 267
  in cancer, 70
  cold, 17
  of colds, 274
  influenza, 280
  (See also specific diseases)
Viscera. The various internal organs of the cavities of the body.
Vision, 201ff.
  in aging, 348
  mechanism of, 206–207
  night, 209
  poisons, 205
  (See also Eye)
Vitamin A, 164, 348
Vitamin B group, 164–165
Vitamin C, 165–166, 348
  for colds, 277
Vitamin D, 164, 191, 220
Vitamin E, 164
Vitamin K, 164
Vitamins. Chemical substances present

  in natural foods and necessary for health, 159, 163–168
  and colds, 277
  in treating psychoses, 148
Volstead Act, 121
Voluntary health organizations, 403ff.
Vomiting, 18, 178, 179, 184
Vulva, 302

Waldeyer's ring, 217
Warts, 228
Washington, abortion, 26
Wasserman test, 316
Wastes, disposal of, 31
Water, 161–162
  drinking, 2
  purification system, 300
  shortages, 29
Water Pik, 226
Water Quality Act, 395
Water supplies, 29
  sterilization, 30
  underground, 30
Wave lengths, 208
Weather in arthritis, 86
Weight, 192
  in aging, 348
  average, 172–173
  desirable, 172–173
  ideal, 172–173
  reduction, 294
Westoff, Charles P., 25
Wetzel grid, 382
Whooping cough, 261, 265
Wind chill, 190
Windpipe (see Trachea)
Withdrawal, 134
Women:
  attitudes toward family planning, 23
  heart disease, 60
  ratio to men, 2
Women's liberation, 300
Wood's light, 229
Workmen's compensation, 82
World Health Organization, 203, 254, 398–400
World Population Year 1974, 416
Worm, 182
Worry, 133
Wrinkles, 228
Wyoming, accident death rate, 80

Xeroderma pigmentosa, 191
Xerophthalmia. Extreme dryness of the conjunctiva, which loses its luster and becomes skinlike in appearance; due to a deficiency of vitamin A. 164

X-rays. Roentgen rays; very short ethereal rays which will pass through solid bodies, cause destructive changes in living tissue, and affect a photographic plate.
in cancer, 76

hazards, 38
in leukemia, 75
technicians, 44
(*See also* Radiation; *and* specific diseases)
XYY pattern, 147

Youth, psychological problems, 12

Zero population growth, 24–25, 319, 335, 417
Zinc, 163, 180
Zoonoses, 248–250